GENERAL MEDICINE PRACTICE HANDBOOK
VOLUME 1

CORE CONCEPTS AND CLINICAL SYSTEMS IN GENERAL MEDICINE

Dr. Kashieca Yap

ALLIED HEALTH PRESS

General Medicine Practice Handbook Volume 1

Core Concepts and Clinical Systems in General Medicine

Authors: **Dr. Kashieca Yap**

Allied Health Press
4164 Lakeshore Road
Burlington ON L7L 1A4
Canada
www.alliedhealthpress.com
Email: orders@arclereducation.com

ISBN: 978-1-77956-856-4

Allied Health Press publishes wide variety of books and eBooks. For more information about Allied Health Press and its products, visit our website at www.alliedhealthpress.com

ABOUT THE AUTHOR

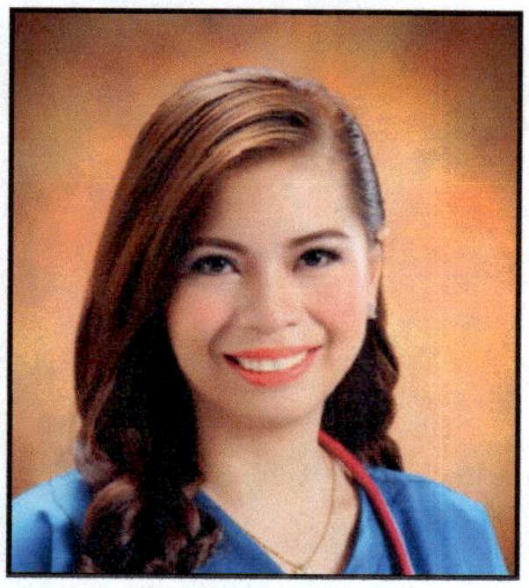

Kashieca Yap, M.D., is a devoted medical doctor and medical writer. She currently works as a general practice physician in a rural town, where she handles adult and pediatric cases, infectious diseases, and chronic medical conditions. Kashieca also lectures on mental health, clinical pharmacology, physiology, and psychiatry and is an enthusiastic researcher and medical writer.

She obtained her medical degree from Cebu Doctor's University College of Medicine and further developed her clinical skills at a large public hospital. Alongside her professional endeavors, Kashieca dedicates her time to volunteering at NGOs and medical missions, reaching out to people in geographically isolated areas. Her unwavering passion for medicine and her strong desire to serve people is a testament to her compassion and skill as a healthcare professional.

Brief Table of Contents

Getting Started with This Book

Chapter Openers

A list of Chapter Outline is presented providing a brief Introduction to what will be covered in the chapter.

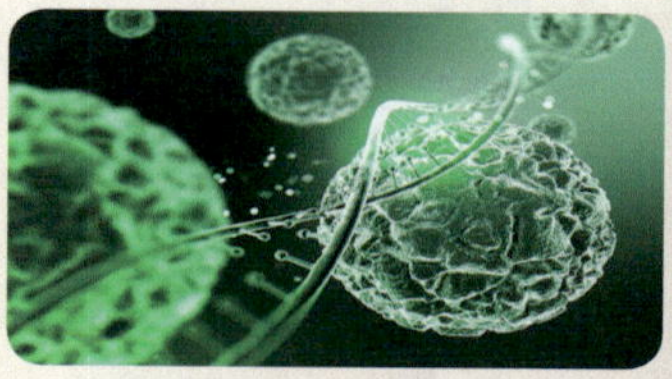

Introduction

Often referred to as the science of life, biology is a broad field of study aimed at comprehending the several kinds of life on Earth, from tiny creatures to sophisticated multicellular entities. Comprising several subfields, including molecular biology, ecology, and evolutionary biology, each of which advances our knowledge of living systems, this field clarifies the mechanisms controlling life events, including development, reproduction, and interaction with the surroundings, which is the central goal of biology. Moreover, biology fills in the void between the natural sciences and medicine by offering a necessary understanding of health, illness, and the interactions between organisms and their environments. Dealing with urgent global issues such as climate change, biodiversity loss, and new diseases depends on an awareness of these complex biological interactions, therefore highlighting the critical part biology plays in modern civilization. Fundamentally, biology explores and tests ideas about the living world using the scientific method. Through methodical observation and experimentation,

LEARNING OBJECTIVES

After studying this chapter, you will be able to:

1. Discuss the scientific method in biology;
2. Explain the cell theory;
3. Discuss the genetics and heredity;
4. Evolution and natural selection;
5. Focus on ecology and ecosystems;
6. Learn about human biology;
7. Evaluate the plant biology;
8. Explain the microbiology;
9. Focus on current trends in biology.

1.1. The Scientific Method in Biology

Learning Outcome

1. Describe the steps of the scientific method;
2. Focus on hypothesis formation;
3. Learn about experimental design.

Learning Outcomes

The beginning of each section of every chapter contains a set of Learning Outcomes that inform students of concepts they should understand. These outcomes help students understand what they should be able to do if they have mastered the material in that section.

Test Your Knowledge

Throughout each chapter, Test Your Knowledge cues you to note which topics have been covered and to self-test your understanding of the material presented.

Test Your Knowledge

1. Explain why correlation does not imply causation in scientific experiments.
2. How does the scientific method help reduce the influence of personal opinions in research?

Chapter Summary

The Summary Section appear at the end of each chapter and summarize main concepts covered throughout the chapter. These points provide key concepts in an engaging and meaningful way.

Summary

The investigation of biological principles highlights the importance of a comprehensive view of life by reflecting the intricate interactions that occur within living systems. The complexity of biology goes beyond individual species or systems, as this essay highlights; it also includes the interactions that mold ecosystems and affect biodiversity. Researchers can conduct in-depth analyses of metabolomic data using sophisticated technologies like MetaboAnalyst, which offer insights into the molecular mechanisms underlying these interactions. As demonstrated by the developments in MetaboAnalyst, for example, the integration of diverse omics data promotes a thorough understanding of metabolic pathways and helps identify important biological markers necessary for research on development and disease (Chong et al., 2018). Additionally, the phenomenon of ecological invasions is a key component of biological research and a vital field of study. The introduction of non-native species into unfamiliar habitats has significant ramifications and calls for multidisciplinary management strategies. Examining the origins and effects of these biological incursions, invasion science has become a crucial field that highlights the need to comprehend ecological dynamics and community interactions. As interest in biological invasions increases, new findings are emerging that put conventional ecological theories and practices to the test. The importance of incorporating various scientific viewpoints is shown by this developing discipline, which also highlights how invasive species shape ecosystems and advances our knowledge of ecological resilience (David et al., 2013). When taken as a whole, these discoveries from invasion science and metabolomics highlight the value of multidisciplinary biology research. Fostering cross-disciplinary collaboration and utilizing technological breakthroughs to improve our comprehension of intricate biological interactions are crucial as we look to the future of biological research. In addition to deepening our understanding of the complexities of life, this method lays the groundwork for tackling urgent environmental issues. Future studies can ensure the continued relevance of biology in a world that is constantly changing by acknowledging the interconnection of biological systems and opening the door to creative solutions that support sustainability and biodiversity conservation. We might imagine a thorough comprehension of life that serves both academia and society at large through ongoing investigation and integration of scientific knowledge.

Knowledge Assessment

The chapter includes material designed to review and reinforce each content. It includes Critical Thinking Questions to help test of your understanding of information presented in the chapter and Short answer Questions to review your understanding of the key concepts presented in the chapter.

Critical Thinking Questions

1. **Who is known as the "Father of Modern Biology"?**
   a. Aristotle
   b. Charles Darwin
   c. Gregor Mendel
   d. Louis Pasteur
2. **What is the basic unit of life?**
   a. Atom
   b. Molecule
   c. Cell
   d. Organism
3. **Which branch of biology studies the interaction of organisms with their environment?**
   a. Genetics
   b. Ecology
   c. Physiology
   d. Botany
4. **Which macromolecule is the main source of energy for living organisms?**
   a. Proteins
   b. Lipids
   c. Carbohydrates
   d. Nucleic acids
5. **DNA is primarily responsible for which function in living organisms?**
   a. Energy production
   b. Protein synthesis
   c. Storing genetic information
   d. Regulating body temperature

Short Answer Questions

1. What is biology, and why is it important to study biology?
2. What are the three main domains of life, and how are they different from one another?
3. Define homeostasis and give an example of how it works in living organisms.
4. What is the cell theory, and why is it fundamental to biology?
5. How do autotrophs and heterotrophs differ in the way they obtain energy?
6. What is the scientific method, and how is it applied in biological research?
7. Discuss how biology helps address global challenges such as climate change, disease, and food security.
8. Explain the levels of biological organization from the smallest unit to the largest. Provide examples at each level.
9. Describe the relationship between structure and function in biology, giving specific examples from cells or organs.
10. How has the discovery of genetics shaped our understanding of inheritance and variation among organisms?

Supplementary Materials

Key Terms: A list of key terms is given for quick reference

KEY TERMS FROM THIS CHAPTER

Annotation enrichment analysis	Biological structure	Cell
Cell theory	Cellular structure	Ecology
Ecosystems	Genetics	Human biology
Microbiology	Natural selection	Organism
Plant biology		

Further Resources: Recommendations for additional readings, websites, and multimedia resources.

References

1. Argelaguet, R., Velten, B., Arnol, D., Dietrich, S., Zenz, T., Marioni, J. C., Buettner, F., et al. (2018). Multi-omics factor analysis—A framework for unsupervised integration of multi-omics data sets. *Molecular Systems Biology, 14*. https://doi.org/10.15252/msb.20178124.
2. Bacher, S., Blackburn, T. M., Essl, F., & Genovesi, P. (2017). *Socio-Economic Impact Classification of Alien Taxa (SEICAT)*. https://core.ac.uk/download/286567949.pdf (accessed on 8th March 2025).
3. Barnett, R., Brace, S., Cucchi, T., & Dobney, K. (2013). *Divergent Evolutionary Processes Associated with Colonization of Offshore Islands*. https://core.ac.uk/download/20664364.pdf (accessed on 8th March 2025).

Detailed Table of Contents

CHAPTER 3

Common Investigations in Medicine 71

CHAPTER 4

Pharmacology in General Practice 107

CHAPTER 5

Cardiovascular System: Diseases, Risk Factors, Diagnostic Approaches, and Treatment Modalities 143

CHAPTER 6

Respiratory System: Common Respiratory Disorders, Diagnostic Tools, and Pharmacological Treatments 179

CHAPTER 7

Gastrointestinal System: Disorders, Diagnostic Approaches, and Treatments 213

CHAPTER 8

Endocrine and Metabolic Disorders 245

CHAPTER 9

Renal and Genitourinary System: Disorders, Diagnostic Approaches, and Treatment Options 279

CHAPTER 10

Hematology and Oncology 311

CHAPTER 11

Rheumatology and Musculoskeletal Disorders 345

LIST OF FIGURES

PREFACE

The art and science of medicine are inextricably bound with the clinician's ability to analyze, diagnose, and manage a wide array of conditions presented by patients over the course of life. From managing a common cold to a chronic condition, the clinician's clinical judgment is based on proper knowledge, systematic thinking, and prudent interpretation of investigative findings. Medical practice is dynamic and expansive, requiring continuous learning, adaptability, and an unrelenting commitment to evidence-based practice. The foundation of this care is rooted in general medicine, where primary and secondary prevention meet with diagnostic precision and therapeutic decision-making.

General medicine is the foundation for the majority of clinical encounters. It is the first point of contact with patients and the manifestation of the diversity of symptoms and diseases that can affect any organ system. From initial history-taking and examination to choosing proper investigation and planning treatments, the family physician serves as both gatekeeper and navigator. The responsibility is great: early detection of life-threatening illness, chronic disease management, and sometimes life-saving interventions are launched here. Systematic understanding of medical principles, therefore, constitutes a vital prerequisite for all clinicians who wish to provide adequate, and timely care in practice.

The *General Medicine Practice Handbook: Volume 1* is designed to guide clinicians, medical students, and other healthcare providers in the development of a practical and sound general medicine foundation. Composed with clarity and relevance in view, the volume harmoniously interweaves the theoretical concepts that are essential with the practical clinical considerations. The volume divides intricate medical information into manageable components, enabling readers to care for patients with confidence and logic. Whether used with clinical postings, licensing exam prep, or day-to-day reference, the information is intended to meet the education and professional needs of those at the patient's bedside.

Chapter 1 has a general introduction to the scope and philosophy of general medicine. It gives the context by outlining the primary responsibilities, skills, and roles of general practitioners in modern healthcare systems. The merits of continuity of care, holistic care, and multidisciplinary teamwork are set out.

Chapter 2 covers the underlying clinical assessment and diagnostic reasoning processes. Readers will be guided through patient interaction—taking history, physical examination, and clinical sign interpretation—preceded by logical decision-making strategies to assist in arriving at a differential diagnosis.

Chapter 3 illustrates the investigations that are routinely employed in medical practice. Hematological, biochemical, microbiological, and imaging modalities are covered, and their indications, limitations, and interpretation are mentioned. Stress is given to the choice of correct tests based on clinical presentation.

Chapter 4 discusses the principles of pharmacology that are relevant to general practice. It discusses drug classification, mechanisms of action, pharmacokinetics, side effects, and rational use of drugs. It further discusses frequent prescribing scenarios and safety concerns, such as drug interactions and monitoring parameters.

Chapter 5 is dedicated to the cardiovascular system. It addresses common disorders such as hypertension, ischemic heart disease, heart failure, and arrhythmias. Diagnostic techniques such as ECG interpretation, echocardiography, and stress testing are covered, as well as both non-pharmacological and pharmacological approaches.

Chapter 6 deals with the respiratory system. It provides information regarding diseases like asthma, chronic obstructive pulmonary disease, pneumonia, and interstitial lung disease. The chapter also addresses techniques in spirometry, imaging, and arterial blood gas determination, and how to select and use inhaled drugs and systemic therapy.

Chapter 7 covers gastrointestinal system disease. From gastroesophageal reflux disease and peptic ulcers to inflammatory bowel disease and hepatic dysfunction, the chapter provides systematic approaches to diagnosis and treatment, including the utilization of endoscopy, imaging, and tests based on laboratory results.

Chapter 8 covers endocrine and metabolic disorders like diabetes mellitus, thyroid disease, adrenal disease, and metabolic syndrome. The chapter mentions clinical features, right hormone assays, imaging techniques, and current management suggestions for acute as well as chronic disorders.

Chapter 9 covers the renal and genitourinary systems. Conditions like acute kidney injury, chronic kidney disease, urinary tract infections, nephrotic syndrome, and benign prostatic conditions are discussed. Diagnostic methods like urine studies, imaging, and renal function monitoring are described, as well as treatment paradigms for both inpatient and outpatient care.

Chapter 10 describes hematological and oncologic disorders that occur in general practice. Anemias, coagulation disorders, leukemia, and common malignancies are covered with attention to identification, initial workup, and early referral. Supportive care and screening strategies are also listed.

Chapter 11 discusses rheumatologic and musculoskeletal conditions such as osteoarthritis, rheumatoid arthritis, gout, and connective tissue disorders. Diagnostic challenges and criteria, the role of serological assessment and imaging, and medical vs. rehabilitative management are illustrated.

Chapter 12 deals with neurological disorders. Common presentations such as headache, epilepsy, stroke, neuropathies, and movement disorders are covered. Clinical signs, noteworthy investigations such as neuroimaging and nerve conduction studies, and the use of drugs and non-pharmacologic measures are explained.

Chapter 13 concludes the book with an overview of infectious diseases, an area of highly active concern in both inpatient and outpatient practice. The bacterial, viral, fungal, and parasitic infections are considered, with descriptions of their pathophysiology, common signs and symptoms, diagnostic testing, therapeutic principles, and public health issues.

This guidebook is designed for heterogeneous readers who work in healthcare. The guidebook will be useful for medical students as a stepping stone from textbook learning to clinical practice. Practicing clinicians and general practitioners can refer to the book for systematic assistance in diagnosing and treating routine conditions. Nursing professionals, physician assistants, and allied healthcare staff can also benefit from the detailed but not too technical descriptions of systems and conditions.

INTRODUCTION TO GENERAL MEDICINE

1

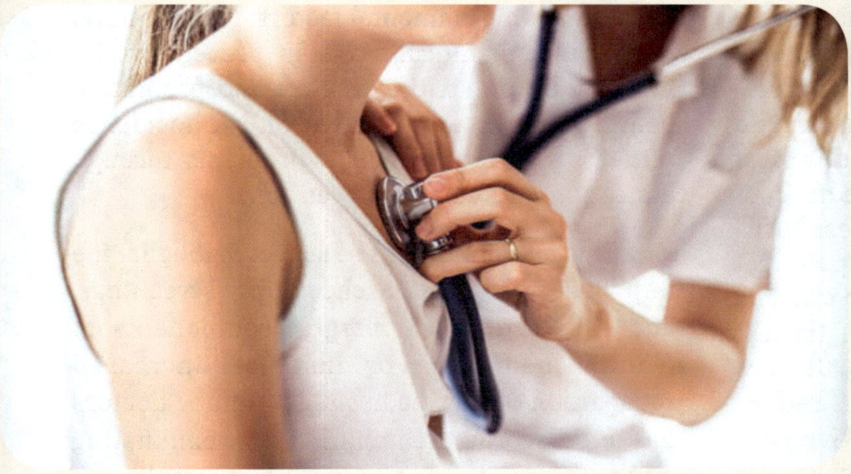

LEARNING OBJECTIVES

After studying this chapter, you will be able to:

1. Understand the role of general practitioners
2. Describe common medical conditions treated
3. Explain diagnostic techniques in general medicine
4. Discuss treatment approaches in general medicine
5. Deal with challenges in general medicine
6. Focus on the future of general medicine

Introduction

General medicine is one of the fundamental pillars of medical healthcare. It provides extensive and holistic care to patients across various age groups and diseases. It includes assessment, diagnosis, and treatment of a wide range of diseases, providing an integrative practice in patient care. As general medicine-trained doctors, general practitioners (GP) need to be aware of how one system relates to another, recognizing the nuances of different conditions, and examining their interactions. The concept of interdisciplinary practice is vital; GPs integrate their practice with other specialists in fields of surgery, dermatology, gynecology, or cardiology. This collaboration enhances patient outcomes and promotes comprehensive treatment plans sensitive to unique health requirements. The practice of general medicine has evolved significantly in the last few decades, prompted by medical research and technological advancements. Diagnoses and treatment protocols have been transformed with advances in diagnostic equipment and treatment protocols. This has enhanced precision for complex conditions as well as the creation of tailored therapeutic plans. Translational research, for instance, on utilizing laboratory findings in clinical practice, has bridged the gap between basic research and clinical practice (Gooneratne et al., 2019). This dynamic exchange promotes continuous updating of healthcare practice, enabling GPs to adapt new information and approaches that improve patient care and enhance disease understanding. Constant commitment to science ensures that general medicine takes the lead in responding to contemporary health challenges. Moreover, general medicine plays a particularly significant role in managing congenital diseases, such as congenital anemia, which present unique challenges in the diagnosis and treatment of patients (Zaplatnikov et al., 2022). The delicate interplay of such a condition necessitates complete knowledge of patient history, potential risk factors, and the latest diagnostic criteria, all of which rest on the shoulders of the GP. With early detection and intervention, GPs are uniquely positioned to improve outcomes, reduce perinatal losses, and carry out effective care strategies. Additionally, the integrative character of the strategy devised by general medicine allows comprehensive patient education and advocacy while promoting preventive health measures, and early treatment that may prevent complications caused by congenital disorders. Therefore, general medicine not only cures present illnesses but also supports broader medical programs in the community aimed at well-being and prevention.

Definition and Scope of General Medicine

The practice of general medicine encompasses a broad area of health activities engaged in the promotion, maintenance, and restoration of wellness across various populations. It is the foundation of medical practice, which involves gathering the entire body of knowledge from all disciplines to provide patient-focused care. It is not just the treatment of specific conditions; rather, it encompasses individuals' overall well-being by addressing physical as well as mental issues. Doctors in this specialty call upon evidence-based guidelines and clinical acumen to diagnose and manage a variety of health conditions, from acute illnesses to chronic illnesses. The holistic character of such a regimen ensures that patients receive personalized treatment, considering the complexity of their health cases as well as the multifaceted interactions of numerous biological, social, and environmental factors. Furthermore, it carries a significant role in prevention. By focusing on preventing disease and promoting health, it seeks to cut down on the incidence of a wide variety of health problems through education and early intervention.

This prevention-based aspect highlights the importance of routine check-ups, screenings, and vaccinations as integral components of overall medicine. For instance, increased recognition of vaccine hesitancy among doctors has underscored the importance of eliminating myths about vaccines and once again establishing immunization as a means of prevention (Gadoth et al., 2021). By educating patients with facts and instruments, family doctors not only help individuals make more informed decisions but also contribute to improving public health outcomes on a population level. Its boundaries reach beyond the individual patient. It is interconnected with public health, community medicine, and global health initiatives. The interconnectedness is representative of the call to a more integrated model of healthcare in the pursuit of equity. The GPs are increasingly called on to grasp the social determinants of health, which directly affect health outcomes. Further, technological innovation and data analytics present the potential of better patient management and individualized treatment plans. As healthcare environments evolve, the position of GPs becomes more important, with the necessity for continuous education and adaptability in an effort to deliver effective care to the diverse and constantly changing needs of their patient base (Matthew et al., 2021). This dynamic attribute recycles the essential importance of general medicine in shaping future trends of healthcare delivery systems (Figure 1.1).

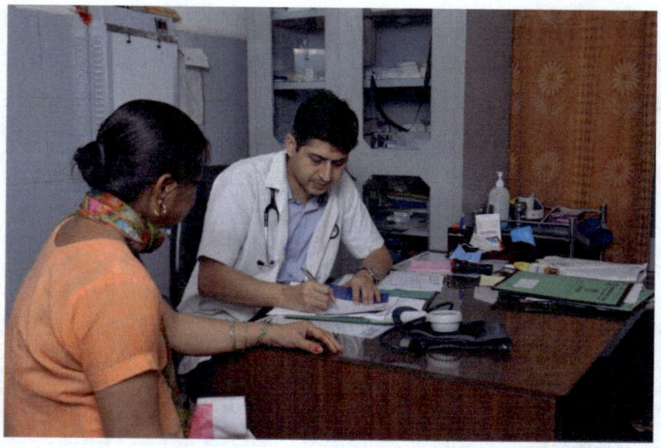

Figure 1.1. A doctor prescribing medicine to a patient.

Source: https://sacredhearthospitaljal.in/wp-content/uploads/2020/01/general_medicine.jpg.

Historical Development of General Medicine

The course of general medicine has been significantly influenced by multiple historical events, which have given rise to its modern-day practice and principles. Its early origins date back as far as ancient civilizations, where healers utilized a combination of natural remedies and spiritual routines to treat ailments. In ancient Egypt, for instance, medicinal herbs and various surgical procedures were described on papyrus scrolls, forming the basis of future medical progress. Greece also formed medical philosophy, most notably through Hippocrates, "Father of Medicine," whose emphasis on clinical observation and ethical practice is summarized in the Hippocratic Corpus. This text pre-dated and dictated medical practice for centuries. Medicine in earlier times was a combination of empirical knowledge and philosophical thought. Over the course of history, it would eventually evolve into a more formal and scientific method. The Middle Ages were a critical turning point in this evolutionary process. The interaction of cultural interchange and major progress in medical understanding defined this period. The disintegration of the Western Roman Empire in the 5th century led to the fragmentation of the practice of medicine in Europe. At the same time, Islamic doctors maintained and developed the medical works of the ancients. Avicenna (Ibn Sina) composed authoritative treatises such as The Canon of Medicine, which fused ancient Greek, Roman, and Persian medical sciences. When European universities began to emerge in the 12th century, they incorporated such Islamic medical texts and spurred a revival of medical schooling. This period also sprang up the concept of hospitals as establishments for care, demonstrating a trend towards organized medical care that would flower into the studies of anatomy and pathology during the Renaissance. This period laid the foundations for contemporary medicine. The Enlightenment and subsequent centuries saw the emergence of general medicine as a distinct discipline solidly rooted in empirical fact and scientific investigation. The 19th and 18th centuries saw revolutionary developments, such as the discovery of vaccines by Edward Jenner and Germ theory by Louis Pasteur and Robert Koch. These scientific advances transformed the idea of the etiology of disease and opened a new era in public health interventions. Advances in surgery and anesthesia have also significantly improved patient care. Through the merging of clinical practice and rigorous scientific methodologies, the new model of general medicine began to form, characterized by evidence-based practices (EBPs) and patient-centered care, eventually revolutionizing the profession and paving the way for contemporary healthcare systems.

Importance of General Medicine in Healthcare

The place of general medicine in the provision of healthcare cannot be overestimated. It forms the foundation of maximum patient management and disease prevention. GPs are most often the first point of contact for individuals obtaining healthcare. They are therefore well-positioned to identify ill health signs and refer patients to a specialist, if necessary. This first function introduces a more integrated provision of healthcare and promotes continuity of care, which does not exist in partitioned healthcare systems. With chronic disease on the increase, there has never been a greater need for accessible general medical care. GPs are equipped with a wide array of skills to deal with various health problems, from acute issues to long-term conditions, and hence deliver integrative care for diverse populations (Gadoth et al., 2021). GP training not only prepares healthcare workers to handle a vast array of disorders but also encourages the importance of integrative patient care. GPs are tasked with assessing patients' physical, mental, and social states, and this demands an intimate understanding of how all these elements correlate. Comprehensive assessments of this nature are essential in the identification of hidden elements that contribute to health outcomes. Moreover, due to the rise in mental health issues blamed on global issues like the COVID-19 pandemic, GPs are increasingly being called upon to address such problems alongside physical ailments. As a focus through various studies, quality mental healthcare in general practice medicine has proven to have actual potential in alleviating psychological distress, further attesting to the role of general medicine in an overall health strategy (Zhou et al., 2020). The support of general medicine is therefore imperative in solving not only immediate healthcare problems but even long-term public health goals. By improving overall access to general medical services, healthcare systems can enhance preventive intervention in care and, therefore, ease the burden of preventable illnesses. Education programs aimed at increasing the number of healthcare workers in general medicine can create a more robust workforce that can handle the diversified health needs in communities. Moreover, with a shift to more patient-centered healthcare, the role of general medicine practitioners in advocacy of patients' needs, lifestyle adaptation counseling, and health literacy becomes more crucial. Increased funding for general medicine is therefore an investment in healthier futures for societies since the practice directly correlates with improved health outcomes and overall population well-being (Zhou et al., 2020; Gadoth et al., 2021).

1.1. The Role of General Practitioners

Learning Outcome

1. Explain the responsibilities of general practitioners
2. Understand the patient-doctor relationship
3. Discuss the impact on community health

The role of GPs goes beyond the initial consultation. GPs play a focal point in the entire continuum of patient care, particularly managing chronic diseases such as diabetes or cardiovascular disease (CVD). GPs not only diagnose and treat disease, but also educate patients in preventive health behaviors, lifestyle modification, and regular health check-ups. This dual function promotes a greater understanding of patients' backgrounds, which is vital in formulating individualized treatment plans. With the evolution of healthcare systems, collaboration between GPs and specialists has increasingly become indispensable. Early referral and effective communication ensure that patients receive holistic treatment, highlighting the value of GPs as care coordinators (Boutros et al., 2024).

GPs also play an essential role in the recognition and management of situations requiring intervention from specialists – for example, oncologists, dermatologists, or surgeons. The expanding role of remedies for skin cancers such as melanoma is a clear demonstration of the requirement for a liaison system in general medicine. GPs are positioned to watch patients for the entire treatment process, detecting side effects and toxicities associated with therapies. Their exposure to immunotherapy-associated complications, for example, allows them to initiate prompt management and facilitate timely referral to oncologists, so that patients receive quality, timely care during their treatment course (Boutros et al., 2024). Such shared care not only enhances patient satisfaction but also optimizes the utilization of healthcare resources.

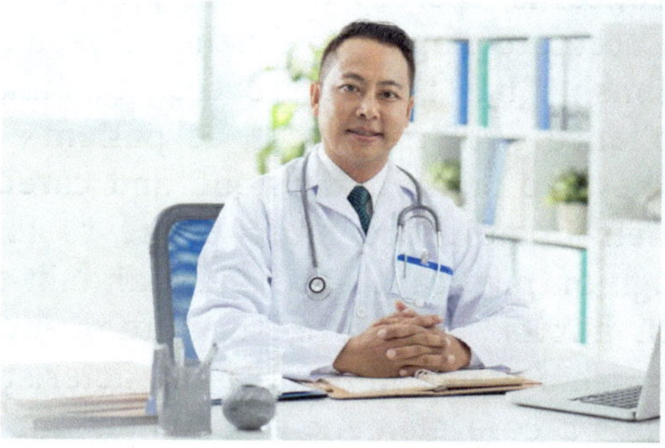

Figure 1.2. General practitioner (GP).

Source: https://cdn-asse ts-eu.frontify.com/s3/frontify -enterprise-files-eu/eyJw YXRoIjoiaWho LWhlYWx0aGNhcm UtYm VyaGFkXC9hY2N vdW50c1wvYzNc LzQw MDA2MjRcL3Byb2plY3Rz XC8yMDlcL2Fzc2V0c1wv OTNcLzM4MTA2XC8wZjdhMmE0MzQ w ZjBhN GQ4YmQzYTM4MzQ4 OWU1NjNjNi0xNjU4MzAxMD MwLmpw Zy J9:ihh-healt hcare-berhad:nYMJB5Lu uXfSBJcG-_Q0t1kYG wm69-ssAPGgKR YpLH M?format=webp.

The creation of general practitioners with extended roles (GPwER) has introduced new efficiencies to the healthcare system. For instance, experiences at independent spinal care centers demonstrate that specialist-trained GPs in spinal disorders can determine the urgency of surgical referral for conditions like low back pain or neck pain after a thorough screening and assessment of such patients. By streamlining the process of patient referral and correctly identifying those patients who actually need surgical treatment, the GPwER cuts unnecessary waiting times, relieving the demand on surgical wards and freeing up greater access to the relevant treatment. Therefore, the evolving role of GPs illustrates the ever-present requirement for general medicine to be flexible and adaptable (Figure 1.2).

1.1.1. Role and Responsibilities of General Practitioners

The working contribution of GPs extends considerably beyond clinical treatment and diagnosis; it also involves responsibilities that have a direct effect on patient outcomes and overall community health. GPs are often the first point of entry into the healthcare system, thereby allowing them to build trusting relationships with their patients. This is essential to frank communication around sensitive matters of health, lifestyle change, and preventive care. GPs are in a unique position to induce behavioral changes in their patients, a skill that maximizes not only their educator role but also emphasizes the necessity of creating an environment for initiating and maintaining healthier lives (Baky et al., 2025). GPs play a pivotal role in public health promotion.

In balancing the duties associated with the risks of over-medicalizing patient care, GPs are confronted with the consequences of medical decisions. Most GPs feel uneasy about the pressures exerted by different forces within society and through technology that tend to shape clinical practices. Such unease tends to foster skepticism regarding their social functions, especially in terms of how they should strike a balance between medical intervention and the conditions of patient experiences. After a qualitative study, the researchers noted that GPs prioritized effective doctor-patient interaction, listening to clinical instinct, and reliance on EBPs over various aspects of their practice (Michaël et al., 2024). These suggestions express a realization of relational processes in healthcare as required, allowing GPs to cope with complexity more authentically and with compassion. Thus, the challenge of being empathetic without over-medicalizing is intrinsic to their work.

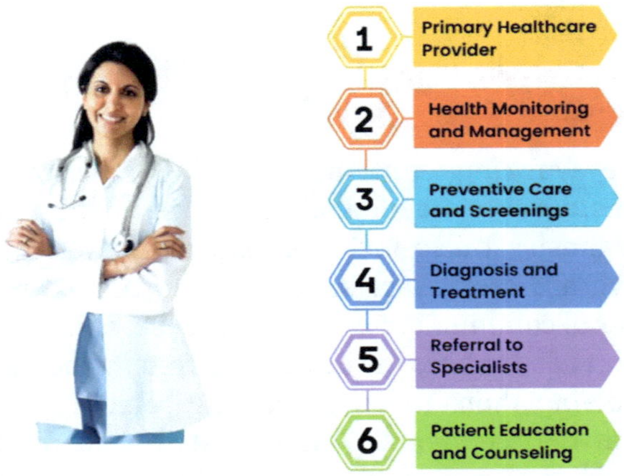

Figure 1.3. Role of general practitioners.

Source: https://deepahospital.b-cdn.net/wp-content/uploads/2024/10/Role-of-General-Physicians-1024x655.webp.

They must also recognize the overlapping vulnerabilities that the patients and they themselves share. In dealing with the problems caused by over-medicalization, the GPs' recognition of their own vulnerabilities can give a clearer image of the patient's needs and the care. By involving an open dialogue of such vulnerabilities, GPs collaborate with patients to develop adaptive, personalized care plans that consider unique circumstances and choices. This collaborative effort encourages co-decision-making and encourages patients to become more active participants in their own healthcare experiences. Meanwhile, GPs are also driven to partake in continuing professional development and leadership programs that address such problems on a community scale. Thus, GPs not only perform their roles when meeting patients but also contribute inputs to broader debates on healthcare practice and ethical concerns in general medicine overall (Figure 1.3).

1.1.2. Patient-Doctor Relationship

The doctor-patient relationship is a fundamental aspect of effective healthcare delivery. The foundation of this relationship is built on trust, communication, and respect. A sound relationship allows patients to freely express their symptoms and concerns, thereby allowing physicians to make accurate diagnoses. Furthermore, a good relationship has been discovered to enhance compliance with treatment, as patients who feel they are being understood and cared for by their doctors are more prone to follow through on medical advice and maintain their health habits. Therefore, the patient-doctor relationship is not an adjunct characteristic of care but a core element that fosters the rest of the medical interaction and results in better health outcomes.

Various factors including cultural competence and the recognition of sex and gender differences in the healthcare experience influence the dynamics of the patient-physician relationship. Clinicians must be aware that these differences have a significant impact on diagnostic and therapeutic responses, as reported in today's medical literature. Understanding how sex and gender influence health behavior and response to treatment is one of the most critical areas for enhancing the quality of care. Through consciously integrating these factors into their practice, healthcare workers can work towards offering more individualized and equitable care. Such a responsive approach not only improves the patient-doctor relationship but also aligns with the broader goals of precision medicine, which is to tailor interventions to consider the unique needs of an individual patient, as detailed by Mauvais et al. (2020).

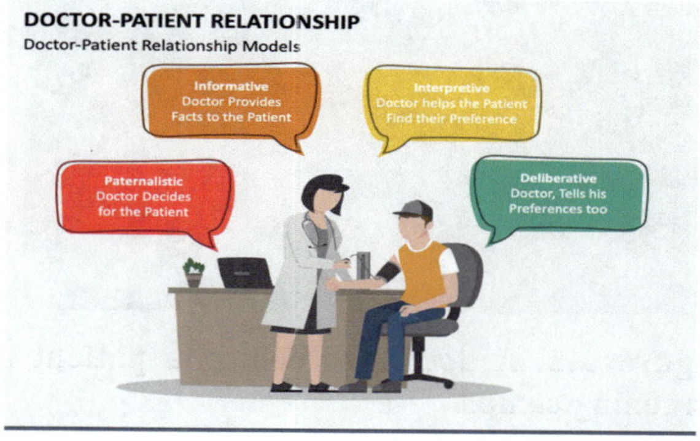

Figure 1.4. Doctor–patient relationship.

Source: https://i.ytimg.com/vi/2tEHjZp3E1c/hq720.jpg?sqp=-oaymwEhCK4FEIIDSFryq4qpAxMIARUAAAAAGAElAADIQj0AgKJD&rs=AOn4CLB2FbhRsg2dX_4SFrOIwYH13_YcDA.

Finally, the evolution of medical science, particularly the microbiota-gut-brain axis, again underscores the need for strong patient-physician relationships. Emerging studies illuminate the intricate mechanisms of how gut microbiota affect not only gut health but also neurological and psychiatric diseases. Intimate communication about lifestyle, diet, and therapeutic approaches is essential in understanding these connections. Effective communication is crucial, as it enables the GP to educate the patient on the significance of aspects such as stress management and nutrition, which have a direct impact on the microbiota and consequently overall health. Through this interaction, healthcare professionals can deliver comprehensive care that addresses physical as well as psychological well-being, illustrating the evolution of cooperation in the practice of medicine today, as observed by John et al. (2019) (Figure 1.4).

1.1.3. Impact on Community Health

In recent years, the impact on community health has increasingly become noticed within the scope of overall medicine, particularly in terms of control of chronic disease. Understanding how geographic disparities influence health outcomes is essential for health practitioners. For example, there have been significant variations in treatment and care for such chronic illnesses as diabetes and hypertension between urban and rural populations. Rural patients also have unique challenges like older age and higher visit frequency, and these need to be catered to with modified healthcare measures. This scenario highlights the impact of socioeconomic factors and the availability of resources on health outcomes within the community, particularly in the case of public health emergencies like the COVID-19 pandemic, which further escalated the inequities. Satisfying these unique needs is required to improve healthcare delivery and optimize health interventions in diverse communities (Duda-Sikuła et al., 2024).

Food insecurity has emerged as a significant public health issue and is a pivotal element that impacts the well-being of the population in the context of internal medicine. It affects millions of individuals across the nation. Although healthcare professionals recognize more and more the necessity of screening patients for food insecurity, the practice falls short all too frequently. Many GPs report screening infrequently, primarily due to concerns of time and other clinical priorities while those at more rural locations cite limited community resources as one of the barriers. These barriers not only affect patient outcomes but also indicate more profound systemic issues contributing to health inequities. Healthcare providers can, by acknowledging and addressing these barriers, work to build more integrated strategies for addressing food insecurity as a critical component of community health interventions (Bunt et al., 2024). Ultimately, the convergence of chronic disease management and food insecurity highlights the importance of multidisciplinary strategies to enhance community health. These are related to each other; those having difficulty with food security are typically at a higher risk for chronic disease, which requires constant management and access to appropriate healthcare services. Thus, this calls for promoting community health interventions with a multiple-approach strategy involving healthcare providers, policymakers, and community organizations. Designing specific interventions for addressing chronic disease management and food insecurity can help build healthier communities. By laying extra stress on the special requirements of mixed populations and eliminating existing barriers, improved health outcomes and quality of life (QoL) might be facilitated among the communities, confirming the resilience of an integrated view of health in general medicine (Bunt et al., 2024; Duda-Sikuła et al., 2024) (Figure 1.5).

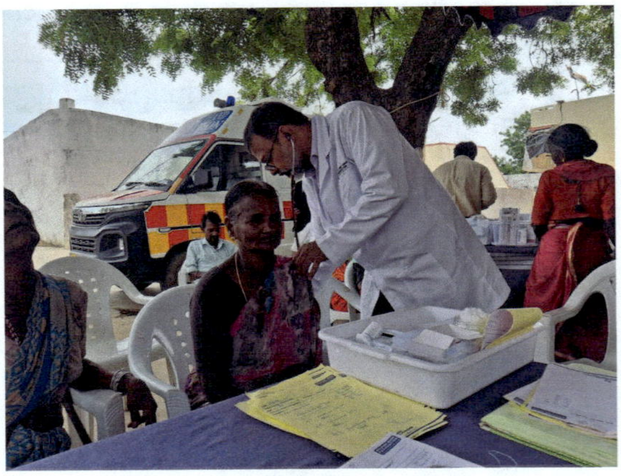

Figure 1.5. A doctor screening a patient at screening camps.

Source: https://th-i.thgim.com/public/incoming/h1ov5b/article68659803.ece/alternates/FREE_1200/IMG-20240919-WA0012.jpg.

Test Your Knowledge

1. What are the primary responsibilities of a General Practitioner?
2. How does the patient-doctor relationship foster trust and improve the overall effectiveness of healthcare delivery in primary care?

1.2. Common Medical Conditions Treated

Learning Outcome

1. Describe chronic diseases
2. Understand acute illnesses
3. Focus on preventive care and health screenings

In general practice, practitioners most often manage a wide range of common medical conditions that need to be addressed and treated quickly and correctly. Among them, headaches are persistent and present in various ways, from tension-type to migraine. A study in EDs in the past revealed that over 86% of non-urgent headaches were treated with predominantly Chinese medicine alongside Western medicine. This two-modality approach not only offers choices for the patient but also can be helpful for improved global outcome of treatment, particularly chronic diseases that are unresponsive to traditional pharmacologic regimens (Mao et al., 2025). Practitioners should be aware of the extent of possible treatments available for headache so that patients' wants and tailored clinical needs may be met.

CVD is another prevalent condition in general practice, characterized by a range of presentations including hypertension, heart failure (HF), and arrhythmias. Such typically occur in older patients who possess complex medical histories, presenting problems in diagnosis and treatment. Multiple challenges arise in the care of these patients. For instance, consider the following scenario: A 66-year-old man with HF and atrial fibrillation (AF) on anticoagulation with apixaban developed chest pain and dizziness. He was soon discovered to have a hemopericardium, a potentially life-threatening complication, which necessitated emergency surgery. This case brings into focus the role of monitoring high-risk patients and also the importance of developing greater awareness among clinicians regarding the role of anticoagulation in the setting of multiple comorbidities (Latif et al., 2024). The case brings into focus not only the nuances of cardiovascular care in the setting of general medicine but also emphasizes the importance of a comprehensive treatment approach. Further, diabetes care has also emerged as another pillar in the practice of general medicine due to the rising pattern of this chronic complication. Diabetes mellitus, particularly type 2, has a strong correlation with lifestyle factors such as physical inactivity and obesity. Disease control often necessitates a multivariant intervention with glycemic control, lifestyle modification, and patient education. Clinicians routinely employ pharmacologic treatments alongside dietary and physical activity interventions to improve patient outcomes. In recent years, advancements in diabetes management have introduced novel therapies that target both metabolic control and cardiovascular risk, enhancing the overall care framework (Mao et al., 2025). As GPs struggle to understand the complexities of diabetes control, they need to remain open to making multiple adjustments in treatment recommendations based on the fluctuating needs of patients, hence maintaining the tenets of general medicine practice.

1.2.1. Chronic Diseases (e.g., Diabetes, Hypertension)

Chronic conditions such as diabetes and high blood pressure are significant public health issues affecting millions of individuals worldwide. Diabetes, a condition characterized by elevated blood levels of glucose, can lead to severe complications such as heart disease, kidney failure, and neuropathy, primarily when poorly managed. This chronic condition has been on a steady rise due to the prevalence of physical inactivity, poor diets, and increased levels of obesity. Similarly, high blood pressure or hypertension can lead to long-term issues such as stroke and heart disease. These long-term ailments require frequent medical care and lifestyle changes to minimize their impact on individuals' QoL.

With increased global awareness of such illnesses, the healthcare systems must adapt to provide comprehensive management plans that emphasize prevention, early detection, and patient education, hence achieving a reduction of the cost burden of healthcare due to chronic diseases (Baum et al., 2020). Management of chronic diseases such as diabetes and hypertension has experienced significant expansion in transformations through the inclusion of technological innovation and patient-centered care. Diabetes care has globally embraced telehealth alternatives, especially during the COVID-19 pandemic, when in-person visits were strictly regulated. Baum et al. (2020) recognized a significant trend in healthcare provision with a dramatic increase in telehealth consultations that allowed uninterrupted follow-up without ever compromising patient care. Similarly, technology-facilitated health platforms currently facilitate personalized care plans based on the individual's needs and comorbidities. Optimal hypertension control is generally achieved with alterations in lifestyle and in conjunction with medication.

The therapy based on this two-prong approach not only impacts blood pressure control but also the associated risk factors. It indicates the importance of a comprehensive approach in treating chronic disease. Physician interaction is also essential in adding value to the outcome of patients with chronic illness. An interdisciplinary approach, where primary care physicians, specialists, and allied health professionals work together, ensures all aspects of a patient's situation are addressed. For instance, a patient-specific care plan, put into practice with the patient collaboratively, can lead to better treatment and lifestyle adherence. As emphasized in the continuous support and education can allow patients, particularly in at-risk populations, to be actively involved in their own healthcare. This multimodal strategy is crucial given the complex interaction of physical, emotional, and social factors surrounding chronic disease care, culminating in disease progression elimination and enhancement of patients' QoL (Figure 1.6).

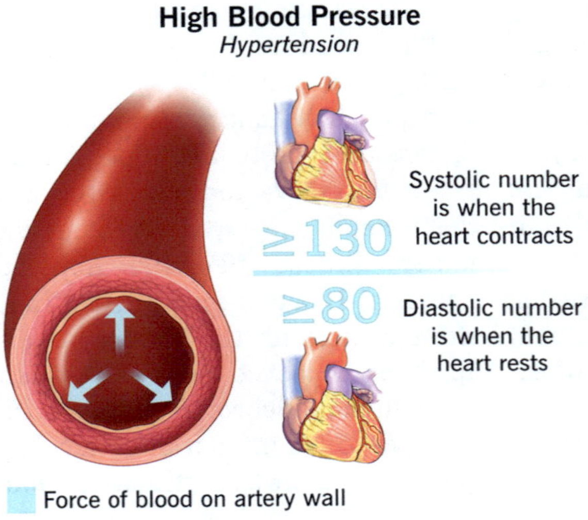

Figure 1.6. High blood pressure illustration.

Source: https://my.clevelandclinic.org/-/scassets/images/org/health/articles/4314-high-blood-pressure-illustration.

1.2.2. Acute Illnesses (e.g., Infections, Injuries)

Acute diseases, particularly trauma and infections, are among the most significant challenges in the field of general medicine. As soon as these patients are encountered, healthcare providers must conduct detailed examinations in a brisk and timely manner to arrive at a plausible working diagnosis and provide appropriate treatment. Acute illnesses may be life-threatening. Management of these diseases is challenged not only by the immediate physiological effects on the body but also by the psychosocial factors, which can influence recovery. For instance, an acute infection, such as meningitis or pneumonia, may rapidly compromise hemodynamics and respiratory status. Precise early diagnosis and treatment are critical; any delay can lead to serious complications, including organ dysfunction or loss of life. Treatment of the underlying pathophysiology of these acute ailments is paramount. Therefore, an effective strategy for the treatment of acute diseases demands a holistic approach considering both situational and clinical elements.

Accidental injuries and falls constitute another big category of acute diseases. Their treatment commonly demands immediate medical care, emphasizing the provision of an efficient emergency response system. Acting on proper management protocols based on EBPs is integral to patient safety and optimal outcomes. Revolutionary practices in clinical management, as illustrated in the literature of emergency medicine, focus on interventions of timely action coupled with proven methods, such as proper sedation and injury stabilization. Quality of care in such life-moment decisions not only impacts immediate recovery but also subsequent QoL.

A multidisciplinary approach, involving the expertise of a team of healthcare professionals, is called for to enhance the outcomes of patients, particularly in complicated cases where injuries could endanger multiple organ systems. The understanding of the interconnection between acute injuries and their long-term consequences remains a crucial part of general medical training. Recent advances in the management of acute illness have changed perspectives on the treatment regimes, particularly intensive care. Old practices, such as liberal sedation and protocol-directed transfusions, have been criticized in critical illness (Singer et al., 2010). Recent research confirms a more refined understanding of patient treatment that prioritizes individualized care. This development follows heightened sensitivity to the vital role played by medical professionals in avoiding undesirable outcomes, such as secondary infection formation and prolonged hospital stay. Aside from these, the criteria outlined through the system of emergency care underscore the importance of addressing acute disorders through a cautious, researched manner (Lowry, 2009). With health practitioners continually improving the way they treat acute diseases, ongoing education and collaboration are essential in responding to the diverse demands of patients effectively (Figure 1.7).

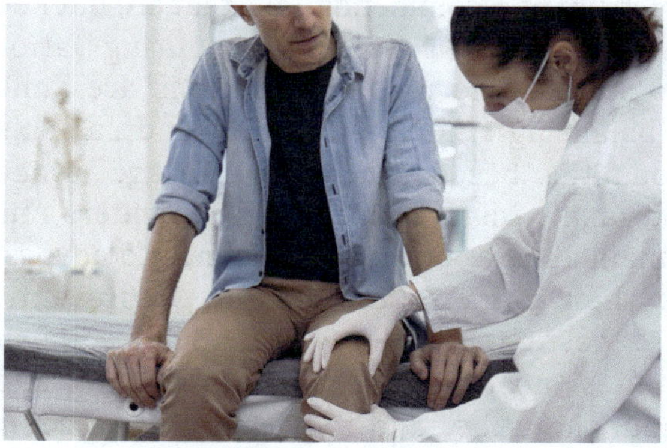

Figure 1.7. Doctors treating patients leg injuries.

Source: https://motionorthopodiatry.com/wp-content/uploads/2025/02/ACL-Injury-Checkup-by-doctor-scaled.jpg.

1.2.3. Preventive Care and Health Screenings

Preventive treatment and health screening cannot be overstressed. Early diagnosis is at the forefront of better patient outcomes. Preventive care is composed of numerous services that entail immunizations, routine check-ups, and screenings that are utilized to identify potential ailments before evolving into serious illnesses. Through such interventions, healthcare workers effectively relieve the burden caused by chronic diseases, eventually enhancing the QoL of the patients. Repeated health checks, such as hypertension, diabetes, and cancer, become an essential means for early diagnosis. Early intervention through these checks significantly enhances prognosis as well as greatly reduces the mortality rates of several diseases. As shown by the evidence available, individuals who receive preventive care tend to live healthier lives, and that serves to reinforce the imperative for mass health education and awareness of these necessary services. Evidence-based guidelines should also be included in the routine practice of preventive care to ensure screening procedures are effective, practical, and efficient. The U.S. Preventive Services Task Force (USPSTF) has set guidelines for a broad spectrum of recommendations that are intended to screen specific populations during various life stages. The recommendations are aimed at balancing risks and benefits, and screening modalities based on factors like age, gender, and family history. Healthcare providers must remain abreast of these guidelines to advocate for their patients and encourage preventive care most appropriate to individualized health profiles, most effectively. Good communication about the utility and importance of screening can facilitate patients' engagement as active partners in their health, cutting through access barriers and encouraging an active attitude toward well-being. This is particularly important in cases where socioeconomic conditions may deter the utilization of such essential preventive care services. Finally, a more detailed investigation of health disparities also highlights the necessity for intervention-focused preventive care and screening services. Racial and ethnic minorities, as specific groups, are disproportionately affected by chronic illness and are typically faced with barriers to accessing healthcare services. Focused interventions on cultural, socioeconomic, and geographic factors are required to move health equity forward. For instance, focused public health campaigns in response to specific community issues can raise awareness and encourage uptake of preventive screening. By applying culturally tailored interventions, health systems bridge gaps in preventive service use between the underserved and those in need. As healthcare provision is in the limelight in this contemporary era, the push towards equity becomes essential. From the discussions around preventive interventions and access barriers, health inequity is central to creating a healthy society via inclusive preventive care interventions (Nicolaidis, 2007; Zupo et al., 2023) (Figure 1.8).

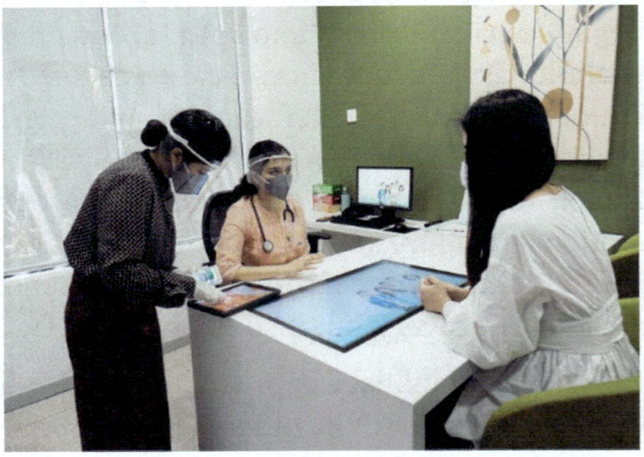

Figure 1.8. Health screenings.

Source: https://nura.in/wp-content/uploads/2025/02/NuraC_15.jpg.

Test Your Knowledge

1. What are the most common chronic diseases managed by General Practitioners?
2. How do General Practitioners balance the treatment of both chronic conditions and acute illnesses in a single patient?

1.3. Diagnostic Techniques in General Medicine

Learning Outcome

1. Describe physical examination methods
2. Understand laboratory tests and imaging
3. Explain the importance of accurate diagnosis

The diagnostic techniques employed in general medicine continually enhance with each revolutionary stride, allowing conditions to be diagnosed earlier and with greater accuracy. The traditional methods of physical examination and radiologic imaging have experienced a phenomenal enhancement, enhancing their diagnostic worth and effectiveness. For instance, synergistic integration of deep machine learning techniques has allowed for intricate analysis of clinical data, leading to improved predictive understanding of patient outcomes. This innovation marks the shift from symptomatic treatment in isolation to precision medicine, allowing clinicians to tailor interventions based on personalized patient data. The application of high-level artificial intelligence (AI) methods in diagnostic applications not only streamlines the process but also optimizes the decision-making platform, establishing a new standard in the field of diagnosis (Mizera et al., 2025). In addition to AI technology, hybrid nanomaterials are also being established as prominent contributors in diagnostic medicine, especially in nanomedicine and regenerative medicine. These composites combine the beneficial properties of different constituents to generate functionalities superior to the sum of their components. Their applications range from enhancing the sensitivity of imaging modalities in bioimaging to advancing point-of-care diagnostic technologies. Hybrid nanostructures, for example, are increasingly used to develop contrast agents and biosensors, which play a vital role in the real-time detection of diseases. The novel advantages of such nanomaterials are the ability to target specific biomarkers preferentially, and this leads to enhanced diagnostic accuracy and precision-based therapeutic regimens. These advances highlight the essential roles played by material science in advancing the practice of diagnosis in general medicine (Zhang et al., 2024). The deployment of these advanced diagnostic techniques not only improves patient management but also reflects significant challenges and opportunities for worldwide healthcare systems. One of the greatest concerns is the way in which the medical practitioners are adequately trained to view and interpret the complex information that such new technologies generate. Furthermore, ethical considerations about confidentiality of data and the role of AI on clinical judgments are ongoing challenges that must be addressed. On the other hand, the ability of these approaches to reduce health costs and improve patient outcomes cannot be overstated. By maximizing the efficacy and specificity of therapies, advanced diagnostic procedures pave the way to an integrated healthcare system, highlighting the contribution of continuous innovation and adaptability to the field of general medicine (Zhang et al., 2024; Mizera et al., 2025).

1.3.1. Physical Examination Methods

The application of physical examination methods is a pillar in general practice, playing essential roles in diagnosis. The practices allow physicians to establish patient health through visual inspection and talk. There are various examination practices, including inspection, palpation, percussion, and auscultation, which complement each other for complete patient evaluation. For instance, inspection can reveal prominent signs of disease, and palpation can identify pathology not immediately apparent. Systematic application of these methods enables clinicians to effectively gain fundamental information guiding the rest of the diagnostic and therapeutic process, thereby emphasizing the central importance of physical examination in clinical practice. Adoption of evidence-based models for physical examination methods can optimize their efficiency, particularly in domains such as child health promotion. Interventions seeking to alter the physical, social, or emotional surroundings of a child may have varied timeliness regarding demonstrating their effectiveness. Practitioners can extend the scope of their diagnostic methods to include broader contextual determinants of patient health by adopting such strategies.

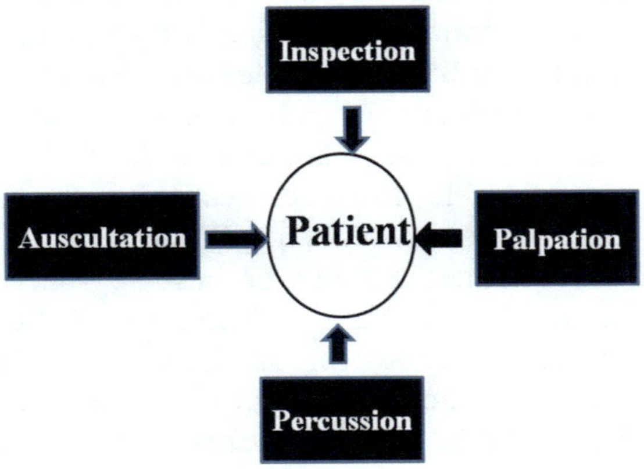

Figure 1.9. Various methods of physical examination of a patient.

Source: https://www.researchgate.net/profile/Rajani-Singh-4/publication/336531710/figure/fig1/AS:960055897776139@1605906571717/Various-methods-of-physical-examination-of-a-patient.png.

This nuanced approach not only produces more precise diagnoses but also facilitates the creation of individualized treatment plans. A child's physical examination can involve examinations of both environmental and physical state, demonstrating how additional contextual layers are required for the full understanding of a patient's general well-being (Vos et al., 2010). Moreover, continuous medical technological and practice advancement has influenced the evolution of physical examination methods. Imaging and telemedicine are specific novel tools and technologies, which are augmenting the traditional examination protocols to facilitate better patient assessment and monitoring. Integration of technology increases the accuracy of diagnosis as well as the chances of greater patient engagement. For instance, the use of portable ultrasound scanners in clinical settings is a fine example of how technology can facilitate detailed exams without compromising patient comfort. Since medicine is constantly developing, health professionals must stay current with advances so that physical examination methods are still valid and effective in an evolving healthcare environment (Araujo-Soares et al., 2010) (Figure 1.9).

1.3.2. Laboratory Tests and Imaging

The role of imaging and laboratory investigations in general medicine is paramount because they provide vital information regarding a patient's health condition, which guides clinical decision-making. Laboratory investigations such as blood chemistry, hematology, and microbiology enable clinicians to detect abnormalities that may signal the presence of underlying disease. These tests are employed in monitoring disease progression, evaluating the efficacy of treatment, and predicting prognoses. For instance, a complete blood count (CBC) will show evidence of low hemoglobin in anemia or increased white cell counts in bacteremia. Metabolic panels delve deeper into the function of organs. As detailed in recent studies, judicious interpretation of laboratory tests supports early interventions that can significantly improve patient outcomes and guide the course of therapy (Holiuk et al., 2025).

Imaging modalities, such as X-ray, ultrasound, and magnetic resonance imaging (MRI), complement laboratory findings by providing pictorial information of internal structures. Not only do they enhance the sensitivity and specificity of diagnosis, but they also help in staging disorders, thus enabling appropriate therapeutic interventions. To illustrate, in osteoarthritis (OA), high-technology imaging can show the extent of joint degeneration, which can uncover intra-articular and periarticular abnormalities of utmost significance to tailor treatment individually. The integration of imaging results and laboratory results presents a more detailed image of conditions, particularly in complex conditions such as multiple sclerosis (MS), where disease monitoring and early detection through MRI are essential for disease control (Lorenzut et al., 2025). The integration of laboratory testing and imaging improves clinical assessment and enables practitioners to develop more informative, personalized modes of patient management. With ongoing innovations in technology, the general medicine field of imaging and laboratory testing is evolving, which leads to innovation that improves diagnostic capabilities.

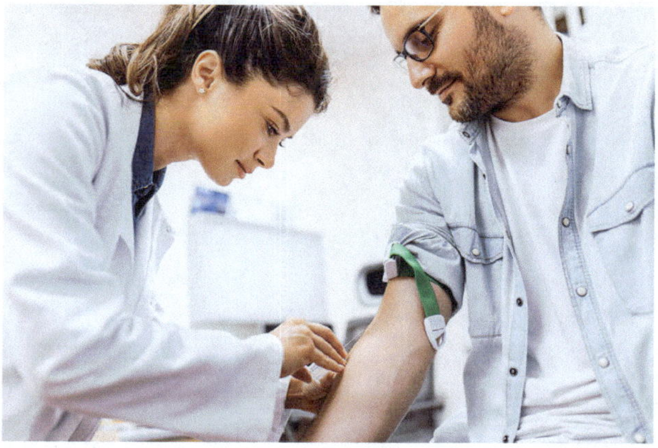

Figure 1.10. A doctor is taking a blood sample for laboratory testing.

Source: https://www.mainlinehealth.org/-/media/images/blog/2023/07/blood-test.jpg.

The creation of biomarkers—molecules found in blood or other body fluids that are associated with disease processes—has the potential to revolutionize the diagnosis and monitoring of disease. For example, some microRNAs were identified to be potential disease biomarkers of OA that enable tailoring treatment strategy (Holiuk et al., 2025). This trend towards incorporating state-of-the-art diagnostics in medicine is indicative of the importance of embracing classical and advanced approaches. The continuous merging of imaging and laboratory testing will definitely shape the future of general practice, with more ability to combine disease surveillance and tailored treatment programs for each patient. With ongoing research and ongoing development in technology, so too will the accuracy of diagnostics improve, and treatment of patients lead to improved results (Figure 1.10).

1.3.3. Importance of Accurate Diagnosis

Precise diagnosis is the foundation of successful general medicine in that it directly affects treatment plans and outcomes in patients. Difficulty in presenting symptoms from patients could frequently result in misdiagnosis, which entails heavy consequences for effectiveness and safety in treatment as well as patient outcome. As an example, evaluation of otolaryngologic complaints that are frequent in general practice requires careful history taking and comprehensive physical examination. As noted by Gilani (2022), the majority of the diagnostic tools needed to make an accurate assessment, such as nasal endoscopy or flexible laryngoscopy, are not usually available in general medicine clinics. Such a limitation requires that GPs employ evidence-based approaches to history taking, asking the right questions, and being sensitive to otolaryngologic illnesses. Such work is critical in the process of excluding likely diagnoses, which will eventually culminate in more efficient management to suit the patient's needs. The repercussions of incorrect diagnosis go beyond treatment delays; they also pose serious threats to patient safety. One of the clearest examples is found in an instance involving misdiagnosis of an infant as dehydrated after a careless administration of diphenoxylate-atropine for diarrhea, according to Khan et al. (2019). It was a result of a lack of knowledge regarding appropriate dosages of drugs in different age groups that led to the infant's development of toxic levels. The subsequent interventions in the ED merely emphasized the importance of accurate clinical assessments. The quick identification of miosis led to the discovery of diphenoxylate-atropine poisoning, in which immediate intravenous administration of naloxone reversed the condition successfully. This case offers a site of demonstration about how important accurate diagnosis processes are in ensuring patient safety and delivering the appropriate interventions in general medicine. In addition to patient safety and effectiveness in treatment, correct diagnosis is also essential to the overall effectiveness of the healthcare system. Misdiagnosis could lead to unnecessary medical expenditure, extended patient suffering, as well as excessive consumption of healthcare resources, hence overburdening the system. They could also create a cycle of mismanagement, as the patients receive treatment for incorrect diagnoses, hence further complicating their medical conditions. When GPs are adequately equipped to make correct evaluations with comprehensive history-taking and physical examination, as emphasized by Gilani (2022), they set a proper platform for follow-up care trajectories. Proper first-time diagnoses thus ensure better allocation of healthcare resources and enhance the quality of provided care. Overall, emphasis on astute and informed diagnostic processes is an essential cornerstone in the landscape of general medicine, ultimately benefiting patients and the healthcare system comprehensively.

Test Your Knowledge

1. What are the key physical examination techniques that General Practitioners use to identify common medical conditions?
2. What is the role of differential diagnosis in general medicine?

1.4. Treatment Approaches in General Medicine

Learning Outcome

1. Understand pharmacological treatments
2. Focus on non-pharmacological interventions
3. Discuss patient education and self-management

In general medicine, treatment models are further shaped by EBPs that integrate new diagnostic technologies and therapeutic protocols. A case in point is the treatment of respiratory pathogens, such as the human metapneumovirus (HMPV), improved with the development of molecular diagnosis. HMPV is among the significant respiratory pathogens responsible for severe morbidity, particularly in susceptible populations like children and older patients. Despite the apparent clinical impact, treatment is primarily focused on supportive care because no particular antiviral drug or vaccine is available. The search for potential therapeutic agents to mitigate the effects of HMPV in future studies is urging a concerted effort toward addressing newly emerging infectious diseases. Thus, the GP must remain updated with evolving practices in treatment to enhance patient care and reduce hospitalization from respiratory infections (Ansori, 2025). Furthermore, the integration of traditional therapies and modern medical practice is more common in general medicine. A good example of this is the use of Traditional Chinese Medicine (TCM) in managing gut microbiota in cancer therapy. A bibliometric analysis further indicates a systemic boost in interest in this area, particularly from 2018, and China is leading the research productivity and collaboration field. Core research areas such as the importance of short-chain fatty acids and their impact on the tumor microenvironment denote a move towards understanding molecular interactions underpinning treatment efficacy. These integrative approaches herald a larger movement in broad medicine, as practitioners are being challenged to explore multi-dimensional treatment models grounded in both traditional herbal medicine and modern scientific data. This emerging specialty not only augments the therapeutic options available but also promotes interdisciplinary correlations that result in enhanced patient outcomes for complex disease (Lei et al., 2025). Increased interdisciplinary endeavors and technologies will presumably complement future therapeutic approaches in general medicine. Emerging scientific disciplines, such as metabolomics and immune checkpoint blockade therapy, pave the way for precision medicine that individualizes treatment according to patient profiles. Such new disciplines can be anticipated to treat significant medical challenges, particularly about chronic and multifactorial conditions. As the field develops, general medicine professionals will need to possess an adaptive and flexible practice that incorporates new research findings into the realm of clinical practice. Professionals can get ready for dealing with the adaptive challenges posed by evolving medical conditions by creating a culture of continuous learning and engagement. Emphasizing a general comprehension of older and newer treatment methodologies will eventually serve a more comprehensive approach to medical care in general medicine (Ansori, 2025; Lei et al., 2025).

1.4.1. Pharmacological Treatments

Pharmacological interventions have emerged as integral components of modern medicine, a broad array of solutions to cure several health conditions. The treatment of psychiatric illnesses, such as bipolar disorder, is one significant area where pharmacological intervention is crucial. Lithium, for example, is well established for stabilizing mood and reducing the frequency of attacks of mania. Despite its proven effectiveness, there is a concerning trend of declining lithium prescriptions throughout the world, as many clinicians overlook its usefulness, inclined instead to fall prey to myths about its safety and dosing in treatment regimens. Addressing these myths can reinvigorate its utilization, thereby enhancing the care of patients at psychiatric clinics. This highlights the importance of clinicians keeping themselves informed of the latest pharmacological treatments and incorporating evidence-based guidance suitably into their treatment plans (Winkelman et al., 2024). Aside from psychiatric care, pharmacological treatment is also essential in treating conditions like restless legs syndrome (RLS) and periodic limb movement disorder (PLMD). The American Academy of Sleep Medicine (AASM) has released some guidelines for the management of these disorders, emphasizing individualized pharmacotherapy based on patient profile. Gabapentin and pregabalin treatments have been provided with strong recommendations due to their moderate level of certainty of evidence in alleviating symptoms. In addition, the role of iron supplementation, guided by serum iron tests, demonstrates the need for a comprehensive treatment approach that incorporates pharmacologic therapies coupled with diagnostic knowledge. These complex management patterns delineate how pharmacologic treatments can significantly improve patient outcomes when combined with clinical guidelines and patient-related variables (Fiorillo et al., 2023). The dynamic nature of pharmacologic treatment necessitates ongoing research and development (R&D) in clinical practice. With each new evidence base, healthcare clinicians must weigh the benefits and risks of pharmacological therapies on an individual basis.

This is particularly germane where various drugs do have conflicting recommendations; e.g., whereas some RLS therapies are favorably viewed, others, like levodopa and pramipexole, are generally recommended against due to side effects. Continuing education, as supplemented by evidence-based guidelines, will enable medical professionals to make informed choices that maximize therapeutic outcomes. Through it, the integration of pharmaceutical treatments into holistic health models will have the twofold advantage of symptom reduction, as well as enhancing the overall QoL for patients with complex medical diseases (Fiorillo et al., 2023; Winkelman et al., 2024) (Figure 1.11).

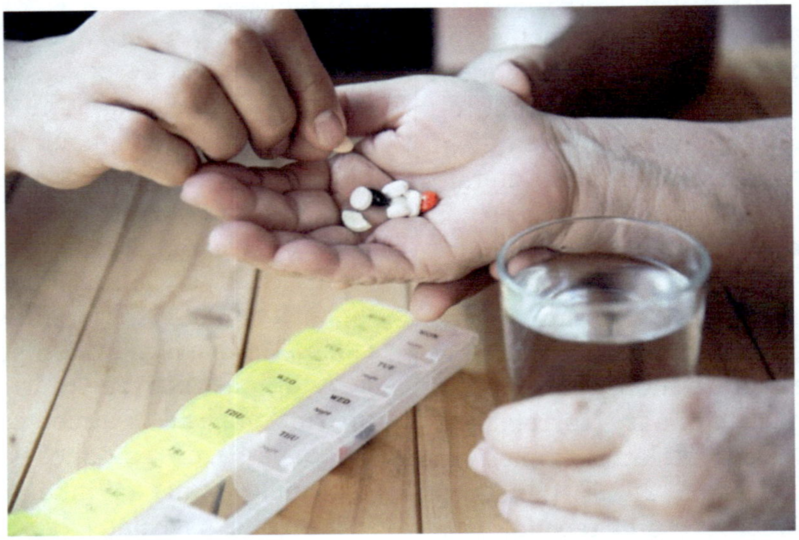

Figure 1.11. Patient taking medicine.

Source: https://nirvanhospital.com/wp-content/uploads/2023/12/Integrating-Medication-Management.png.

1.4.2. Non-Pharmacological Interventions

Non-pharmacological interventions play a significant role in patient treatment in general medicine, particularly the management of chronic diseases. They are based on a spectrum of interventions that extend from behavior modification to lifestyle modifications aimed at improving outcomes without the use of medication. Cessation programs for smoking are a good case in point since it has been found through research that smoking cessation improves responses in most conditions, including cancer. Studies discovered that offering extensive cessation programs that encompass counseling and follow-up has a higher success rate compared to minimal intervention. This alteration not only translates to better health outcomes but also contributes to lower healthcare costs associated with the re-emergence of disease, further outlining the role of more extensive non-pharmacological interventions in clinical work (Cameron et al., 2018). Also, incorporation of non-pharmacological care extends to prevention and management of osteoporosis, a disease of particular importance in old age. In accordance with a systematic review of the literature, structured exercise and fracture liaison multidisciplinary services by non-physician health professionals were found to be effective. Resistance training progression, specifically, was shown to decrease the incidence of falls in patients who had experienced a hip fracture. This is a strategy that prioritizes the application of tailored exercise protocols that are sensitive to the specific patient needs, in addition to creating a culture of a multidisciplinary team. The outcomes of this review highlight not only the efficacy of these interventions but also the need for further research into identifying more methods for fracture prevention as well as overall health improvements among the at-risk populations (Adams et al., 2020). The integration of non-pharmacological interventions within general practice is another challenge to the classical biomedical model, promoting a whole-person approach to healthcare. The interventions usually focus on the education and self-management of the patients, allowing them to be active participants in their health. In making this possible, resources and assistance are provided by the healthcare givers so that the individuals can make appropriate decisions on changes in lifestyles and compliance with the preventive measures. This model of educational and collaborative care builds a stronger patient-provider relationship, trust, and effective communication. With the changing healthcare landscape, ongoing evaluation and integration of these interventions remain significant in the development of comprehensive treatment plans that incorporate patient QoL in addition to conventional medical treatments. With this paradigm shift, general medicine as a discipline can further continue towards improved and more patient-centered care approaches.

1.4.3. Patient Education and Self-Management

In the field of general medicine, patient self-management and education become key elements that enable individuals to manage their own health. Successful educational interventions not only provide patients with appropriate knowledge but also build patients' confidence in self-managing chronic diseases. For example, culinary medicine (CM) is a revolutionary model that incorporates nutrition education into medical education for healthcare providers. With structured programs like CALM, which offer cancer risk reduction skills, medical students show a substantial improvement in valuing the role of nutrition in patient care and in personal health behavior. These curricula emphasize diet's contribution to preventing and managing disease and foster a milieu of healthy empowerment in contrast to treatment-focused reactivity. Indeed, encouraging a deeper understanding of health via education can lead to successful self-management behaviors on the part of patients and greater competency on the part of healthcare providers (Stephanie et al., 2025). Additionally, the use of genomic medicine in healthcare highlights yet another dimension of patient education and self-management. With an increasing number of non-geneticist healthcare providers providing genetics-informed care, knowledge of genomic testing and understanding its implications are now essential. Recent pediatrician surveys reflected a strong need to enhance their expertise in genetic testing for neurodevelopmental disorders (NDDs). While most pediatricians acknowledge the importance of studying genetic services, ignorance and lack of resources hinder them from effectively using these tools. Closing these gaps with targeted educational interventions can ultimately allow healthcare providers to lead to better-educated families well-positioned to make decisions regarding genetic testing and its consequences. This illustrates an unmistakable chain of causation between education for providers and patient empowerment, which implies the necessity of ongoing education in general medicine (Szuto et al., 2024). Patient education and patient self-management are inextricably linked to adequate provision of healthcare, affecting not only the outcome of patients but also the use of resources by the healthcare system. Patients who are well-educated to become active agents for their care have improved reported satisfaction and QoL. Interventions that target patient education on self-management skills such as decision-making, self-monitoring, and communication with healthcare providers enhance participation and compliance with treatment regimes. Moreover, these programs can reduce the cost of healthcare by preventing complications through better management of disease. The message is clear: establishing a solid foundation for patient education and self-management can have a profound effect on patients and healthcare systems and position them in an invaluable position in the future of general medicine. Hence, healthcare professionals must emphasize learning themselves as they facilitate patients with resultant effective self-management (Szuto et al., 2024; Stephanie et al., 2025) (Figure 1.12).

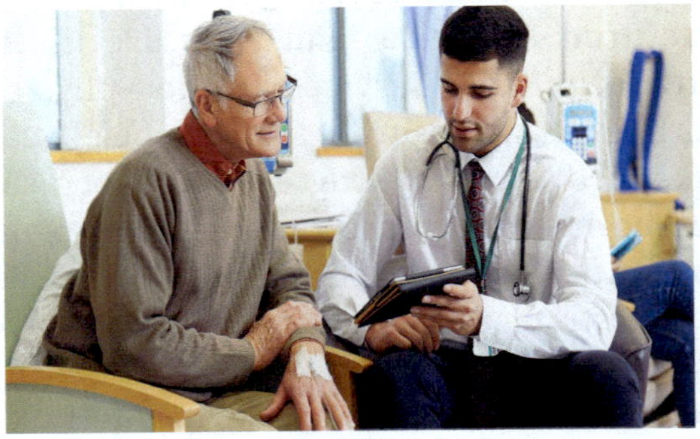

Figure 1.12. Enhancing patient education through video-based solutions.

Source: https://www.enghousevideo.com/wp-content/uploads/2024/08/the-importance-of-patient-engagement-and-education.jpg.

Test Your Knowledge

1. What role do pharmacological treatments play in the management of common conditions?
2. How do General Practitioners incorporate non-pharmacological interventions, such as lifestyle modifications, physical therapy, or dietary changes, into a patient's treatment plan?

1.5. Challenges in General Medicine

Learning Outcome

1. Focus on the challenge of access to healthcare services
2. Manage patient expectations
3. Keep up with medical advancements

The field of general medicine is riddled with intricate challenges that have an impact on both patients and professionals. One of the significant challenges is the standardization of treatment procedures, particularly in the field of novel therapies such as extracellular vesicles (EVs). These biological particles have emerged as effective therapeutic agents due to their roles in intercellular communication. However, the absence of standardized protocols for their isolation, characterization, and delivery has led to variability in findings across experiments. Organizations such as the International Society for Extracellular Vesicles (ISEV) have recognized this issue, urging the adoption of standard frameworks to improve clinical application reliability. With a greater application of new modalities in general medicine, it is necessary to develop strong guidelines for guaranteeing efficacy of treatment and patient safety, making this an immediate challenge within the current medical scene (Haghighitalab et al., 2025). Another extremely critical challenge for general medicine is the application of advanced technologies, i.e., medical Vision-Language Models (Med-VLMs). These computer vision-driven models also have the potential to transform healthcare as they combine visual and textual information, hence strengthening clinical interventions. Nevertheless, their implementation using Med-VLMs is challenged by significant obstacles. There is the constraint of data availability and limited generalizability across different patient groups, constraining their usage. Ethical considerations of fairness, accountability, and patient confidentiality also add complexities to be navigated by clinicians. Stringent mechanisms for evaluation and inclusive regulatory schemes are called for to introduce these technologies safely into healthcare operations. Resolution of these problems is central to the ethical integration of AI innovation into regular medicine (Kalpelbe et al., 2025). In addition to technological integration and standardization, healthcare professionals are challenged with resolving the socioeconomic disparities that impact patient access to medical care. Disparities in health results are often linked to a greater number of social determinants of income, education, and place, thereby making it even more challenging to provide equal healthcare. General medicine must evolve to cope with such challenges, which will require practitioners to adopt a holistic philosophy and consider the social aspect of health. Initiatives to combat health literacy, community participation, and the distribution of resources could mitigate such disparities and bring about better health outcomes. By addressing socio-economic concerns as well as clinical ones, general medicine can pioneer the path to a more effective and equitable health system that ultimately benefits patients from all walks of life.

1.5.1. Access to Healthcare Services

Availability of healthcare services is a central issue that significantly impacts public health outcomes. The foundation of universal health coverage, as the United Nations' sustainable development goals define it, is rooted in the imperative to limit out-of-pocket expenditure (OOPE) incurred by patients when they receive medical care. Excessive OOPE deters patients from seeking healthcare services, leading to adverse health outcomes and increased medical impoverishment. The relationship between public government expenditure on health and OOPE is complex; whereas more investment leads to higher availability of services, it may also lead to higher direct expenditure for the consumer. Hence, a multi-faceted approach to reduce OOPE is needed, such as government health schemes and mandatory insurance schemes to lower the financial burden on patients (Kaladharan et al., 2024). Further, fair access to medical services is often limited by structural inequalities in the healthcare system, as in the case of the inclusion of mental healthcare services in general care units. Legislatively, Gauteng province in South Africa aims at fair access to cognitive, neurological, and substance use disorders. However, drug procurement for the disorders has notable inequalities in service delivery. General health units source the majority of the drugs, but their availability in municipalities and levels of service differ significantly. This inconsistency underscores the importance of examining not only the level of provision but also the equitable distribution, as this dictates the extent to which quality care is accessible to various populations (Robertson et al., 2024). Addressing these imbalances remains a requirement in a bid to enhance the overall access to integrated healthcare services. Finally, improving access to health requires combined efforts to establish strong public health systems and promote preventive practices. Countries need to adopt entirely holistic approaches, prioritizing health intervention that saves lives and education in a bid to improve living habits. By adopting measures such as the increase in comprehensive health insurance and the control of medicine prices, countries will overcome the economic barriers that are often attached to healthcare access.

Additionally, improved healthcare delivery to vulnerable populations, such as those with chronic diseases or lower socio-economic status, is required. By promoting an integrated system that supports preventive care as much as treatment options, policymakers can work towards a more equitable healthcare system that is in line with the general goals of health equity and universal coverage (Kaladharan et al., 2024; Robertson et al., 2024) (Figure 1.13).

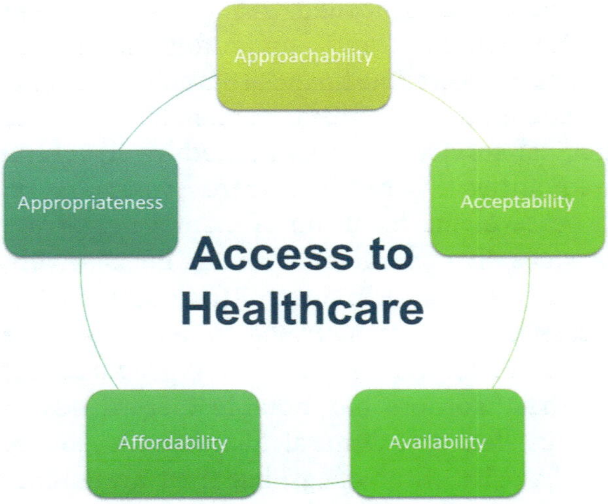

Figure 1.13. Access to healthcare.

Source: https://static.wixstatic.com/media/a27d24_fa4f38042031443bb56065209d9bb748~mv2.jpg/v1/fill/w_568,h_528,al_c,q_80,usm_0.66_1.00_0.01,enc_avif,quality_auto/a27d24_fa4f38042031443bb56065209d9bb748~mv2.jpg.

1.5.2. Managing Patient Expectations

Successful management of patient expectations is a critical component of healthcare delivery in general medicine. Knowledge of the psychological determinants underlying patient experiences can contribute significantly to treatment outcomes and satisfaction. By embracing effective communication strategies, health workers are capable of reconciling patient expectations with the reality of their medical condition and treatment plan. For instance, the incorporation of facilities such as visual presentations of patient data and patient-specific treatment goals facilitates constructing a more accurate interpretation of anticipated outcomes.

From evidence, clinicians remarked that dashboards, which amalgamate key patient and outcome information, not only serve as tools for providing information but also enable meaningful conversations between patients and providers, enhancing the patient-clinician relationship (van Kooij et al., 2025). Finally, these strategies reshape the patient experience, minimizing anxiety and unpredictability, as well as optimizing treatment protocol compliance. The use of technology, particularly the employment of AI and robotic assistance, has introduced new dimensions to managing patient expectations. While these technologies usher in increased efficiency and improved care, they also generate varied responses from patients, ranging from enthusiasm to skepticism. Most patients develop apprehension that is correlated with their expectation of technology's potential in the healthcare industry. Negative attitudes arise from fear of the unpredictability of technology as well as the emotional incompetence of AI systems (Smola et al., 2025). To reverse this challenge, healthcare professionals must take steps to to educate patients on the limitations and benefits of such technology. This way, providers can have more faith and reliance, hence making the way to a more technologically advanced health arena smoother. Moreover, medical practitioners have to acknowledge the broader picture of patient needs outside the technical details. In most instances, patients battle emotional and psychological issues related to their health conditions, which carry a unique bearing on the way they view treatment results. The use of empathetic communication and active listening allows clinicians to detect such underlying issues and, hence, modify their approach to meet specific patient requirements. Integration of clinical knowledge with emotional intelligence creates a platform where patients are dealt with as human beings and not just as cases, eventually paving the way for better management of expectations. Achieving this balance is crucial because it directly impacts patients' willingness to engage in their treatment plans, creating an egalitarian approach that enhances health outcomes and fosters a deeper exploration of their health experiences (van Kooij et al., 2025) (Figure 1.14).

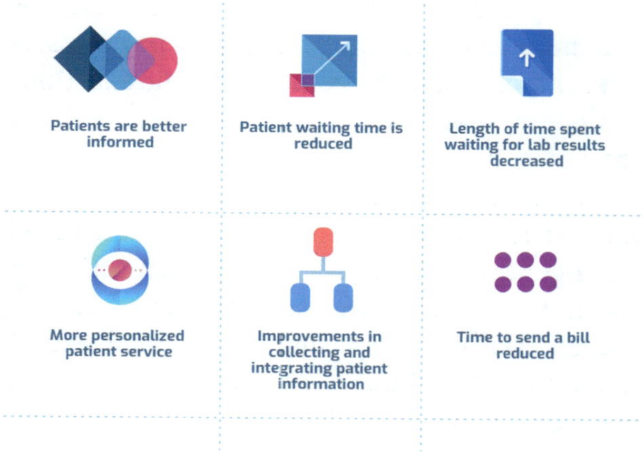

Figure 1.14. Benefits in managing increased patient expectations in healthcare.

Source: https://www.predictiveanalyticstoday.com/wp-content/uploads/2020/01/What-are-the-Benefits-in-Managing-Increased-Patient-Expectations-in-Healthcare.png.

1.5.3. Keeping Up with Medical Advancements

In the constantly changing landscape of general medicine, it is essential to keep abreast of developments in medical technologies to provide outstanding patient care. The speed at which new drugs are being developed, especially in dermatology, illustrates how innovation can contribute directly to better therapy outcomes. For example, the development of sophisticated topical gel preparations has revolutionized psoriasis treatment. These formulations take advantage of novel gelling agents that enhance drug efficacy as well as patient comfort and compliance by making treatment administration more straightforward and more convenient. According to recent patent discussions, such innovative delivery systems' safety and efficacy effectiveness underscore their ability to transform dermatology disease treatment and improve patient compliance and well-being (Bahmani et al., 2025). This advancement forms part of a broader trend in medicine where patient-focused practice and technological development are increasingly intertwined, shaping the future face of health management. Likewise, the application of AI in diagnostic imaging is an even more compelling illustration of the medical practice's necessity to remain responsive to technological advancements. Most prominently in breast cancer diagnosis, AI has demonstrated considerable potential in enhancing the accuracy and efficiency of mammography screening. The mammography screening with artificial intelligence trial (MASAI) illustrated how modalities with AI support could attain equivalent detection rates but with a considerable reduction in the workload of radiologists. Supported by such research, AI has emerged as an effective tool that minimizes false positives and false negatives, hence enabling rapid and accurate diagnoses (Nasr et al., 2025). By integrating such technology into routine clinical practices, health systems can address the care of prevalent diseases such as breast cancer, thus improving patient outcomes and optimizing the use of available resources in the health facility. Integration of new technologies and treatment is essential, particularly in regions with serious health problems. Countries such as Pakistan, which suffer from high levels of diseases such as breast cancer, can benefit immensely from developments in medical technology. Since most of the population is rural-based and requires quality diagnostic services, AI-validated screening methods can bridge the gap in healthcare provision. The use of the above technologies not only addresses the problem of high case fatality rates due to late presentations but also offers a cost-effective and scalable solution to mass screening programs. Emphasizing the necessity for healthcare leaders to adopt such innovation can make system-wide change in terms of prioritization and management of disease. Last but not least, continued discovery and integration of progress in overall medicine will be essential for improving healthcare provision, patient outcomes, and QoL in populations with many varied diseases (Nasr et al., 2025).

Test Your Knowledge

1. What are the main barriers to access to healthcare services in general medicine?
2. What are patient expectations?

1.6. The Future of General Medicine

Learning Outcome

1. Describe integration of technology in practice
2. Understand evolving roles of general practitioners
3. Focus on trends in patient care and public health

Looking to the horizon of broad medicine, the intersection of cutting-edge technologies is the key to determining the future of patient care. Advances in AI, telemedicine, and precision medicine are drivers of leadership in this innovation. These technologies not only enhance diagnostic accuracy but also increase accessibility to care, allowing healthcare providers to deliver tailored treatment plans according to individual patient needs. For instance, AI-based diagnostic tools have also shown potential for the detection of diseases at a more advanced stage, which is particularly relevant for managing complex conditions. Once again, however, there are attendant ethical concerns, roll-out expense, and the need for strict regulatory guidelines, as highlighted in some recent research. These must be addressed intelligently so that technology integration in medicine serves both patient care and the overall healthcare system to an equal extent (Memon et al., 2025). Moreover, the advent of large language models (LLMs) into general medicine is also expected to revolutionize aspects of clinical documentation and patient interaction. With healthcare becoming more and more data-driven, the LLMs can streamline administrative tasks, making it more efficient, as well as allowing medical personnel to devote more time to face-to-face patient care. The new natural language processing arena is particularly notable, as it not only enhances communication between the patient and provider but also helps to assimilate properly complex medical information. Recent bibliometric evidence implies a growing corpus of literature devoted to the applications of LLMs across various medical specialties, including internal medicine and oncology. This trend emphasizes a broader realization of the prospective benefits of such technologies, further attesting to the notion that the future of general medicine will be inextricably linked to advancements in data analytics as well as patient management tools (Gülcan et al., 2025). The future of general medicine will undoubtedly rely on continuous innovation and the conversion of new technologies into instruments to meet evolving patients' needs. Prioritizing personalized medicine, facilitated by genomic data and AI, is a shift from the old one-size-fits-all solution to medicine. But for these innovations to prevail, all the efforts need to go into dismantling the barriers that could forestall widespread adoption. Continued training and education of healthcare professionals are required to ensure they are better placed to utilize the most out of these advanced tools. There should be a symbiosis among medical professionals, policymakers, and technology developers in creating a sustainable model that encourages the ethical use of emerging medical technologies. In the end, adjusting to this future will lead to improved healthcare outcomes and a fairer healthcare system for all (Memon et al., 2025).

1.6.1. Integration of Technology in Practice

Application of technology in the practice of medicine is a revolutionary shift towards enhanced patient care and overall clinical effectiveness in general medicine. Development of new drug products such as extended half-life factor concentrates and novel bi-specific antibodies is a classic example of such a shift. These advancements also reduce the severity and frequency of bleeding, allowing patients to lead everyday lives without fear (Srivastava et al., 2020). Moreover, standardization of therapies by improved laboratory monitoring equips healthcare providers with the resources they require for tailored patient management. The organized and systematic philosophy advocated by updated clinical guidelines prioritizes the adoption of technology in planning robust treatment protocols, resulting in enhanced patient health outcomes within the clinic. Telemedicine has emerged as a fast-growing player in the utilization of technology in overall medicine, particularly in the era of world health crises. COVID-19 demonstrated the value of telehealth services as it offered an alternative to in-person consultations. Telemedicine allowed for ongoing monitoring and treatment of patients while being under social distancing measures (Rashid et al., 2020). Telemedicine's expansion at warp speed brought increased access for patients, especially from underserved or rural communities. This convergence reduces travel loads and facilitates timely interventions, thereby leading to proactive healthcare. With the medical fraternity embracing these online platforms, challenges of technology adoption, such as varying levels of patient familiarity and proper training of the healthcare professionals, need to be addressed. The destiny of technology assimilation in overall medicine is left to the creation of harmonized policy and ethics structures that support equity of access to care. Telerehabilitation process standardization through education and resource allocation can help fill gaps, facilitating an integrated healthcare system. Leveraging evidence from patient registries and accrued data can help inform best practices and enhance evidence-based decision-making (Srivastava et al., 2020). As the healthcare landscape continues to evolve, technological innovation will play a key role in guiding patient-centered models of care and improving overall health outcomes. By facilitating communication among care providers, policymakers, and technology vendors, adoption of these systems can ensure that advances in medical practice are effective and equitable, ultimately benefiting the global population (Figure 1.15).

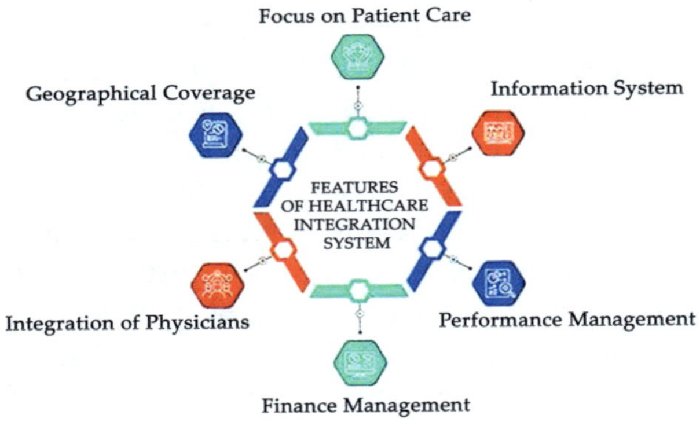

Figure 1.15. Features of the healthcare integration system.

Source: https://cdn-lipbd.nitrocdn.com/NmtxoNywbwrhgCusRjwzXqAEjXRnHzOa/assets/images/optimized/rev-a4fdd8a/www.osplabs.com/wp-content/uploads/2020/11/Features-of-Healthcare-Integration-System.jpg.

1.6.2. Evolving Roles of General Practitioners

The evolving roles of the GPs are more applicable when understood in the context of contemporary healthcare requirements. As patients' initial points of contact, GPs must now navigate challenging medical landscapes that require them to assume other roles beyond traditional practice. This revolution includes the adoption of technological innovation, particularly through the mechanisms of electronic health records (EHRs) and telemedicine. These technologies enable more efficient patient management and greater access to services. Furthermore, GPs are now more likely to be members of multidisciplinary teams, collaborating with specialists and allied health professionals to deliver integrated care. This transformation demands GPs to have comprehensive clinical expertise along with working with technology, ultimately enhancing their capacity to provide personalized and timely healthcare services as patient requirements get more sophisticated and diverse. To challenge the intricate problems lurking within modern healthcare systems, GPs also have key roles to play in health promotion and preventative care. Their activities are more than basic diagnosis and cure, becoming proactive management of health through lifestyle modification and prevention of chronic illness. This adaptation is most pertinent with rising lifestyle-related conditions, which require GPs to create targeted health strategies for their patients. Public and clinician education to heighten awareness of the importance of preventive care is needed. Thus, GPs are positioned not just as clinicians but as health literacy champions, confronting patients with education outreach. This role switch redefines the GP not just as a caregiver but as an essential educator in the continuum of healthcare, thus ensuring improved population health outcomes. Additionally, as the healthcare systems become more inclined toward innovative technology, the GPs' role will also have to change drastically. With the inclusion of AI and other digital resources in clinical practice, the GPs will have to update their skill sets to utilize these innovations productively. The new bright hospital concept captures this change, with the GPs embracing data-driven decision-making and utilizing AI to enhance patient care. The transition is not without challenges, however, fighting off staff shortages and ensuring ethical use of technology will continue to be paramount. Evolution of the GP's role is an indication of broader changes in healthcare, calling on practitioners to be adaptable, responsive, and informed enough to make sense through an increasingly dynamic landscape of medical treatment, following development outlined in relevant studies illustrating the co-occurrence of technology and human-centered practices in healthcare delivery (Alhashim et al., 2024; Jovy-Klein et al., 2024).

1.6.3. Trends in Patient Care and Public Health

The patient care and public health scenario is transforming at a rapid rate due to technological advancements and greater attention to preventive care. The integration of telemedicine has been a significant trend, which was again highlighted with the pandemic due to COVID-19. There is greater availability for patients to access healthcare providers without the need to visit them physically, allowing for timely consultations and ongoing monitoring of chronic diseases. This transformation not only increases the accessibility of care to patients in remote or underserved populations but also promotes continuity in treatment protocols. With these transformations in healthcare systems, education of healthcare professionals in digital resources becomes increasingly essential for maintaining quality and equitable patient care. Thus, this focus on technology-aided care is one aspect of a larger development towards innovation and efficiency in patient health outcomes in the realm of general medicine. Furthermore, health disparities among populations have inspired growing trends in public health to address inequities. Social determinants of health, including socioeconomic status, environment, and education, profoundly influence access to care and overall outcomes. By integrating the determinants of public health interventions, practitioners to build interventions that can increase marginalized groups' health outcomes. With community participation and culturally appropriate care, health programs aimed at reducing disparities are picking up pace. Educational programs and preventive health measures are being tailored to address specific community requirements, as with studies into diseases like Bartholin gland abscesses, where early diagnosis and effective treatment have been linked with better outcomes in 25–35-year-old women (Hamidi, 2025). This tailoring mirrors the necessities of interprofessional working in healthcare and public health. Apart from these advances, an increasing need exists for robust surveillance networks and investigation of newly emergent pathogens such as the HMPV. As a medically serious cause of respiratory illness, HMPV is a prototype of what public health agencies have to deal with in detecting and controlling outbreaks. With its capacity to cause severe disease in vulnerable populations, including children and the elderly, such agents' epidemiology and clinical manifestations must be thoroughly understood to ensure adequate public health measures (Ansori, 2025). Trends in current times point towards a necessity for research in vaccine and therapeutic development, pointing towards an international collaboration among researchers, healthcare practitioners, and policymakers. This joint initiative aims to lower respiratory diseases' impact on public health and enhance readiness for upcoming public health emergencies, ultimately leading to improved patient care for general medicine.

Test Your Knowledge

1. How is the integration of digital health technologies transforming the practice of General Medicine?
2. What are the most significant trends in healthcare today?

SUMMARY

In general medicine, discoveries from large-scale studies provide deep analysis of the efficacy of treatment protocols and outcomes in patients. By extensive critical analysis of clinical observations, clinicians can utilize findings to make evidence-based optimum practices that enhance patient care. As an example, research on cocaine abuse cases among patients who come in with chest pain demonstrated dominant trends that can influence ED guidelines. These findings stress integrating the evaluation of substance use into standard medical assessment, thereby establishing a direct relationship between comprehensive patient histories and improved clinical outcomes, as shown in the case of a specific correlation with emergency conditions (Bandeeri et al., 2004). Accordingly, the field of general medicine is fortified by these well-educated conclusions and eventually drives the refinement of health promotion and disease prevention activities. Additionally, the integrity of postgraduate medical examination and education processes forms a foundation for care quality delivered in the specialty—postgraduate medical exams, such as the MRCP (UK) Part 1. Examination comes under high-level scrutiny that indicates problems around standardization and long-term consistency. Evidence of the efficacy of marker questions across varying examination diets indicates a continued imperative to maintain standards of education in accordance with evolving medical knowledge and practice environments. As the evidence suggests, procedures applied in standard-setting are vital to maintaining the validity of medical education (Anonymous et al., 2005). Therefore, a valid conclusion in medical education reflects the need to construct flexible systems that adapt to advances in both medical practice and pedagogy. In essence, combining research findings and educational rigor in general medicine reflects a solid template for enhanced healthcare service delivery. The findings of studies that emphasize drug abuse and examination uniformity reinforce the use of an integrated method in medical practice. By the marrying of empirical evidence and educational integrity, the profession of general medicine can develop a culture of continuous improvement, ultimately readying practitioners adequately to meet the evolving needs of patient care. It is this union that supports the highest value of decision-making informed by research, which goes far beyond impacting clinical practice to also affecting the paradigms upon which medical professionals are trained and assessed. It imposes a culture of excellence within the healthcare industry, providing scope for enhanced patient outcomes and affirming general medicine's vital role.

In general medicine, understanding the variation of healthcare practice across nations is essential for improving patient outcomes. One of the significant findings is the variation in the rate of hospital transfer among nursing home residents within Germany and the Netherlands. Research indicates that the patients in German nursing homes are much more frequently sent to the hospital compared to their counterparts in the Netherlands, with 26.5% of visits to the ED reported versus mere 7.9% in the Netherlands ($p < 0.0001$). This sharp contrast reflects the influence of health systems on managing patients and justifies the requirement of a robust primary care system. Physician roles in the decision-making regarding hospital transfers also underscore systemic variation. GPs are less involved in these essential transfer decisions in Germany than elder care physicians are in the Netherlands, where they have a strong gatekeeping position within the healthcare system. Such a variation is essential as it underscores how comprehensive care and physician involvement shape the pathways of patients in healthcare systems. Comparing these variations, health policymakers could easily find that there are implications of their decisions on patient care and resource utilization. In addition, arguments regarding the certainty and admissibility of expert opinion in medical cases reveal more complexity in general medicine. As seen in debates in meetings following the

Summit organized by the Victorian Chapter of the Australian Academy of Forensic Sciences, the gatekeeper role of judges regarding the validity of expert evidence in medical cases has significant practice standard implications. The debates emphasized the necessity of continuously reevaluating forensic techniques of evidence to continue to assure their reliability. This call for rigorous analysis resonates deeply with broader challenges in mainstream medicine for EBP, patient protection, and the standards by which practitioners operate within clinical and forensic contexts (Ross, 2020).

KEY TERMS FROM THIS CHAPTER

- Acute diseases
- Chronic diseases
- Diabetes mellitus
- General medicine
- Gynecology
- Health strategy
- Healthcare operations
- Acute injuries
- Dermatology
- Extracellular vesicles (EVs)
- General practitioners (GP)
- Health challenges
- Healthcare delivery
- Healthcare services

CRITICAL THINKING QUESTIONS

1. **What is the primary role of a general practitioner (GP)?**
   a. Specializing in the treatment of a single organ system
   b. Performing surgeries for complex conditions
   c. Providing primary care, diagnosing and treating common illnesses, and referring patients to specialists when necessary
   d. Prescribing medication only for mental health issues
2. **Which of the following is considered a common condition treated by general practitioners?**
   a. Heart transplants
   b. Diabetes mellitus
   c. Brain tumors
   d. Organ rejection in transplant patients
3. **Which diagnostic technique is commonly used by general practitioners to assess a patient's overall health?**
   a. MRI scans
   b. X-rays
   c. Physical examination and patient history
   d. Blood transfusions
4. **Which of the following is a common treatment approach in general medicine for chronic conditions such as hypertension or diabetes?**
   a. Immediate surgery
   b. Pharmacological treatment and lifestyle modifications
   c. Radiotherapy
   d. Immunization
5. **What is one of the major challenges faced by general practitioners in the field of general medicine?**
   a. Managing only a small number of patients
   b. Not having access to modern diagnostic equipment
   c. Dealing with patients who prefer over-the-counter treatments instead of prescribed medications
   d. Overcoming the complexity of rare diseases that require highly specialized care

Short Answer Questions

1. What are the key responsibilities of a general practitioner (GP) in the healthcare system?
2. How do general practitioners collaborate with specialists in patient care?
3. What are some of the most common medical conditions that general practitioners encounter in their practice?
4. How do GPs prioritize treatment for patients with multiple coexisting conditions?
5. What diagnostic tools and techniques are typically used by general practitioners to assess common medical conditions?
6. How do general practitioners decide when to refer patients for specialized diagnostic tests or imaging?

Answers to Critical Thinking Questions

1. (c) 2. (b) 3. (c) 4. (b) 5. (d)

REFERENCES

1. Wilson, N., Hurkmans, E., Adams, J., Bakkers, M., Balážová, P., Baxter, M., Blavnsfeldt, A., Briot, K., Chiari, C., Cooper, C., Dragoi, R., Gäbler, G., Lems, W., Mosor, E., Pais, S., Simon, C., Studenic, P., Tilley, S., De La Torre, J., & Stamm, T. A. (2020). Prevention and management of osteoporotic fractures by non-physician health professionals: a systematic literature review to inform EULAR points to consider. *RMD Open*, *6*(1), e001143. https://doi.org/10.1136/rmdopen-2019-001143Aldhafiri, M. F., Saleh, S., Saqer, A., Almutairi, A., Saadi, J., Almutrfi, et al. (2024). Electronic medical records: Impacts, outcomes, challenges, and opportunities. *The Medical Journal of Cairo University*. https://www.semanticscholar.org/paper/848d608261d096cdbaa5f86c20ad7195edad2198 (accessed on 27th June 2025).
2. Alhashim, M., Aladel, F., Bukhamseen, M., & Alhariqi, A. (2024). Awareness of interventional radiology and the associated radiation exposure risk among the public population and primary care physicians in Saudi Arabia. *Saudi Journal of Radiology*. https://www.semanticscholar.org/paper/7d6144e120effccb9b91f28a5d74ab85a1921bf6 (accessed on 27th June 2025).
3. Anonymous, De Gruijter, D. N. M., Ghiselli, E. E., General Medical Council, David, H. A., et al. (2005). Changes in standard of candidates taking the MRCP(UK) Part 1 examination, 1985 to 2002: Analysis of marker questions. https://core.ac.uk/download/1704288.pdf (accessed on 27th June 2025).
4. Ansori, A. (2025). Human metapneumovirus (HMPV): A brief overview. *Svāsthya: Trends in General Medicine and Public Health*. https://www.semanticscholar.org/paper/da13772d8457793e9c6c79fa5711ed7388bfb8d6 (accessed on 27th June 2025).
5. Araujo-Soares, V., Avenell, A., Dombrowski, S. U., Johnston, et al. (2010). Identifying active ingredients in complex behavioral interventions for obese adults with obesity-related co-morbidities or additional risk factors for co-morbidities: A systematic review. https://core.ac.uk/download/11303997.pdf (accessed on 27th June 2025).
6. Bahmani, K., Rani, N., Nasa, P., & Devi, S. (2025). Recent innovations in gelling agents and topical gel formulations for psoriasis treatment: A patent review. *Current Physical Chemistry*. https://www.semanticscholar.org/paper/67699a91c1718062eecf1433980ef2f68823bdf9 (accessed on 27th June 2025).
7. Baky, I., Bourke, A., Byrne, C., MacDonagh, J., Clifford, A., Niranjan, V., & O'Regan, A. (2025). How do doctors manage physical activity advocacy for patients and their own self-care? A qualitative interview study of general practitioners in Ireland. *BMJ Open, 15*. https://www.semanticscholar.org/paper/c4f39bd454b6a9f3e7001fa6ece19dd1e89dcb01 (accessed on 27th June 2025).
8. Bandeeri, N., Henry, J. A., Meredith, C., Treacy, et al. (2004). The prevalence of cocaine-associated chest pain in a London hospital. https://core.ac.uk/download/5230488.pdf (accessed on 27th June 2025).
9. Bashshur, R. L., Doarn, C. R., Frenk, J., Kvedar, J. C., & Woolliscroft, J. O. (2020). Telemedicine and the COVID-19 pandemic, lessons for the future. *Telemedicine Journal and e-Health, 26*, 571–573. https://doi.org/10.1089/tmj.2020.29040.rb (accessed on 27th June 2025).
10. Baum, A., Kaboli, P. J., & Schwartz, M. D. (2020). Reduced in-person and increased telehealth outpatient visits during the COVID-19 pandemic. *Annals of Internal Medicine, 174*, 129–131. https://doi.org/10.7326/m20-3026 (accessed on 27th June 2025).

11. Boutros, A., Carlino, M. S., & Menzies, A. M. (2024). Melanoma medicine: New drugs for melanoma and the role of the general practitioner. *Australian Journal of General Practice, 53*(9), 619–624. https://www.semanticscholar.org/paper/5917b4a3bb2b868f4c36dd47308 49705a0e324d5 (accessed on 27th June 2025).

12. Bunt, S., Traxler, M., Zimmerman, B., Rosenbaum, M., Heaberlin, S., Cronholm, P. F., Kinsey, E. W., et al. (2024). Family medicine clinician screening and barriers to communication on food insecurity: A CERA general membership survey. *The Journal of the American Board of Family Medicine, 37*, 196–205. https://www.semanticscholar.org/paper/50c1c693b7bd7ff9 ac97971393f08d18244bd997 (accessed on 27th June 2025).

13. Cameron, E., Chan, K., Djalalov, S., Evans, et al. (2018). Economic evaluation of smoking cessation in Ontario's regional cancer programs. https://core.ac.uk/download/323068286.pdf (accessed on 27th June 2025).

14. Cordey, M., Chatelard, S., Widmer, D., Ouvrard, P., & Herzig, L. (2024). Ordinary defensive medicine: In the shadows of general practitioners' postures toward (over-)medicalization. *Philosophy, Ethics, and Humanities in Medicine: PEHM, 19*. https://www.semanticscholar.org/paper/ca220d34441a0bc17c79d964602656b66cb6dacf (accessed on 27th June 2025).

15. Cryan, J. F., O'Riordan, K. J., Cowan, C. S. M., Sandhu, K. V., Bastiaanssen, T. F. S., Boehme, M., Codagnone, M. G., et al. (2019). The microbiota-gut-brain axis. *Physiological Reviews, 99*, 1877–2013. https://doi.org/10.1152/physrev.00018.2018 (accessed on 27th June 2025).

16. De Vos, E., & Sege, R. D. (2010). Evidence-based healthcare for children: What are we missing? https://core.ac.uk/download/71351227.pdf (accessed on 27th June 2025).

17. Duda-Sikuła, M., & Kurpas, D. (2024). Enhancing chronic disease management: Personalized medicine insights from rural and urban general practitioner practices. *Journal of Personalized Medicine, 14*. https://www.semanticscholar.org/paper/4de3e3d9ccee41addab742d122f58a7 52a635fc4 (accessed on 27th June 2025).

18. Fassmer, A., Zuidema, S., Janus, S. I. M., & Hoffmann, F. (2024). Differences in emergency department visits and hospitalization between German and Dutch nursing home residents: A cross-national survey. *European Geriatric Medicine, 15*, 787–795. https://www.semanticscholar.org/paper/e731624aac91d371bd0c44f98a200d5f7794a8f0 (accessed on 27th June 2025).

19. Fiorillo, A., Sampogna, G., Albert, U., Maina, G., Perugi, G., Pompili, M., Rosso, G., et al. (2023). Facts and myths about the use of lithium for bipolar disorder in routine clinical practice: An expert consensus paper. *Annals of General Psychiatry, 22*. https://www.semanticscholar.org/paper/60a87301781fd01a2e6170c8f5f8fc9d316d65b1 (accessed on 27th June 2025).

20. Gadoth, A., Halbrook, M., Martin-Blais, R., Gray, A., Tobin, N. H., Ferbas, K. G., Aldrovandi, G. M., et al. (2021). Cross-sectional assessment of COVID-19 vaccine acceptance among healthcare workers in Los Angeles. *Annals of Internal Medicine, 174*, 882–885. https://doi.org/10.7326/m20-7580 (accessed on 27th June 2025).

21. Gann, G. D., McDonald, T., Walder, B., Aronson, J., Nelson, C. R., Jonson, J., Hallett, J. G., et al. (2019). International principles and standards for the practice of ecological restoration. Second edition. *Restoration Ecology, 27*. https://doi.org/10.1111/rec.13035 (accessed on 27th June 2025).

22. Gencer, G., & Gencer, K. (2025). Large language models in healthcare: A bibliometric analysis and examination of research trends. *Journal of Multidisciplinary Healthcare, 18*, 223–238.

https://www.semanticscholar.org/paper/e957f1f98f18adcded31fbaaa7844c23e044cf07 (accessed on 27th June 2025).

23. Ghany, M. G., & Morgan, T. R. (2019). Hepatitis C guidance 2019 update: American Association for the Study of Liver Diseases–Infectious Diseases Society of America recommendations for testing, managing, and treating hepatitis C virus infection. *Hepatology, 71*, 686–721. https://doi.org/10.1002/hep.31060 (accessed on 27th June 2025).

24. Gilani, S. (2022). Seven cardinal questions for the patient with ear, nose or throat complaints: Review. *Medicine, 101*. https://www.semanticscholar.org/paper/e653aa4840947b1aa23cfd311efd8d05a607af5f (accessed on 27th June 2025).

25. Gooneratne, T., & Atturu, G. (2019). Introduction to translational research in vascular surgery/medicine. *Indian Journal of Vascular and Endovascular Surgery, 6*, 162–170. https://www.semanticscholar.org/paper/d18221bbf60ea1bd8935bf7d002f2529a5365acd (accessed on 27th June 2025).

26. Haghighitalab, A., Kazemi Noughabi, M., Hassanzadeh, H., Shekari, F., Moghadam Matin, M., Lim, R., Bidkhori, H., et al. (2025). Developing a general checklist for the effective administration of extracellular vesicles in biomedical and clinical research. *Cell Journal, 26*(11), 656–668. https://www.semanticscholar.org/paper/63e879e7ca7d3b70a1a6b2acea69c8e30b8a6f30 (accessed on 27th June 2025).

27. Hamidi, H. (2025). Frequency, clinical presentation, and management of Bartholin's abscess: A case study at Rabia Balkhi Hospital, Afghanistan in 2022. *Svāsthya: Trends in General Medicine and Public Health*. https://www.semanticscholar.org/paper/1cc03beece838a04db059cb0436d03f59b6c12a6 (accessed on 27th June 2025).

28. Harris, S. R., Borawski, E., Lachman, R., Malone, L., DePalma, J., & Barkoukis, H. (2025). Culinary medicine in medical education: A pilot study targeting cancer risk reduction strategies through culinary and lifestyle medicine education. *Frontiers in Nutrition, 12*. https://www.semanticscholar.org/paper/a1cdb163eeeda3d23311678472b8b64974ebba14 (accessed on 27th June 2025).

29. Holiuk, Y., & Strafun, I. (2025). Development of a personalized approach concept for the application of regenerative technologies in patients with osteoarthritis and aseptic necrosis of the hip and knee joints. *Cell and Organ Transplantology*. https://www.semanticscholar.org/paper/eb5b78eb805117b199631a3da9b5c1de3aeb0ab2 (accessed on 27th June 2025).

30. Jack, C. R., Bennett, D. A., Blennow, K., Carrillo, M. C., Dunn, B., Budd Haeberlein, S., Holtzman, D. M., et al. (2018). NIA-AA research framework: Toward a biological definition of Alzheimer's disease. *Alzheimer's & Dementia, 14*, 535–562. https://doi.org/10.1016/j.jalz.2018.02.018 (accessed on 27th June 2025).

31. Jovy-Klein, F., Stead, S., Salge, T., Sander, J., Diehl, A., & Antons, D. (2024). Forecasting the future of smart hospitals: Findings from a real-time Delphi study. *BMC Health Services Research, 24*. https://www.semanticscholar.org/paper/eaadf238d593013413421941d5041395ef97c4fc (accessed on 27th June 2025).

32. Kaladharan, S., & Manayath, D. (2024). Out-of-pocket healthcare expenditure in emerging economies: Evidence from panel data analysis. *The Journal of Medicine Access, 8*. https://www.semanticscholar.org/paper/64eb79a384f32b41f6a21d9535f5978a6745bfaf (accessed on 27th June 2025).

33. Kalpelbe, B. C., Adaambiik, A. G., & Peng, W. (2025). Vision language models in medicine. *ArXiv, abs/2503.01863*. https://www.semanticscholar.org/paper/6e2ef61b9f81e1cdff0869b25ef208d3d148be0d (accessed on 27th June 2025).

34. Khan, H., Asghar, S. A., Kanwal, S., Qadar, L., & Qadri, K. (2019). Diphenoxylate-atropine (Lomotil) toxicity in infantile diarrhea: A case report of therapeutic failure. *Cureus, 11*. https://www.semanticscholar.org/paper/edc7ad7145a2f21a08475eaf3e1bd8ee21e038f8 (accessed on 27th June 2025).

35. Latif, R., Aloqaily, M., Rabadi, A., Arshad, K., Kurian, A. I., Obeidat, I. A., & Al-Sanouri, I. (2024). Apixaban-induced hemopericardium in a post-TAVR patient: A case report highlighting diagnostic and management challenges. *The American Journal of Case Reports, 25*, e944173-1–e944173-5. https://www.semanticscholar.org/paper/b79e10a7875b496d0483238cc0cb87695fb245b4 (accessed on 27th June 2025).

36. Lei, Y., Shan, Y., Zhou, D., & Chen, C. (2025). The bibliometric analysis of research on traditional Chinese medicine regulating gut microbiota for cancer treatment from 2014 to 2024. *Hereditas, 162*. https://www.semanticscholar.org/paper/15680ea9d6e53ed06a3371802fdcbc4e8e62b9de (accessed on 27th June 2025).

37. Lorenzut, S., Del Negro, I., Pauletto, G., Verriello, L., Spadea, L., Salati, C., Musa, M., et al. (2025). Exploring the pathophysiology, diagnosis, and treatment options of multiple sclerosis. *Journal of Integrative Neuroscience, 24*(1), 25081. https://www.semanticscholar.org/paper/2381862f6d0210a66b03150611c574e89a15269e (accessed on 27th June 2025).

38. Lowry, J. (2009). Lecture notes: Emergency medicine (3rd edn). *Annals of the Royal College of Surgeons of England, 91*, 446–447. https://www.semanticscholar.org/paper/e3624f284faf8da950f5fc08daf770040654ffc9 (accessed on 27th June 2025).

39. Mao, Z., Wu, S., Fan, Y., Sun, J., Lyu, S., & Su, Q. (2025). Chinese medicine for headaches in emergency department: A retrospective analysis of real-world electronic medical records. *Frontiers in Neurology, 15*. https://www.semanticscholar.org/paper/46744fdaf44070b0bd58227c0f726adb0ec8e215 (accessed on 27th June 2025).

40. Mauvais-Jarvis, F., Bairey Merz, C. N., Barnes, P. J., Brinton, R. D., Carrero, J. J., DeMeo, D. L., De Vries, G. J., et al. (2020). Sex and gender: Modifiers of health, disease, and medicine. *The Lancet, 396*, 565–582. https://doi.org/10.1016/s0140-6736(20)31561-0 (accessed on 27th June 2025).

41. Memon, Z., Memon, Q. Z., Iqbal, H., Haider, S. J., Devi, R., & Maheen, M. (2025). Innovative approaches in pediatric medicine: Emerging trends and future perspectives. *Journal of Medical & Health Sciences Review*. https://www.semanticscholar.org/paper/744e7a451386de5168df76b51c2faf5dc775888b (accessed on 27th June 2025).

42. Mizera, J., Pondel, M., Kepinska, M., Jerzak, P., & Banasik, M. (2025). Advancements in artificial intelligence for kidney transplantology: A comprehensive review of current applications and predictive models. *Journal of Clinical Medicine, 14*. https://www.semanticscholar.org/paper/3e75555b649c72afd7508e657ef8ea2b6c020016 (accessed on 27th June 2025).

43. Nasr, M. U., & Saleem, M. K. (2025). Embracing innovations to fight breast cancer: A letter to the editor. *JPMA. The Journal of the Pakistan Medical Association, 75*(4), 682. https://www.semanticscholar.org/paper/bc89808ae00d7be18b40c311096bee87834a3716 (accessed on 27th June 2025).

44. Nicolaidis, C. (2007). Partner interference with healthcare: Do we want one more piece of a complex puzzle? *Journal of General Internal Medicine, 22*, 1216–1217. https://www.semanticscholar.org/paper/50f5893f76450042768c4dceff3bc89c848e65ea (accessed on 27th June 2025).

45. Page, M. J., Moher, D., Bossuyt, P. M., Boutron, I., Hoffmann, T., Mulrow, C. D., Shamseer, L., et al. (2021). PRISMA 2020 explanation and elaboration: Updated guidance and exemplars for reporting systematic reviews. *BMJ*. https://doi.org/10.1136/bmj.n160 (accessed on 27th June 2025).

46. Rabady, S. (2024). The future of general practice and family medicine in Austria. *Wiener Klinische Wochenschrift, 137*, 105–108. https://www.semanticscholar.org/paper/df33ec87bb322dc99246007c4298540236168f2d (accessed on 27th June 2025).

47. Robertson, L., & Bouwer, J. C. (2024). Mental health services in Gauteng, South Africa: A proxy evaluation using pharmaceutical data. *The South African Journal of Psychiatry: SAJP: The Journal of the Society of Psychiatrists of South Africa, 30*. https://www.semanticscholar.org/paper/8c92636813f62619570d4fd155916f6a6851b554 (accessed on 27th June 2025).

48. Ross, A. (2020). The reliability and validity of expert evidence: Law, science and medicine in summit. The rapporteur's view. *Australian Journal of Forensic Sciences, 52*, 246–248. https://www.semanticscholar.org/paper/b57e644b80d09b74be3797e6af81f0cc91038595 (accessed on 27th June 2025).

49. Sabharwal, P., & Singh, I. (2024). Anticipating tomorrow: Future trends and predictions in Ayurveda entrepreneurship. *Future Health*. https://www.semanticscholar.org/paper/7321c0da1166d3e95033a1adf53a8129788437a8 (accessed on 27th June 2025).

50. Singer, M., & Matthay, M. (2010). Thinking outside the box: Introduction. *Critical Care Medicine, 38*(10 Suppl), S511. https://www.semanticscholar.org/paper/742f3471f333b1ecf3118bae1dfecb3460ce0301 (accessed on 27th June 2025).

51. Smola, P., Młoźniak, I., Wojcieszko, M., Zwierczyk, U., Kobryn, M., Rzepecka, E., & Duplaga, M. (2025). Attitudes toward artificial intelligence and robots in healthcare in the general population: A qualitative study. *Frontiers in Digital Health, 7*. https://www.semanticscholar.org/paper/1208df5ae32de82a9adf5db44349a5daba184064 (accessed on 27th June 2025).

52. Srivastava, A., Santagostino, E., Dougall, A., Kitchen, S., Sutherland, M. L., Pipe, S. W., Carção, M., et al. (2020). *WFH Guidelines for the Management of Hemophilia, 3rd edition. Hemophilia, 26*, 1–158. https://doi.org/10.1111/hae.14046 (accessed on 27th June 2025).

53. Szuto, A., Dickson, M., Baribeau, D., Carroll, J. C., Carter, M. T., Chad, L., Costain, G., et al. (2024). 25 Genomic medicines in pediatric care for neurodevelopmental disorders: An assessment of practices, attitudes and education needs of Ontario pediatricians. *Pediatrics & Child Health*. https://www.semanticscholar.org/paper/fb793259cf7cf21c201d663926d96a0c338b7703 (accessed on 27th June 2025).

54. van Kooij, Y. V., Loos, N., Arends, G. R., Tabeau, K., Slijper, H., Veltkamp, J., Selles, R. W., et al. (2025). How do clinicians use, experience, and value applications of outcome information in daily care? A mixed-methods study. *Journal of Rehabilitation Medicine, 57*. https://www.semanticscholar.org/paper/ac82790fa34ab85a5a14297b86850e260e8e4cbb (accessed on 27th June 2025).

55. Whittle, I., Yull, D., Yee, J., Czechowicz, G., Murphy, P., Clausen, E., & Yau, Y. H. (2023). Using general practitioners with an extended role in spinal practice for the initial assessment of patients referred to spinal surgeons: Preliminary experience and challenges. *Primary Healthcare Research & Development, 24.* https://www.semanticscholar.org/paper/57075167e65c56bb1d7e0fef29d0d89cfc9944b4 (accessed on 27th June 2025).

56. Winkelman, J. W., Berkowski, J., Delrosso, L., Koo, B. B., Scharf, M. T., Sharon, D., Zak, R. S., et al. (2024). Treatment of restless legs syndrome and periodic limb movement disorder: An American Academy of Sleep Medicine clinical practice guideline. *Journal of Clinical Sleep Medicine: JCSM: Official Publication of the American Academy of Sleep Medicine.* https://www.semanticscholar.org/paper/fc1f025503c38f4861557d6378e77103348416cf (accessed on 27th June 2025).

57. Zaplatnikov, A., Podzolkova, M. N., Ponimanskaya, M. A., Denisova, Y. V., Dmitriev, A. V., Dement'ev, A. A., Chabaidze, Z., et al. (2022). Congenital anemia: A diagnostic algorithm. *Russian Journal of Woman and Child Health.* https://www.semanticscholar.org/paper/f478d747eadfab944bdd73f0210ecbf0e10b23dc (accessed on 27th June 2025).

58. Zhang, D., Chen, Y., Hao, M., & Xia, Y. (2024). Putting hybrid nanomaterials to work for biomedical applications. *Angewandte Chemie (International Ed. in English), 63,* e202319567–e202319567. https://www.semanticscholar.org/paper/e5e3fac801c98bffe343f8c0f2f34fe8d095cc65 (accessed on 27th June 2025).

59. Zhou, J., Liu, L., Xue, P., Yang, X., & Tang, X. (2020). Mental health response to the COVID-19 outbreak in China. *American Journal of Psychiatry, 177,* 574–575. https://doi.org/10.1176/appi.ajp.2020.20030304 (accessed on 27th June 2025).

60. Zupo, R., Moroni, A., Castellana, F., Gasparri, C., Catino, F., Lampignano, L., Perna, S., et al. (2023). A machine-learning approach to target clinical and biological features associated with sarcopenia: Findings from northern and southern Italian aging populations. *Metabolites, 13.* https://www.semanticscholar.org/paper/dc42b48c24b31c64a6693677d386c2957a52ffdc (accessed on 27th June 2025).

CLINICAL ASSESSMENT AND DIAGNOSTIC REASONING

2

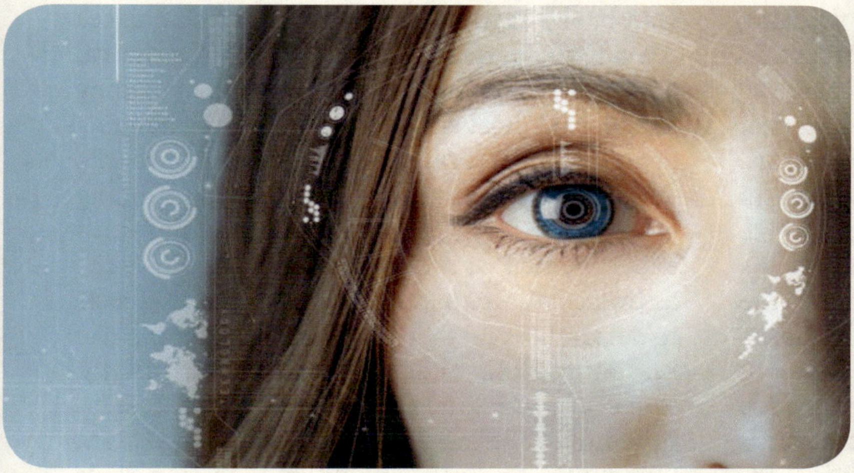

LEARNING OBJECTIVES

After studying this chapter, you will be able to:

1. Describe the clinical assessment process
2. Explain the types of clinical assessments
3. Describe diagnostic reasoning models
4. Define the role of clinical guidelines
5. Focus on challenges in clinical assessment
6. Understand the impact of technology on assessment

Introduction

The importance of clinical assessment and diagnostic reasoning in healthcare cannot be overstated, as it is the central pillar of effective patient management and intervention strategies. With increasing sophistication in healthcare, practitioners need to develop analytical and clinical competencies to navigate different cases of successful patients successfully. Clinical assessment is an inclusive exercise that involves patient history taking, physical examination, and the application of diagnostic aids. These factors not only update the practitioner's understanding of the patient's condition but also facilitate the application of EBP. New frameworks, such as the PARiHS framework, offer practical frameworks for valuing and applying knowledge translation within clinical settings, highlighting the need for context and evidence in diagnosis (Grandos et al., 2008). Moreover, diagnostic thinking takes more than gathering information; it is based on synthesizing and making clinical judgments that influence treatment selection. By finding patterns and interpreting clinical information, clinicians engage in a cognitive process that significantly impacts patient outcomes. Patient values and clinical judgment interact to shape individual treatments meaningfully. Most notably, initiatives such as the European Breast Guidelines identify the position that expertise and stakeholder engagement have in building effective diagnostic protocols as expressing faith that clinical guidelines must evolve through joint feedback (Massimo et al., 2017). This fusion of knowledge and collaboration is the basis for crafting the diagnostic thinking process. At the final analysis, the intersection of clinical assessment and diagnostic reasoning compels the necessity of continuous education and adjustment in medicine. Clinicians are tasked with keeping abreast with advances in medical research and technology to maximize their diagnostic capabilities. As health systems encourage patient-centered approaches, the value of nuances in diagnostic processes becomes increasingly necessary. Advances in clinical assessment models and collaborative guidelines in the future can guide practitioners in navigating the complexity of patient care while having their approach grounded firmly in evidence-based procedures. The continuous evolution of clinical assessment and diagnostic reasoning not only contributes to improving patient outcomes but also further promotes the entire health sciences profession for many years to come.

Definition of Clinical Assessment

The definition of clinical assessment is marked by a comprehensive approach that includes the assessment of a patient's health status in various ways. The procedure entails integrating a number of factors, including taking medical history, physical examination, test ordering, and an interview with the patient. Clinical assessment serves as the beginning of clinical reasoning, whereby it enables health issues to be recognized as well as informing future choices. Practical clinical assessment is not merely a procedural exercise; it demands critical thinking and analytical skills to decipher information and understand the patient's condition. Since human health is multi-dimensional, practitioners would look for standard assessment tools and guidelines to optimize their assessment's validity to get acomplete picture of the patients' needs and situation. In addition, integrating technology into clinical assessment has revolutionized the traditional approach by adding to its new practices such as virtual patients (VPs). These web-based simulations of actual clinical cases provide the perfect platform for training clinical reasoning competence, satisfying the ongoing need for medical education to adapt to changing healthcare delivery patterns. In this regard, the VPs' design might be crucial in making training programs effective. For instance, studies have experimented with various design features, such as branched case paths and sequenced feedback, to determine whether they can influence clinical reasoning skills (Adebajo et al., 2012). Lastly, these innovations highlight the necessity to combine traditional clinical assessment techniques and contemporary education tools to optimize learning and patients' outcomes. As clinical assessment grows increasingly permeated with advanced technological solutions, there is an imperative need for a unifying solution that enhances both usability and accuracy. One of the leading challenges of transforming intensive care unit (ICU) data into useful information is the extremely large quantity of information presented by patient monitoring equipment, so efficient data prioritization and clustering techniques are necessary (Allart et al., 2012). By using analysis methods that prioritize relevant information, clinicians can make their clinical assessments easier to navigate so that there is a simpler and more natural experience. This change is an important essential not only in terms of the functionality of assessments but also to create quick decision-making within high-stress scenarios. The ongoing development of clinical assessment practices highlights the need to integrate strong traditional methods with new technological innovation, ultimately culminating in better clinical outcomes and care for the patient (Figure 2.1).

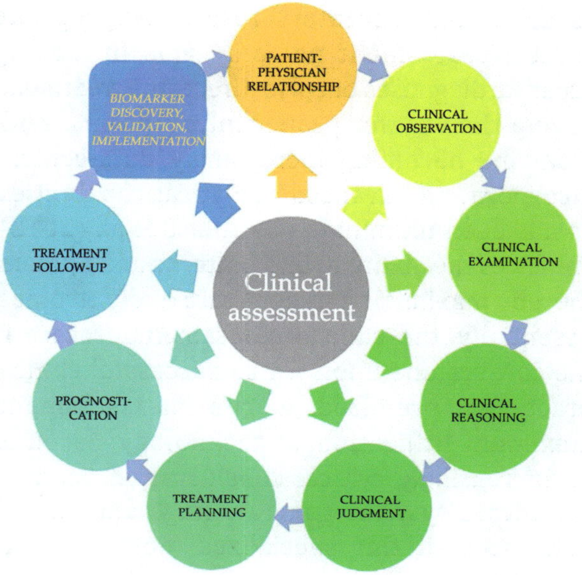

Figure 2.1. Clinical assessment.

Source: https://media.springernature.com/lw685/springer-static/image/art%3A10.1007%2Fs13311-023-01410-3/MediaObjects/13311_2023_1410_Fig1_HTML.png.

Importance of Diagnostic Reasoning

The role of diagnostic reasoning in clinical evaluation cannot be overemphasized. Proper diagnostic reasoning enables healthcare providers to correctly diagnose an illness in a patient, facilitating timely interventions whose impact can greatly influence health outcomes. For example, diagnostic mistakes may lead to ineffective treatments, extended stays in the hospital, and even higher mortality rates. A study highlighted that in 12.3% of the instances, inconsistencies between discharge and admission diagnoses might be due to errors in diagnostic reasoning. The finding highlights that an understanding of patients' presenting features, as well as context-sensitive intuition, is essential. Awareness of new presentations by diagnosticians is a key component in preventing errors and thus the importance of doctors critically considering their diagnostic approach to enhance patient quality of care and safety (Birrenbach et al., 2019). Furthermore, the growing sophistication of modern medicine and research also complicates diagnostic reasoning. Despite the enormous volume of medical literature being created annually, transposing research findings into practice is typically an arduous endeavor. Evidence suggests that the relationship between clinical presentation and treatment outcome is typically provisional, leading to potential cases of overtreatment and undertreatment. This reality underscores the necessity for robust diagnostic reasoning, considering not just the best available evidence but also working knowledge of a patient's unique circumstance. Employing a systematic approach, such as the cybernetic cycle of nosology, semeiology, pathophysiology, and therapy, promotes reproducibility and predictivity of clinical decision-making. Clinical techniques such as these can allow clinicians to guide the fundamentals involved in medical evidence so that diagnostic reasoning is maintained in accuracy and contextuality (Journois et al., 2009). Interestingly, the improvement of diagnostic reasoning also involves ongoing education and reflective practice for health professionals. As medical practice evolves, clinicians must be adaptable and receptive to enhancing their diagnostic skills. This is done through continuous learning, e.g., engaging in continuing medical education and inter-professional educational partnerships that can provide the ability to feed and enhance diagnostic knowledge. Cultivating an inquiry-based and critical thinking culture within healthcare systems can make this more likely to allow providers to be active in effective,practical diagnostic reasoning. Ensuring that practitioners can recognize when evidence is not available will enable them to be more alert and reactive in their manner of handling patient care. Prioritizing the building of diagnostic reasoning, ultimately, yields improved patient outcomes while also making clinical assessment techniques more accurate and effective overall in an evolving medical world (Figure 2.2).

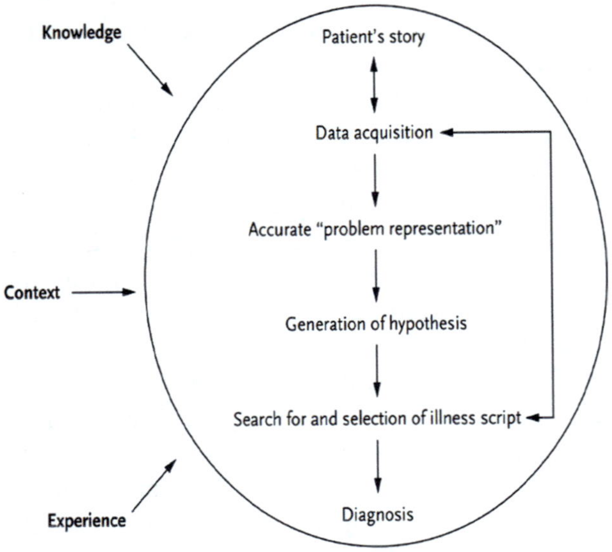

Figure 2.2. Key elements of the clinical diagnostic reasoning process.

Source: https://www.researchgate.net/profile/Judith-Bowen-2/publication/6674220/figure/fig1/AS:341162536783873@1458350895088/Key-Elements-of-the-Clinical-Diagnostic-Reasoning-Process.png.

2.1. The Clinical Assessment Process

Learning Outcome

1. Understand the basics of initial patient evaluation
2. Gather patient history
3. Describe physical examination techniques

Clinical assessment is an essential part of healthcare because it becomes the foundation upon which diagnostic reasoning evolves. It is a systematic process that involves history, physical examination, and pertinent diagnostic tests. Clinicians gather information to create an overall picture of the patients' state of health, which is essential for identifying potential health issues. The process requires critical thinking and the ability to synthesize various data sources, such as EHRs and laboratory results. Appropriate clinical assessment not only aids in making accurate diagnoses but also directs the treatment, paving the way for proper interventions. With medicine becoming increasingly data-centric, incorporating advanced analytical capabilities, as has been illuminated by Allart et al. (2012), enhances the ability to find patterns and outliers, thereby maximizing patient care and outcomes. Essentially, the clinical assessment process is the cornerstone upon which successful clinical practice is premised. In clinical assessment, maximum utilization of technology becomes an increasingly critical consideration. Modern healthcare systems generate huge amounts of data, necessitating specialized tools to create transparency and comprehensibility of the information. Data overload is often a problem for clinical professionals; however, such innovations as knowledge-based and machine learning approaches, as cited by Allart et al. (2012), are robust solutions. These approaches enable healthcare workers to incorporate sophisticated information efficiently, with the outcome that valuable medical points are not lost or misinterpreted. User interaction with advanced graphical user interfaces can also enhance clinical decision-making, enabling practitioners to adjust analytical parameters in real-time. Through sense-making of compound data sets, health practitioners are better placed to identify significant events and call upon the interventions necessary in a timely fashion, demonstrating the revolutionary possibilities of technology for the clinical assessment process. Besides, effective clinical evaluations transcend the direct application of diagnosis; they are critical in the review of new medical technologies and new procedures. Physician-manufacturer interaction can enhance clinical evaluation for new devices, demonstrating the importance of cooperation in the clinical environment. Cost-effectiveness analysis methods that simplify the process of assessing new medical devices, as described in, allow medical professionals to economically evaluate innovation, consequently affecting clinical practice directly. These evaluations use models that compare new procedures' clinical and economic performance against established standards to facilitate informed decision-making. Thus, integrating new evaluation technologies with paradigms in clinical practice not only progresses patient care but also guarantees that new technologies converge with economic imperatives. This joint process, highlighting the worth of data in clinical evaluation, strengthens the diagnostic reasoning process, ultimately benefiting patients and healthcare systems.

2.1.1. Initial Patient Evaluation

The initial assessment of the patient is an important starting point in diagnostic thinking and clinical reasoning. At this step, it is necessary to collect detailed information regarding the patient's medical history, current symptoms, and other social concerns that affect their well-being. Initial assessments conducted well not only serve to create a basis for comparison for ascertaining the patient's current status but also assist in forming the therapeutic relationship between the patient and the clinician. This interaction's quality can significantly impact diagnostic performance and therapeutic success. While traditional means of appraisal are under threat, there is greater recognition that novel approaches, such as simulation and reflective coaching, will be able to enable learning and transfer in real-world clinical settings, thereby making up for the limitations of conventional approaches to comprehending dynamic clinical judgments (Loving et al., 2010). Incorporation of sophisticated technologies into initial patient evaluations encourages improved handling of data and analytical power. Adoption of sophisticated information systems facilitates the consolidation of fragmented data streams, thereby providing a broader picture of the patient's condition. Sophisticated systems can rank important data and categorize information, which assists clinicians in recognizing relevant patterns that may otherwise remain unnoticed. Incorporating technology is fundamental, especially in high-pressure departments like ICUs, where the density of data can be daunting to healthcare practitioners.

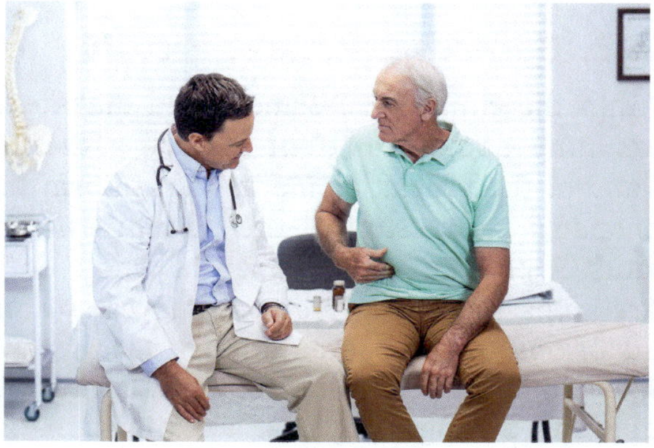

Figure 2.3. Initial assessment.

Source: https://dam.northwell.edu/m/a67d28427ce7f78/Drupal-web_AdobeStock_136188586.jpg.

Increased interfaces that bring together analytical and visual strategies directly play a role in clinical decision-making by improving the detection of life-threatening disorders (Allart et al., 2012). Hence, incorporating these technologies in initial evaluations can accelerate the evaluation process towards quick and accurate interventions. Furthermore, successful initial patient evaluations are critical not only for clinical diagnosis but also for ensuring patient safety and enabling successful health outcomes. Utilizing a methodical process incorporating open communication and empathetic listening, healthcare providers can uncover underlying conditions that are not immediately apparent. That first encounter sets the tone for follow-up evaluations and care plans, making an established rapport essential. By complementing the assessment process with reflective practice and modern technological tools, clinicians can bridge the divide between outdated practice and new expectations of patient care. Finally, an adequate initial evaluation responds to short-term diagnostic needs and sets up a basis for extended clinical participation, prioritizing accuracy and vigilance in the clinical setting (Loving et al., 2010) (Figure 2.3).

2.1.2. Gathering Patient History

Within the clinical assessment and diagnostic reasoning domain, patient history gathering is one of the crucial elements that inform the clinician's impression of the patient's health status. A patient history taken in whole or in part helps identify current health conditions and brings to fore potential risk factors and underpinning causes that may not be readily apparent through physical examination. By using a systematic history-taking process, clinical practitioners can gather relevant facts regarding the patient's medical history, lifestyle, and psychosocial parameters. Comprehensive evaluation is crucial in developing patient-tailored treatment plans and enhancing patient involvement in their healthcare process. As errors in clinical judgment have profound health implications, it cannot be overemphasized that meticulous history-taking places in prominence a central aspect of high-quality clinical practice in contemporary healthcare (Loving et al., 2010). Also, patient history gathering is maximized by synergizing technology and simulation-based learning. New trends in the pedagogic strategy have been promising in upgrading clinical skills and refining diagnostic insight. For instance, high-fidelity simulation (HFS) sessions allow students to practice history-taking in virtual settings where they can immediately use feedback to enhance performance. Not only does this real-world experience strengthen the applicability of patient communication, but it also promotes closure of the gap between theory and practice. Using video recordings of simulated interviews, teachers can support reflective practice for students, where they can critically reflect on their approach to taking patient histories. This structured reflection improves a deeper understanding of the nuances of successful communication with patients and, therefore, high-quality care that is delivered (Escota et al., 2020). Moreover, acknowledging the challenge healthcare providers face in obtaining patient histories, especially from diverse populations, is of paramount significance in enhancing diagnostic reasoning.

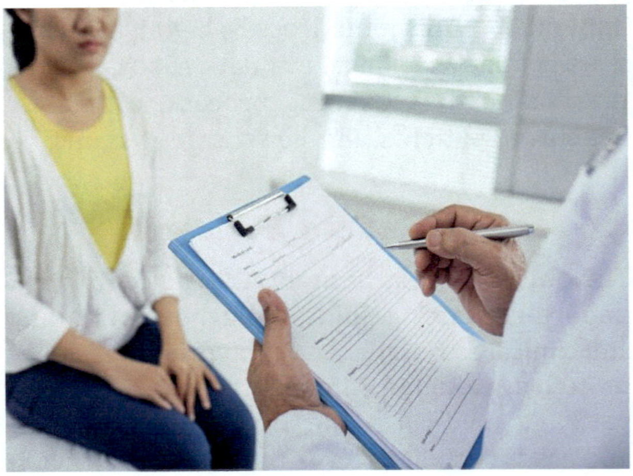

Figure 2.4. Taking medical histories.

Source: https://cdn-clhbh.nitrocdn.com/NPcSlZqrCJzJITEGsuXNhCkoWmIrfjFP/assets/images/optimized/rev-a3140de/www.unitekcollege.edu/wp-content/uploads/2022/01/shutterstock_454645918-768x513.jpg.

Health literacy variability, language discordance, and variation in levels of health literacy may hamper effective communication and result in incomplete histories. While the healthcare system grapples with these complexities, there exists an urgent need for training models that promote cultural competence and empathetic listening in taking histories. By incorporating discussion and training on these dimensions, healthcare professionals can better understand the patient's individual comprehension and better engage the patient in an informed conversation about their health. In essence, the continuous process of creating patient history-taking methodologies is pivotal not only for clinical evaluation and academic success but also for improved patient outcomes and clinician-patient relationship trust (Loving et al., 2010) (Figure 2.4).

2.1.3. Physical Examination Techniques

The contribution of physical examination skills to clinical assessment cannot be overemphasized since the skills are the fundamental instruments health practitioners employ to detect patient problems. These skills, including inspection, palpation, percussion, and auscultation, enable clinicians to gather critical information and formulate early hypotheses regarding a patient's well-being. Both techniques require rigorous training and practice to mastery since the precision of the outcome directly affects the diagnosis and plans for management that follow. An example is practical auscultation of heart sounds; it will be the difference between , regular, or pathological status and thus determine further investigative action. Optimal technique and a keen eye for detail are needed since they help clinicians identify concealed evidence that might represent underlying disease states, thereby aiding in diagnostic reasoning. Moreover, regular application of these techniques promotes a methodical patient evaluation that can be done in various clinical practices. The harmony between technology and traditional physical examination techniques has transformed clinical practice so that health professionals remain proficient in a dynamic environment. For example, web-based tutorial sites customized for medical education have been made available to supplement training for new and seasoned practitioners alike. Such sites attempt to reflect the pedagogical standards promoted by organizations such as the European League Against Rheumatism, focusing on an integrative learning of core rheumatology knowledge. By offering flexible, accessible educational material, such sites facilitate informal learning, allowing users to construct their physical examination skills at their own rate. Adaptive features of such sites can also offer personalized learning experiences, enhance individual strengths, and address weaknesses. Here, technology integration in physical examination education complements traditional approaches and enables future clinicians with the realities of today's medical environments (Armstrong et al., 2005). Effective remediation techniques for underperforming students in the field of physical examination skills are imperative to ensure proficiency in clinical practice.

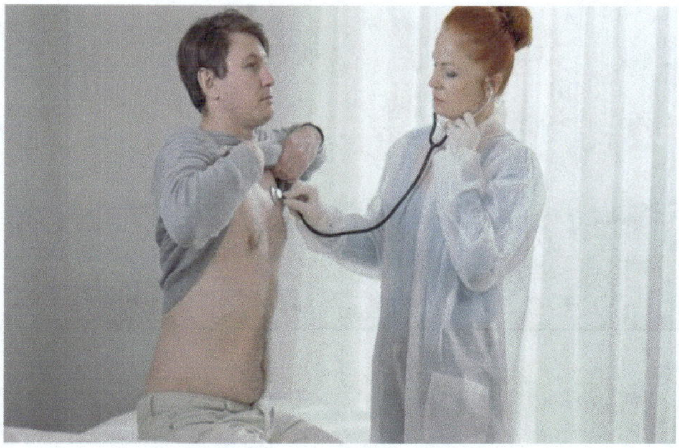

Figure 2.5. Auscultation of a man.

Source: https://t4.ftcdn.net/jpg/04/20/61/89/360_F_420618940_pVtKQTbwMcVw4KB1aDjJBLoHuBh0AkMq.jpg.

It is mostly teachers who cannot make trainees move from underperformance to competency. The framework professional associations, such as the Infectious Diseases Society of America, provide is also helpful in guiding for overcoming some of the most prevalent learning barriers clinicians-in-training (Escota et al., 2020). The competency-based model encourages educators to focus on concrete building blocks of the physical examination, including skills mastery and knowledge application to clinical scenarios. By using tailored feedback and individualized performance assessment, educators can create a supportive learning environment that promotes growth and resiliency in learners. Ultimately, good remediation directly benefits the individual practitioner's skill set but also, more importantly, patient care outcomes because well-trained professionals are more proficient at performing thorough, accurate assessments, which inform diagnostic reasoning (Figure 2.5).

Test Your Knowledge

1. What are the key components of an adequate initial patient evaluation in clinical practice?
2. What are the main questions used during patient history taking, and how do they contribute to diagnosis?
3. How can clinicians use findings from the physical exam to guide further diagnostic testing or treatment decisions?

2.2. Types of Clinical Assessments

Learning Outcome

1. Understand psychological assessments
2. Discuss physical health assessments
3. Define functional assessments

A comprehensive understanding of clinical evaluations is crucial within the area of diagnostic reasoning, as they can directly influence patients' results. One of the most typical forms is physical evaluation, which involves a reasoned patient assessment through observation, palpation, percussion, and auscultation. These measures allow practitioners to obtain significant physiological data and recognize abnormalities. To this, laboratory investigations—such as blood tests, urinalysis, and imaging reports—are likewise pivotal to excluding or confirming probable diagnoses. The: The synthesis of data from physical and laboratory examinations enhances the clinician's ability to develop an even-handed diagnostic picture, eventually leading to more aware clinical decision-making. This totalistic approach emphasizes the importance of mechanically integrating the two evaluation forms to inform patient care and treatment plans. Psychosocial assessments are another essential clinical assessment category that entails evaluating a patient's social, emotional, and mental health. These assessments may involve formal interviews, self-report questionnaires, and observational measures to relieve an individual's psychological status and relationship with the environment. By employing tools such as the Beck Depression Inventory or the various anxiety scales, clinicians can measure emotional distress objectively and provide a framework for diagnosis. Furthermore, awareness of a patient's social determinants of health—socioeconomic status to family functioning—substantially affects diagnosis and treatment plans. The overlap of physical and mental health further boosts the necessity for psychosocial assessments, which can further reveal issues hindering recovery. This multi-dimensional analysis then increases a more intimate knowledge of the patient and his or her trajectory of health. Technological advancements have introduced novel types of clinical assessments, combining data analysis and machine learning techniques in clinical practice. For instance, advanced monitoring systems enable the collection of real-time data, enhancing the diagnostic process through detecting anomalies and providing predictive analytics. These systems support detecting important events in patient care, facilitating clinicians in the timely decision-making process. As termed in existing literature, there is equally a need for greater integration of analytical methods into healthcare technology to address mounting patient complexity and volume of data (Allart et al., 2012). Cost-effectiveness analysis has also evolved as a significant instrument for evaluating new medical device innovation, enabling well-informed decisions by both healthcare professionals and innovators (Craven et al., 2009). This blending of methodology and technology not only enhances the validity of clinical measurement but also assists in aligning clinical interventions with optimal patient outcomes.

2.2.1. Psychological Assessments

Psychological assessment tests are core to clinical practice and are a valuable resource for clinicians to evaluate mental illness and guide treatment. Throughout the assessment process, various methodologies are employed, including interviews, observation techniques, and population-specific standardized measuring tools. Through the integration of structured interviews and psychometric testing, a comprehensive understanding of a patient's cognitive, emotional, and behavioral functioning is possible. This multi-faceted approach enhances diagnostic validity and aids in monitoring treatment progress and outcome. While the psychological evaluator navigates the intricate landscape of psychological testing, he or she must be sensitively aware of these tests' impact, particularly on decision-making capacity (DMC) and clinical judgment. Perhaps one of the most crucial aspects of psychological testing is its ability to evaluate the DMC of psychiatrically complex patients. Research has indicated that the appreciation and reasoning functions play significant roles in DMC judgments across various patient populations. For example, Anderson et al. (2013) note that in competent patients, to understand treatment options, appreciation was a stronger predictor of DMC in psychiatric patients, while reasoning was emphasized in medical patients. This distinction emphasizes the importance of placing the assessments within the individual's unique clinical context since application of DMC with a single evaluative criterion can lead to misestimates of consent to treatment. Acknowledgment of variability in DMC assessments enhances clinicians' ability to individualize interventions and uphold ethical standards in patient care. Moreover, the employment of screening tools like the child and adolescent intellectual disability screening questionnaire (CAIDS-Q) indicates the significant role that psychological tests can play, but in specific populations, in this instance, in young offenders. According to Curtis et al. (2012), the CAIDS-Q demonstrated sound predictive validity, which enabled practitioners to identify intellectually disabled young offenders correctly. The ability to differentiate among individuals with and without intellectual disabilities based on such measures is a significant move forward in clinical testing, a foundation for individualized treatment. Finally, ongoing evaluation and refinement of psychological testing are required not only for proper diagnosis, but for optimal therapeutic alliance and successful treatment outcomes in a wide range of clinical settings.

2.2.2. Physical Health Assessments

The significance of physical examination of health in practice cannot be overestimated, as it is a critical component employed in the diagnosis and planning of care for patients. Through systematic examination of physical signs and symptoms of the body and the patient's medical history, clinicians can gather important information that influences clinical decision-making. The process not only helps identify real health issues but also assists in the detection of possible health threats that may need to be prevented. The evolving complexities of healthcare, including higher medical errors and shortages of trained personnel, necessitate a robust system for conducting these assessments. As determined through new simulation technologies, the traditions of gaining clinical judgment may need to adapt to more contemporary protocols to achieve an improved quality of care (Loving et al., 2010). Regarding diagnostic reasoning, physical health examination is essential to achieving an informed perception of a patient's status. Physical examination can include subjective and objective evaluation, allowing physicians to better understand the patient's status. Detailed evaluations can vital signs, physical examinations, and individual laboratory testing that lead to an accurate diagnosis. The ability to conduct these evaluations effectively is achieved by comprehensive training and familiarity with the foundations of clinical assessment. Remediation of skill, particularly for underperforming students in clinical settings, emphasizes the importance of well-designed feedback and assessments and professional development along these lines (Escota et al., 2020). Moreover, integrating novel learning pedagogies in conducting physical health assessment can redefine learning outcomes in the health field. HFS provides a differentiated platform for learners to experience experiential, hands-on learning exercises in tandem with real-time feedback. It is more feasible for increased reflective practice of learners, in that they can critically reflect on their performance in a safe and controlled environment. By employing such modern pedagogy, educators are not only able to foster students' clinical competencies but also diagnostic thinking skills. Given the emphasis on competency-based models, the competence to conduct accurate and valid physical health assessments will prove essential in preparing future healthcare practitioners for challenges in current medical practice (Loving et al., 2010) (Figure 2.6).

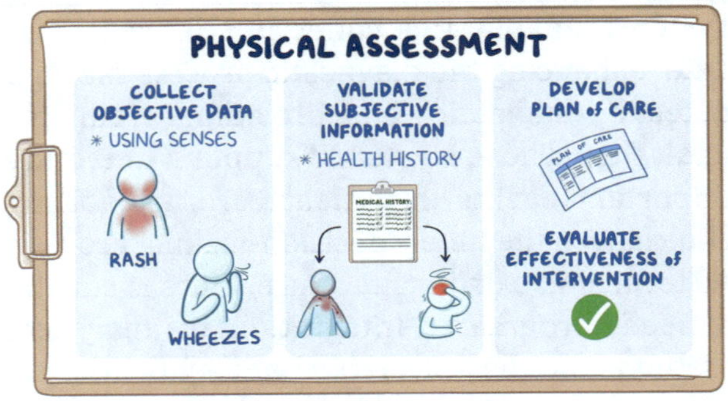

Figure 2.6. Physical assessments.

Source: https://d16qt3wv6xm098.cloudfront.net/ke2ckj7qQEGpQ0AIsRDb6sEYQZ2mmK9P/_.jpg.

2.2.3. Functional Assessments

Functional evaluations are the core of clinical assessment and diagnostic thinking through evaluating how well people function across various domains of their lives. Functional evaluations surpass typical diagnostics by providing a more nuanced observation of the person's capability and struggles in day-to-day functioning. They use a variety of standardized tests and techniques to accumulate data about behavior, cognitive function, and emotion, and end up proposing a comprehensive treatment plan. For instance, within autism spectrum disorder populations, functional assessments can highlight profiled strengths and deficits in cognitive processing, which is critically important when providing interventions, particularly suited to each individual. Such a sensitive assessment increases the value placed on context in understanding the needs of an individual, enhancing the quality of care offered by health professionals. Furthermore, functional assessments allow proper diagnostic reasoning through the real living functioning of patients in their own setting, rather than solely relying on formal diagnostic criteria. This personalized process promotes a dynamic perception of how some conditions manifest themselves in day-to-day life, revealing patterns that are not observable with standardized testing. For example, by assessing for daily living skills, social skills, and emotional regulation, clinicians can construct a more detailed description of an individual's functioning. Further, in recent research, the use of cluster analyses has identified distinct cognitive patterns among high-functioning autism individuals. It has been used to argue that one diagnosis may be ignoring heterogeneity among this population (Wagner et al., 2014). These findings justify the worth of functional assessments in yielding proper and effective treatments. Functional assessments are also utilized in forensic institutions, where it is necessary to recognize a person's functional abilities to make legal judgments. As structural neuroimaging has emerged more significantly in the legal process, adding functional assessments is necessary to attain an evidence-based approach to the evaluation of mental states for legal judgment. The subtle cues yielded by functional assessments can be utilized to corroborate neuroimaging results, which, while being increasingly involved in courts, are subject to cognitive biases that can cause aberrant interpretations (Ferracuti et al., 2018). As the clinical evaluation landscape shifts, it becomes increasingly important to create cohesive approaches that integrate functional evaluation and neuroimaging to guide strong, objective diagnostic reasoning in clinical and forensic contexts (Figure 2.7).

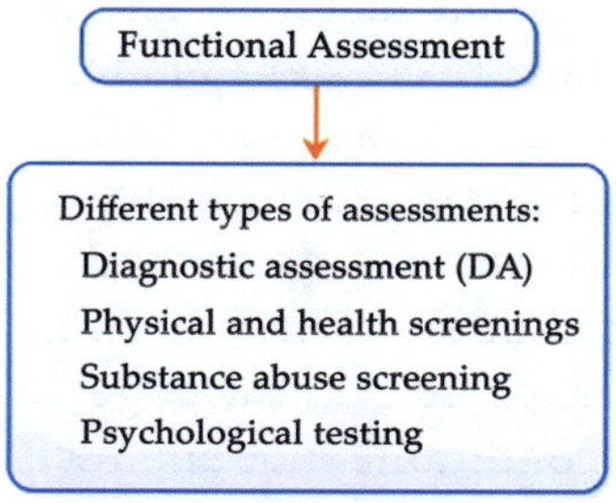

Figure 2.7. Functional assessment.

Source: https://pathlore.dhs.mn.gov/courseware/AdultMentalHealth/FA/images/01_07.jpg.

Test Your Knowledge

1. What are the primary purposes of psychological assessments in clinical practice, and what tools are commonly used?
2. How do physical health assessments differ from psychological assessments in terms of methods and objectives?
3. What key components are evaluated during a functional assessment, and why is this important for patient care?

2.3. Diagnostic Reasoning Models

Learning Outcome

1. Describe the hypothetico-deductive model
2. Understand the concept of Bayesian reasoning
3. Define pattern recognition

In clinical assessment, diagnostic reasoning models are the underlying frameworks that guide health practitioners to come to a diagnosis of the patient. Models of a systematic strategy and clinical expertise, which facilitates thorough analysis of patient histories and symptoms. A few of the most prominent models include the hypothetico-deductive model, which encourages practitioners to formulate hypotheses using initial patient data, and the pattern recognition model, in which clinicians apply past experience and knowledge to recognize patterns of conditions that align with provided symptoms. By blending these models, medical professionals can construct a robust diagnostic strategy, maximizing the possibility of timely and accurate diagnoses. It is particularly vital in emergency settings, where effective condition identification can contribute significantly to patient outcomes and the course of care. New research has shown the prevalence of diagnostic error within clinical practice, particularly in emergency settings, where initial findings may not necessarily align with final diagnoses. One influential study found that approximately 12.3% of cases for patients had notable admission and discharge diagnosis inconsistencies, demonstrating the critical need for effective diagnostic reasoning models (Birrenbach et al., 2019). Such inconsistencies increase hospital stay lengths and correlate with increased patient mortality. Specifically, the data indicated that those patients who had diagnostic errors had , more extended hospital stays and higher rates of in-hospital mortality, and, therefore, the importance for clinicians to enhance their reasoning skills repeatedly. This research places context in diagnostic models in perspective, suggesting that the clinician's comprehension of patient presentation plays a vital role in predicting and preventing discrepancies. To enhance clinical decision-making strategies in medical education better, it is immediately necessary to establish the underpinnings of clinical decision-making strategies. Deliberate clinical inertia or choosing not to intervene as an act of last resort response strategy signifies that clinicians need to undergo critical thinking and reflective practice (Croskerry et al., 2018). Educational programs to create these skills must join medicine curricula to resist widespread cognitive biases corroding sound diagnosis. A clear focus on temperate, evidence-based approaches can potentially redirect 'more is better' culture into one of critical evaluation and discrimination. By establishing a situation that encourages deliberation over impulsivity in diagnostics, healthcare facilities allow novice practitioners to gain the skills needed for efficient and reliable clinical measurement, ultimately leading to improved patient care outcomes.

2.3.1. Hypothetico-Deductive Model

The hypothetico-deductive model is an underlying framework in clinical diagnosis and diagnostic thinking that closely resembles research principles in the scientific realm. The model aims to generate hypothesis from preliminary patient data and clinical symptomatology, leading healthcare practitioners to generate differential diagnoses. Through this framework, clinicians apply these hypotheses to subsequent data gathering and patient history in a systematic fashion and progressively narrow their differential diagnoses based on further information. This repeated cycle enhances critical thinking and renders clinical judgments more trustworthy. A complete understanding of the hypothetico-deductive model is vital for practitioners seeking accurate diagnoses since it facilitates a methodical approach to uncertainty in clinical practice. Clinicians, based on the hypothetico-deductive model, also have to consider the internal constraints related to hypothesis formation. Clinical presentations are usually complicated and require a combination of systematic reasoning and an intuitive clinical approach to diagnosis. The literature on clinical decision-making acknowledges the interaction between the two approaches, and the hypothesized diagnoses must be reevaluated continuously against changing patient information. Incidentally, although systematic methods promote objectivity, the intuitive-humanistic model recognizes experiential knowledge and contextual insight in clinical reasoning, as presented in clinical decision-making literature. Integrating both models facilitates greater understanding of patient care with improved outcomes through clinical knowledge harmonization and patient individual variation. Combined with the hypothetico-deductive framework, new theories propose a cognitive continuum offering greater comprehension of decision-making procedures. Such a vision would assert that analytical and intuitive reasoning, traditionally binary, rather exist on a continuum. Keeping this in mind, more flexible diagnostic thinking on the part of clinicians is achievable through switching between logical methods and intuitive flashes of insight freely. Such flexibility is particularly critical in dynamic clinical environments where one has to make rapid and accurate decisions. Opening oneself to this cognitive range, healthcare professionals maximize their clinical reasoning abilities, leading to more effective diagnostic procedures and richer patient care experiences. The combined use of the hypothetico-deductive model with this continuum approach will help clinicians more effectively address the intricacies of patient presentation, improving both decision-making and patient outcomes (Figure 2.8).

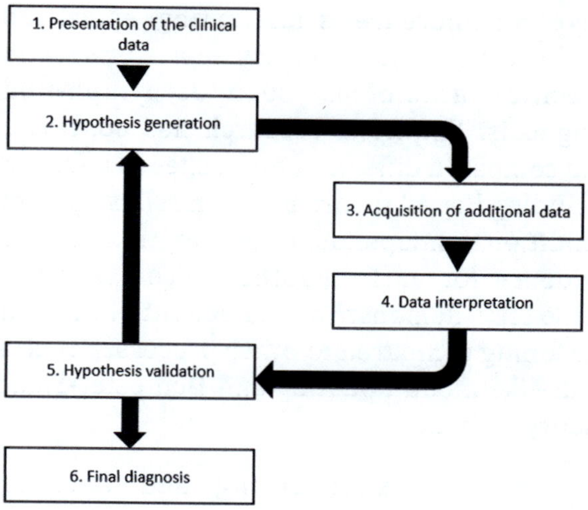

Figure 2.8. The hypothetico-deductive reasoning process.

Source: https://www.researchgate.net/profile/Imene-Jraidi/publication/322856617/figure/fig6/AS:631595987898395@1527595626725/The-hypothetico-deductive-reasoning-process.png.

2.3.2. Bayesian Reasoning

Bayesian reasoning is a dominant model in clinical assessment and diagnostic reasoning in which healthcare providers can make inferences when there is uncertainty. Probabilistic thinking revolves around the revision of initial beliefs by utilizing new evidence, and this allows for a more advanced understanding of a patient's condition. Bayesian reasoning enhances decision-making in diagnostic imaging, particularly in radiology. For instance, radiologists apply this method when interpreting mammograms, analyzing micro-calcifications using symbolic reasoning and advanced image processing methods. By constructing models mimicking radiologists' decision-making, such as in CADMIUM II, doctors can apply Bayesian reasoning in everyday practice to improve diagnostic accuracy and outcome for patients (Alberdi et al., 2004). In the diagnostic reasoning context, the evaluation of different approaches to inference is critical to enhancing clinical decision-making.

Bayesian inference is fascinating, specifically in the context of expert systems for treating specific pathologies, such as lymph-node diagnosis. Empirical research has contrasted and compared different approaches to inference, including Bayes' theorem, which relies upon the conditional independence assumption between evidence for each hypothesis. The results of these tests demonstrate the benefit of Bayesian reasoning compared to other processes such as odds-likelihood updating and Dempster-Shafer theory of belief.

Through expert-rating and decision-theoretic estimates, medical experts can determine the value of Bayesian reasoning in clinical settings, thereby enhancing the overall validity of diagnostic systems (Heckerman et al., 2015). Moreover, integrating Bayesian reasoning in clinical guidelines is a step towards evidence-based medicine, where decisions are made on quantifiable evidence and probabilistic grounds. This approach is beneficial in situations of uncertainty, such as rare disease diagnosis or uncertain presentations. Using Bayesian rules, clinicians can rationally evaluate the likelihood of potential diagnoses, thereby directing appropriate investigations and therapy. The iterative nature of the Bayesian method allows continuous refinement of diagnostic skill as patient data become more readily available. Finally, Bayesian thinking in clinical testing favors a rigorous scientific approach, allowing more thoughtful and personalized patient treatment. As clinical diagnosis becomes increasingly complex, the application of Bayesian thinking will expand, shaping the future of clinical decision-making.

2.3.3. Pattern Recognition

Within clinical assessment and diagnostic reasoning, pattern recognition is essential for clinical professionals, enabling them to identify vital signs and symptoms from incongruous medical data. As clinicians struggle with patients who have complex and diverse health issues, the ability to select patterns among patient presentations becomes significant. In so doing, it often entails the use of clinical experience and knowledge, which facilitates the selection of pertinent information and enhances diagnosis. Systematic pattern recognition among frequent themes in patient cases supports better decision-making since practitioners can leverage established clinical heuristics to optimize their evaluation. Such cognitive shortcuts are not just convenient; they can influence patient outcomes when practitioners recognize patterns typical of emergent or urgent health conditions.

The issue of managing large amounts of data in clinical environments complicates pattern detection in diagnosis reasoning. Due to emerging medical technologies, clinicians face condensed information presentations produced by monitoring devices, particularly in ICUs. Under such conditions, applying analytical methods such as temporal data abstraction and principal component analysis becomes necessary to address this overload and achieve efficient patient care. As by Allart et al. (2012), the inclusion of facilities for visual analysis enables practitioners to recognize prominent patterns that can be used as indicators of worsening health.

Apart from this, these tools enable real-time decision-making and enhance the user's capacity to detect anomalies via an orderly graphical interface, speeding up and making clinical evaluations more effective.

Pattern recognition is not only found in the clinical environment but is also ubiquitous in the educational environment, where it is a key element in the education of the next generation of healthcare professionals. A case study of the type of resource, such as the web-based learning tool described by Armstrong et al. (2005), shows the manner in which pedagogically scaffolded materials can build the skills of pattern recognition among both medical professionals and students. By providing access to case histories and personalized learning paths, such projects submerge knowledge within a working environment so that users can explore realistic clinical conditions. This strengthens their capacity to recognize patterns of patient presentation and promotes informal learning, allowing development of clinical reasoning essential at diagnosis. By strengthening theoretical knowledge concerning practical application, healthcare education can enhance future clinicians' diagnostic competence and patient care outcomes.

Test Your Knowledge

1. How does the hypothetico-deductive model guide clinicians through the diagnostic process?
2. What role does Bayesian reasoning play in updating diagnostic probabilities based on new clinical information?
3. How does pattern recognition enable experienced clinicians to make rapid diagnoses?

2.4. The Role of Clinical Guidelines

Learning Outcome

1. Understand evidence-based practice
2. Describe standardized assessment tools
3. Discuss clinical decision-making frameworks

Clinical guidelines are essential for clinical assessment and diagnostic thinking, providing evidence-based frameworks that guide practitioner decision-making—clinical guidelines condense research evidence to provide recommendations that clinicians can use to guide patient care. The complexity of modern healthcare also necessitates guidelines, as doctors have to contend with an overload of clinical information and diverse patient presentations. By providing standardized diagnostic and treatment methods, clinical guidelines reduce variability in care, thereby improving patient outcomes and guaranteeing best practice among practitioners. They also foster uniformity in healthcare settings, which is essential in maintaining a high standard of care in today's diverse medical environments. Furthermore, the inclusion of clinical guidelines in healthcare practice has also gained more importance, particularly addressing the evolving environmentalclimate of clinical errors and deficits in clinical judgment. As stated in other research work, traditional teaching and assessing clinical reasoning methods have been unsuccessful in preparing competent healthcare practitioners. New curricular frameworks incorporating clinical guidelines facilitate the building of problem-solving and critical thinking skills required for sound diagnostic reasoning. For instance, methodologies such as high-resolution simulation acknowledge the equilibrium between theoretical knowledge and clinical practice in a pragmatic approach. This facilitates students in navigating clinical decision-making more effectively (Loving et al., 2010). This multi-dimensional approach conforms to the recent perception that clinical competence is not merely a process of applying knowledge but also one of situational sense of patient-specific situations. Further, using clinical guidelines offers a forum for continuous improvement in the quality and safety of patients. By following strict evidence-based guidelines, healthcare providers can systematically track and improve their clinical practices based on outcomes and feedback. This process is particularly relevant in the face of growing examination of medical mistakes, which have been linked to preventable adverse patient outcomes. Criticism of healthcare practice calls for a shift to EBP that supports patient safety and effectiveness (Aspiuynall et al., 2007). Clinical guidelines, in this case, not only provide the foundation for informed clinical decisions but also serve as aids for ongoing professional development. By encouraging a learning and thinking culture, clinical guidelines challenge health practitioners to implement EBP, resulting in improved patient care and outcomes.

2.4.1. Evidence-Based Practice (EBP)

Evidence-based practice (EBP) is a cornerstone in clinical assessment and diagnostic reasoning, guiding healthcare providers to make decisions based on the best available evidence. The very essence of EBP lies in the meticulous integration of clinical expertise, patient values, and the best available research evidence. This three-way relationship is where professionals can apply sound evaluation processes to assess their clinical interventions. By emphasizing critical thinking, EBP supports the evaluation of the validity and applicability of various sources of information before they are implemented in practice. Continuous development of the critical thinking ability of nurse prescribers also highlights the imperative for agreement regarding effective teaching strategies and assessment measures for enhancing such skills (Adams et al., 2006). Finally, EBP enhances patient care quality and fosters an environment of inquiry and EBP within healthcare settings. The intricate processes of clinical decision-making models further enable the application of EBP to clinical assessment and reasoning. Historically, two simple models—the information processing model and the intuitive-humanist model—have shaped how clinical decisions are reached. Information processing model demands an analytically arranged strategy, whereas the intuitive-humanist model is founded on intuitive experience-based insights. The recent developments placed a multidimensional model bringing together elements of both, making EBP more applicable by incorporating patient-specific factors necessary to enable cue and pattern recognition (Aspiuynall et al., 2007). This shift towards decision-making models calls for practitioners to consider more influences, thereby increasing their clinical thinking process and improving patient outcomes through a better understanding of applying evidence to practice. Incorporating EBP into clinical assessment and diagnostic thought calls for commitment to continuous learning alongside collaboration among medical professionals.

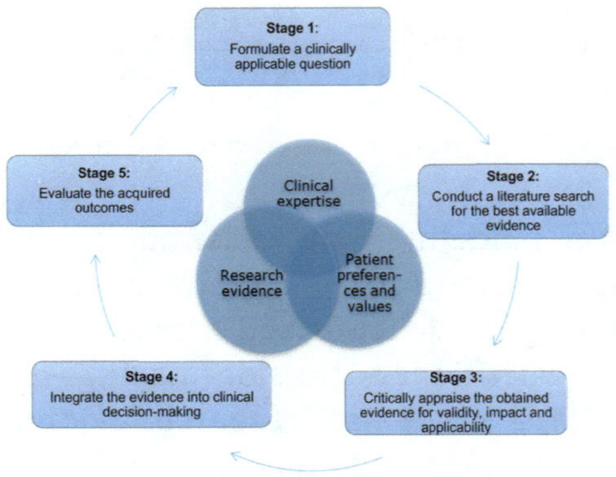

Figure 2.9. Evidence-based practice cycle.

Source: https://www.researchgate.net/profile/FerdouzRamazan/publication/358843222/figure/fig1/AS:11431281085794244@1663885498646/Evidence-based-practice-cycle-5-7.png.

As clinical environments evolve, practitioners must remain conversant with applying the newest research and adaptive learning strategies. Engagement in interdisciplinary teams has the potential to facilitate the sharing of diverse perspectives and insights that supplement the employment of evidence in practice. Moreover, sustaining a culture that values ongoing education and critical reflection has the potential to elicit meaningful change in the delivery of care. By making EBP an integral component of clinical judgment, healthcare providers are better positioned to meet patient care demands, that diagnostic and treatment options are scientifically valid and tailored to each patient's circumstances, thereby leading to improved health outcomes and patient satisfaction (Figure 2.9).

2.4.2. Standardized Assessment Tools

Using standardized tests in clinical practice is essential to obtain reliable and consistent appraisals of patient abilities, particularly in decision capacity. The MacArthur Competence Assessment Tool for Treatment (MacCAT-T) and the Competence Assessment Tool for Psychiatric Advance Directives (CAT-PAD), for instance, are assessment tools that measure systematic aspects like Understanding, Appreciation, Reasoning, and Expression of a decision. This allows accurate and reliable measurement of these key aspects to inform clinical decision-making and direct treatment planning. Their application helps healthcare providers assess patients' capacities and gives a uniform mode to compare.

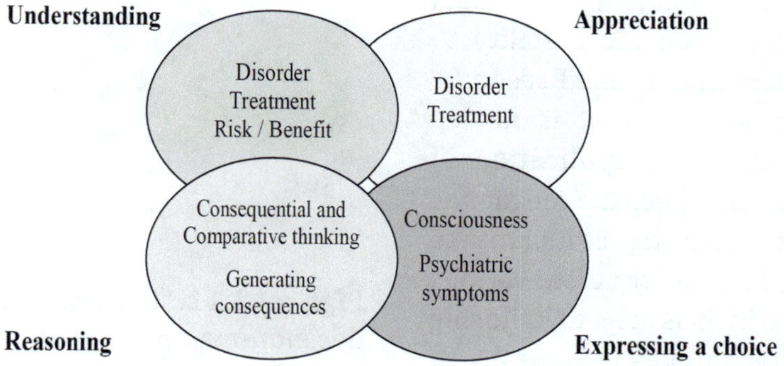

Figure 2.10. Key elements of the MacArthur competence assessment tool.

Source: https://www.researchgate.net/publication/332384308/figure/fig1/AS:11431281244736195@1715994974000/Key-elements-of-the-MacArthur-Competence-Assessment-Tool.tif.

Through their implementation, clinicians improve consistency when examining mental capacity, pivotal in clinical evaluation and diagnostic reasoning, especially when complex treatment decisions are being made. Using these structured tools enhances clinician confidence and patient care quality, as assessment becomes more uniform and less subject to individual bias. The efficacy of standard instruments also transfers to clinical education as an instructional tool for clinical reasoning. Implementing VPs in medical education is the best example of this integration, with web-based simulations that enable a real learning process for students. Effectiveness studies of VPs by different designs highlight structured clinical reasoning feedback and branching case paths as imperative features, demonstrating positive correlation to improved clinical reasoning skills. For instance, one study assessing multiple VP designs indicated that those with structured feedback significantly enhanced students' performance on standardized clinical reasoning tests. This highlights the crucial role that standard tools play in educational settings and clinical practice, providing a bridge between theoretical knowledge and clinical application in actual practice, enriching learning, and augmenting diagnostic reasoning abilities.

Additionally, the meta-analytic analysis of the DMC in various patient groups further documents the function of standardized assessments in clinical diagnosis. Comparing schizophrenia spectrum disorders (SSD) and bipolar disorders (BD) individuals using standardized measures, researchers not only identified differences in performance but also in the subtle understanding of mental ability by diagnosis. Results showed BD patients scored marginally higher in specific domains, providing clinicians with evidence supporting individual patient assessment. However, the inability to find differences in Understanding and Reasoning domains points to how critical it is not to overgeneralize. This rigorous application of standardized measures enhances the diagnostic reasoning process by alerting clinicians to nuances of differences in capacity across various patient populations, which is key to tailoring effective therapeutic techniques (Figure 2.10).

2.4.3. Clinical Decision-Making Frameworks

In clinical assessment and diagnostic reasoning practice, clinical decision-making models offer scaffolding critical to supporting healthcare professionals in their work through complex patient cases. Models facilitate systematic decision-making, ensuring convergence of clinical knowledge, patient data, and interdisciplinarity. Underpinning their operation is the assumption that standardized protocols can reduce variability in practice and enhance patient outcomes. As highlighted in the research on ICU physiotherapists, another crucial factor in sound decision-making is teamwork between physicians and maintaining an atmosphere of mutual knowledge and thorough management strategies (Hanekom et al., 2017). Such a team-based organization is particularly imperative in high-pressure settings like the ICU, where accurate and timely decisions can directly affect patient safety and recovery. Additionally, clinical decision-making paradigms may be applied through formal guidelines, wherein expert opinion is combined with evidence-based information for informing clinical practice. Bodies such as the European Commission have developed systematic guidelines, including the European Breast Guidelines for diagnosing breast cancer and screening, as an example of the worth of a systematic process to clinical decision-making (Massimo et al., 2017).

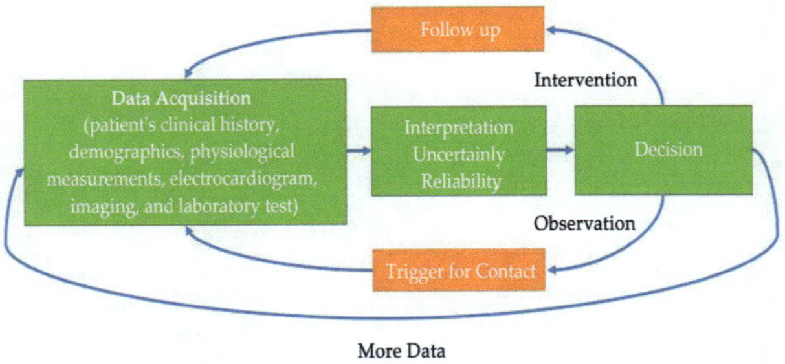

Figure 2.11. General framework of clinical decision-making.

Source: https://www.researchgate.net/profile/Nematollah-Saeidi/publication/367009099/figure/fig1/AS:11431281114076321@1674221975391/General-framework-of-clinical-decision-making.png.

By incorporating views of various stakeholders into guidelines, such guidelines render frameworks current and practical to implement. By this ongoing enhancement of clinical standards, decision-making is not only of better quality, but clinical practice also conforms to evolving evidence-based studies to allow continuing professional development and patient-centered care. Finally, clinical decision-making models are key to bridging the theoretical information and its practice in the real clinical field. In the dynamic patient care environment, the models allow clinicians to operate with uncertainty and make knowledge-based decisions that constitute current best practices. By accommodating the integration of individual clinical expertise and the aggregation of experience from various disciplines, healthcare systems can optimize patient outcomes and uphold safety standards. As is evident from the controversy regarding minimum standards of care for ICU physiotherapists, formalized guidelines are key to advancing enhanced clinical thinking and safe patient care (Hanekom et al., 2017). Hence, the demand for precise clinical decision-making guidelines remains a prime concern in the movement towards enhancing healthcare quality and efficacy (Figure 2.11).

Test Your Knowledge

1. How do clinical guidelines support evidence-based practice in healthcare?
2. What are the benefits of using standardized assessment tools in clinical evaluations?
3. How do clinical decision-making frameworks help practitioners apply guidelines in complex patient cases?

2.5. Challenges in Clinical Assessment

Learning Outcome

1. Focus on subjectivity in patient reporting
2. Deal with the integration of cultural considerations into clinical assessment and diagnostic reasoning
3. Discuss the limitations of diagnostic tests

The clinical assessment landscape is plagued by numerous challenges that can significantly impact diagnostic reasoning. Such challenges include the complexity of seeing epistemic activities as part of the assessment. Epistemic activities comprise a wide range of cognitive processes necessary for effective diagnosis, including generating hypotheses and evaluating evidence. Manual observation of such activities is not only time-consuming but also open to personal bias, which makes the results of an assessment invalid. The latest advances in automated detection of such activities offer a way to eliminate the above drawbacks; however, there are significant hurdles. For instance, precisely demarcating the limits of epistemic activities and distinguishing between similar activities are indispensable issues that, if not resolved, can complicate the effectiveness of computer-aided solutions (Bauer et al., 2018). Therefore, applying technology in medical assessments should be carried out with caution so that it enhances and does not impede the diagnostics process. Another pressing clinical assessment issue is the inadequacy of traditional models to train and evaluate clinical judgment. The current healthcare crisis, with high rates of medical mistakes and staff vacancies, highlights the importance of new techniques for assessment. Traditional, experiential evaluations often overlook the complexity of clinical decision-making and thus render clinicians incompetent. Health professions educators are increasingly turning to web-based technologies and HFS as new choices to close this gap. These new methods are designed to provide a more rigorous assessment than simple observation. While these tools promise much toward the development of learning and evaluation, they are best applied with attention to ensure that they reflect a clinician's diagnostic reasoning abilities (Loving et al., 2010). Lastly, the incorporation of reflection in clinical evaluation can pose its own challenges. Guided reflection, specifically after simulated practice, is intended to support learning among students and help uncover areas for improvement. Although of pedagogical value, guided reflection lacks reliability in implementation. For example, students may struggle to provide meaningful feedback on their video-recorded performance due to nervousness or inadequate debriefing training. Further, if not anchored in a robust structure that encourages reflective contemplation on the material, the reflection exercise will become redundant rather than an enriching, productive learning experience. Therefore, it is crucial to work in an environment that fosters effective self-assessment and critical reflection to enhance the development of clinical reasoning skills among prospective health professionals (Loving et al., 2010).

2.5.1. Subjectivity in Patient Reporting

Patient subjectivity plays a significant role in diagnostic thinking and clinical evaluation because patients' perceptions and conceptions of their illnesses differ significantly from what clinicians can observe. Several factors, including personal experience, state of mind, and cultural background, give rise to these subjective accounts. For instance, a patient might rate symptoms of pain that are mood- and insight-dependent and may lead to discrepancies between what the patient reports and what the clinician notices. This discrepancy can affect the diagnostic process since clinicians will often apply the patient's report to approximate symptoms and set out treatment plans. Thus, medical professionals need to identify subjectivity to gain the skill of interpreting, validating, and synthesizing patient-reported data with clinical data to enhance the validity of diagnoses as well as enhance patient care. Bias as a phenomenon also plays a role in making patient reporting subjective. Research indicates that cognitive biases, such as confirmation bias and context bias, can color patients' understanding and report of symptoms, unconsciously influencing clinical judgments. For instance, patients may only listen to what they believe are relevant symptoms, excluding others or magnifying them in light of preconceived notions regarding their sickness.

Cognitive biases tend to distort the clinical picture, which complicates diagnosis. Furthermore, healthcare professionals may inadvertently reinforce these biases when they interpret patient reports through their personal lenses. To deal with these issues, there needs to be a method of clinical training involving awareness and control over bias, a process wherein both patients and professionals play a part in a more objective and interactive diagnostic thinking mechanism. Incorporation of strategies for ensuring objectivity in assessing the patient is needed to maximize diagnostic precision. Training healthcare professionals in applying structured interview methods, valid assessment tools, and patient-centered communication can reduce the effects of subjectivity. This has been supported in ongoing recommendations in clinical literature to minimize clinical bias. Using standardized scales to measure pain, for example, can provide a less subjective measurement that is added to patient-reported symptoms. In addition, interdisciplinary collaboration can ensure that several sources of knowledge guide the diagnostic process, hence anchoring it in a broader context than patient self-reporting. This is a step towards increasing diagnostic reliability and creating a setting where patients are validated and understood, eventually bringing about improved health outcomes. The conflict is to apply such practices uniformly in clinical practice, ensuring the interaction between subjectivity and objectivity is well acknowledged and managed well in the context of diagnostic reasoning (Figure 2.12).

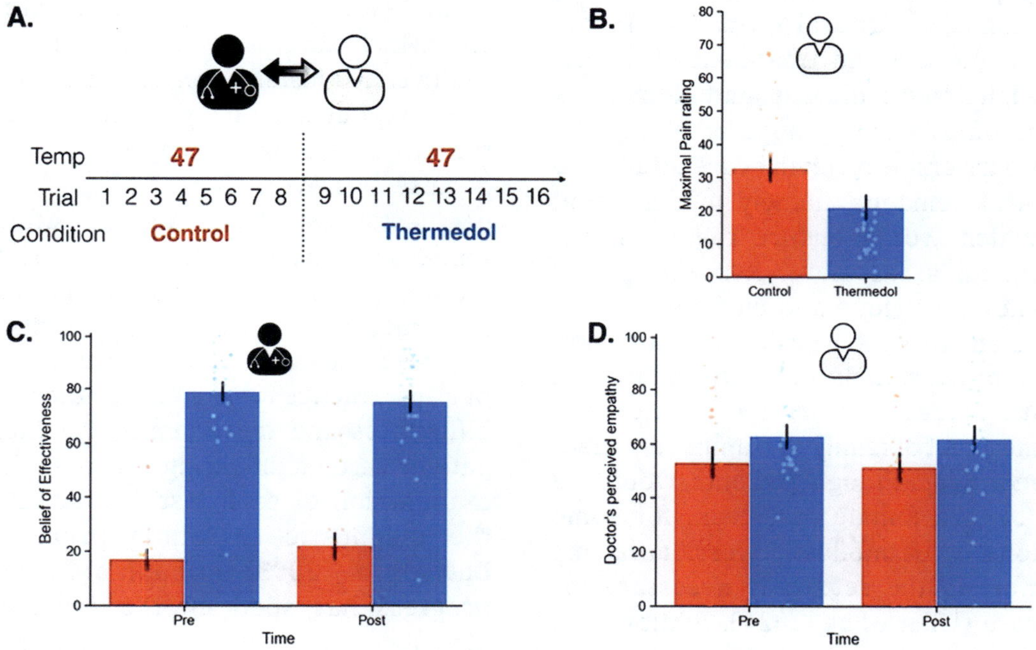

Figure 2.12. Subjective reports from doctors and patients during the doctor–patient interaction phase. (A) A demonstration of the experimental design. (B) Patients reported experiencing less pain in the thermedol treatment compared to the control treatment based on their maximal pain level from their continuous pain ratings. (C) Doctors' beliefs formed during the doctor conditioning phase were maintained and did not change after each treatment. (D) Patients reported that the doctors were more empathetic during the thermedol treatment than during the control treatment.

Source: https://www.researchgate.net/publication/336710103/figure/fig2/AS:816670457225238@1571720818437/Subjective-reports-from-doctors-and-patients-during-the-doctor-patient-interaction-phase.jpg.

2.5.2. Cultural Considerations

Integrating generative and cultural factors into clinical evaluation and diagnostic thought is vital for efficient provision of care. Acceptance of various patient backgrounds allows health professionals to modify their approaches to suit specific cultural needs. This is particularly crucial in evaluating the role of generative AI in healthcare, in which ethical considerations and prejudice in training data can disproportionately affect marginalized populations. For instance, response biases in AI can exaggerate health inequalities if patient data reflects societal inequalities. By implementing culturally responsive assessment processes, healthcare providers can combat assumed inaccuracies created by AI and foster patient activation and education. This emphasizes the necessity for ongoing talk about the intersection of technology and cultural competency within the healthcare sector (Al-Akhras, 2024). In minority populations, such as Muslim women, the importance of cultural influences in the diagnosis of disease and treatment of illness, such as Alzheimer's disease and dementias (ADRD), becomes glaringly apparent. They will likely face barriers in receiving care attuned to their cultural demands, namely modesty and privacy, which would ensure their comfort during clinical assessment. Respecting this group's unique religious and cultural practice is critical to enhance their healthcare outcomes. Healthcare professionals need to understand the various stages of spiritual practice and consider the effect of family dynamics on patient interactions. Even though patients would be disposed toward female caregivers for some examinations or be modestly worried, having such comfort in the setting is necessary for effective care (Irfan et al., 2024). Additionally, cultural adaptation is about developing care plans consistent with patients' beliefs and values. For Muslim women with ADRD, it is essential that their end-of-life care and religious practice choices, e.g., organ donation, are known to be used in the building of patient-centered diagnostic reasoning. Using Islamic ethics to guide treatment plans will enable clinicians to build trust and collaboration and ensure that care plans are consistent with patients' family organization and cultural systems. Permission to make such considerations as Halal-friendly medications will also enhance therapeutic compliance. Lastly, encouraging an open debate about cultural values and incorporating these elements in clinical care results in an enhanced, broader care strategy, improving patient outcomes in patients with varied backgrounds and care quality (Irfan et al., 2024).

2.5.3. Limitations of Diagnostic Tests

Diagnostic tests are critical components of clinical assessment, but they are often accompanied by significant limitations that can impact the diagnostic process's validity and reliability. Perhaps the most widely recognized limitation is the test accuracy variability inherent in the test, which can lead to false negatives and false positives. For instance, certain tests may be highly sensitive but not highly specific, complicating the diagnostic process by giving a high rate of false positive results. The performance of diagnostic tests might also be influenced by numerous variables, including the patient's unique physiological status and clinicians' subjective interpretation of test results. As noted in recent research, evaluating decision-making in nursing practice must consider these judgment differences and the potential ramifications to patient care, highlighting the need for critical examination of each test's limitations during the diagnostic reasoning process (Allen-Davis et al., 2003). In addition, technological progress has sped up the development of high-level diagnostic tools; however, such advancements will not necessarily translate to enhanced clinical outcomes. The application of clinical prediction rules (CPRs) illustrates this issue. CPRs are designed to improve clinical reasoning, but they were seen to lack a gap in their application and understanding among students and practitioners, as per studies. A high majority of physiotherapy students, for instance, reported unfamiliarity with CPRs, indicating that learning courses might not effectively incorporate such tools into training (Kelly et al., 2016). This imbalance suggests a greater general constraint in terms of the training and use in practice of diagnostic tests, wherein the lack of appropriate training can disable healthcare professionals from effectively using these rules. The disparity between available diagnostic tools and educational content that facilitates the use of these tools thus represents an important shortfall in advancing clinical assessment approaches. Lastly, interpreting the results of diagnostic tests will often appeal to an educated recognition of their limitations, resulting in a challenge to clinical decision-making. Physicians could be prone to cognitive biases like overdependence on test results, to the detriment of clinical presentation or patient history, to advance toward a more holistic approach to diagnosis. Clinical assessment regulation calls for an integrative thinking system where clinicians must scrutinize the strengths and weaknesses of diagnostic tests critically. In the process, the clinicians can craft a more holistic perspective that considers the patient's personal context, enhancing diagnostic accuracy. By recognizing such limitations, healthcare professionals can make their way through the intricacies of clinical reasoning, ultimately leading to better patient outcomes and improved care delivery (Allen-Davis et al., 2003).

Test Your Knowledge

1. How does subjectivity in patient self-reporting affect the accuracy of clinical assessments?
2. Why is it important to consider cultural factors during clinical assessments, and how can they impact diagnosis and treatment?
3. What are some common limitations of diagnostic tests that clinicians must be aware of during patient evaluation?

2.6. The Impact of Technology on Assessment

Learning Outcome

1. Define electronic health records
2. Discuss telemedicine and remote assessments
3. Explain the role of artificial intelligence in diagnostics

Technology integration into clinical evaluation has transformed traditional methods of evaluating patient care and diagnostic reasoning. VPs, for instance, demonstrate how sophisticated technology can enhance clinical education by offering web-based, realistic cases that challenge students to apply their reasoning skills in simulated environments. Such VPs include some aspects such as structured feedback and branching paths, which have a strongly significant impact on learning outcomes. When these design elements are integrated into the teaching framework, educational institutions can promote critical thinking and improve diagnostic skills among students. These innovations point toward the necessity for the application of technology in developing a robust learning process that enables future clinicians to address clinical decision-making problems in real-world settings (Adebajo et al., 2012). Moreover, data handling systems in the health industry have also revolutionized the assessment process. Modern ICU information systems, when properly developed, can filter and categorize vast volumes of patient data to support better-informed clinical decisions. These systems rely on advanced analytical methods, and therefore, healthcare professionals can synthesize major information effectively and speedily. Machine learning algorithms incorporated within them can assist in recognizing patterns that can indicate arriving medical complications. This technological advancement not only streamlines the task of managing data but also enhances clinicians' diagnostic capabilities and dynamic tracking of conditions, thus ensuring timely interventions that determine pivotal influence over patient outcomes (Allart et al., 2012). The broadening of the implications of these technology advances transcends performance measurement; they redefine clinical competency to understand and measure. With the utilization of emerging technologies like VPs and sophisticated data systems, instructors can now evaluate learners' clinical reasoning in a more inclusive manner than in the past. The focus has been shifted to an experiential model of learning that facilitates practical application and the context of the scenario in the real world. This change is vital in creating a new crop of healthcare professionals who are not only competent to work with technology but also have the capacity for critical thinking and practical problem-solving in crises. Through this, technology adoption becomes critical in constructing whole-person approaches to assessment that fully capture the needs and complexities of clinical practice.

2.6.1. Electronic Health Records (EHRs)

The implementation of EHRs is a paradigm shift in the art of clinical evaluation and diagnostic reasoning. EHRs enable patient data capture in one integrated digital format, enhancing the speed and precision of healthcare delivery. Clinicians can access a patient's medical history, medication list, and laboratory data with unprecedented ease, facilitating more accurate clinical decision-making. In addition, EHRs support embedding sophisticated analytical tools that can assist in detecting patterns and outliers in patient data, thus aiding diagnostic reasoning. Nonetheless, the quality of EHRs relies on their capacity to present relevant information without overloading clinicians, which calls for features to focus and cluster information to make it easier to read and use. The delicate balance between clarity and data richness is necessary to improve patient outcomes and build a more responsive healthcare environment (Allart et al., 2012). Despite all that EHRs can offer, the healthcare industry has been challenged with their effective adoption and utilization. Of concern is the very nature of the health systems that are comprised of diverse specialties and uneven practices, rendering standardization inadvisable. EHR systems will have to evolve with these complexities while guaranteeing that they meet the needs of both patients and providers. The past challenges in bringing information technology to healthcare show us a terrain filled with obstacles, where decision-making tends to be centralized, defeating the decentralized benefits EHRs were supposed to bring. For EHRs to fulfill their potential as facilitators of clinicians, there needs to be a paradigm shift towards developing user-focused systems that enhance decision-making at the point of care. This requires stakeholder alignment across healthcare practitioners and technology developers to create solutions that respect the complexities of clinical practice (Austin et al., 2006).

The impact of effective use of EHRs reaches far beyond isolated patient interactions, however, with an influence on the overall quality of healthcare delivery. As a means of enabling more reasoned diagnosis and automating information management, EHRs can potentially improve patient safety and promote an evidence-based culture. As healthcare continues to evolve, the role of EHRs as a foundation technology grows increasingly significant. Their capacity to facilitate real-time data sharing and multidisciplinary groups facilitates the continuity of care, resulting in better health outcomes. However, as these organizations invest in EHR systems, it is essential to value ongoing training and support for healthcare providers. Ensuring clinicians are adequately trained to optimally leverage such platforms will bridge the gap between technology and practice, transforming EHRs from mere digital repositories into crucial enablers of improved clinical reasoning and evaluation (Allart et al., 2012) (Figure 2.13).

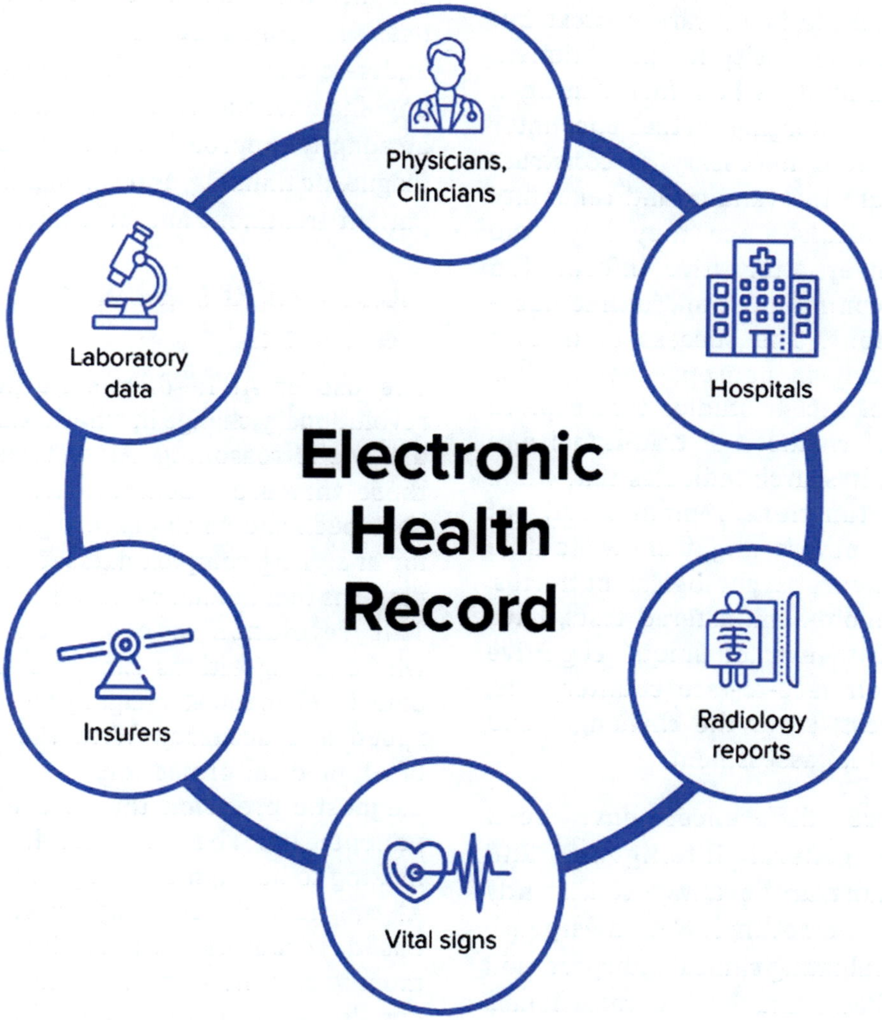

Figure 2.13. Electronic health records (EHRs).

Source: https://appinventiv.com/wp-content/uploads/2022/07/How-to-build-an-EHR-system-02-1.webp.

2.6.2. Telemedicine and Remote Assessments

The application of telemedicine in clinical assessments has revolutionized the medical sector by presenting novel solutions for traditional diagnostic procedures. Remote assessment enables the continuation of critical patient assessment, especially during emergencies, like the COVID-19 outbreak. Medical experts can conduct assessments through technology from the comfort of patients' homes, thereby removing barriers to access and reducing the risk of infectious disease transmission. This shift not only broadens the healthcare context but also highlights the necessity for practitioners to alter their thinking when formulating a diagnosis to meet emerging virtual encounter dynamics. Thus, it is necessary to construct models that ensure the validity and reliability of remote appraisals since they have the potential to convey alternative information and foster miscommunication, unlike face-to-face interactions. The success of distant testing, particularly in neuropsychology, has been the focus of recent studies that explore comparative performances of traditional and teleassessments. Research indicates that while some cognitive functions remain steady at different places, others might show notable variations. Teleneuropsychological batteries, among other remote-administered tests, have been discovered to extract unique cognitive factors from their face-to-face counterparts, and in the process, cover the challenges and intricacies of virtual assessment.

For instance, differences have been established in general intelligence and processing speed that are not always consistently measured in remote settings. This divergence necessitates reevaluating clinical interpretation methods to emphasize that health professionals must be cognizant of such differences while drawing inferences from distant assessments (Datoc et al., 2022). Furthermore, the validity and acceptability of tele-neuropsychology in pediatrics have gained extensive attention and have developed in terms of the possible benefits of incorporating telemedicine into practice. A systematic review highlighted that tele-neuropsychological assessment via video conference or phone was feasible, with minimal difference in behavior during testing (Dimitriou et al., 2023). Overall, the evidence suggests that, despite some drawbacks, remote assessment can provide clinicians with valuable information about a patient's cognitive abilities. However, to enhance the external validity of such research, uses heterogeneous samples and examines under-researched cognitive functions. Lastly, the ongoing advancement of telemedicine requires an adaptive approach in clinical assessment and diagnostic thinking, as it can significantly impact patient treatment and outcomes.

2.6.3. Artificial Intelligence in Diagnostics

The use of AI in diagnostic processes is a revolutionary change in clinical examination and diagnostic reasoning. AI systems, particularly those that use machine learning algorithms, have been shown to possess greater capability for analyzing complex datasets and identifying patterns that human clinicians may not perceive. This revolution is best seen in radiology, where AI algorithms can process and analyze data from medical imaging with breathtaking speed and accuracy. With the incorporation of AI, medical professionals can enhance their diagnostic precision thus providing improved patient care. The scope for human decision-making to be augmented by AI is enormous, as AI can help clinicians by providing evidence-based recommendations, but also provide them with time to exercise their expertise for detailed analysis of patients. Along with this, the current situation of using AI for diagnosis also has a negative aspect that must be dealt with. Most AI systems operate on the premise of readily available datasets that are not necessarily representative of the variety of patient populations encountered in the field. This bias is problematic to diagnostic algorithm generalizability and performance within various demographic groups.

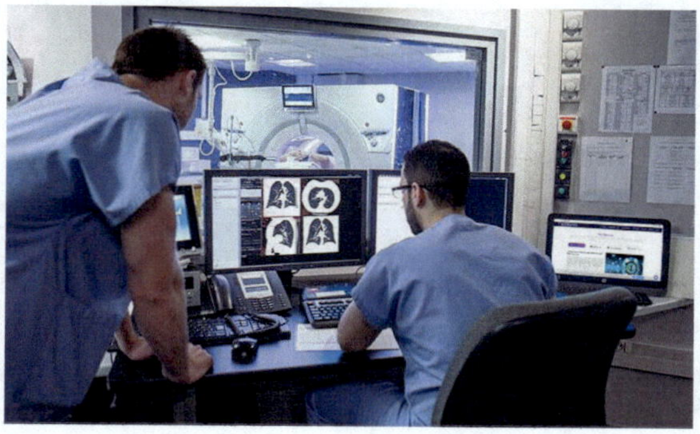

Figure 2.14. Artificial intelligence in medical diagnosis.

Source: https://miro.medium.com/v2/resize:fit:700/1*B7loj1btEtNY5qxLZEtD_Q.jpeg.

Furthermore, employment of AI systems must be balanced against the essential abilities of clinicians, who learn to reason within the framework of patient management. Subsequent studies should focus on crafting hybrid models that synthesize AI-powered insights and human wisdom to produce a collaborative process that augments clinical judgment while preserving patient-centeredness. In selected applications, the prognostic role of AI in predictive analytics is increasingly becoming well-recognized, especially in domains like cancer risk prediction. Early detection significantly increases the likelihood of successful treatment in most cancers, including breast cancer, whereby early treatment can lead to better survival. Under such a scenario, sophisticated AI systems, such as those utilizing artificial neural networks, can evaluate risk factors and predict the likelihood of disease development. For example, to fight breast cancer, algorithms may integrate different risk models for assessing susceptibility to draw a comprehensive picture of patient vulnerability with some level of confidence regarding predictions. Healthcare systems can reinforce diagnosis frameworks through such sophisticated approaches, moving toward personalized care and improved patient treatment (Abelha et al., 2005; Keles et al., 2015) (Figure 2.14).

Test Your Knowledge

1. How have electronic health records (EHRs) transformed the process of clinical assessment and patient data management?
2. What are the advantages and limitations of telemedicine for conducting remote patient assessments?
3. In what ways is artificial intelligence (AI) being integrated into diagnostic processes to improve accuracy and efficiency?

SUMMARY

The systematic practice of clinical analysis and reasoning in diagnosis is the pillar of effective healthcare delivery. This multi-faceted process requires clinicians to synthesize information from various sources, exercise critical thinking, and apply rules of diagnosis and concepts of medical science. Together. Automated tools and AI-based approaches refine such processes via hypothesis generation facilitation and evidence evaluation, with scholarship in educational psychology exploring this area (Bauer et al., 2018). With the increasing complexity of patient cases comes the need for robust diagnostic reasoning frameworks that can adapt to address new challenges in clinical practice. This ongoing evolution highlights the need for healthcare workers to remain current on traditional and new methods of providing high-quality care to their patients.

The impact of innovation in technology on clinical assessment cannot be overstated. Machine-learning-based tools and analytical techniques are being developed to support healthcare personnel not only in understanding patient data but also in making prudent decisions in high-risk environments such as ICUs. The requirements posed by dense data displays require novel responses, such as information prioritization and clustering to optimize user interaction with clinical data systems (Allart et al., 2012). By building user-focused interfaces that maximize clarity and insight, these technologies enable clinicians to counteract potential health threats in patients effectively. Therefore, technology-diagnostic reasoning intersection is a crucial innovation in medical practice that enhances decision-making and communication among clinical teams. Furthermore, the future of clinical assessment and diagnostic reasoning relies on a collaboration model that blends human intelligence with AI. Embracing such hybrid models can make the diagnosis process more efficient, reduce cognitive burden, and ultimately improve clinical performance. The evolving patient care needs the professionals to stay current with the latest technology and apply it practically. Continuous research on automated detection and analysis of diagnostic reasoning tasks will enhance the learning environment for future health professionals and the quality of patient care (Bauer et al., 2018). AsAs clinical diagnosis and reasoning evolve, integrating new technologies and techniques will become essential in achieving excellence in outcomes to ultimately redefine the standards of healthcare practice.

Critical thinking is the most valuable skill in clinical assessment and diagnostic thinking. It entails several cognitive skills like data analysis, synthesizing conclusions, and evaluating the implications of clinical decisions. Adams et al. (2006) have reported that effective healthcare decision-making, particularly for nurse prescribers, heavily relies upon these qualities. Instructors are thus encouraged to use diverse instructional strategies that enable the development of critical thinking competencies among nursing practitioners. Such an instructional focus is crucial as nurse prescribers are increasingly being tasked with having higher clinical reasoning to ascertain whether medicines prescribed in patient care are appropriate. The relevance of models to inform clinical assessment cannot be overstated. The PARiHS model, according to the literature, is a helpful tool for understanding research implementation processes within healthcare. As outlined by Grandos et al. (2008), the model attempts to bridge the gap between theoretical models and practice in actual clinical practice. It focuses on context by suggesting a two-stage approach to assessment and diagnosis—first estimating the evidence factors and context, then determining suitable facilitation approaches relevant to specific situations. This underscores the necessity of a highly sensitive awareness of the clinical environment in which practitioners are working, and the provision of a better quality of care. To continue building the practice of clinical assessment and diagnostic reasoning, ongoing discussion about conceptual frameworks and models used in the practice is essential. In line with the literature, a less explicit typology is needed to group frameworks, theories, and models to achieve further the aim of heightening clarity and operational effectiveness in research and practice. Grandos et al. (2008) offer that the future of frameworks like PARiHS lies in their further refinement and contextualization toward stakeholder engagement. This imperative puts the construction of conceptual models at the center stage in guaranteeing continuous improvement in clinical decision-making processes toward the eventual achievement of enhanced health results and effective best practices delivery across different healthcare settings.

KEY TERMS FROM THIS CHAPTER

- Bipolar disorders (BD)
- Clinical assessment process
- Clinical education
- Clinical guidelines
- Clinical interventions
- Clinical presentation
- Clinical settings
- Cancer risk prediction
- Clinical decision-making models
- Clinical expertise
- Clinical information
- Clinical prediction rules (CPRs)
- Clinical reasoning abilities
- Cognitive biases

CRITICAL THINKING QUESTIONS

1. **Which of the following best describes the primary purpose of the clinical assessment process?**
   a. To prescribe medication for all patients
   b. To gather relevant information for diagnosis and treatment planning
   c. To complete paperwork for insurance purposes
   d. To perform surgical interventions
2. **Which type of clinical assessment primarily involves direct observation of the patient's behavior in a natural setting?**
   a. Psychological testing
   b. Self-report questionnaires
   c. Behavioral assessment
   d. Laboratory tests
3. **The hypothetico-deductive model in diagnostic reasoning primarily involves:**
   a. Generating multiple hypotheses and testing them against clinical data
   b. Using clinical guidelines to confirm a diagnosis without further testing
   c. Making decisions based solely on patient self-reports
   d. Applying a fixed diagnostic algorithm to all patients
4. **What is the central role of clinical guidelines in the diagnostic process?**
   a. To replace clinical judgment entirely
   b. To provide evidence-based recommendations to standardize care
   c. To speed up patient discharge from the hospital
   d. To limit diagnostic options to one approach
5. **Which of the following is a significant challenge introduced by integrating technology in clinical assessments?**
   a. Increased accuracy in all diagnoses
   b. Complete elimination of human clinical judgment
   c. Universal accessibility without any technical issues
   d. Difficulty in maintaining patient privacy and data security

Short Answer Questions

1. What are the essential steps in the clinical assessment process, and why is each important?
2. How do psychological, physical health, and functional assessments differ, and how do they complement each other in patient evaluation?
3. Describe the hypothetico-deductive model of diagnostic reasoning and explain how it guides clinical decision-making.
4. How does Bayesian reasoning improve diagnostic accuracy compared to other reasoning models?
5. What role do clinical guidelines play in supporting evidence-based practice and standardized patient care?

Answers to Critical Thinking Questions

1. (b) 2. (c) 3. (a) 4. (b) 5. (d)

REFERENCES

1. Abelha, A., Alves, V., Machado, J. M., Neves, et al. (2005). Agent based decision support systems in medicine. https://core.ac.uk/download/55603653.pdf (accessed on 27th June 2025).
2. Banning, M. (2005). Measures that can be used to instill critical thinking skills in nurse prescribers. *Nurse Education in Practice, 6*(2), 98–105. https://doi.org/10.1016/j.nepr.2005.10.001Adebajo, A., Montgomery, A. A., Round, A. P., Wilson, A. S., Friedman, C. P., Moher, D., Cook, D. A., et al. (2012). Virtual patients design and its effect on clinical reasoning and student experience: A protocol for a randomized factorial multi-center study. https://core.ac.uk/download/9561512.pdf (accessed on 27th June 2025).
3. Al-Akhras, M. (2024). Editorial: Evaluating generative AI-based models in healthcare. *Jordan Medical Journal*. https://www.semanticscholar.org/paper/3b212070acb5b2d98ccad8e9f566d764e188ee5d (accessed on 27th June 2025).
4. Alberdi, E., Lee, R., & Taylor, P. (2004). Elicitation and representation of expert knowledge for computer aided diagnosis in mammography. https://core.ac.uk/download/9559371.pdf (accessed on 27th June 2025).
5. Allart, L., Hubert, H., Kamsu-Foguem, B., Lemdani, et al. (2012). User-centered visual analysis using a hybrid reasoning architecture for intensive care units. https://core.ac.uk/download/12043821.pdf (accessed on 27th June 2025).
6. Allen-Davis, D., Aspinall, M. J., Baron, R., Buckingham, C. D., Thompson, C., Considine, J., Cooksey, R., et al. (2003). Measuring the quality of judgement and decision-making in nursing. https://core.ac.uk/download/60160.pdf (accessed on 27th June 2025).
7. Ambrosio, M., Bocchi, G., Bramesfeld, A., Deandrea, S., Dimitrova, N., Lerda, D., Neamtiu, L., et al. (2017). Report on the call for feedback about the scope of the European guidelines for breast cancer screening and diagnosis: European Commission Initiative on Breast Cancer. https://core.ac.uk/download/84886790.pdf (accessed on 27th June 2025).
8. Anderson, A. S. D., Appelbaum, P. S., Bartlett, P., Berg, J. W., Freyenhagen, F., Folstein, M. F., et al. (2013). Decision-making capacity for treatment in psychiatric and medical in-patients: Cross-sectional, comparative study. https://core.ac.uk/download/17197976.pdf (accessed on 27th June 2025).
9. Armstrong, R., Hall, W., Maier, P., Ng, L., et al. (2005). JointZone: Users' view of an adaptive online learning resource for rheumatology.
10. Aspiuynall, M. J., Benner, P., Carnevali, D., Carnevali, D., Gerrity, P., Gordon, M., Harbison, J., et al. (2007). A review of clinical decision-making: Models and current research. https://core.ac.uk/download/334115.pdf (accessed on 27th June 2025).
11. Austin, T., Darlison, M. W., Ingram, D., Kalra, D., et al. (2006). Towards an interoperable healthcare information infrastructure – Working from the bottom up. https://core.ac.uk/download/1670855.pdf (accessed on 27th June 2025).
12. Bauer, E., Fischer, F., Fischer, M. R., Gurevych, I., et al. (2018). Challenges in the automatic analysis of students' diagnostic reasoning. http://arxiv.org/abs/1811.10550 (accessed on 27th June 2025).
13. Birrenbach, T., Exadaktylos, A. K., Hautz, S. C., Hautz, W. E., et al. (2019). Diagnostic error increases mortality and length of hospital stay in patients presenting through the emergency

room. https://core.ac.uk/download/219690184.pdf (accessed on 27th June 2025).

14. Craven, M. P., Crowe, J. A., Lu, B., Morgan, H. J., et al. (2009). Deploying a spreadsheet tool for early economic value assessment of medical device innovations with healthcare decision makers. https://core.ac.uk/download/9703990.pdf (accessed on 27th June 2025).
15. Croskerry, P., Cullen, L., Egerton-Warburton, D., Fatovich, D. M., et al. (2018). Deliberate clinical inertia: Using meta-cognition to improve decision-making. https://core.ac.uk/download/196606885.pdf (accessed on 27th June 2025).
16. Curtis, J., McKenzie, K., Michie, A., Murray, C., et al. (2012). Screening with young offenders with an intellectual disability. https://core.ac.uk/download/41069887.pdf (accessed on 27th June 2025).
17. Datoc, A. (2022). A comparison of tele neuropsychological and traditional neuropsychological battery factor structures. https://core.ac.uk/download/534378712.pdf (accessed on 27th June 2025).
18. Delogu, G., Di Fazio, N., Fineschi, V., Frati, P., et al. (2024). Capacity to consent in healthcare: A systematic review and meta-analysis comparing patients with bipolar disorders and schizophrenia spectrum disorders. https://core.ac.uk/download/621402116.pdf (accessed on 27th June 2025).
19. Dimitriou, D., Hood, A. M., Kirkham, F. J., Stotesbury, H., et al. (2023). Tele-neuropsychological assessment of children and young people: A systematic review. https://core.ac.uk/download/567877137.pdf (accessed on 27th June 2025).
20. Escota, G., Melia, M. T., et al. (2020). The struggling infectious diseases fellow: Remediation challenges and opportunities. https://core.ac.uk/download/322802240.pdf (accessed on 27th June 2025).
21. Ferracuti, S., Miolla, A., Sartori, G., Scarpazza, C., et al. (2018). The charm of structural neuroimaging in insanity evaluations: Guidelines to avoid misinterpretation of the findings. https://core.ac.uk/download/188827245.pdf (accessed on 27th June 2025).
22. Grandos, A., Kitson, A., Loftus-Hills, A., Oxman, A., Titchen, A., Titchen, A., Van de Ven, A. H., et al. (2008). Evaluating the successful implementation of evidence into practice using the PARiHS framework: Theoretical and practical challenges. https://core.ac.uk/download/48947.pdf (accessed on 27th June 2025).
23. Gur, A. G., Gur, A. E., Gur, O. M., Gur, R. E., et al. (2016). A perspective on the potential role of neuroscience in the court. https://core.ac.uk/download/144231732.pdf (accessed on 27th June 2025).
24. Hanekom, S., Patman, S., Plani, N., van Aswegen, H., et al. (2017). Developing minimum clinical standards for physiotherapy in South African ICUs: A qualitative study. https://core.ac.uk/download/213606949.pdf (accessed on 27th June 2025).
25. Heckerman, D. (2015). An empirical comparison of three inference methods. http://arxiv.org/abs/1304.2357 (accessed on 27th June 2025).
26. Irfan, B., Ankouni, G., Reader, J. M., Seraji-Bozorgzad, N., Giordani, B., Bakulski, K., Bhaumik, A., et al. (2024). Faithful approaches: Considering Islamic tenets in ADRD care for Muslim women. *Alzheimer's & Dementia, 20*. https://www.semanticscholar.org/paper/c94326f0fce9ed7be7820c7a93cfb07ba14b99b7 (accessed on 27th June 2025).

27. Journois, D., & Squara, P. (2009). Intelligence-based medicine. https://core.ac.uk/download/pdf/288471.pdf (accessed on 27th June 2025).
28. Keles, A., Kalteh, A. A., Caldeira, A. T., Rodrigues, B., Salvador, C., Jacobi, C. E., Carneiro, D., et al. (2015). Logic programming and artificial neural networks in breast cancer detection. https://core.ac.uk/download/55639222.pdf (accessed on 27th June 2025).
29. Kelly, D., Knox, G., Rivett, D., Snodgrass, S. J., et al. (2016). Physiotherapy students' perceptions and experiences of clinical prediction rules. https://core.ac.uk/download/84111168.pdf (accessed on 27th June 2025).
30. Loving, G., McPherson, M. A., & Shortridge, A. (2010). Using web-based reflection with video to enhance high fidelity undergraduate nursing clinical skills education.
31. Skellern, C. (2015). Minimizing bias in the forensic evaluation of suspicious paediatric injury. https://core.ac.uk/download/43374514.pdf (accessed on 27th June 2025).
32. Thompson, C. (1999). A conceptual treadmill: The need for 'middle ground' in clinical decision-making theory in nursing. https://core.ac.uk/download/60172.pdf (accessed on 27th June 2025).
33. Wagner, A. E. (2014). Neurocognitive profiles in autism spectrum disorder. https://core.ac.uk/download/211347908.pdf (accessed on 27th June 2025).
34. Williams, I. L. (2017). At the pillar of the proverbial golden calf: Sacrificing the need for 'responsible knowing' on the altar of a compliance-based ethic. https://core.ac.uk/download/127631208.pdf (accessed on 27th June 2025).

COMMON INVESTIGATIONS IN MEDICINE

3

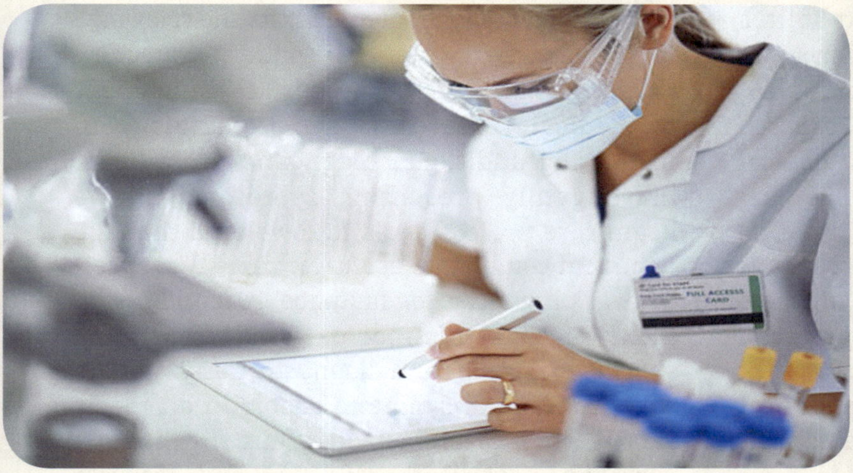

LEARNING OBJECTIVES

After studying this chapter, you will be able to:

1. Understand blood tests
2. Describe imaging techniques
3. Explain the fundamentals of biopsies
4. Discuss endoscopic procedures
5. Define genetic testing and urinalysis

Introduction

The health profession is characterized by an endless pursuit to understand and diagnose various afflictions affecting human health. Lying at the center is routine questioning doctors employ to assess, diagnose, and manage numerous medical conditions. These questions are central to medical practice, which provides clinicians with data to support informed treatment decisions. General medical tests consist of laboratory, imaging, and clinical tests, each providing unique information to create an inclusive patient review. While new technologies have changed the diagnostic process, traditional methods remain highly effective in primary healthcare services, pointing towards the blending of established procedures with latest technologies in medical tests. Inborn errors of metabolism (IEMs) provide a clear example of the complexity of diagnostic tests in the medical sciences. These genetic conditions result from mutations in genes that disrupt metabolic pathways, leading to various clinical presentations that make timely diagnosis puzzling. The pathophysiology of IEMs highlights the significant role of screening and evaluation in identifying early metabolic dysfunctions, particularly in neonates. Early and accurate diagnosis, as described in recent literature, is crucial to managing IEMs because it plays a decisive role in influencing long-term health outcomes. Traditional screening protocols rely on targeted assays that may sometimes overlook the full extent of possible metabolic disorders. Thus, research into untargeted metabolomics is an intriguing opportunity for the widening and specificity of IEM diagnostics, whereby the possibilities of numerous metabolites that suggest varying metabolic pathways can be examined simultaneously (Fiehn et al., 2019). The evolution of qualitative research methods continues to push the art of medical investigations, particularly those involving intricate patient experience and results. Narrative and qualitative systematic reviews have gained popularity for integrating intricate literature about investigations into perfectly interwoven findings. The method can offer insightful information regarding the implications of various diagnostic procedures, including their efficacy and challenges encountered in their application within the clinical environment. The use of narrative approaches, highlighted by recent studies, can also offer more insight into medical research's social and cultural contexts. By emphasizing qualitative methods alongside quantitative data more, healthcare practitioners can better value patients' experiences and the effectiveness of investigative interventions, paving the way towards improved clinical practice and policy (Jones et al., 2004).

Definition of Medical Investigations

The term medical investigations refers to the broad category of diagnostic tests employed to evaluate patient health. Medical investigations are designed to identify the presence, absence, or extent of medical conditions and inform clinical decisions. Key modalities include laboratory testing, imaging testing, and clinical examination, each adding valuable information to the diagnostic process. Accuracy and reliability in this research are critical, as they dictate treatment strategies and affect outcomes. Regardless, variation in coding behaviors could complicate understanding EHRs, impairing the development of cut-and-dry clinical guidelines. The addition of inflammatory markers, signs, and other markers can be used to support disorder case definitions, as in rheumatoid arthritis (RA), in which appropriate coding is delayed relative to symptom presentation, as evidenced by recent studies that demonstrate the relevance of such marker systems to patient trajectory (Hansell et al., 2013). Another key component of medical research is symptomatology in instigating additional diagnostic procedures. Investigating presenting symptoms allows healthcare professionals to develop a timeline of patient complaints useful for rapid diagnoses. In ovarian cancer, for instance, research using EHRs revealed distinct patterns associating specific symptoms and diagnostic delay. Median time from initial symptom report to diagnosis can be very heterogeneous, thus highlighting variation in early identification and accurate recording of symptoms. Delays not only increase patient morbidity but also may add complexity to the treatment and prognosis options. Secondly, using various definitions of diagnosis can expose the potential discrepancies in EHR data and support the argument that standardized symptom documentation methods are a precursor to meaningful analysis. This research supports the need for extensive investigations to enhance patient care at an individual level and data integrity at a general practice level (Majeed et al., 2009). Finally, medical investigations extend beyond testing; they are a scientific process to analyze patient data to improve health outcomes. Good medical investigations synthesize a mix of sources of information, including clinical assessment, laboratory test results, and imaging tests, into a unified plan of action for patient care. With greater EHR usage, optimizing how to define and interpret medical investigations is increasingly essential. Advances such as the development of indicator markers, which can capture nuances of patient trajectories of health before formal diagnoses, are characteristic of the evolving context of medical research. Not only does an interest in comprehensive data collection and analysis enable timely and accurate diagnoses, but it also enhances the quality of medicine. These investigations, therefore, form the pillar of contemporary medicine, guiding evidence-based interventions and continuous improvement in the patient care process (Figure 3.1).

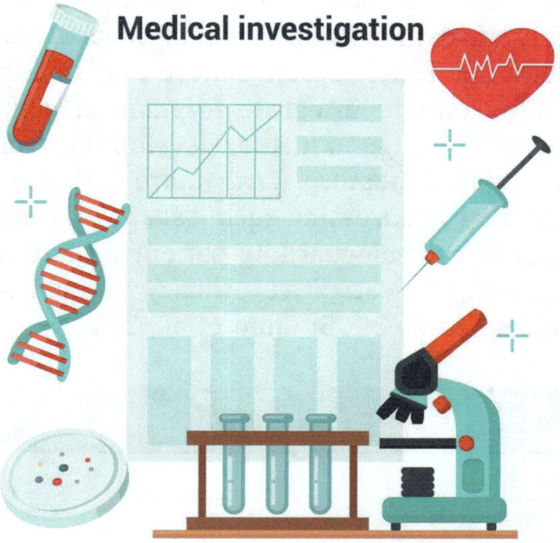

Figure 3.1. Illustration of medical investigation.

Source: https://static.vecteezy.com/system/resources/previews/043/188/754/non_2x/medical-investigation-a-form-with-the-results-of-laboratory-tests-laboratory-equipment-dna-test-tube-petri-dish-microscope-vector.jpg.

Importance of Investigations in Diagnosis and Treatment

Investigations are pivotal in the proper diagnosis and effective management of medical diseases. They provide crucial information that can influence clinical decisions, thus ensuring that patients receive the most appropriate care for them. For instance, in the case of interstitial lung disease (ILD), various diagnostic procedures such as pulmonary function tests (PFTs) and computed tomography (CT) scans are performed to assess lung function and identify fibrotic changes underlying the disease. Not only do these tests assist in classifying the disease, but they also facilitate the selection of optimal management strategies, thereby establishing the importance of meticulous investigative measures in substantially improving patient outcomes (Fenech et al., 2012). By making a definite diagnosis through proper measurements and images, physicians can avoid trial-and-error therapy, and ultimately more effective and prompt interventions. In addition, the roles of investigations extend beyond the aim of diagnosis; investigations are necessary in monitoring disease progression and evaluating treatments' impact. As an example, in dermatology, skin biopsies are frequently performed to establish the nature of skin lesions and direct subsequent management plans. Recent research showed that a vast majority of new referrals to dermatology had their condition probed appropriately, enabling early diagnosis and personalized treatment regimens (Amato-Gauci et al., 2005). This correlation between robust probing procedures and better treatment regimens is a significant aspect of patient care, wherein ongoing follow-up probes will reveal the effectiveness of the treatments administered so that changes can be instituted accordingly and without wasting time. The integration of investigations into the practice of current patient care ensures that healthcare providers can respond in an adaptable manner to changing clinical situations. Finally, integrating investigative protocols into practice ensures standardized care across multiple medical specialties. Standardization helps not only improve the precision of diagnostic procedures but also ensure communication among healthcare providers. For instance, in the case of referral notes containing a diagnosis, like in the case of a dermatology study, referring physician-specialist correlation could significantly impact patient management. The study revealed that 65% of the referrals contained a diagnosis, with high correspondence comparable to dermatologist assessments (Amato-Gauci et al., 2005). Such correspondence enhances the significance of adequate communication enabled by standardized investigational practices in ensuring patients benefit from integrated care pathways. Therefore, the functions of investigations in diagnosis and treatment cannot be exaggerated; they form the cornerstone upon which successful and concerted healthcare provision is founded.

Overview of Common Types of Investigations

Within the field of medicine, various types of investigations play a crucial role in evaluating patients and guiding therapeutic strategies. Diagnostic investigations like imaging studies, laboratory tests, and biopsies are necessary for a definitive diagnosis. Imaging techniques like X-rays, MRIs, and CT scans provide helpful information regarding structural defects, while laboratory tests examine body fluids for biochemical defects. Apart from this, biopsies enable histological examination, which is essential in diagnosing cancer and other pathological conditions. All these modalities contribute to clinical findings and enable further diagnosis refinement, ultimately directing the patient's management plan. The second broad category of investigations includes epidemiological studies, which direct public health policies and preventive measures. These investigations attempt to identify patterns, causes, and effects of disease and health conditions within specified populations. For example, correlational research can establish risk factors and disease associations and yield preventive measures. Cohort as well as case-control studies are also capable of providing information regarding the progression of the disease and the efficacy of therapy and, in turn, contributing to advances in medical science. Synthesis of findings from such studies is crucial for policy making in healthcare and improving patient outcomes across diverse healthcare environments and therefore necessitates community-based studies. Lastly, technological advancement is redefining the landscape of medical investigations by integrating medical cyber-physical systems (MCPS). MCPS integrates technology and healthcare delivery to support advanced data collection and processing. However, the complexity of MCPS poses extra concerns regarding data integrity and security within the investigation. Compromises have immense implications for impacting patient safety and data availability, making investigations reliant upon these systems more challenging. It is important to integrate forensic principles into MCPS design to further develop the overall investigative posture. With more reliance on technology, addressing such issues will remain important in safeguarding patient welfare and improving investigative efficacy in medicine (Bourne et al., 2005; Choo et al., 2017).

3.1. Blood Tests

Learning Outcome

1. Discuss complete blood count (CBC)
2. Understand blood chemistry panels
3. Describe coagulation tests

Blood tests are a priceless diagnostic tool in modern medicine, allowing physicians to assess various physiological and disease states. By examining blood samples, clinicians can evaluate organ function, detect infections, follow chronic illness, and even diagnose metabolic disorders. The information from these tests can not only be utilized to diagnose diseases but also to guide therapy and follow up on patients' responses to therapies. For example, a CBC can show anemia, leukocytosis, or thrombocytopenia, and each would indicate underlying disease processes that must be investigated further. These general blood analyses underscore growing reliance on laboratory testing in developing individualized and effective patient management strategies. Blood testing is also essential in the early diagnosis of most diseases, which would strongly influence patient outcomes. Early diagnosis is especially crucial in conditions such as diabetes, where routine blood sugar tests can provide information regarding a person's metabolic status. The need for early interventions cannot be overstressed since earlier treatment reduces the threat of long-term complications. Yet, while diagnostic testing of metabolic disorders by means of blood checks can show imbalance, diagnosis of certain disorders can remain undetected even with alarming laboratory results. This emphasizes the importance of using a multi-dimensional patient assessment approach.

Results of laboratories have to be always viewed in the overall clinical situation, taking physical exam and patient history as an integral component of quality care. Besides, innovation in blood test techniques has introduced new methods that enhance the accuracy of diagnosis. Traditional approaches have utilized progressively more advanced technologies such as mass spectrometry and genomic screening to provide increased understanding of metabolic pathways and disease susceptibility. Interestingly, IEMs will most likely be overlooked during initial analyses, highlighting the necessity for rigorous screening protocols.

In a certain way, untargeted metabolomics can identify a wider set of abnormalities than routine testing protocols, as it is not solely dependent on pre-established lists of analytes. Following implementing these new technologies, the medical community has seen the potential of more accurate and enhanced diagnostic capabilities, which leads to enhanced targeted treatments and better patient outcomes, especially for complex diseases where conventional methods are insufficient (Fiehn et al., 2019). Thus, as blood tests continue to advance, they will assume an increasingly pivotal role in the clinical research and management setup.

3.1.1. Complete Blood Count (CBC)

Complete blood count (CBC) is a simple but time-tested and potent tool in the medical profession. It yields important information about a patient's general hematologic status. This collective test examines several parameters: red blood cells, white blood cells, hemoglobin, and platelets. Interpreting each value and its relationship gives the GP an overall picture of multiple ailments. Each part of the CBC plays a distinct role.

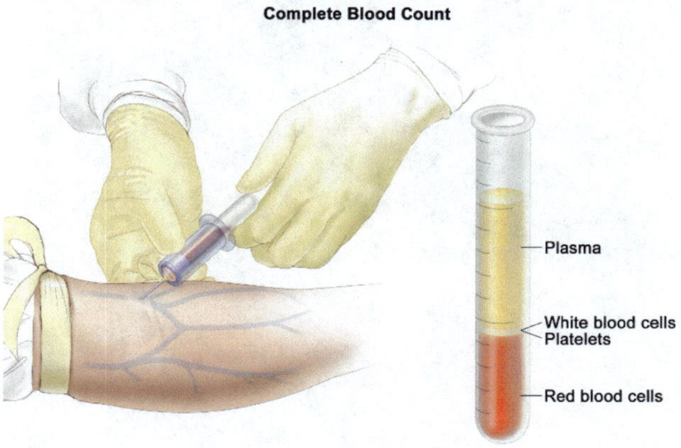

Figure 3.2. Complete blood count (CBC).

Source: https://nci-media.cancer.gov/pdq/media/images/526546.jpg.

Red cell counts will indicate either anemia or polycythemia, white counts may indicate infection or neoplastic disease, and the differential counts can point towards the source of infection, whether viral, bacterial, or parasitic. Given the common occurrence of blood disorders, the CBC is widely applied in routine and diagnostic assessment of frequent presentations, e.g., fatigue to acute febrile illnesses, reflecting its role as a bread-and-butter investigation in coming to a diagnosis and guiding therapy. In clinical practice, the CBC is vital because it is inexpensive and time-saving. Results from this test can lead to follow-up laboratory tests and direct clinical management plans. For example, a low hemoglobin level detected by a CBC may lead a clinician to evaluate possible causes of anemia, such as iron deficiency or chronic disease. Similarly, white blood cell count abnormalities may require additional testing to rule out infection or blood disease (Figure 3.2).The use of CBC is also established in acute care settings, where timely decision-making is critical.

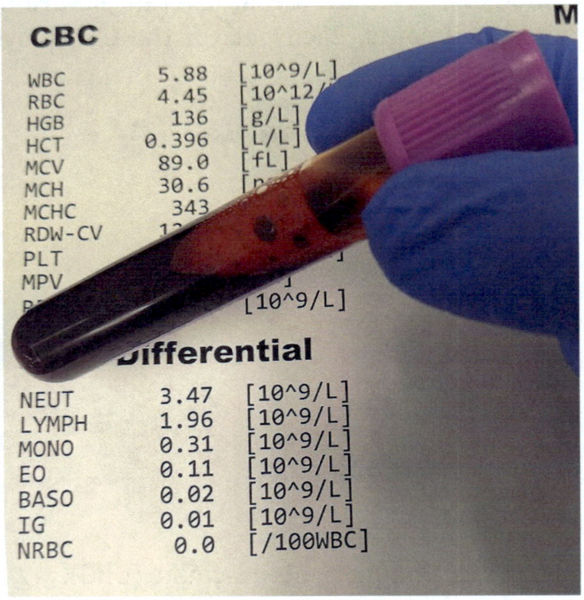

Figure 3.3. A CBC specimen in front of a printout displaying CBC and differential results.

Source: https://upload.wikimedia.org/wikipedia/commons/thumb/c/cf/Complete_blood_count_and_differential.jpg/800px-Complete_blood_count_and_differential.jpg.

It is often incorporated into the initial examination of acute-symptomatic patients, as demonstrated in guidelines advocating for incorporation alongside other tests, such as blood gas analysis and chest radiography in emergency cases (Biagioli et al., 2007). Besides, the instrumentation and technique of the CBC have also been enhanced, and thus, the findings are more precise and trustworthy. Automated hematology analyzers are now available, which can provide a definite breakdown of blood cell types and streamline the diagnosis process. Further, better laboratory procedures allow for the detection of less subtle hematological abnormalities that would have otherwise been missed in manual counts. These technologies are essential, especially when it comes to diagnosing such a complicated illness as leukemias or thrombocytopenia, where small changes have grave implications on a clinical level. The CBC is thus not a solitary test; it is an avenue to further understand a patient's health status and how it can enable timely and helpful medical interventions (N/A, 2010) (Figure 3.3).

3.1.2. Blood Chemistry Panels

Blood chemistry panels are a valuable tool of contemporary medicine, enabling health practitioners to gain clear information regarding a patient's metabolic status and organ function. Organized panels consist of tests on the concentration level of different substances in the blood, such as electrolytes, enzymes, hormones, and metabolites. The outcomes can help clinicians identify disorders, monitor the course of disease, and determine the effectiveness of treatment. Particularly, panels reveal abnormalities that exist in kidney and liver function, details crucial to the control of diseases like diabetes, liver disease, or chronic kidney disease (CKD). By providing a snapshot of the biochemical environment in the body, blood chemistry panels are an essential component of preventive medicine and early detection of potential health issues. The interpretation of blood chemistry panel results should be rooted in a sophisticated knowledge of the interrelationship between various biochemical markers. For example, elevations in liver enzymes such as alanine aminotransferase (ALT) and aspartate aminotransferase (AST) may be indicative of hepatic inflammation or injury. Still, they can also be secondary to disease elsewhere in the body, so further evaluation is warranted. Similarly, abnormal glucose can suggest metabolic disease, but must be interpreted within the context of a patient's history and concomitant clinical presentations. Integrating such discoveries into the broader clinical context is crucial for making well-informed medical decisions. Advanced imaging technology, such as coherent Raman imaging (CRI), could enhance diagnostic accuracy and blood chemistry and convert subjective ratings into more quantifiable measures, bridging gaps in histopathological diagnoses (Camp et al., 2017).

Table 3.1. The Blood Chemistry Panel

Total Cholesterol	Alkaline Phosphatase	Sodium
HDL cholesterol	ALT	Potassium
Non-HDL cholesterol	AST	Calcium
Chol/HDL ratio	Albumin	Fasting Blood Sugar
LDL cholesterol	Bilirubin, total	Glycosylated hemoglobin
Triglycerides	BUN/ creatinine ratio	Bilirubin (Total and direct)

Source: https://www.researchgate.net/publication/294257344/figure/tbl2/AS:670328019759124@1536830062870/The-blood-chemistry-panel.png

Aside from this, as medical science advances, blood chemistry panels that consider advancements in technology and disease process understanding are becoming updated. Emerging studies have explored the use of metabolic profiling in identifying not only diseases but also the susceptibility of individuals to specific diseases. By referencing blood chemistry results to genetic and environmental factors, doctors can offer more personalized forms of treatment and prevention. The identification of distinctive metabolites linked to disorders such as autism spectrum disorder makes accuracy in diagnosis imperative, suggesting a significant paradigm shift in medical professionals' understanding of blood chemistry (Alger et al., 2012). Therefore, the ongoing evolution of blood chemistry panels affirms their central role in standard medical practice and the drive towards personalized health interventions (Table 3.1).

3.1.3. Coagulation Tests

Coagulation assays are invaluable diagnostic tests in the clinical assessment of hemostasis, allowing doctors to evaluate the patient's capacity to coagulate blood. Tests are particularly valuable in bleeding disorders because they can diagnose platelet function, clotting factor deficiency, or both. Prothrombin time (PT) and activated partial thromboplastin time (aPTT) are the assays most used for measuring separate pathways of the coagulation cascade. The results of these tests contribute to clinical judgments surrounding further diagnostic workup and guide therapeutic intervention, such as anticoagulation treatment or the administration of clotting factor concentrates. In essence, coagulation testing is a component of preoperative risk assessment and the management of most hematologic diseases and considerably impacts patient outcomes and clinical management practice. Coagulation test interpretation requires a general understanding of underlying physiology and potential pathologies. Abnormalities of PT or aPTT can be due to a vast spectrum of disorders, ranging from vitamin K deficiency to the effect of anticoagulant drugs, such as warfarin or heparin. Diseases such as liver disease, disseminated intravascular coagulation (DIC), and genetic clotting disorders, such as hemophilia, can significantly influence coagulation profiles. Therefore, it is crucial that clinicians in the interpretation of such tests consider the whole clinical setting. This comprehensive approach not only maximizes diagnostic accuracy but also helps deliver appropriate therapeutic modalities that may minimize the risk of serious complications, such as uncontrolled bleeding or thromboembolic events, enhancing patient safety and effectiveness of care. Furthermore, advances in laboratory techniques have improved the accuracy and speed of coagulation testing, but standardization and interpretation are still difficult. Advances in point-of-care testing instruments allowed for real-time assessment of coagulation, especially in critical care units, where quick decision-making is needed. However, these technologies may not be applicable to broad use due to variations in local practices and the capabilities of equipment. Second, contextual interpretation of findings is paramount since coagulation tests can be influenced by medication use, acute conditions, and patient comorbidities. Therefore, while coagulation tests are a valuable asset in the clinician's arsenal, these have to be interpreted against a personalized context, taking into consideration the peculiar conditions in which the health status of each patient presents to the clinician and the potential for concomitant ailments that could confound findings (Figure 3.4).

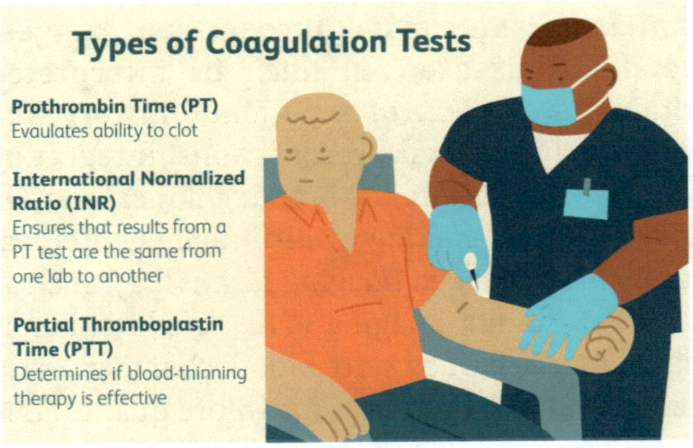

Figure 3.4. Types of coagulation tests.

Source: https://www.verywellhealth.com/thmb/AQMRhHC490BeGXtDvvZ06gZtIrE=/1500x0/filters:no_upscale():max_bytes(150000):strip_icc()/what-do-your-pt-ptt-and-inr-results-mean-3157005_V2-012-a23ffe57b301411fa13d2d3a3e32c630.png.

Test Your Knowledge

1. What components are measured in a Complete Blood Count (CBC)?
2. How do blood chemistry panels assess organ function, and which key markers are typically included in these tests?
3. What is the clinical significance of coagulation tests, and in what scenarios are they most commonly used?

3.2. Imaging Techniques

Learning Outcome

1. Understand the application of X-rays in medicine
2. Explain the concept of magnetic resonance imaging (MRI)
3. Discuss computed tomography (CT) scans

Imaging technology occupies a central position in modern medicine, playing a key role in diagnosis and treatment planning across all branches of medicine. Adopting advanced imaging modalities has transformed clinical medicine to enable medical professionals to obtain detailed anatomical and functional data about the human body. X-ray radiography is one of the most widely utilized imaging technologies, mainly because it excels in imaging bone structures and in fracture diagnosis. However, newer imaging modalities such as optical coherence tomography (OCT) are becoming increasingly popular due to their higher specificity and resolution for evaluating soft tissues, particularly in dentistry. Studies indicate that OCT is a preferable alternative to standard X-ray processes for assessing dental condition and the success of treatments. However, its low penetrability can restrict its application in some instances, for example, in bone imaging where deeper penetrations are needed (Bradu et al., 2020). In abdominal imaging, ultrasonography and CT are crucial for determining organ structure and function. Ultrasonography is also valued due to its non-invasive nature and real-time image, with immediate feedback during clinical assessment. CT scans are much more detailed cross-sectional images and are best suited for the diagnosis of tumors and internal trauma. Advanced technology utilizes complementary tests like nuclear medicine to assess organ function and systemic disease. These procedures, which include radionuclides and gamma cameras, allow medical professionals to detect dynamic functional information, raising their diagnostic efficiency far higher than in traditional imaging (Sadeleer et al., 2011). This integration of multiple imaging modalities reflects the requirement for an integrative method of medical research. Lastly, this collaboration between different imaging modalities is a step forward in medical diagnosis, which increases the early and correct detection of diseases. With the ever-growing role of technology in medicine, clinicians are equipped with an increasingly vast toolkit for studying structural and functional aspects of disease states. Such imaging modalities are also successful as they apply to new areas such as personalized medicine, where personalized imaging results guide tailored treatment protocols based on the patient. Despite benefits, new imaging modalities bring issues, including cost-effectiveness and patient access. Continued R&D is required to enhance these technologies to where they can provide on their potential for providing quality care in a variety of clinical scenarios.

3.2.1. X-Rays

The medical application of X-rays has revolutionized diagnostic imaging to make it possible for medical professionals to visualize the internal body structures effectively. Unlike other imaging modes, X-rays employ ionizing radiation to produce contrast images that are critical in diagnosing a wide range of conditions, from fractures to infections. The procedure functions through the passage of rays via the body, which are either absorbed or passed through by different tissues and generate a distinct image on the film or digital detector. This potential not only facilitates the detection of acute illnesses but also aids in monitoring the progress of the disease and the efficacy of treatment. However, even given the utility of X-ray technology in medicine, the associated risks of ionizing radiation exposure require its deployment to be used cautiously, particularly in repeated imaging in specific populations, such as children and those requiring continuous monitoring. Despite their essential role in medicine as a diagnostic tool, X-rays have generated concerns regarding potential injury, primarily that of cancer risk from ionizing radiation. Experiments assessing low-dose radiation exposures generally exhibit a sophisticated correlation between radiation doses and cancer risk. It has been found that most better-quality studies do not observe any appreciable causal link between oncogenesis and low-dose radiation, including medical X-ray doses (Doss et al., 2020).

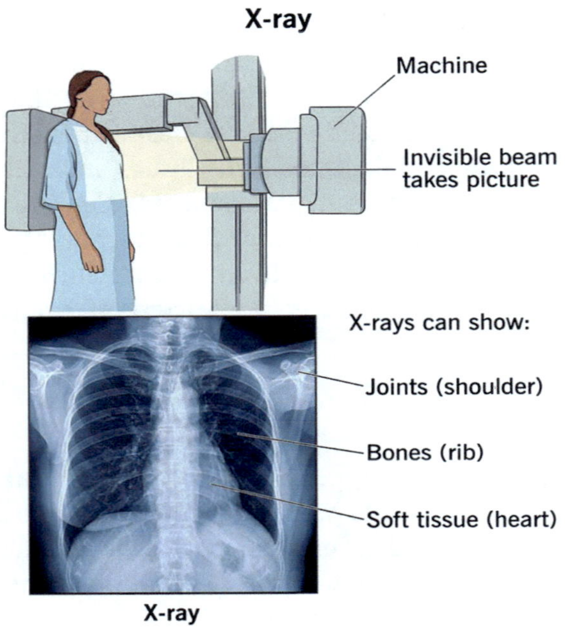

Figure 3.5. X-ray.

Source: https://my.clevelandclinic.org/-/scassets/images/org/health/articles/21818-x-ray.

This reservoir of evidence highlights the necessity for ongoing risk assessment and stringent guidelines to restrict exposure while still allowing for requisite diagnostic imaging. Awareness of these possible risks can promote healthcare providers' and patients' informed decision-making regarding proper use of X-rays in clinical practice. Apart from that, technological advances have also led to improved imaging techniques to enhance the diagnostic quality of X-rays with reduced exposure to radiation. Advances such as digital radiography and dose management systems have made it possible to achieve higher resolution images at lower doses of radiation. Further, using cognitive engineering principles in designing imaging systems can help improve the interpretation of the data generated through X-rays by doctors. For instance, monitoring systems that focus on significant physiological trends and improve decision-making efficiency can reduce misinterpretations, thus increasing patient safety (Alberdi et al., 2001). Through these developments, prioritization and their integration into clinical practice, the medical community can enhance X-rays' diagnostic capabilities while adequately controlling associated risks (Figure 3.5).

3.2.2. Magnetic Resonance Imaging (MRI)

Magnetic resonance imaging (MRI) has been an essential modality in contemporary medicine and widely utilized because of its ability to image soft tissues with unparalleled resolution. Unlike previous technologies, MRI employs strong magnetic fields and radio waves to produce detailed images of organs and structures in the body, rendering it very effective in imaging the brain, spinal cord, joints, and internal organs. The advantages of MRI extend beyond mere visualization; it offers a non-invasive method that does not employ ionizing radiation, thus being more patient-friendly for patients requiring multiple imaging tests. This is of greater significance in pediatrics and patients requiring extensive tracking of chronic conditions, where radiation exposure has significant long-term effects. In addition to its use in diagnosis, MRI also plays a growing role in guiding treatment interventions in medicine. Today's advances include the integration of fusion imaging, where ultrasonography is combined with MRI to optimize diagnostic accuracy, particularly in hepatology and urology. Using such hybrid methods, physicians can obtain comprehensive information about complex conditions, improving the accuracy of interventions such as biopsies or precise treatments. While MRI has been promising in other areas, more studies are needed to realize its capabilities to the full extent. For instance, clinical research evaluating the impact of novel MRI technology, including fat and water imaging, shows that these new technologies have the potential to radically change pain mechanism understanding and improve clinical outcomes, particularly in musculoskeletal conditions and spinal injury (Crawford et al., 2018).

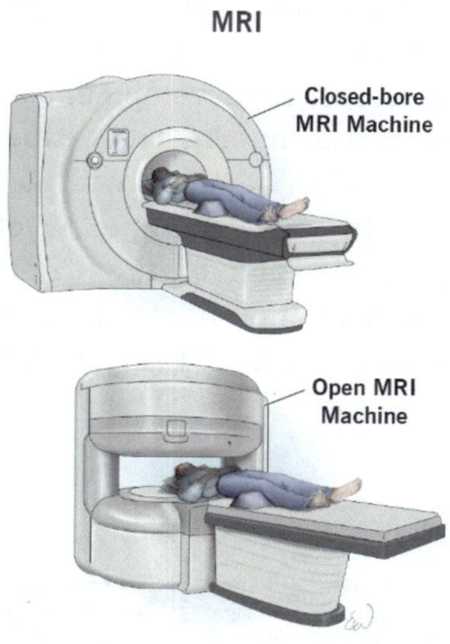

Figure 3.6. Magnetic resonance imaging (MRI) illustration.

Source: https://my.clevelandclinic.org/-/scassets/images/org/health/articles/4876-mri.

MRI flexibility is also exemplified by its application in emerging fields such as obstetrics and gynecology. Enhanced imaging capability could potentially enable early detection of conditions as benign pathologies to cervical cancer. Notably, the potential application of fusion imaging in such domains has been contemplated, with implications for its entire assessment in handling utility in prenatal diagnosis and gynecologic conditions that need to be evaluated systematically in the future. As medical imaging technology continues to advance, medical professionals must update themselves with the latest developments. With the uptake of advanced techniques, such as fusion imaging, the medical community can significantly advance diagnostic capability, thereby enhancing treatment outcomes and patient care (Bellati et al., 2018) (Figure 3.6).

3.2.3. Computed Tomography (CT) Scans

Computed tomography (CT) scans have transformed medical imaging through precise cross-sectional images of body internals. The non-surgical technique utilizes X-ray technology that allows clinicians to visualize complicated anatomical areas in a manner not accessible with standard X-rays. The ability to produce high-resolution images rendered CT scans an essential tool in the diagnosis of illnesses like tumors and internal injuries, as well as infectious diseases.

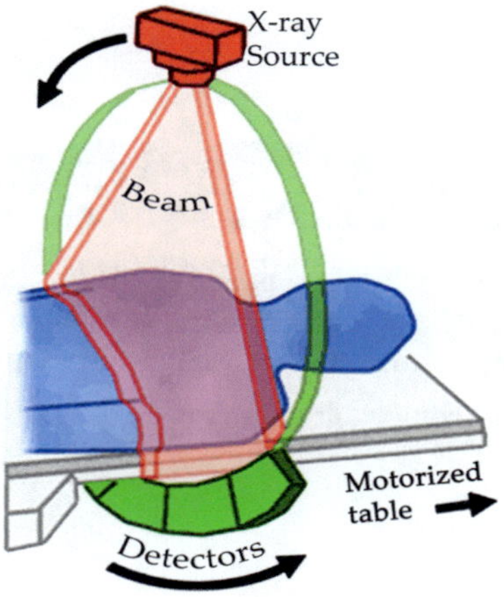

Figure 3.7. Drawing of the CT fan beam and the patient in a CT imaging system.

Source: https://upload.wikimedia.org/wikipedia/commons/d/d2/Drawing_of_CT_fan_beam_%28left%29_and_patient_in_a_CT_imaging_system.gif.

With advanced algorithms, modern CT scanners create intricate three-dimensional reconstructions of scanned areas, enhancing a physician's capacity to examine information and formulate treatment plans. As such, the integration of CT imaging in daily clinical practice has significantly improved diagnostic accuracy and efficiency in numerous clinical scenarios, demonstrating its critical role in modern medicine. Although they are valuable, the use of CT scans also raises issues regarding the safety of patients in terms of radiation exposure. Although the ionizing radiation of CT scans is necessary to produce diagnostic images, it may result in an increased cancer risk in vulnerable populations, including children and pregnant women. Consequently, physicians must weigh the need for a CT scan against damage, a maxim often governed by the ALARA (as low as reasonably achievable) concept. In addition, advances in other imaging modalities, e.g., MRI and ultrasound, offer alternative methods for specific disease processes, potentially limiting over-reliance upon CT scans. Later on, the medical field is always stressing the judicious utilization of CT scans in a manner that benefits would surpass risk factors, thereby ensuring patient safety. CT scans also play a key role in guiding interventional procedures, facilitating diagnosis as well as treatment by physicians. For instance, in the case of biopsies, real-time imaging using CT scans allows accurate positioning of needles into presumptive lesions, increasing the likelihood of obtaining successful samples. Moreover, their ability to visualize blood vessels with angiographic techniques will enable them to better plan surgery, such as vascular interventions or tumor resections. The information provided by CT imaging greatly supports multidisciplinary treatments for complex diseases. As development is ongoing in research and technology, it is expected that enhancement of CT imaging will go to refine diagnosis ability and therapeutic outcomes, ensuring the position of the CT scan as a standard medical investigation (Esler et al., 2007; Ahmed et al., 2017) (Figure 3.7).

Test Your Knowledge

1. What types of medical conditions are best diagnosed using X-rays?
2. How does Magnetic Resonance Imaging (MRI) differ from Computed Tomography (CT) in terms of imaging technology and clinical application?
3. In what clinical situations is a CT scan preferred over an MRI or X-ray, and why?

3.3. Biopsies

Learning Outcome

1. Explain the types of biopsies
2. Understand the role of biopsies in cancer diagnosis
3. Discuss the risks and benefits of biopsy procedures

Biopsies are a part of the diagnostic evaluation of most medical disorders, and an opportunity to recover tissue samples for histologic examination. The primary target is establishing the extent or the presence of cancers, infections, or autoimmune disorders. With techniques like needle biopsies, surgical excision, and endoscopic procedures, physicians can retrieve definitive samples that supply valuable information about cell alterations. The advancement of imaging modalities like ultrasound and MRI has also enhanced the accuracy of biopsies by enabling better localization of lesions and lowering the risk of complications. As with continuous developments in medical science, the application of fusion imaging techniques has increased in some areas by improving diagnostic accuracy in gynecological and urological procedures, altering the features of biopsy performance and interpretation in clinical practice (Bellati et al., 2018). Evolution in biopsy techniques has been underscored by the emergence of newer modalities such as cryobiopsy, primarily in assessing lung disease. Cryobiopsy has specific merits, including procuring tissue greater than usual with preservation of architectural elements without generating significant artefacts, as seen with standard biopsy methods. Comparative studies have demonstrated a remarkable enhancement in diagnostic yield using cryobiopsy for both cancer diagnosis and ILD. Besides, the evidence shows that cryobiopsy is as reliable as flexible thoracoscopy in assessing pleural lesions, thus widening its clinical application. These new techniques are a step towards more precise diagnostic tools for advancing higher patient outcomes through better disease characterization (Griff et al., 2019). Despite the development in biopsy techniques, clinical practice also has some issues and challenges. Choice between biopsy methods is most often determined by lesion site, patient anatomy, and the patient's general health status. Moreover, the risk of complications such as bleeding and infection necessitates careful patient selection and pre-procedure assessment. As such, practitioners must remain abreast of the literature and guidelines in biopsy indications and methods to best serve their patients. Furthermore, integrating multidisciplinary approaches, including clinical management, pathology, and radiology, is also important in facilitating effective assessments and treatment guidelines from biopsy findings. The ongoing interaction between the experts brings about an interdisciplinary environment, eventually leading to enhanced quality of care for those undergoing biopsy (Bellati et al., 2018; Griff et al., 2019).

3.3.1. Types of Biopsies (e.g., Needle, Excisional)

In clinical research, biopsies play an integral role in diagnosing numerous ailments, particularly malignancies. Biopsies can be categorized broadly into various forms, varying in their methodologies and applications. Needle biopsies, including fine needle aspiration (FNA) and core needle biopsies, are increasingly favored for their least invasive nature. FNA allows for sampling of cells from pathological masses with rapid diagnoses that are highly significant in diseases such as lymphadenopathy. Cytological examination based on needle biopsies helps in early diagnosis. However, challenges continue to be faced, particularly in differentiating malignancy and benignancy, as seen in the literature on the problems related to lymph node examinations (Geddie et al., 2012). Hence, the selection of an appropriate biopsy technique has a direct impact on diagnosis accuracy and is thus crucial for clinical practice. Excisional biopsies are different from their needle counterparts in that they involve surgically removing a complete lesion or significantly larger pieces of tissue. The technique is beneficial where an unambiguous diagnosis is required or the lesions are large. Doctors can obtain valuable information regarding tumor nature such as type, grade, and potential stage by subjecting removed tissue to histopathological examination. In malignancies, such as oral squamous cell carcinoma, thorough analysis is crucial since accurate tissue diagnosis is the core of proper treatment plan planning (Torras et al., 2015).

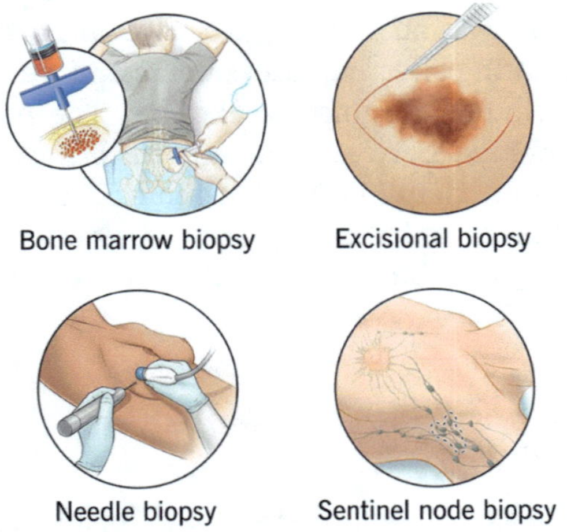

Figure 3.8. Types of biopsies.

Source: https://my.clevelandclinic.org/-/scassets/images/org/health/articles/15458-biopsy.

The excisional biopsy's advantage of providing a generous tissue specimen not only aids in diagnosing cancer but also assists in planning treatment, mirroring its key role in contemporary medical assessment and oncologic management. The choice of biopsy method also the outcome of the patient and the risk of the procedure. While needle biopsies are associated with less pain and recovery, they do not always yield sufficient tissue for a definitive diagnosis in complex cases requiring sophisticated morphological analysis. Excisional biopsies, however, are more invasive and entail greater surgical hazards, including infection and scarring. The selection of the two procedures must nevertheless consider clinical goals, patient factors, and the specific nature of the case. Understanding the benefits and drawbacks of both approaches not only guides practitioners into the proper decision and allows patients to receive optimum diagnostic treatment. Ultimately, the variability in biopsy procedures accentuates the vital role of histopathology in diagnosis and the treatment of various medical conditions (Figure 3.8).

3.3.2. Role in Cancer Diagnosis

The function of investigations during cancer diagnosis is fundamental since proper disease diagnosis can significantly impact patient management and treatment protocols. Diagnostic modalities such as imaging technologies like CT and MRI offer critical information about tumor size, location, and metastasis. Histopathological analysis via biopsies provides a definitive diagnosis since pathologists can evaluate tissue samples for malignancy. Furthermore, improvement in molecular screening, such as genetic screening, is increasingly being utilized to identify specific biomarkers associated with unique cancers. These technologies assist in establishing a diagnosis of cancer but also tailor medicine by identifying the optimal treatment modalities in accordance with one's genetic makeup. Thus, this research highlights the need for an integrated cancer diagnosis based on complementary strategies that can facilitate focused interventions to maximize therapeutic response. Cancer diagnosis today also encompasses, besides traditional diagnostic tests, prognostic models that forecast a patient's likelihood of future health status beyond disease classification. It has been suggested that, based on diagnostic labels alone, significant influences that impact prognosis and QoL can be overlooked. In turn, illnesses that do not easily fit into well-defined disease categories, like chronic fatigue syndrome, illustrate the shortcomings of historical classification. Prognostic models, conversely, enable clinicians to integrate a range of information, including genetic, biological, and psychosocial information, to inform clinical management. With a broader view of patient health, clinicians can provide better predictions and tailor interventions to improve overall therapeutic regimens.

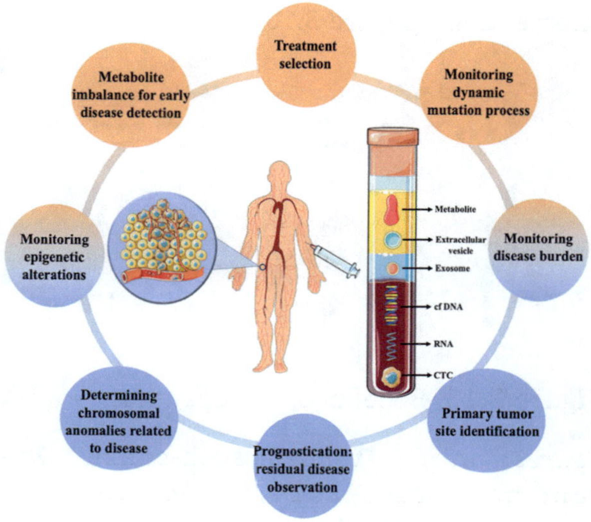

Figure 3.9. Applications of liquid biopsy in cancer diagnosis, along with the different biomarkers commonly targeted using the technique.

Source: https://www.researchgate.net/publication/367157687/figure/fig1/AS:11431281395191071@1745472971774/Applications-of-liquid-biopsy-in-cancer-diagnosis-along-with-the-different-biomarkers.tif.

This change in paradigm from stringent diagnostic categorization to a broad definition of patient prognosis mirrors the evolving face of cancer diagnosis and treatment in contemporary medicine. Moreover, the interplay between diagnostic testing and patient education cannot be overstated, particularly when examining the psychological impact of a cancer diagnosis. The patients will often grapple with uncertainty and anxiety following diagnostic testing, and therefore, open communication must be provided by medical caregivers. Effectively conveying the meaning of diagnostic findings, either to confirm cancer or to consider other options, is of fundamental importance to patient expectation management and patient and provider trust. Furthermore, education initiatives that provide counseling interventions can empower patients to be actively involved in their own care decision-making and treatment planning. As highlighted in current discussions regarding clinical practice, emphasis on prognosis and not mere disease diagnosis can revolutionize patient-clinician debate and decision-making. Thus, a on open communication and care support maximizes overall experience in individuals with the challenges of cancer diagnosis and treatment (Figure 3.9).

3.3.3. Risks and Benefits of Biopsy Procedures

Biopsy procedures are an essential component of modern-day diagnostic practice within medicine, providing vital information capable of being utilized for the direction of treatment. However, deciding to perform a biopsy must weigh the benefit of the clinical intervention against the risks involved. Risks of biopsies can include bleeding, infection, and damage to overlying structures or organs. Such side effects may be even more severe among those patients who have comorbidities or poor performance status, reducing their general health and recovery capacity. Thus, physicians have an ethical responsibility to engage extensively with patients in relation to such risks and at the same time establish the advantages of tissue sampling in arriving at a precise diagnosis and treatment, particularly in controversial cases, such as lung cancer among patients with performance status 3 and 4 (Farley et al., 2017). The benefits of biopsy interventions are significant in that they allow clinicians to make definitive tissue diagnoses that can dramatically alter management plans. For instance, in oncology, the ability to diagnose individual tumors and their molecular characteristics makes it possible to design tailored treatment plans, thereby improving patient outcomes. Though only 5% of the poor performance status patients received treatments that necessitated tissue diagnosis, a few of those who did show enhanced survival, again emphasizing the significance of biopsies in deciding on a treatment plan (Farley et al., 2017). Moreover, attaining a correct diagnosis can eliminate doubts regarding a patient's condition, reduce anxiety, and allow subsequent personalized follow-up plans. Ultimately, carefully balancing these numerous factors can direct the clinical decision-making process to whether or not to undertake a biopsy. In situations where there are complex medical cases, such as lung cancer with heterogeneous performance statuses, the decision as to whether or not to perform a biopsy depicts the nuances of risk and benefit. The study on North Glasgow's lung cancer patients indicates that while a high rate of lower performance status patients undergo biopsies, they do not receive continuous treatment as anticipated. It raises some serious questions about the usefulness of biopsies in increasing survival rates, as most of the patients who were put through them did not experience noticeable changes in their prognosis (Farley et al., 2017). Therefore, even as the inherent risks of biopsy procedures must be carefully controlled, their therapeutic potential—especially with respect to individualized therapies—should not be ignored. Selection of patients and carefully considering individual health conditions are critical for maximizing the efficacy of biopsy interventions (Figure 3.10).

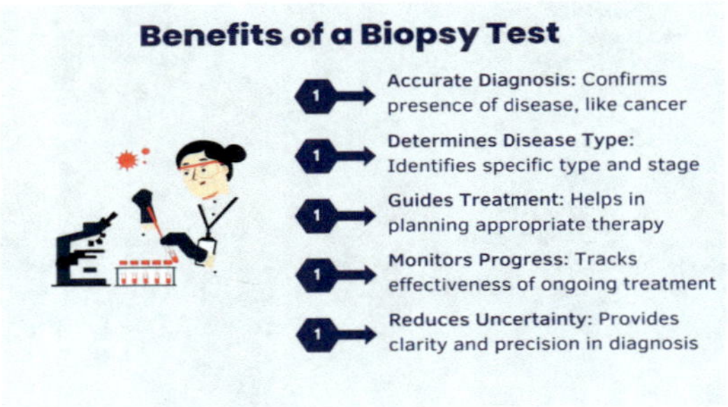

Figure 3.10. Benefits of a biopsy test.

Source: https://vshospitals.b-cdn.net/wp-content/uploads/2024/07/Benefits-of-a-Biopsy-Test-1024x671.webp.

Test Your Knowledge

1. What are the main types of biopsies, and how is the choice of method determined?
2. How does a biopsy contribute to the diagnosis and staging of cancer?

3.4. Endoscopic Procedures

Learning Outcome

1. Explain the types of endoscopies
2. Understand diagnostic and therapeutic uses of endoscopy
3. Discuss preparation and recovery for patients

Endoscopic procedures have revolutionized diagnostic and therapeutic medicine, presenting patients with minimally invasive options. Utilizing an endoscope—a flexible tube with a camera and light source—endoscopic procedures allow health professionals to visualize through to internal organs and structures with breathtaking clarity. Endoscopy applications extend beyond visualization to interventions such as biopsy, polypectomy, and the treatment of gastrointestinal (GI) bleeding. This integration of therapy and diagnosis not only enhances patient safety and comfort but can also lead to shorter recovery periods, thereby significantly reducing hospital stays. With advancing technology in the medical sector, endoscopic interventions continue to evolve, bringing new solutions to complex medical conditions, underscoring their significance in modern medicine. Endoscopic interventions, among other benefits have immensely supported the management of urological diseases. For instance, treatment of giant staghorn renal stones, which are categorically difficult due to the rates at which they recur, is now able to employ a laparoscopic pyelolithotomy and endoscopic pyelolithotripsy combined procedure. This procedure has been found to possess a high rate of stone clearance, similar to more invasive procedures, yet it highlights the effectiveness of endoscopic procedures in urology. Of note, open surgery complications are being avoided, thus this option becomes a better choice for experienced laparoscopic surgeons. Applying this combined strategy represents an essential step forward in treating urological pathologies, emphasizing the need for ongoing investment in endoscopic technology and education to provide the best possible patient outcomes (Salhi et al., 2015). Additionally, the endoscopic procedure's role carries over into the treatment of comorbidities commonly linked with such pathologies as obesity. The World Health Organization (WHO) highlights the rising levels of obesity and its related medical complications, like type 2 diabetes, CVDs, and certain cancers, which impose a significant burden on health systems. To this end, endoscopic bariatric procedures like sleeve gastrectomy and gastric bypass have been found effective in achieving a dramatic weight loss. These procedures not only minimize surgical trauma but also allow patients to have an all-encompassing approach to the prevention of obesity-related complications. In light of the global obesity epidemic, endoscopic interventions are poised to become an essential weapon in the fight against this public health crisis and the improvement of the QoL of individuals afflicted by it (Agius et al., 2014) (Figure 3.11).

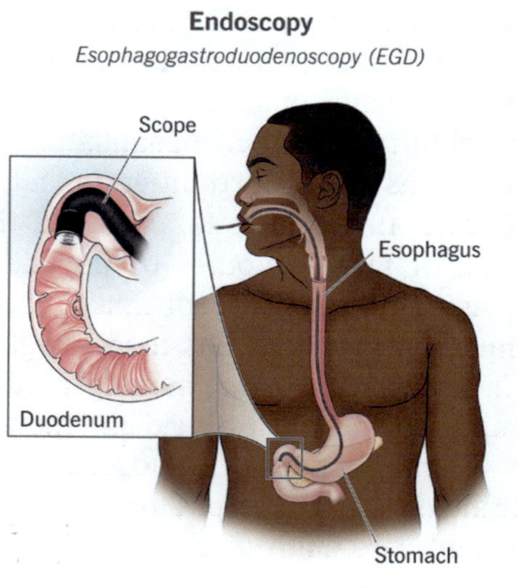

Figure 3.11. Endoscopy.

Source: https://my.clevelandclinic.org/-/scassets/images/org/health/articles/25126-endoscopy.

3.4.1. Types of Endoscopies (e.g., Gastrointestinal, Bronchial)

Endoscopy is a vital medical diagnostic technique to examine the internal body anatomy, primarily the GI tract and the respiratory system. GI endoscopy is a group of procedures, including esophagogastroduodenoscopy (EGD), colonoscopy, and sigmoidoscopy, designed to diagnose and treat various digestive system ailments. EGD, for instance, provides direct visualization of the esophagus, stomach, and duodenum to recognize abnormalities such as ulcers or tumors. Conversely, colonoscopy examines the large bowel, providing pointers to conditions such as colorectal carcinoma and inflammatory bowel disease (IBD). Biopsies, polypectomy, and cauterization can generally be performed simultaneously, making GI endoscopy a diagnostic and therapeutic procedure. Bronchial endoscopy, or flexible bronchoscopy as it is sometimes referred to, is another serious type of endoscopy, and this involves the airways and the lungs. That is how physicians can visualize the bronchial tubes and obtain tissue samples that can be significant in diagnosing respiratory illnesses, including infections, cancers, and chronic obstructive pulmonary disease (COPD). The possibility of direct visualization of the bronchi opens up opportunities for advanced therapeutic interventions, such as forced expulsion of foreign bodies or deposition of drugs. As knowledge in bronchial endoscopic techniques increases, it has increasingly been used in association with imaging modalities, thus enhancing diagnostic yield and therapeutic effect. Overall, bronchial endoscopy's role is significant in managing respiratory complications and patient care. Multidisciplinary application of endoscopy is available in various medical specialties, substantiating its global applicability beyond GI and bronchial examinations. Specifically, endoscopic interventions are frequently considered in the prudent treatment of patients with atherosclerotic coronary heart disease (CHD). For instance, when elective GI endoscopy in patients is complicated by the temporary withdrawal of platelet-directed pharmacotherapy, it is necessary to evaluate the risk of both their cardiac disease and the scheduled endoscopic study. Integrating risk assessment methods in clinical practice is essential in preventing adverse effects during such procedures. Such versatility of endoscopy, along with prudent management strategies in comorbid patients, once again solidifies its place as a routine investigation in medicine, resulting in better diagnosis, treatment, and safety of patients (Abraham et al., 2009; Brouwers et al., 2015) (Figure 3.12).

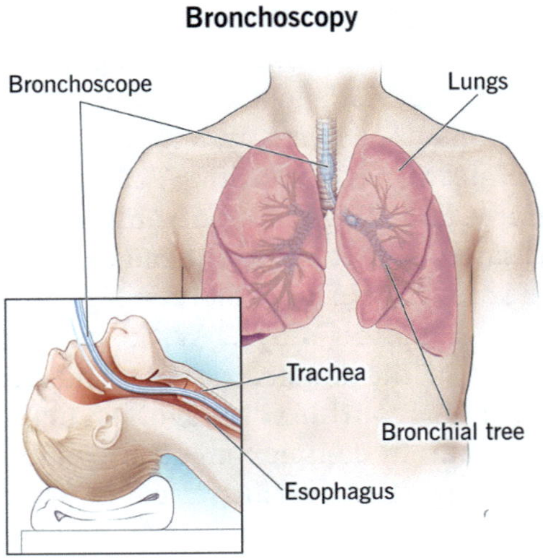

Figure 3.12. Bronchoscopy.

Source: https://my.clevelandclinic.org/-/scassets/images/org/health/articles/bronchoscopy.

3.4.2. Diagnostic and Therapeutic Uses

Diagnostic medicine relies significantly on advances in technology and methodology for research to enhance patient care by providing timely and accurate diagnoses. Investigations such as blood studies, imaging tests, and biopsies define conditions that underlie health. An excellent example would be the evaluation of hypereosinophilia, which involves distinguishing between probable etiologies, such as infections, allergy, and malignancy. The diagnostic criterion of hypereosinophilic syndrome (HES) suggests the intricacies of the case, given that patients can present with elevated eosinophil levels with no cause being established. This creates challenges for clinicians, who need to assess eosinophil levels and utilize imaging and histopathological examination to establish possible underlying neoplasms or reactive disorders (Brys et al., 2015). Thus, a successful diagnosis lies in examining numerous features that assist in providing appropriate therapeutic interventions. Following proper diagnosis, conditions revealed by diagnostic investigations are of significance for their therapeutic management. Treatment regimen for HES, for example, is complex and requires individualization based on the specific pathophysiology underlying the patient's condition. Management strategies may range from corticosteroids and immunosuppressive therapies to targeted biologic agents, depending on whether the condition is identified as idiopathic or secondary to some other cause, such as malignancies. This highlights that the condition should be diagnosed by thorough diagnostic processes and clinical judgment should be exercised in their treatment (Brys et al., 2015). The interface of laboratory diagnosis and therapeutic intervention mirrors the paramount need for a synthesized medicine model, whereby diagnostics inform treatment protocols, leading to improved patient care and QoL. Second, the ongoing refinement of diagnostic and treatment techniques is progressive in developing medical practice. New technologies, such as genetic testing and advanced imaging technologies, provide new perspectives on polydiseases like HES. The interaction with precision medicine enables tailor-made interventions based on patients' genetic profiles, maximizing therapeutic responses and minimizing toxicities. For instance, therapy for HES is increasingly being individualized based on meticulous scrutiny of patient-specific information to enable more targeted treatment (Brys et al., 2015). In addition, the continuing development of minimally invasive diagnostic equipment has the potential to bring disorder identification earlier on, a scenario that will ultimately have a positive effect on treatment outcomes. The symbiotic existence of diagnostics and therapy thus not only helps exhibit the intricacy of modern medicine but also provides patients with timely and advantageous interventions, enhancing clinical practice care quality.

3.4.3. Preparation and Recovery for Patients

The most important components of patient care are good preparation and recovery, particularly following surgical or invasive medical procedures. Proper patient preparation enhances the likelihood of a successful outcome while reducing anxiety and uncertainty. The most critical components of such an initiative are extensive pre-operative assessment, adequate communication about the procedure, and building a conducive environment that listens to the patients' concerns. Using formal instruments such as the readiness for hospital discharge scale (RHDS) can help quantify patients' readiness for discharge, focusing on areas where additional support may be needed to ensure patient confidence and safety. This progressive approach makes transitions from the hospital to the home easier and dramatically impacts the recovery timelines, promoting overall health results through emphasis on continuity of care and patient engagement along the medical pathway (Piacentine et al., 2006). Recovery from surgery often necessitates multifactorial examination beyond the post-operative environment. Age, overall health, and socio-economic status may influence the recovery process. In patients with rotator cuff tears, a perfect recovery regimen involving both operative and non-operative interventions is crucial. The decision to treat will go a long way in determining recovery, with conservative treatment such as platelet-rich plasma (PRP) injections being a classic example of the strength to enhance healing. Educating patients about recovery expectations and rehabilitation requirements must be incorporated into patient preparation since learning inherently increases compliance with follow-up and rehabilitation. Patient-specific problems are addressed through individualized recovery strategies and enable quicker rehabilitation, reducing the risks for post-operative complications while building the therapeutic alliance between patient and care provider (Loccisano et al., 2016). Additionally, the incorporation of follow-up care and reinforcement of self-management strategies can exert an appropriate impact on long-term recovery pathways. It is more patient-empowering for patients when they are actively involved in their recovery plans, showing the importance of patient education and support throughout recovery. Interventions such as physical therapy, medication management, and lifestyle changes must be clearly explained to patients before discharge, providing them with ways of managing their health independently. Such a care continuum, especially for patients with more than one need, is necessary to help them access resources and support systems as soon as they are back home. Successful recovery is contingent upon this tension of preparation and ongoing monitoring, facilitating improved health status and lowering the chance of hospital readmission due to complications (Piacentine et al., 2006).

Test Your Knowledge

1. What are the main types of endoscopic procedures, and what areas of the body do they examine?
2. How are endoscopic procedures used both diagnostically and therapeutically in clinical practice?
3. What conditions can be detected or treated through gastrointestinal endoscopy?

3.5. Genetic Testing

Learning Outcome

1. Explain the types of genetic tests
2. Focus on genetic testing implications for personalized medicine
3. Describe ethical considerations in genetic testing

In the past few years, genetic testing has become a mainstay of contemporary medicine, revolutionizing how illnesses are diagnosed, treated, and prevented. By analyzing an individual's DNA, doctors can detect genetic variations that may cause many health issues. This capability not only enhances preventive therapy through the identification of disease-associated risks at an early stage but also enables individualized treatment regimens as a function of the patient's unique genetic profile. Genetic testing has thus emerged as a highly beneficial instrument in oncology, cardiology, and genetic disorders, facilitating more targeted interventions directly linked to the etiologic basis of disease. This growing emphasis on personalized medicine increases the call for ongoing innovation and research into genetic testing technology to ensure accuracy in detection and management strategies. Moreover, the inclusion of genetic testing into more general diagnostic settings has provided insight into diseases once little understood. With the information from numerous omics technologies, including proteomics and genomics, researchers can now investigate the intricate biological processes responsible for conditions such as cardiometabolic diseases. Existing evidence suggests that combining different omics data facilitates the identification of stable biomarkers, which can significantly affect disease management and patient outcomes. Specifically, proposed interventions using gender medicine may illuminate the interaction of biological sex with genetic components and eventually yield more efficient and patient-focused lines of care. Such developments in the use of genetic testing to guide clinical care mirror the shift toward an expanded definition of health and illness, highlighting genetics's role in shaping patient care models (Argano et al., 2019). In addition to clinical application, ethical considerations in genetic testing are becoming increasingly important as technology advances. Privacy, informed consent, and possible discrimination based on genetic information are just a few of the concerns that raise fundamental questions regarding the responsible use of genetic data. Biomolecular technology and bioinformatics developments have further enriched the complexity by making detailed genetic profiling possible, but equally demand strict surveillance and regulatory norms to safeguard patient rights. There is a need for ethical guidelines due to the genuine possibility of misuse of genetic information in various areas of life, such as employment and insurance. Therefore, with genetic analysis continuously evolving and expanding in scope, the medical community must remain vigilant for such ethical considerations so that the benefit of this forceful questioning is derived in the interest of enhancing patient care without trespassing on individual rights or social justice (Calfee et al., 2017) (Figure 3.13).

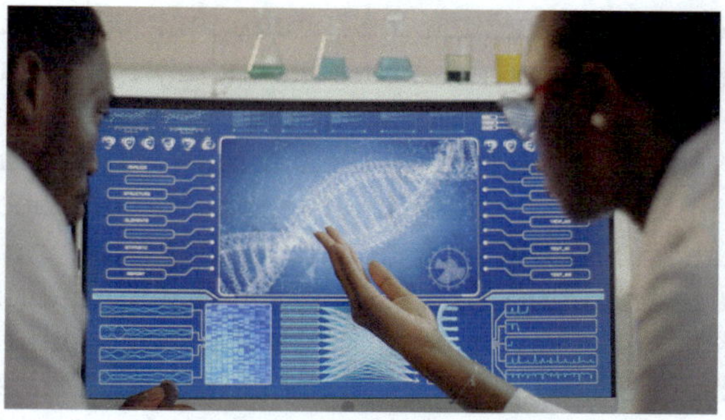

Figure 3.13. Genetic testing.

Source: https://www.cdc.gov/genomics-and-health/media/images/gen_testing.jpg.

3.5.1. Types of Genetic Tests (e.g., Carrier Testing, Diagnostic Testing)

In contemporary medicine, genetic testing is an integral component of understanding and coping with most medical conditions, used with differences dependent on the test's purpose. Carrier testing helps identify the carriers of a gene mutation associated with an inherited illness free from disease. Such testing is of most use to prospective parents since it allows them establish the likelihood of passing genetic disorders to their children. Screening for conditions such as cystic fibrosis or sickle cell disease informs couples about reproductive decisions, thus influencing health in the family. As knowledge about genetics and technology improves, the role of carrier testing becomes increasingly significant. This paves the way for more personalized healthcare approaches. In contrast, diagnostic testing is to confirm or rule out a specific genetic disorder in an individual already experiencing symptoms or with the likelihood of inheriting an inherited disease. This type of testing is critical in the diagnosis of the appropriate treatment regimen and can have a significant impact on patient management. An example is the case of suspected muscular dystrophies, where genetic testing provides definitive diagnoses that guide therapy. By detecting specific mutations, clinicians can tailor treatments to match the genetic composition of the disease, for instance, gene therapies or drug therapy. Through diagnostic testing, patients are given knowledge about their conditions, making it possible for timely interventions and proper management of their health, leading to a better QoL. The ethical, legal, and social implications of genetic testing cannot be excluded either. The effects of genetic information exceed those on the individual's health, reaching into family relationships, privacy, and insurance. ALRC reports have identified the need for broad frameworks to address these sensitive issues, which would show that genetic information is handled responsibly without impeding progress in medical research. As more genetic tests are conducted, debates surrounding their social effects are always necessary. Physicians and lawmakers must join forces to conquer the complex circumstance of genetic testing, which will be a focal point of future medical research, guaranteeing innovations that preserve private and family rights (Opeskin et al., 2025). Thus, the awareness of the multilateral character of genetic tests, from carrier testing to diagnosis, is still essential in contemporary clinical practice.

3.5.2. Implications for Personalized Medicine

Personalized medicine is an evolutionary leap that extensively enhances patient management with directed therapeutic intervention. One of the peculiarities of this paradigm is the fusion of several 'omics' technologies, particularly proteomics, capable of illuminating the unique molecular pathways underlying individual diseases. By identifying precise protein profiles, clinicians cannot only trace disease progression but also predict treatment response and enhance therapeutic intervention. This approach is especially critical in oncology, where the very high heterogeneity of cancers necessitates individually oriented strategies to optimal treatment. Studies indicate that proteomics-based interventions are capable of allowing earlier and more efficient decision-making regarding treatment to meet the urgent need for new therapies in diseases such as bladder cancer treatment, where standard options remain few. Consequently, proteomic data integration has the potential to advance personalized medicine for better patient stratification and prognostication, which can revolutionize clinical outcomes (Frantzi et al., 2017). In addition, the implications of personalized medicine also address biological aspects, but they have to integrate gender considerations in medical practice. Gender medicine, as the primary foundational element of customized care, emphasizes the vital interplay of biological markers and psychological or cultural behaviors that affect health outcomes. The importance of distinguishing sex from gender cannot be overstated because of its general applicability to clinical manifestations and treatment responses. The identification of some sex/gender differences permits enhanced prevention measures, improves the sensitivity for clinical symptom detection, and aids optimization of therapy. In this respect, the application of omics technologies is a key to the identification of the sex- and gender-specific disease markers. These innovations have the potential to lead to better provision of care and alleviation of inequalities, which ultimately result in the ultimate goal of personalized care to individuals' individual characteristics (Bellini et al., 2019). As the customized medicine paradigm transforms, the accommodation of both the biological and sociocultural is ever more crucial. The influence of the patient's genetic makeup, environmental factors, and psychosocial processes demonstrates the complexities of disease and health. Personalized medicine pathway must be concerned with multidisciplinary alliances that address diseases' genetic origins and gender-influenced and otherwise sociocultural behavior. This integrated perspective allows health professionals to establish individualized diagnostic assessments and therapy plans that better meet the diverse needs of patients.

Moreover, recognition of the significance of patient-centered care has the potential to increase motivation towards healthcare. By leveraging future technologies and creating an inclusive model of gender medicine, the healthcare industry can move towards more comprehensive personalized medicine that will improve overall patient outcomes and healthcare equity (Frantzi et al., 2017; Bellini et al., 2019) (Figure 3.14).

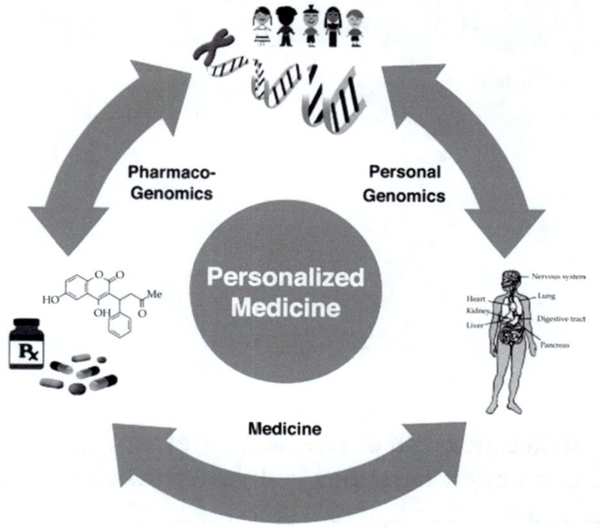

Figure 3.14. Personalized medicine.

Source: https://www.researchgate.net/publication/51150639/figure/fig1/AS:202611224518660@1425317688478/Personalized-medicine-Personal-genomics-connect-genotype-to-phenotype-and-provide.png.

3.5.3. Ethical Considerations in Genetic Testing

The growing prominence of genetic testing within contemporary medicine has also bequeathed us an array of ethical concerns that need to be scrutinized. Perhaps the most fundamental of these ethical concerns is genetic discrimination, particularly in terms of employment and insurance. As more genetic information is made available, there is also the very real risk of individuals being judged discriminatorily based on their susceptibility as per their genes, rather than their actual state of health. This concern raises vital questions about the effectiveness of existing legal safeguards, which may not be appropriate for the complexities and fluidities of the genetic information environment. Moreover, as the distinction between prenatal screening and genetic screening comes more clearly, the necessity of informed consent becomes more evident. Individuals must be fully cognizant of the limitations and implications of such tests, generally including unexpected results that could alter relationships within families or cause emotional distress, thereby cementing the necessity of ethical guidelines in the practice of genetic testing (Alderson et al., 2001). The second significant aspect of the ethical framework of genetic testing is the issue of privacy and confidentiality. The fragile nature of genetic data necessitates robust safeguards against unauthorized access or exploitation. However, the same technologies that enable genetic testing can create risks, particularly when data are processed in centralized databases or exchanged across numerous medical and research platforms. The threat of confidentiality violations poses legitimate cause for alarm about the effects on individuals, as such violations threaten to place them at risk by subjecting them to stigmatization or social isolation. To counteract these risks, it is paramount that healthcare providers and policymakers develop sufficient frameworks that uphold patient confidentiality while making room for applicable research advancement. Also, public discourse concerning the ethical implications of genetic testing must transform to include diverse perspectives and in policy development to consider the views of suffering patients (Haimes et al., 2014). In addition, the ethical implications expand to the influence of genetic testing on family dynamics and societal expectations. The concept of relatedness becomes of overriding importance when genetic data informs choices surrounding childbearing and medical intervention. For instance, the revelation of unexpected inherited diseases is likely to bring about emotional pain for families because the subjects grapple with the acceptance of their genetics and how it will impact their relatives. This underscores the need for genetic counseling to help individuals and families understand genetic studies' challenges. Counselors can help lead the discussion on the social and ethical dimensions of the test outcomes, hence ensuring informed decision-making. Ultimately, the ethical landscape of genetic testing is multifaceted, with ongoing discussion and education of healthcare providers, patients, and the community at large to work through the nuances involved in this ever-evolving area (Haimes et al., 2014).

Test Your Knowledge

1. What are the main types of genetic tests, and what is each used for?
2. How does genetic testing contribute to the development and application of personalized medicine?

3.6. Urinalysis

Learning Outcome

1. Explain the components of urinalysis
2. Describe common conditions diagnosed through urinalysis
3. Understand the limitations of urinalysis

Urinalysis is a fundamental diagnostic method employed in the majority of clinical specialties that provides valuable information about the patient's health status. Urinalysis involves the examination of urine for the content of certain substances, which may indicate underlying health issues or disease processes. Physical, chemical, and microscopic analysis of the urine are the usual elements of urinalysis, and each contributes to an overall picture of the patients' condition. Physical examination analyzes the color, transparency, and smell of urine, while chemical testing tests for pH, protein, glucose, and ketones, and others. Moreover, microscopic examination identifies cellular structures such as red blood cells, white blood cells, and crystals, signifying infections, metabolic disorders, or kidney damage, thereby justifying the critical role of urinalysis in disease diagnosis at an early stage. In the practice of veterinary medicine, urinalysis has become a valuable tool for evaluating urinary tract infections (UTIs) in canine patients. Recent studies confirm the utility of urine culture evaluation, showing the presence of bacteria in typical concentrations of uncomplicated UTIs (Chew et al., 2012). For instance, in a clinical trial comparing antimicrobial regimens, some regimens were shown to have comparable efficacy in achieving microbiologic and clinical cure rates. The ability to determine the species and number of bacteria present in a urine specimen not only aids diagnosis but also directs therapeutic decision-making, which can ultimately lead to beneficial results for animal patients and owners. Thus, urinalysis is a critical diagnostic weapon in human and veterinary medicine. Secondly, urinalysis may also shed light on systemic diseases that are not necessarily detectable with perceivable symptoms at the outset. As an example, the occurrence of glucose in the urine typically indicates possible diabetes mellitus, while proteinuria may indicate kidney disorders or systemic diseases such as hypertension or HF. Daily analysis can thus facilitate early treatment and management of chronic diseases, and therefore act effectively in preventive care. Moreover, advances in diagnostic technology have improved the sensitivity and specificity of urinalysis, so it is now a reliable component of routine medical check-ups. With continued advancements in medicine, even more refinement of urinalysis procedures will still be crucial in the ongoing quest for better diagnostic performance and patient care, and in emphasizing its continued importance among general medical investigations (Figure 3.15).

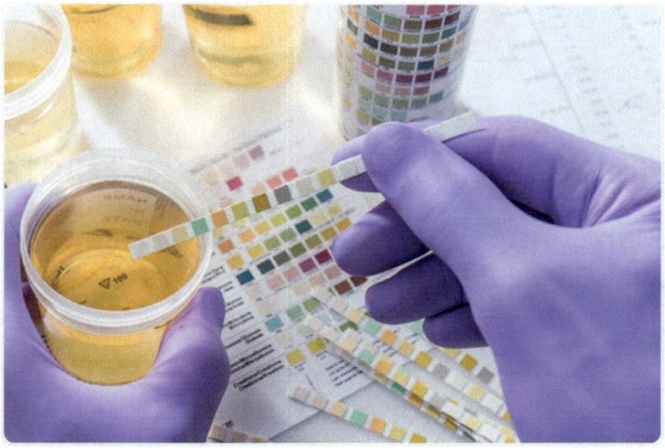

Figure 3.15. Urinalysis.

Source: https://www.news-medical.net/image-handler/picture/2021/3/shutterstock_1245033115.jpg.

3.6.1. Components of a Urinalysis

Urinalysis is a bedrock tool in the practice of diagnostic medicine that has several significant elements that collectively provide a patient's health status. In particular, a urinalysis is usually made up of three primary analyses: physical examination, chemical analysis, and microscopic examination. Physical examination checks the urine's color, odor, and appearance, allowing gross abnormalities like hematuria or cloudiness to be identified. These results may indicate underlying conditions such as renal stones or UTIs. As a group, the chemical test employs dipsticks to measure specific gravity, pH, and the presence of certain substances such as protein, glucose, and ketones. This biochemistry profile is critical in diagnosing renal function or metabolic disease, addressing the multifaceted nature of urinalysis as a diagnostic tool in routine medical screening. Microscopic examination of urine sediments is the third element that augments the two others with specific cellular and acellular elements to assist in clinical decision-making. The a technician or trained pathologist who carries out the stage using a microscope to scan the urine for red and white blood cells, epithelial cells, bacteria, crystals, and casts. All of these findings are of diagnostic significance; for example, the finding of significant white blood cells could be a sign of infection, whereas findings of casts can suggest glomerular damage. Furthermore, the presence of urine crystals can help determine potential nephrolithiasis. Overall, these microscopic findings add information to the context that may corroborate suspicions generated by physical and chemical inspection or lead healthcare providers toward alternative diagnoses, emphasizing the unifying nature of an entire urinalysis. Although the strength of urinalysis elements is significant, there are challenges in ensuring the accuracy and reliability of its results. Variation in the collection, handling, and analysis of specimens can introduce variability that becomes the cause of spurious clinical interpretations. Furthermore, a systematic review revealed concerns regarding the methodological quality of studies evaluating diagnostic tests, specifically in the case of UTIs among children, in which poorly reported studies can skew the evidential basis for clinical guidelines (Biggi et al., 2005). With medical professionals increasingly relying on urinalysis for informed choice, resolving these problems of quality control is vital. Therefore, ongoing education and standardization of laboratory tests are essential in an attempt to optimize the diagnostic value of urinalysis so that it remains a cornerstone of the armamentarium of routine investigative modalities in medicine.

3.6.2. Common Conditions Diagnosed Through Urinalysis

Urinalysis is a routine diagnostic aid employed in modern medicine to permit clinicians to identify several common conditions. UTI is one of the primary diseases that is diagnosed through urinalysis and diagnosed by the detection of bacteria, white blood cells, or red blood cells in the urine. They indicate urinary tract inflammation and infection. Urinalysis also hints towards diseases such as diabetes mellitus, in which high glucose concentrations in urine can be detected. The presence of ketones in the urine may suggest inefficient glucose metabolism, thus indirectly hinting towards metabolic derangement. Overall, urinalysis is a cheap, non-invasive first-line test that can provide us with crucial information for detecting underlying health issues in patients. Another frequently detectable disease by urinalysis-is kidney disease. Protein in the urine (proteinuria) is usually a sign of damage to the glomeruli, the kidneys' filtering units. It is a dangerous sign because it could be an indicator of CKD or renal failure. High creatinine or blood urea nitrogen (BUN) levels can also indicate compromised kidney function. Hematuria, or the presence of blood in the urine, is another foreboding finding that can be due to a collection of etiologies, ranging from renal stones to malignancies. With the utilization of information gained through the use of urinalysis, physicians can initiate timely treatment and further investigation, hence significantly increasing patient outcomes. Finally, urinalysis also facilitates the diagnosis of metabolic and systemic diseases. For instance, in patients with liver diseases, the presence of bilirubin in urine may indicate widespread liver failure or bile duct blockage. Also, urinalysis may be helpful in determining hydration level by establishing the concentration levels of specific gravity, useful in conditions such as dehydration. Although diversified in its applications, urinalysis sometimes can require confirmation by other investigations to establish the nature of a found abnormality. Thus, while urinalysis is invaluable in diagnosis, in most instances it is a stepping stone to more in-depth investigation, and ultimately increases diagnostic accuracy and patient management (Figure 3.16).

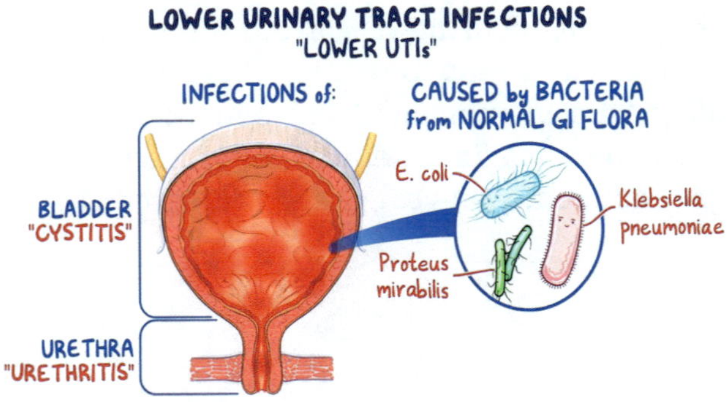

Figure 3.16. Lower urinary tract infection (UTI).

Source: https://d16qt3wv6xm098.cloudfront.net/s9lNBu8STVCWbeDn94U2Zw6WTiGe-stZ/_.jpg.

3.6.3. Limitations of Urinalysis

Urinalysis is a valuable medical diagnostic tool, but limitations have an extraordinary impact on the diagnosis and treatment of patients. One of the major issues is that it cannot provide definitive diagnostic information. For instance, although urinalysis can detect the presence of proteins, glucose, or blood, it cannot determine the origin or cause of these abnormalities. This deficit of specificity necessitates further testing to ascertain the underlying condition, i.e., renal disease or diabetes, lending credence to the argument that urinalysis is often a first step in the workup and not a diagnosis. In studies using congestive heart failure (CHF), for example, only 13% of patients received urinalysis, calling attention to its limited application towards the diagnosis of conditions with complicating factors and need for supplementation with alternative methods of diagnosis (Camilleri et al., 2004). A significant limitation of urinalysis is also that it is susceptible to pre-analytical and analytical errors. Pre-analytical factors like improper collection and storage can produce variable test results. For example, sample contamination or delay in processing can alter the chemical composition of the urine, producing false positives or false negatives. Once again, variations in the analytical procedure, including differences in reagent quality or instrument calibration, make consistency in test results difficult. A diabetic ketoacidosis case study in the management revealed these pitfalls, with deviations from recommendations seen in monitoring of parameters across several cases (Abela et al., 2008). These errors highlight the need for standard procedures to enhance the reliability and dependability of urinalysis. Furthermore, urinalysis is limited in its interpretative value, considering the influence of numerous extraneous variables on its results. All three will considerably alter urine composition and potentiallypotentially mislead clinical impressions. For instance, a patient's fluid intake can dilute or concentrate the urine and affect the detectability of many solutes. Certain foods, such as beets or asparagus, can result in urine color or odorous changes that can be confused with pathology. This needs careful monitoring of a patient's history concerning urinalysis results. In conclusion, while urinalysis is a widespread investigation in medicine, its limitations necessitate the use of complementary diagnostic approaches to confirm the correct clinical findings.

Test Your Knowledge

1. What are the main components of a routine urinalysis, and what does each component assess?
2. Which common medical conditions can be diagnosed or monitored using urinalysis?
3. What are the limitations of urinalysis in diagnosing medical conditions?

SUMMARY

In summarizing the findings of many studies that are habitually done in medicine, it is evident that the effects of ordering test habits greatly influence clinical practice and healthcare costs. One study conducted on medical students and doctors found that several participants ordered tests not recommended by an expert panel, indicating a notable disparity between clinical guidelines and clinical decision-making. The implications of such behaviors are multiple, piling unnecessary healthcare costs estimated at approximately $17,000 and potentially resulting in patient injury through inappropriate treatment or misinterpretation of laboratory results. Thus, greater education of medical practitioners on proper test ordering is of critical importance in an effort to curtail these disparities and optimize patient care outcomes. Furthermore, the predominance of drug abuse, such as cocaine, in patients presenting with chest pain, complicates the terrain of standard medical investigations. Identification of abuse is part of avoiding misdiagnosis and treatment methods. The necessity for an extended insight into a patient's history and presentation symptoms, particularly in acute settings, may determine what kind of tests should be requested as well as the resulting management protocols.

This helps to support the necessity for an integrated patient assessment, whereby investigations are not merely symptom-driven but context-driven, thereby making clinical decision-making relate to best practice and reducing the risk of inappropriate interventions. Overall, a critical appraisal of routine medical investigations helps to illustrate that patient factors and professional practice both have an overarching influence on test ordering behavior. Misconception- or social norm-based studies can lead to over-testing, which is not always linked to improved patient outcomes. As indicated by study outcomes examining test ordering practice and drug abuse in clinical presentations, there is a need for ongoing research and education to maximize these practices. Future action must be to establish an environment where clinical decisions are based on evidence-based guidelines and complete awareness of the patients' context, so that both resources are used effectively and patient care is optimized.

Medical investigations are a crucial cornerstone in diagnosing and treating disease, directly affecting the patient's outcome. Medical investigations cover a variety of assessments, from imaging scans and laboratory tests to clinical examinations that provide valuable information about a patient's health. Proper deployment of these investigations in a timely fashion allows medical professionals to diagnose conditions accurately and permit suitable treatment mechanisms. For instance, identifying malignancy-associated hypercalcemia (HM) by routine laboratory exams can lead to an immediate intervention that can alter the prognosis for malignancy patients such as lymphoma or adenocarcinoma (Aguila et al., 2022). Therefore, tests not only enhance diagnostic precision but also enable clinicians to monitor disease development and evaluate the efficacy of therapy, making their importance evident in the medical field. In an acute environment, the role of investigations becomes even more pivotal, particularly in neurologic emergencies, which can pose a high rate of medical admission. In such a situation, timely and definitive assessment is mandatory because it allows rapid decision-making and intervention strategies. For instance, acute neurological disorders can be responsible for 10–20% of these types of admissions, and hence, there is a need for quicker investigation techniques that will improve patient outcomes (Aminoff et al., 2018). The inclusion of investigations such as neuroimaging and neurological examination into acute pathways will enable clinicians to enhance interdisciplinary collaboration between emergency services and neurology specialties and encourage a multi-specialty pathway with shorter treatment delays as well as hospital length of stay. Furthermore, the worth of investigations extends beyond immediate clinical applications; they play an essential role in contemporary medical research and developing new treatment modalities. Ongoing diagnostic method innovations guide evidence-based care and lead to personalized medicine, wherein treatments are tailored to specific patient profiles based on detailed investigation results. This development is observed in recent studies related to conditions such as HM of malignancy, where identifying underlying biological mechanisms can lead to breakthrough treatments (Aguila et al., 2022). This, therefore, means that systematic application of questions enhances individual-patient therapy and contributes to the broad medical body of information, solidifying their tremendous place in today's medicine.

KEY TERMS FROM THIS CHAPTER

- Advanced imaging technology
- ALRC reports
- Biochemical markers
- Blood chemistry panels
- Chronic kidney disease (CKD)
- Clinical management plans
- CT scans
- Alanine aminotransferase (ALT)
- Automated hematology
- Blood cells
- Blood tests
- Chronic obstructive pulmonary disease (COPD)
- Concomitant ailments
- Data availability

CRITICAL THINKING QUESTIONS

1. **A core needle biopsy is typically used to obtain tissue from which of the following?**
   a. Solid organs or masses
   b. Blood vessels
   c. Bone marrow
   d. Skin lesions
2. **Which of the following endoscopic procedures is used to visualize the interior of the large intestine?**
   a. Laparoscopy
   b. Gastroscopy
   c. Colonoscopy
   d. Bronchoscopy
3. **Which blood test is most commonly used to assess kidney function?**
   a. ALT
   b. Creatinine
   c. Troponin
   d. Bilirubin
4. **Which component most indicates anemia in a complete blood count (CBC)?**
   a. Platelet count
   b. Hemoglobin
   c. WBC count
   d. Neutrophil percentage
5. **Which imaging technique involves ionizing radiation?**
   a. MRI
   b. Ultrasound
   c. PET scan
   d. CT scan

Short Answer Questions

1. What information can a Complete Blood Count (CBC) and blood chemistry panel provide, and how do these tests assist in diagnosing systemic conditions?
2. Compare the uses and limitations of X-rays, CT scans, and MRI in diagnosing internal abnormalities.
3. What are the different types of biopsy procedures, and how are they selected based on the clinical context?
4. In what ways are endoscopic procedures diagnostic and therapeutic, and which conditions commonly require endoscopy?
5. How does genetic testing support personalized medicine, and what types of conditions are most frequently evaluated using this method?
6. What are the key components of a routine urinalysis, and which conditions can it help detect or monitor?
7. How can the results of multiple investigations (e.g., blood tests, imaging, and urinalysis) be integrated to arrive at a comprehensive diagnosis?

Answers to Critical Thinking Questions

1. (a) 2. (c) 3. (b) 4. (b) 5. (d)

REFERENCES

1. Côté, E., Edwards, N. J., Ettinger, S. J., Fuentes, V. L., MacDonald, K. A., Scansen, B. A., Sisson, D. D., & Abbott, J. A. (2015). Management of incidentally detected heart murmurs in dogs and cats. *Journal of the American Veterinary Medical Association*, *246*(10), 1076–1088. https://doi.org/10.2460/javma.246.10.107Abela, A. G., Azzopardi, J., Calleja, N., Debono, M., et al. (2008). An audit of the management of diabetic ketoacidosis at St Luke's Hospital. https://core.ac.uk/download/46602182.pdf (accessed on 27th June 2025).
2. Abraham, N. S., Becker, R. C., Chan, F., Dauerman, H. L., et al. (2009). Management of platelet-directed pharmacotherapy in patients with atherosclerotic coronary artery disease undergoing elective endoscopic gastrointestinal procedures. https://core.ac.uk/download/pdf/82100823.pdf (accessed on 27th June 2025).
3. Agius, R. (2014). An evaluation of the bariatric surgical patient. https://core.ac.uk/download/46602470.pdf (accessed on 27th June 2025).
4. Ahmed, F., & Maisano, J. (2017). ToScA North America (6–8 June 2017, The University of Texas, Austin, TX) program. https://core.ac.uk/download/211334283.pdf (accessed on 27th June 2025).
5. Al Salhi, Y., Autieri, D., Carbone, A., Fuschi, A., et al. (2015). Combined laparoscopic pyelolithotomy and endoscopic pyelolithotripsy for staghorn calculi: Long-term follow-up results from a case series. https://core.ac.uk/download/54522245.pdf (accessed on 27th June 2025).
6. Alberdi, E., Lyon, A., Azevedo, B., Barnard, A., Boshuizen, H. P. A., et al. (2001). Expertise and the interpretation of computerized physiological data: Implications for the design of computerized monitoring in neonatal intensive care. https://core.ac.uk/download/9559372.pdf (accessed on 27th June 2025).
7. Alderson, P., Aro, A. R., Dragonas, T., Ettorre, E., et al. (2001). *Prenatal screening and genetics*. https://core.ac.uk/download/pdf/83462.pdf (accessed on 27th June 2025).
8. Alger, J. R., Bejjani, A., Frew, A. J., Kim, H. S., et al. (2012). Elevated glutamatergic compounds in pregenual anterior cingulate in pediatric autism spectrum disorder demonstrated by 1H MRS and 1H MRSI. https://core.ac.uk/download/323080471.pdf (accessed on 27th June 2025).
9. Amato-Gauci, A. J., Aquilina, S., & Boffa, M. J. (2005). A cross-sectional survey of a dermatology outpatient service in Malta. https://core.ac.uk/download/46601918.pdf (accessed on 27th June 2025).
10. Aminoff, M. J., Inouye, S. K., Pearce, J. M. S., Rabinstein, A. A., & Weatherall, M. W. (2018). Acute neurology: A suggested approach. https://core.ac.uk/download/195329417.pdf (accessed on 27th June 2025).
11. Aquilina, J., Cefai, E., & Mallia, M. (2015). A review on the investigation of peripheral neuropathy at Mater Dei Hospital. https://core.ac.uk/download/46603552.pdf (accessed on 27th June 2025).
12. Argano, V., Balistreri, C. R., Giarratana, R. M., Lio, D., et al. (2019). On the road to accurate biomarkers for cardiometabolic diseases by integrating precision and gender medicine approaches. https://core.ac.uk/download/268910274.pdf (accessed on 27th June 2025).

13. Bandeeri, N., Henry, J. A., Meredith, C., Treacy, K., et al. (2004). The prevalence of cocaine-associated chest pain in a London hospital. https://core.ac.uk/download/5230488.pdf (accessed on 27th June 2025).

14. Becker, R. C., Blanco, A., Blomback, M., Cambas, B., Chantarangkul, V., Chantarangkul, V., Chitolie, A., et al. (2003). Guidelines on fibrinogen assays. https://core.ac.uk/download/9349786.pdf (accessed on 27th June 2025).

15. Bellati, F., Caserta, D., Costanzi, F., De Marco, G., et al. (2018). Real-time virtual sonography in gynecology & obstetrics: Literature's analysis and case series. https://core.ac.uk/download/195777140.pdf (accessed on 27th June 2025).

16. Bellini, T., Bonaccorsi, G., Bramanti, B., Carè, A., et al. (2019). "Bridging the gap": Everything that could have been avoided if we had applied gender medicine, pharmacogenetics and personalized medicine in the gender-omics and sex-omics era. https://core.ac.uk/download/286075866.pdf (accessed on 27th June 2025).

17. Biagioli, F. E., Hamilton, A., & Warren, J. (2007). Evaluation of apparent life-threatening events in infants. https://core.ac.uk/download/62760030.pdf (accessed on 27th June 2025).

18. Biggi, A., Fretzayas, A., Gervaix, A., Haberlik, A., Hitzel, A., Hitzel, A., Hoberman, A., et al. (2005). How does study quality affect the results of a diagnostic meta-analysis? https://core.ac.uk/download/57953.pdf (accessed on 27th June 2025).

19. Bourne, J., Firman, E., Mottram, C., Round, R., et al. (2005). A safer place for patients: Learning to improve patient safety. https://core.ac.uk/download/105328.pdf (accessed on 27th June 2025).

20. Bradu, A., Dobre, G. M., Duma, V. F., Erdelyi, R., et al. (2020). Dental diagnosis and treatment assessments: Between X-rays radiography and optical coherence tomography. https://core.ac.uk/download/341624142.pdf (accessed on 27th June 2025).

21. Brodbelt, D. C., Charalambous, M., & Volk, H. A. (2016). The evidence behind the diagnostic investigation of canine idiopathic epilepsy. https://core.ac.uk/download/36779228.pdf (accessed on 27th June 2025).

22. Brodbelt, D. C., Charalambous, M., & Volk, H. A. (2016). The evidence behind the treatment of canine idiopathic epilepsy. https://core.ac.uk/download/36779227.pdf (accessed on 27th June 2025).

23. Brouwers, A., Links, T., & van der Horst-Schrivers, A. N. A. (2015). Somatostatin receptor scintigraphy in medullary thyroid cancer. https://core.ac.uk/download/pdf/157691621.pdf (accessed on 27th June 2025).

24. Brys, A. K., Sheth, M. R., Sohn, D. D., Sweidan, R., et al. (2015). Diagnostic and therapeutic considerations in idiopathic hyper eosinophilia with warm autoimmune hemolytic anemia. https://core.ac.uk/download/323075654.pdf (accessed on 27th June 2025).

25. Calfee, C. S., & Meyer, N. J. (2017). Novel translational approaches to the search for precision therapies for acute respiratory distress syndrome. https://core.ac.uk/download/323074546.pdf (accessed on 27th June 2025).

26. Cameron, P., Cooke, M., & Schull, M. (2011). A framework for measuring quality in the emergency department. https://core.ac.uk/download/1385753.pdf (accessed on 27th June 2025).

27. Camilleri, N., Sammut, D., & Schembri, S. (2004). An overview of the management of congestive heart failure in Malta. https://core.ac.uk/download/46601876.pdf (accessed on 27th June 2025).

28. Camp Jr, C. H., & Cicerone, M. T. (2017). Histological coherent Raman imaging: A prognostic review. http://arxiv.org/abs/1709.07325 (accessed on 27th June 2025).

29. Carreras Torras, C., & Gay Escoda, C. (2015). Techniques for early diagnosis of oral squamous cell carcinoma: Systematic review. https://core.ac.uk/download/71042585.pdf (accessed on 27th June 2025).

30. Chauffard, A., Vickers, A., Hingorani, A. D., Timmis, A., Vickers, A. J., Hay, A. D., Mar Del, C., et al. (2015). The science of clinical practice: Disease diagnosis or patient prognosis? Evidence about "what is likely to happen" should shape clinical practice. https://core.ac.uk/download/19747711.pdf (accessed on 27th June 2025).

31. Chew, D. J., Daniels, J. B., Irom, S., Keil, M., et al. (2012). Evaluation of the efficacy and safety of high dose short duration enrofloxacin treatment regimen for uncomplicated urinary tract infections in dogs. https://core.ac.uk/download/323068657.pdf (accessed on 27th June 2025).

32. Choo, K. K. R., Glisson, W. B., & Grispos, G. (2017). Medical cyber-physical systems development: A forensics-driven approach. http://arxiv.org/abs/1708.05374 (accessed on 27th June 2025).

33. Crawford, R. J., Elliott, J. M., Hancock, M. J., Smith, A. C., et al. (2018). Advancing imaging technologies for patients with spinal pain: With a focus on whiplash injury. https://core.ac.uk/download/161704527.pdf (accessed on 27th June 2025).

34. Creighton, E. K., Keating, M. K., Lyons, L. A., Sisó, S., et al. (2016). Characterization of an inherited neurologic syndrome in Toyger cats with forebrain commissural malformations, ventriculomegaly and interhemispheric cysts. https://core.ac.uk/download/323069548.pdf (accessed on 27th June 2025).

35. D'Souza, E., Jiwa, M., Krejany, C., Meng, R., et al. (2018). How are junior doctors managing patients with self-limiting illnesses at their first presentation? A video vignette study. https://core.ac.uk/download/213607031.pdf (accessed on 27th June 2025).

36. De Sadeleer, C., Dobbeleir, A., Ham, H., Peremans, K., et al. (2011). Nuclear medicine: Investigation of renal function in small animal medicine. https://core.ac.uk/download/55842771.pdf (accessed on 27th June 2025).

37. Delaney, A., Laupacis, A., Liberati, A., Weale, A. R., Kulkarni, A. V., Lokker, C., Moher, D., et al. (2013). Bibliometrics of systematic reviews: Analysis of citation rates and journal impact factors. https://core.ac.uk/download/16664987.pdf (accessed on 27th June 2025).

38. Doss, M., Fairley, R., Murphy, K., et al. (2020). The risk of cancer from CT scans and other sources of low-dose radiation: A critical appraisal of methodologic quality. https://core.ac.uk/download/305124024.pdf (accessed on 27th June 2025).

39. Esler, J., Harrison, K., Jeffrey, R., Kirby, J., et al. (2007). Oocyte cryopreservation as an adjunct to the assisted reproductive technologies. https://core.ac.uk/download/12759048.pdf (accessed on 27th June 2025).

40. Farley, J. M. B., Maclay, J. D., McCowan, C., Milroy, R., et al. (2017). Obtaining tissue diagnosis in lung cancer patients with poor performance status and its influence on treatment and survival. https://core.ac.uk/download/77601615.pdf (accessed on 27th June 2025).

41. Fenech, M., Gouder, C., & Montefort, S. (2012). Interstitial lung disease in Malta. https://core.ac.uk/download/46602323.pdf (accessed on 27th June 2025).

42. Fiehn, O., Ismail, I. T., & Showalter, M. R. (2019). Inborn errors of metabolism in the era of untargeted metabolomics and lipidomic. https://core.ac.uk/download/323068986.pdf (accessed on 27th June 2025).

43. Fortina, P., Kricka, L. J., Park, J. Y., & Polsky, T. G. (2015). The future of laboratory medicine–A 2014 perspective. https://core.ac.uk/download/54509579.pdf (accessed on 27th June 2025).

44. Frantzi, M., Latosinska, A., Merseburger, A. S., Mischak, H., et al. (2017). Clinical proteomics for precision medicine: The bladder cancer case. https://core.ac.uk/download/111557480.pdf (accessed on 27th June 2025).

45. Geddie, W. R., & Schwock, J. (2012). Diagnosis of B-cell non-Hodgkin lymphomas with small-/intermediate-sized cells in cytopathology. https://core.ac.uk/download/pdf/8736640.pdf (accessed on 27th June 2025).

46. Griff, S. (2019). Infuses der Art der Materialgewinnung auf die Diagnosefindung in der Lungenpathologie. https://core.ac.uk/download/222573993.pdf (accessed on 27th June 2025).

47. Haimes, E., & Toom, V. (2014). Hidden in full sight: Kinship, science and the law in the aftermath of the Srebrenica genocide. https://core.ac.uk/download/41069578.pdf (accessed on 27th June 2025).

48. Hansell, A., Tate, A. R., Nicholson, A., Tate, A. R., Tate, A. R., Lovis, C., Edwards, C. J., et al. (2013). Optimizing use of electronic health records to describe the presentation of rheumatoid arthritis in primary care: A strategy for developing code lists. https://core.ac.uk/download/9837008.pdf (accessed on 27th June 2025).

49. Jones, K. (2004). Mission drift in qualitative research, or moving toward a systematic review of qualitative studies, moving back to a more systematic narrative review. https://core.ac.uk/download/76770.pdf (accessed on 27th June 2025).

50. Kitsiou, A., Caforio, A. L. P., Porta-Sanchez, A., Vahanian, A., Iung, B., Carrera, C., Szymanski, C., et al. (2013). ESC core curriculum for the general cardiologist (2013). https://core.ac.uk/download/55756305.pdf (accessed on 27th June 2025).

51. Loccisano, A. (2016). Platelet-rich plasma for the treatment of partial rotator cuff tears. https://open.bu.edu/bitstream/2144/14355/9/Loccisano_bu_0017N_10415.pdf (accessed on 27th June 2025).

52. Majeed, A., Tate, A. R., Verdecchia, A., Ryerson, A. B., Martin, A. G. R., Rachet, B., Yawn, B., et al. (2009). Determining the date of diagnosis–is it a simple matter? The impact of different approaches to dating diagnosis on estimates of delayed care for ovarian cancer in UK primary care. https://core.ac.uk/download/2709969.pdf (accessed on 27th June 2025).

53. N/A. (1985). *Focal Spot, Fall 1985.* https://core.ac.uk/download/129069250.pdf (accessed on 27th June 2025).

54. N/A. (2010). *A Research Documentation on Men's Sexual Health Disclosed.* https://core.ac.uk/download/pdf/18491829.pdf (accessed on 27th June 2025).

55. Opeskin, B., Weisbrot, D., & Breen, K. (2025). *Essentially Yours: The Protection of Human Genetic Information in Australia.* https://core.ac.uk/download/pdf/30672952.pdf (accessed on 27th June 2025).

56. Pedescoll Aguila, C. (2022). *Hypercalcemia of Malignancy in The Dog* (Bachelor's thesis, Universitat Autònoma de Barcelona. Facultat de Veterinària). https://core.ac.uk/download/532375199.pdf (accessed on 27th June 2025).

57. Piacentine, L., & Weiss, M. (2006). Psychometric properties of the Readiness for Hospital Discharge Scale. https://core.ac.uk/download/213077027.pdf (accessed on 27th June 2025).

58. Zammit, E. (2009). *The Irritable Bowel Syndrome.* https://core.ac.uk/download/46602223.pdf (accessed on 27th June 2025).

PHARMACOLOGY IN GENERAL PRACTICE

4

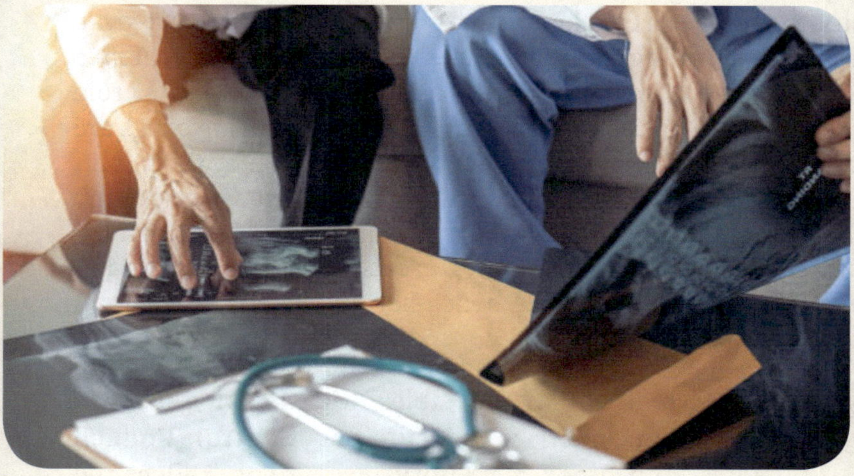

Introduction

Pharmacology is a critical area of practice, with the greatest significance of integrating drugs into the treatment of patients. Pharmacology gives healthcare providers the knowledge to formulate informed treatment decisions. This subject entails the pharmacology of drug action and physiological responses of the body, which are crucial for building effective therapeutic regimens. Because patients present with a wide array of conditions, clinicians must navigate the subtleties of pharmacokinetics (PK) and pharmacodynamics (PD) to tailor therapies to the patient's individual needs. Regulation schemes, such as the establishment of the South African Health Products Regulatory Authority (SAHPRA), demonstrate the necessity for efficient drug approval mechanisms and strict safety assessments to provide only effective drugs to patients who need them (Antrobus et al., 2018). In addition, the clinical use of pharmacological knowledge depends not only on the clinician's drug knowledge but also on the drugs being available to the patients. An increase in the regulatory backlog

LEARNING OBJECTIVES

After studying this chapter, you will be able to:

1. Understand the historical development of pharmacology
2. Describe the fundamentals of pharmacokinetics and pharmacodynamics
3. Discuss commonly prescribed medications in general practice
4. Explain adverse drug reactions and drug interactions
5. Focus on patient education and medication adherence
6. Define ethical considerations in pharmacology

may hinder the timely therapeutic effect, and thus, robust regulatory structures that can handle the complexity of today's healthcare are crucial (Antrobus et al., 2018). With the application of quality management systems and prioritization of risk-based evaluations, healthcare professionals can enhance practice effectiveness and ensure that they utilize drugs with the optimal safety profiles. In the congruent application of pharmacology and regulatory processes, balancing treatment innovation with patient safety is efficiently played, ultimately strengthening general practice integrity (Antrobus et al., 2018). In conclusion, the significance of pharmacology in general practice cannot be overestimated given its wide-ranging impact on patient outcomes and health provision. With the increased development of the world of drugs and regulatory policy, practitioners need to be astute during their training and application of the concepts of pharmacology. Creating effective treatment regimens requires not only in-depth knowledge of many drugs but also a feeling of worth in the regulatory system that governs their administration. As the field progresses, general physicians must advocate and engage in more proper regulation processes so that patients can be given access to required drugs at the right time. Lastly, an EBP of pharmacology leads to better clinical decision-making and patient care outcomes for general practice overall.

Definition of Pharmacology

Pharmacology, a fundamental branch of medicine, is the science that examines drug action upon biological systems. Pharmacology encompasses drug properties, drug actions, and their pharmacological effect and toxicities. Pharmacology is the bridging science between medical science and clinical practice, providing medical professionals with an integrated view of pharmacodynamics and PK. By outlining the mechanisms through which drugs alter physiological functions, pharmacology informs the prescribing process so clinicians can weigh potential gains against risk. In everyday general practice, this information is vital, where clinicians traditionally manage a variety of illnesses that are responsive to pharmacologic therapy. Knowing pharmacology enables clinicians to anticipate drug interactions and select pertinent therapeutic regimens for patients, thereby enhancing quality care in everyday clinical practice. Pharmacological advancement has been formulated under the influence of regulatory forces shaping drug development and approval. Regulatory bodies, such as the Medicines Control Council, have played an essential role in establishing standards and ensuring drugs are effective and safe for consumption by the public. The regulatory cycle involves extensive scrutiny and comparison among world authorities, which highlights areas of improvement and performance benchmarking.

For instance, substantial variations in registration timetables, for example, between South Africa's Medicines Control Council and other regulatory institutions, reflect the complexity of pharmacological regulation (Banoo et al., 2019). Apart from assuring quality and safety, these regulatory procedures also enhance individuals' trust in pharmacological medication. As practicing physicians navigate the dynamic world of medicine, compliance with regulatory guidelines is essential to maximize patient outcomes and prevent risks from pharmacotherapy.

Further, the advent of novel psychoactive substances has added complexity to the pharmacological domain, presenting new challenges for regulators and healthcare professionals. The Advisory Council on the Misuse of Drugs has been at the forefront of addressing challenges presented by these drugs, urging a multi-faceted approach towards understanding and minimizing potential harm (Advisory Council on the Misuse of Drugs, 2011).

Pharmacology provides the scientific foundation on which to base an understanding of the effects of these drugs on health so that GPs can make informed discussions about their use. This evolving landscape underscores the necessity for continuous education in pharmacology to cope with new drugs effectively and educate patients on their implications. The term pharmacology, therefore, means more than merely the science of drugs; it is a constantly evolving dynamic interaction between science, regulation, and clinical use that practitioners in general practice have to cope with effectively (Figure 4.1).

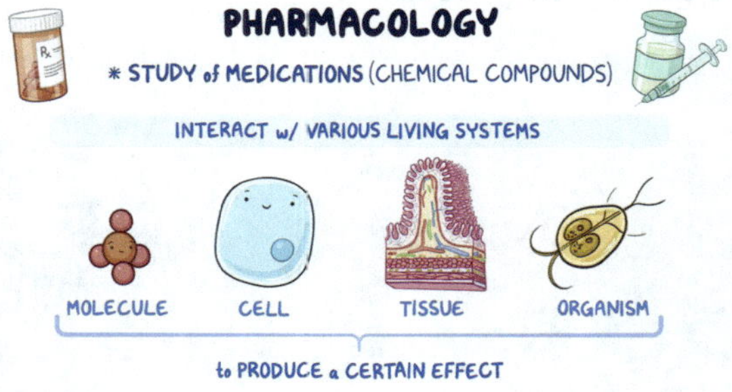

Figure 4.1. Pharmacology.

Source: https://www.osmosis.org/_next/image?url=https%3A%2F%2Fd16qt3wv6xm098.cloudfront.net%2FsPEgvPMUTGqq0LnDc7QQLSQuSkKEC8aN%2F_.jpg&w=3840&q=75.

Importance of Pharmacology in General Practice

The intricate interaction of pharmacology with general practice is brought out by the significant role played by physicians in managing patient treatment regimens. A comprehensive understanding of pharmacology allows GPs to provide informed decisions about medications given to their patients. These include mechanisms of drugs, therapeutic actions, contraindications, and potential drug interactions, which are crucial in tailoring treatment plans to patient requirements. Additionally, professionals must keep themselves informed about evolving guidelines and advancements in the pharmacology field to ensure optimal patient outcomes. For instance, numerous patients in primary care may have chronic conditions that overlap with intricate medication therapies. Thus, a good grounding in pharmacology ensures proper communication between healthcare providers and between healthcare providers and patients to ensure that the treatment is safe and effective. This education ultimately improves the overall standard of care in general practices, resulting in better health outcomes and patient satisfaction.

Pharmacology is also instrumental in impacting patient safety and adverse drug reaction management, which is another crucial matter in general practice. GPs are often the first point of contact for patients with side effects of drugs prescribed by them, hence requiring complete understanding of pharmacovigilance. Pharmacological principles in understanding enable physicians to identify, assess, and reduce risks of drug therapy effectively. By way of example, with around 8 million patients with migraine in the UK, the evolution of migraine drugs, like triptans and new drugs, is an old story of practice professionals needing to be well aware of pharmacological progress that can make a considerable difference in alleviating patient burden.

Staying current with such drug classification and treatment options advances is crucial for primary care physicians. The ability to handle and communicate drug therapy's risks and advantages is thus central to patient health protection and better treatment outcomes (Overy et al., 2014). Besides enhancing patient care, pharmacology use extends beyond that to encompass motivating multidisciplinary teams in healthcare settings to work collectively. Coordination of knowledge between various disciplines, such as nursing, physiotherapy, and pharmacy, is crucial in delivering integrated care. For example, in ICUs, pharmacological principles of drugs assist in efficient collaboration and patient management procedures. Coordination of healthcare workers ensures that each healthcare worker contributes his or her pharmacological knowledge of drugs to avoid errors and improve therapeutic effects. This has been emphasized in recent studies that indicate the importance of synergy in medical information and effective communication in critical care environments (Hanekom et al., 2017). Through collaboration, professionals can combine their expertise, resulting in a more robust healthcare system that can better address the complex needs of patients.

4.1. Historical Development of Pharmacology

Learning Outcome

1. Discuss early medicinal practices and herbal remedies
2. Deal with the evolution of pharmacological science
3. Focus on key milestones in drug discovery

The evolution of drugs throughout history has had a considerable impact on current general practice, highlighting advances in drug discovery and control. Throughout the mid-20th century, the field experienced sudden developments with the discovery of new therapeutic agents as the major driving factor. The Thalidomide catastrophe brought to light the risks involved with inadequate testing of drugs, forcing greater vigilance in strict safety procedures and extensive clinical trials. A Witness Seminar notes that the 1950s and 1960s were an exciting era for clinical pharmacology in the UK, calling for in-depth knowledge of the effect of drugs on humans and the development of proper safety standards. It forced regulatory authorities and pharmaceutical industries to re-evaluate their roles, resulting in enhanced coordination in ensuring drug efficacy and safety, forming the basis of today's pharmacovigilance practices in daily general practice (Reynolds et al., 2008). As pharmacological practice evolved worldwide, regulatory systems kept improving with both public health needs and challenges posed by novel drugs being met. In South Africa, reforms to the drug registration process resulted in the establishment of the SAHPRA, replacing the Medicines Control Council. This change came to address enormous backlogs in the handling of applications while emphasizing accountability and quality in processes.

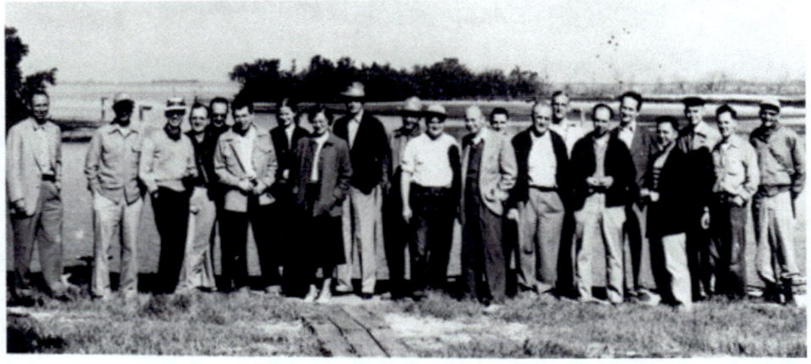

Figure 4.2. Early College of Medicine faculty, including Thomas H. Maren, at Cedar Key in 1955.

Source: https://pharmacology.med.ufl.edu/files/2017/09/EarlyFaculty.png.

Historical reviews reveal that the successful implementation of an effective regulatory environment hinges on incorporating risk-based evaluation methods and quality management systems that foster decision-making and openness. Such innovations feature prominently in today's pharmacology, as they facilitate the confidence of family practitioners to prescribe medication that has undergone rigorous scrutiny (Antrobus et al., 2018). Furthermore, the historical course of pharmacology reflects the ongoing dynamic between innovation, regulation, and practice. Clinical pharmacology's entry into practice has enabled a deeper understanding of drug interactions, side effects, and therapeutic response, fostering a culture of evidence-based prescribing. This background reminds healthcare professionals to keep up with evolving drug regulation and principles of pharmacology so that drugs can be used safely and effectively in patient care. By identifying the lessons learned from past pharmacological challenges and regulation shifts, practitioners can continue to advocate strict patient care standards, based on an intimate familiarity with drug safety and efficacy, integral to today's clinical practice (Figure 4.2).

4.1.1. Early Medicinal Practices and Herbal Remedies

The ancient medical treatments and herbal medicine are integral to pharmacology, having evolved from the centuries-old reliance on nature-derived drugs for therapy. All ancient civilizations across the globe employed various plant-derived materials, suggesting an intimate relationship between human beings and their worlds. The treatments were essentially holistic in principle, treating not only the physical illness but also the individuals' mind and soul. Therefore, herbal medicine was typically administered through complex preparation and use, reflecting a sophisticated understanding of plant traits before modern scientific procedure. The use of these medicines was the basis of contemporary pharmacology by fostering awareness of diversity and laying the groundwork for the scientific study of drug interactions and drug action. The significance of ancient medicinal traditions, particularly in multi-cultural societies such as Africa, cannot be underestimated, wherein 80% of the population is estimated to still rely on African traditional medicine (ATM). ATM is characterized by traditions and conventions deeply rooted in indigenous culture and convention, exemplifying the oral transmission of medicinal plant information. The practices are diverse and complex enough for formal documentation and integration into mainstream healthcare systems. Documentation and codification of this tacit knowledge make it possible for the therapeutic potential of indigenous flora to be more effectively utilized in conjunction with traditional medicine. This syncretic unification can facilitate the development of integrative approaches respectful of modern standards and traditional savoir-faire, ultimately facilitating better care for patients and pharmacological equity in practice (Diallo et al., 2013).

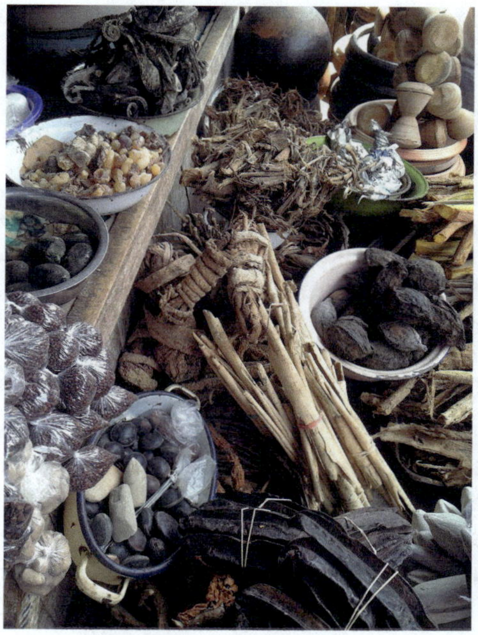

Figure 4.3. Medicinal plants on a market stall, Ghana.

Source: https://upload.wikimedia.org/wikipedia/commons/thumb/7/70/Traditional_Medicine.JPG/800px-Traditional_Medicine.JPG.

As the global medical community continues to appreciate the need for a blend of contemporary pharmacological treatment and traditional herbal treatments, whether safety and efficacy are debated becomes the question. Requests for uniform practice reflect a desire to place herbal remedies on the same criteria as traditional medicines. Advances like the One-World Medicine idea encourage a team approach that integrates traditional and Western medical practice, with patient safety and informed choice taking precedence. While the past practice of herbal medicine shows a wealth of knowledge, today's practice has to emphasize sustainability, quality control, and evidence-based confirmation. In doing so, the embrace of such ancient medical practice by conventional pharmacological practice could enhance overall global health, as seen in legislative frameworks like the Nagoya protocol, aiming to codify benefit-sharing regulation (Abdelfatah et al., 2019) (Figure 4.3).

4.1.2. Evolution of Pharmacological Science

The history of pharmacology is deeply entwined with the pursuit of well-being and health by human beings, as evidenced by archaeological findings pointing towards ancient pharmacological practice dating back to prehistoric ages. Neanderthals purportedly were already utilizing medicinal plants to treat ailments, suggestive of a natural experience of therapeutic medicines in nature. With the advancement of civilizations came the sophistication of their methods of medicine. The Egyptians and Greeks employed plant therapies, like Papaver somniferum, and techniques akin to modern hypnosis in their therapeutic rituals. Such an early intersection of psychology and physical therapy existed before the modern contemporary understanding of mind-body interactions, a fundamental aspect of pharmacology today, particularly in general practice, where patient welfare is always the priority. A sensitivity editor to the historical roots of pharmacological practice reveals how underlying ideas about the treatment of body and mind changed over thousands of years. As pharmacology developed from crude remedies to more formalized scientific practice, the burden of empirical evidence gained increasingly greater significance. The 19th and 20th centuries were the decades of explosive progress, with rigorous scientific probing and the structuring of pharmacodynamics and PK as core branches of the science. Drug development began based on greater knowledge about human physiology and biochemistry. Leading researchers and chemists isolated and synthesized active pharmaceutical ingredients, which enabled targeted therapies to cure specific conditions more effectively than ever before. This revolution was a paradigm shift in medical practice, as physicians began prescribing evidence-based medicine rather than relying mainly on traditional remedies.

Thus, pharmacological science's evolution revolutionized patient treatment and provided the basis for the very demanding drug treatments in modern general practice. Despite remarkable progress, the controversy between conventional pharmacological approaches and alternative therapies such as homeopathy continues to evoke considerable interest among physicians. Historical accounts indicate that homeopathy, despite being founded on principles very different from evidence-based pharmacology, was the dominant force for decades following its discovery in the late 18th century. Certain medical professionals continue to attempt to research the use of homeopathic therapies, especially when conventional therapies have failed or where patients specifically ask for non-pharmacological interventions. The comparison of the two paradigms of treatment side by side raises fundamental issues of efficacy and safety in pharmacology, particularly in the general practice environment. There must be a compromise between scientific proof and practical considerations since health professionals want to provide a more holistic care tailored to individual needs, marking the primary narrative of evolution in pharmacology in delineating contemporary medical practice (Aabel et al., 2017) (Figure 4.4).

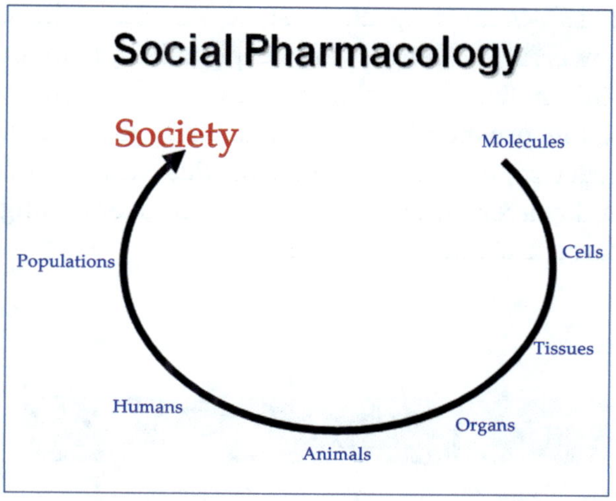

Figure 4.4. Social pharmacology is the ultimate evolution of pharmacological sciences.

Source: https://www.researchgate.net/profile/Margaux-Lafaurie/publication/351963513/figure/fig1/AS:1051669144027138@1627748871801/Different-topics-in-pharmacology-social-pharmacology-is-the-ultimate-evolution-of.jpg.

4.1.3. Key Milestones in Drug Discovery

The landscape of drug discovery has evolved significantly across the decades, with some milestones being standouts that have achieved tremendous progress in pharmacological interventions in mainstream medicine. One is the synthesis and identification of the major drug compounds, which began in earnest in the mid-20th century. This era witnessed the development of sulfa drugs and penicillin, which transformed the treatment of bacterial infection and heralded the advent of antibiotics as a pillar of modern medicine.

The introduction of these drugs changed not just patient outcomes but also impacted the procedures through which new drugs were screened and confirmed. This trajectory of history emphasizes the general shift from the isolation of natural products to the rational design and synthesis of medicines that subsequently came to define the drug discovery landscape. Technology has also played an underlying role in shaping today's drug discovery, particularly through integrating computational approaches and high-throughput screening practices. These technologies, in addition to accelerating the discovery of candidate drugs, have also improved the efficacy and safety profiles before they enter clinical trials. The advancement of product definition companies represents a paradigm shift in translating laboratory results into drugs that can be sold. By acquisition of early-stage results and product development, these organizations create a pipeline connection with pharmaceutical firms, enhancing new drug commercialization (Roth et al., 2010).

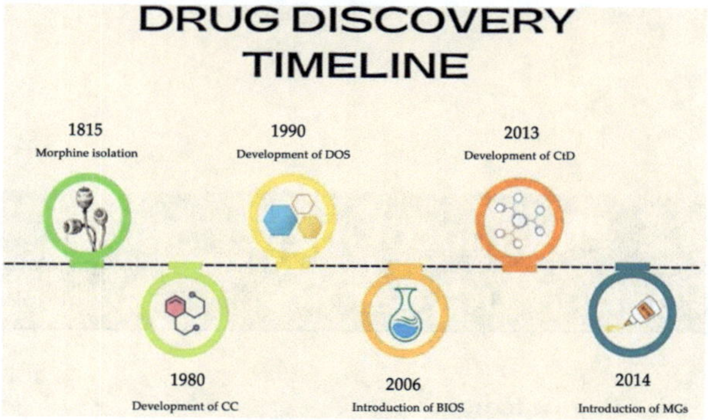

Figure 4.5. Drug discovery field milestones.

Source: https://www.researchgate.net/publication/370490675/figure/fig1/AS:11431281244792397@1715996740329/Drug-discovery-field-milestones.png.

The fusion of scientific discovery with business models thus constitutes a crucial milestone in guaranteeing that new therapeutics consistently transition from concept to clinical use. Despite the advances, the pharma sector continues to struggle with a few foundational issues, primarily productivity and R&D expenditure. Exorbitantly high clinical trial attrition rates capture a dismal pattern of declining efficiency in drug discovery during the past few years, which calls for innovative solutions to reverse this trend. Applying modeling and simulation (M&S) techniques is regarded as one such option. Through creating more profound insight into mechanistic knowledge and encouraging implementable expertise in the R&D pipeline, M&S has pledged to optimize development efficiency (Hunt et al., 2013). With drug discovery confronting these powerful challenges, the perpetual adjustment and makeover within the field is bound to shape prospects for pharmacology in general practice, demanding continuous innovation and concerted working together in overcoming current challenges (Figure 4.5).

Test Your Knowledge

1. What role did early medicinal practices and herbal remedies play in the development of pharmacology?
2. What are some important milestones in the history of drug discovery that marked the transition from natural remedies to synthetic drugs?

4.2. Pharmacokinetics and Pharmacodynamics

Learning Outcome

1. Understand the definition and significance of pharmacokinetics
2. Describe pharmacodynamics and its implications
3. Focus on the interaction between pharmacokinetics and pharmacodynamics

Pharmacokinetics (PK) and pharmacodynamics are essential for effective medication management in primary care. PK examines how a drug is absorbed, distributed, metabolized, and excreted by the body, and it characterizes the time course of drug concentration in terms of the dose administered. Clinicians use the principles of PK to tailor dosage according to patient factors such as age, weight, and renal function. This individualization is especially crucial in pediatrics, where pharmacokinetic models guide recommendations to maximize therapeutic effects while reducing toxicity. Through the use of such models, practitioners can set safe dosing regimens that take into account the heterogeneous physiological responses seen in different patient populations, facilitating improved healthcare practice, particularly in intricate cases of pediatric infectious diseases where there is a high need for accurate dosing (Abdel-Rahman et al., 2014). Pharmacodynamics, on the other hand, addresses the drug's biological activity and mechanisms of action. It explores drugs' interactions with physiologic systems and the association between such interactions and therapeutic or toxic effects. The pharmacodynamic profile of a drug, including potency, is crucial in the computation of the therapeutic window and the maximization of clinical effects. For medications such as stimulants used in attention deficit/hyperactivity disorder (ADHD) therapy, an understanding of both pharmacokinetic and pharmacodynamic interactions can enhance therapeutic outcomes. Empirical data have shown that stimulant medication is effective across the majority of populations but that it might have slight differences by age and gender, which can impact patient outcomes. These nuances underscore the necessity for ongoing research and tailored therapeutic plans in clinical practice daily (Barke et al., 2010). The integration of PK and pharmacodynamics in practice not only enhances clinical decision-making but also allows for the safe and effective use of drugs among fluctuating patient populations. The integration of these two aspects is particularly illustrated with combination drugs, where more than one drug is taken simultaneously. With multiple drugs, it is necessary to know the pharmacokinetic profile to know how drugs will react with one another and how monitoring should be conducted. Moreover, novel model strategies in pharmacodynamics and PK are unveiling prospects for more targeted drug development, especially in infectious diseases and immunology. By accepting such innovations, GPs can improve administration so that they align with evolving therapeutic practices and contribute positively to patient outcomes (Abdel-Rahman et al., 2014).

4.2.1. Definition and Significance of Pharmacokinetics

Pharmacokinetics is an integral discipline of pharmacology involving absorption, distribution, metabolism, and excretion (ADME) of medications by the organism. Multi-aspect research is crucial to drug interaction with biological tissues. By studying how a drug crosses blood-organ barriers to enter the bloodstream, distribute to tissues, is metabolized by the body's enzymes, and ultimately is excreted, PK provides critical information needed to optimize therapeutic utility and safety. Clinicians must consider pharmacokinetic principles when prescribing medicines because variations in these processes can lead to varying therapeutic effects in different patients. Thus, PK is not only a scientific foundation but also a practical method for guiding clinical decision-making in daily practice, delivering customized patient care that maximizes the therapeutic potential of drug therapy. In practice, pharmacology, the relevance of PK is underscored by its capability to explain inter-individual variation in drug response. Age, gender, prior medical conditions, and genetic polymorphisms can profoundly impact pharmacokinetic parameters, thus the drug's concentration and efficacy in patients.

Pharmacokinetic innovations are at the center of precision medicine design, which focuses on tailoring drug therapy to the individual's own characteristics. Recent studies emphasize the importance of drug-metabolizing enzymes and transporters and drug-dietary substance or biologics interaction, highlighting the complexities of pharmacotherapy (Abduljalil et al., 2019). Sensitivity to such differences promotes good prescribing practice, which results in enhanced patient care and minimizes drug-related side effects. Furthermore, continuing advances in pharmacokinetic research are central to enhanced clinical practice. Emerging technologies and methods, such as physiologically-based pharmacokinetic modeling, yield greater insight into drug performance in differing groups and conditions. Studies also explore novel metabolic pathways and the function of novel enzymes, thereby increasing our understanding of drug interactions and treatments (Abduljalil et al., 2019). Clinicians with information regarding these developments can more accurately forecast potential drug-drug interactions and drug pharmacokinetic effects of comorbidities. Therefore, ongoing development and integration of pharmacokinetic practice into the day-to-day routine not only enable safer and more effective prescribing of drugs but also foster an added appreciation for the unique therapeutic landscape of each patient (Figure 4.6).

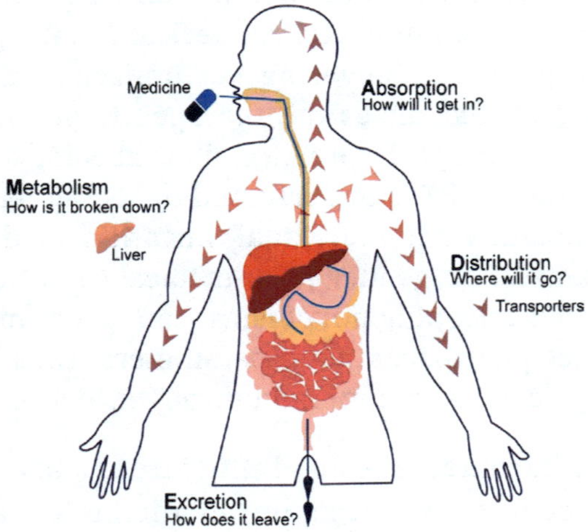

Figure 4.6. Pharmacokinetics.

Source: https://f.hubspotusercontent10.net/hubfs/5802814/image3.png.

4.2.2. Understanding Pharmacodynamics and Its Implications

Pharmacodynamics, the study of how drugs affect biological systems, provides valuable information about mechanisms of action and therapeutic effects of various pharmacologic agents. Knowing the complex interaction between a drug and its target receptors helps health practitioners to predict the safety and efficacy of drugs.

This information is particularly valuable in general practice, as physicians must select the optimal therapeutic interventions among variable patient populations with due consideration to interindividual variability in drug response. The combination of drug concentration and effect, influenced by factors such as receptor affinity and intrinsic activity, forms the foundation for treatment paradigms, helping practitioners optimize dosages to maximize therapeutic effects while minimizing toxicity. Thus, a practical knowledge of pharmacodynamics offers a foundation on which clinicians can make appropriate decisions regarding drug handling in primary care. Beyond efficacy, the impact of pharmacodynamics also extends into the overall fields of safety and therapeutic drug monitoring. Adverse drug reactions can be highly variable from patient to patient based on genetic, environmental, and physiological considerations that affect drug metabolism and excretion. For instance, variations in the activity of cytochrome P450 enzymes can lead to dramatic variations in treatment response, potentially leading to treatment failure or toxicity. Thus, the use of pharmacodynamic principles assists practitioners to identify populations at risk who may require more tailored dosing regimens. Again, the principle of drug interaction, either pharmacodynamic or pharmacokinetic, can lead to a better understanding of how a patient's drug profile impacts treatment efficacy.

These are crucial in everyday practice, as patient treatment regularly involves the co-prescription of a plurality of drugs. Pharmacodynamics becomes important in certain clinical scenarios, e.g., managing chronic inflammatory conditions like psoriatic arthritis (PsA). The introduction of tumor necrosis factor inhibitors (TNFi) revolutionized PsA treatment with stunning clinical performance and the ability to prevent radiographic progression in most patients. However, insight into the drug's pharmacodynamics underscores the value of consideration of patient-specific factors, including immunogenicity, to maximize therapeutic effects. Because some patients will not be successful on TNFi, knowing pharmacodynamic properties allows clinicians to assess the potential for success with such treatment or seek other options, such as biosimilars or other targeted therapy. To effectively cope with issues such in pharmacotherapy, one must apply the principles of pharmacodynamics in day-to-day clinical decision-making, enhancing patient care and overall outcomes in practice (Kraft et al., 2017) (Figure 4.7).

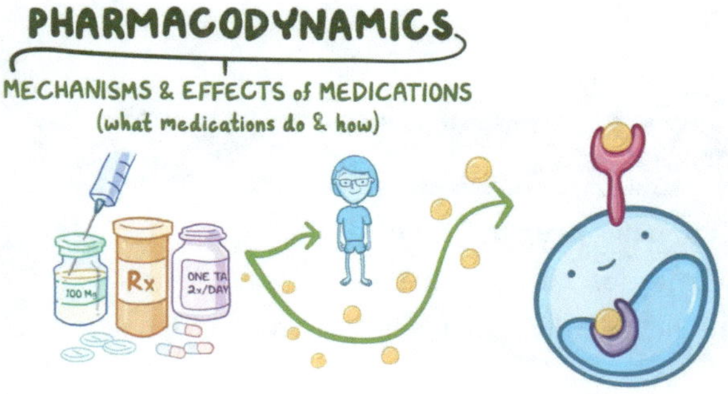

Figure 4.7. Pharmacodynamics.

Source: https://d16qt3wv6xm098.cloudfront.net/e4gT4FRHQg2zJpoR0WO_-K5uQbGiw-1A/_.jpg.

4.2.3. Interaction Between Pharmacokinetics and Pharmacodynamics

The PK and pharmacodynamics (PD) interaction is vital in studying drug effects on the body concurrent with being metabolized and eliminated. PK addresses the ADME of drugs that govern their therapeutic action duration. PD addresses the biochemical and physiological effects of drugs on their sites of action. Integrating these two disciplines allows clinicians to optimize dosing regimens to achieve desired therapeutic outcomes with fewer side effects. Such information garnered through exploring such interaction becomes integral to tailoring pharmacotherapy to individuals, offering efficacy and reducing toxicity. This unified perspective emphasizes the need for clinicians to be well informed about the behavior of drugs in the body and their relationship to clinical response in patients, reiterating the pivotal role of PK and PD in effective general practice (Giovagnoli et al., 2025). Enhanced pharmacokinetic M&S has significantly improved the validity of knowledge about drug interactions and their impact on patient treatment. For instance, simulation approaches allow scientists to model complex systems that mimic reality, making it possible to predict drug behavior without the ethical problems of live trials. Using simulations can thus illuminate the pharmacokinetic properties of novel drugs while preventing potential drug-drug interactions, particularly in polypharmacy cases common in general practice. Besides, integrating high-quality clinical trial data into such models can potentially make more accurate predictions of drug response variability across populations and guide practitioners' medication management choices. With scientists exploring the interface of PK and PD via simulation, there are more opportunities for improved therapeutic strategies (Giovagnoli et al., 2025).

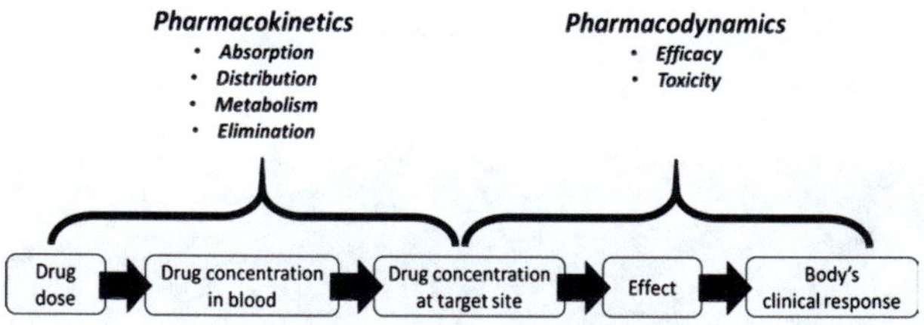

Figure 4.8. The relationship between pharmacokinetics and pharmacodynamics with respect to the effects of drug dose on the body.

Source: https://www.researchgate.net/profile/Nicole-Young/publication/319632558/figure/fig1/AS:616357381021704@1523962459672/The-relationship-between-pharmacokinetics-and-pharmacodynamics-with-respect-to-the.png.

It is critical to appreciate how diseases condition PK in order to customize effective treatment regimens in everyday practice. Liver or renal impairment, for instance, can drastically modify the ADME of drugs such that their efficacy and toxicity are altered. Patients with renal impairment, for example, will need drug dosage adjustment based on impaired clearance of drugs that are primarily excreted by the kidneys. Similarly, comorbid illnesses often necessitate careful management of pharmacodynamic interaction among drugs. This makes personalized medicine paramount, such that the clinician must evaluate a patient's complete medical history and concomitant medications to prevent adverse drug interactions. Hence, ongoing studies on diseases that affect pharmacokinetic processes justify a deeper understanding of inter-individual variability in drug response, reinforcing patient care and outcomes in practice (Abduljalil et al., 2019) (Figure 4.8).

Test Your Knowledge

1. What is pharmacokinetics, and why is it important in understanding drug therapy?
2. Define pharmacodynamics and explain how it relates to the effect of a drug on the body.
3. How do pharmacokinetics and pharmacodynamics differ, and how do they complement each other in clinical pharmacology?

4.3. Commonly Prescribed Medications in General Practice

Learning Outcome

1. Describe categories of medications frequently used
2. Explain the role of antibiotics in general practice
3. Understand the management of chronic conditions with pharmacotherapy

In reality, some drugs tend to be standard drugs because they are prevalent in the treatment of many medical conditions. Antihypertensives, statins, and antidepressants are among the most frequently prescribed medications. Antihypertensives, which have the function of stabilizing blood pressure, are instrumental in reducing the CVD risks. Statins are commonly used in maintaining cholesterol in check and are instrumental in preventing heart attack and stroke. Concurrently, antidepressants are being focused on for a considerable percentage of mental illnesses for improved QoL in patients. Their widespread utilization underscores the importance of learning about their pharmacological action mechanisms, side effects, and the necessity of patient-tailored individual treatment in daily practice. In addition, the efficacy of these medications can affect the patient's adherence to medication as prescribed, a consideration in chronic disease management. Evidence reports that medication compliance has improved outcomes in patients with chronic heart failure (CHF) (Griese-Mammen et al., 2019). Variability in compliance rates demonstrates various factors, such as regimen complexity and individual patient characteristics. Hence, healthcare practitioners must be adequately trained with techniques to encourage compliance, such as streamlining medication regimens and patient education. Screenings of patients' drug experiences can also feed into better management plans, culminating in better overall outcomes in general practice. Lastly, the physician's work does not end with prescription procedures; training and learning pharmacology is critical for effective medicine management in general practice. In the context of mental healthcare, the Medicines with Respect program emphasized the importance of education and training in medicine management among mental health nurses (Hemingway et al., 2014). These programs prepare healthcare providers for managing the complexities of pharmacologic therapies so that they can function competently as prescribers. Encouraging nurses and primary care practitioners to continue training is essential, not just to build their confidence levels but also to strengthen the overall efficacy of the healthcare system. Comprehensive education ultimately supports improved patient care and ensures that drugs most frequently prescribed are utilized maximally for the welfare of varied patient groups.

4.3.1. Categories of Medications Frequently Used

The role of pharmacology encompasses several classes of medications that perform essential roles in everyday practice. Analgesics, the single broad category, share widespread use in pain management. Analgesics, ranging from nonsteroidal anti-inflammatory drugs (NSAIDs) like ibuprofen to opioids like morphine, can truly improve patients' QoL. Although NSAIDs are generally favored due to their safety profile and effectiveness in the management of mild to moderate pain, opioids continue to play a critical role in controlling severe pain, especially in the post-operative patient. Nevertheless, the growing epidemic of opioid abuse is an issue for clinicians, requiring judicious patient evaluation and monitoring to ensure effective relief of pain versus the threat of dependency and adverse effects. Therefore, GPs must keep themselves informed with good prescribing practice and newer substitutes to optimize patient care and safety. Another significant category of drugs prescribed widely in general practice is antihypertensives, which are essential for the management of elevated blood pressure, an important CVD risk factor. This category includes various antihypertensive drug classes, including ACE inhibitors, beta-blockers, and calcium channel blockers, each with unique mechanisms of action to appropriately regulate blood pressure. For instance, ACE inhibitors induce the relaxation of the blood vessels by inhibiting the angiotensin-converting enzyme (ACE), which subsequently lowers blood pressure levels. Individual patient factors, including associated diseases and side-effect tolerance generally determine the choice of specific antihypertensive drugs. As hypertension remains among the leading preventable causes of morbidity and mortality, the importance of effective antihypertensive prescribing and lifestyle change patient education cannot be overstressed to facilitate holistic management of this endemic chronic condition. Antibiotics form another vital class of drugs widely prescribed in general practice, especially for controlling bacterial infections. With a wide variety of agents, such as penicillins, cephalosporins, and macrolides, antibiotics can cure infections as slight as uncomplicated UTIs to as serious as more systemic infections. However, the issue of antibiotic resistance is a significant dilemma, leading to higher healthcare costs and treatment failure. Thus, GPs are responsible for adhering to evidence-based guidelines in antibiotic prescription to create the desired effect while limiting the potential for resistance development. Appropriate education on the use of proper antibiotics is crucial, raising awareness among patients to prevent unnecessary prescription of antibiotics and following prescribed regimens. This complex approach to prescribing antibiotics is essential to preserve the efficacy of these precious medicines in daily practice (Hemingway et al., 2014; Schenk et al., 1959) (Figure 4.9).

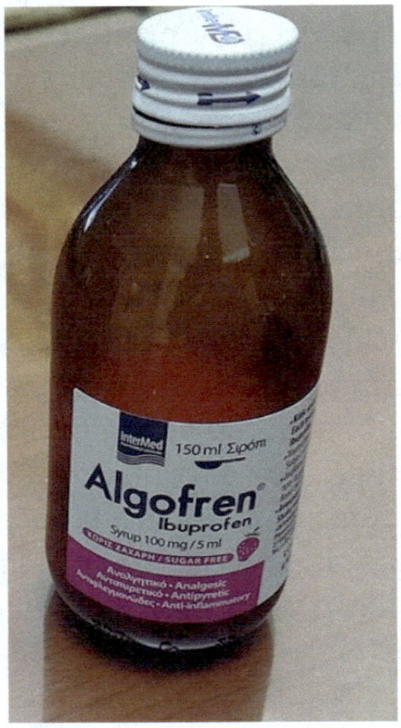

Figure 4.9. A 150 mL bottle (100 mg/5 mL dosage) of ibuprofen.

Source: https://upload.wikimedia.org/wikipedia/commons/thumb/0/0a/Ibuprofen_syrup.jpg/320px-Ibuprofen_syrup.jpg.

4.3.2. Role of Antibiotics in General Practice

Antibiotics are essential in general practice, with the central area of application is treating bacterial infections and preventing secondary complications from such diseases. In the primary healthcare sector, GPs are exposed to a range of infectious conditions that require proper application of antibiotics so that appropriate treatment can be provided. In particular, correct diagnosis is essential as antibiotics do not function for infections caused by viruses. Over-prescription and abuse of the drugs may cause immense public health problems, including antibiotic resistance. Current studies indicate that antibiotic resistance among common pathogens such as Helicobacter pylori is rising significantly, particularly in some regions of the globe where treatment failures are repeatedly happening at a higher rate because of the resistance (Aramin et al., 2016). Therefore, GPs must be prudent in their antibiotic prescribing to reduce the risk of resistance and optimize patient outcomes. Antibiotic resistance represents a significant challenge for general practice, influencing treatment algorithms and empirical therapy selection. Rising rates of resistance globally are encouraging clinicians to stay current with local resistance patterns, which can be highly variable geographically. For instance, resistance rates to clarithromycin in Japan and Italy are very high and influence the treatment of *H. pylori* infections by GPs (Aramin et al., 2016). This disparity emphasizes the importance of local epidemiological data in guiding clinicians in prescribing antibiotics. Furthermore, tailored treatment protocols, based on patient profiles and resistance information, can achieve increased recovery rates and diminished failure in treatment, again testifying to the application of personalized medicine in antibiotic stewardship programs. The evolution of the practice of antibiotic prescription is a direct consequence of changes in clinical roles among practitioners. As nurse prescribers and pharmacists assume greater responsibilities to prescribe across a broader spectrum of medicines, including antibiotics, greater cooperation between these groups and GPs will be necessary. This increased collaboration can further enrich patient care through more extensive assessment and ease of treatment plans. However, transformation also increases controversy regarding the effects of dispersing prescribing rights among various healthcare providers. It is essential to balance expanded access to antibiotics and strong expertise in their judicious use to guard against the dangers of overprescription and resistance. Ultimately, education-based collaboration that emphasizes antibiotic stewardship is a basis for responsible pharmacological practice in general practice.

4.3.3. Management of Chronic Conditions with Pharmacotherapy

The therapy of chronic illnesses through pharmacotherapy requires a rich understanding of the interaction between drug agents and disease physiology. Chronic illnesses such as obesity and diabetes require personalized treatments that address the multi-factorial nature of these illnesses. For example, obesity is now being recognized not only as an issue of overweight but as a complex chronic disease involving many influencing factors like metabolic pathways and behavioral patterns. The treatment of obesity, especially of clinically severe cases, is itself a complex undertaking; standard therapies are only partially effective. Clinicians would do well to carefully consider pharmacotherapy options, such as the FDA-approved drug orlistat for long-term weight managementits potential benefits. They should be aware that many drugs may have the side effect of weight gain, emphasizing the need for collaborative medication management (Ameer et al., 2018).

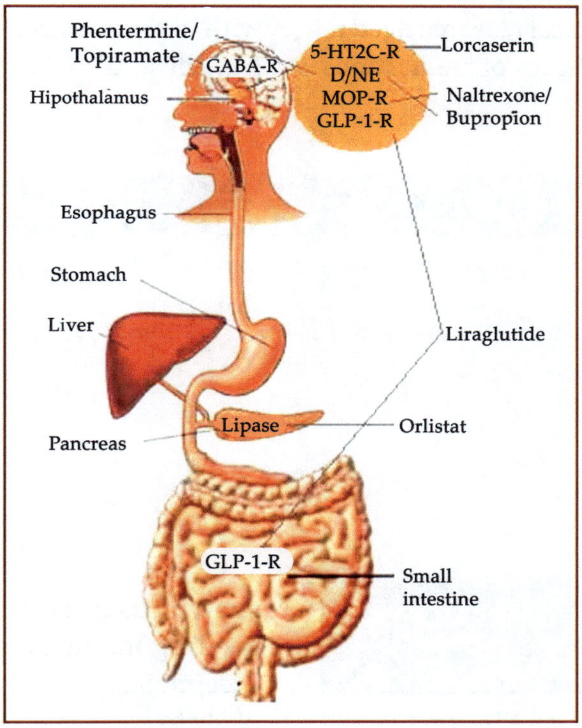

Figure 4.10. Mechanism of action of long-term anti-obesity pharmacotherapies.

Source: https://www.researchgate.net/publication/312567640_Pharmacotherapy_in_the_Treatment_of_Obesity.

Management of chronic disease also needs to take patient demographics into account, particularly with the aging population. In most clinical guidelines, the term "elderly" refers to patients who may have specific pharmacological requirements often overlooked due to imprecise age-related classifications. Most studies have demonstrated that the majority of guidelines are not or exact in defining the elderly, which may result in broad treatment recommendations that do not account for the unique characteristics of each patient. Guidelines will also rest on a chronological age strategy that does not capture the imperceptible phenomenon of frailty and altered PK of aging. These needs are reframing the definition of and application of pharmacotherapy by clinical guidelines in older patients to enable treatment to be optimized on an individual basis to address the individual physiological alterations of aging, as well as the effects of drugs and medications (Bajorek et al., 2014). Additionally, the integration of evidence-based research in pharmacotherapy is necessary for optimal management of chronic illness. With expanding knowledge of the pathophysiology of disease conditions such as obesity, there lies a need to translate new knowledge into practice effectively. Academic and clinical research need to go ahead to establish the efficacy of medications for comorbidities associated with the disease conditions, particularly in the multicultural patient population. For instance, the traditional understanding of obesity as a straightforward fat storage condition is oversimplified and fails to account for the intricate biochemistry involved. Practitioners are thus called upon to adopt a more holistic outlook that takes into account the most current scientific advancements. The incorporation of pharmacotherapy management informed by rigorous research will enhance patient care and align treatment guidelines with current optimal practice in pharmacology (Ameer et al., 2018) (Figure 4.10).

Test Your Knowledge

1. What are the main categories of medications frequently prescribed in general practice, and what conditions do they typically treat?
2. What is the role of antibiotics in general practice, and what are some key considerations to prevent antibiotic resistance?

4.4. Adverse Drug Reactions and Drug Interactions

Learning Outcome

1. Explain the types of adverse drug reactions
2. Understand the importance of monitoring drug interactions
3. Focus on strategies for minimizing risks in prescribing

Adverse drug reactions (ADRs) are a source of great concern in the practice of pharmacology today, particularly in general practice. They can result from several factors, including patient characteristics, the intrinsic pharmacological profile of the drug, and risk for drug interaction. The incidence of ADRs is exceptionally high in elderly patients who are likely to have polypharmacy—the simultaneous use of several drugs. As expounded by Boussery et al. (2015), elderly patients demand increased vigilance in prescribing behaviors, as patients are more susceptible to the risks of both ADRs and the potential for potentially inappropriate prescribing (PIP). Therefore, physicians must initiate a thorough medication review process and regularly screen patients' medication regimens to identify and preempt risks for ADRs, ensuring that patient safety and clinical outcomes are optimized. Drug interaction knowledge is equally essential to the practice of pharmacology, as these drug interactions will either increase the risk for ADRs or diminish therapeutic efficacy. Drug interactions may arise through pharmacokinetic or pharmacodynamic means, whereby an interaction might affect the absorption, metabolism, or excretion of a second drug. Clinicians need to be aware of these kinds of interactions, especially when prescribing treatment regimens to patients who are already on several drugs. Literature identifies the need for systematic screening of PIP in the elderly, as depicted by Boussery et al. (2015). Instruments like GheOP3S can be utilized in assessing relevant PIP in community pharmacies, in a bid to increase the level of awareness regarding potential drug interactions that may not be evident through clinical assessment. By utilizing tools and interventions that address drug interactions, practitioners will be able to better assess their patients for undesirable outcomes. The combined strategy for drug interaction and ADR management is essential to practitioners, as it enhances integrated patient care. It is necessary to consider not only the therapeutic application of drugs but also their potential for toxicity and side effects. A comprehension of historical contexts relating to pharmacology, such as the therapeutic properties of natural products, underscores the complex interaction of drugs with biological systems. As noted, the majority of modern medicines have their origin in plants with both curative and poisonous potentialities. It is thus imperative to be familiar with these double properties, especially in general practice, where patients may show a preference for more natural types of treatment. Extensive training on ADRs, interactions, and the chemistry of drug agents forms the bedrock of effective pharmacological practice, ultimately leading to better and safer patient care in the general practice environment.

4.4.1. Types of Adverse Drug Reactions

Adverse drug reactions (ADRs) are a broad category of adverse drug responses, classifying them into various categories that are relevant to understand in pharmacology. ADRs are typically classified as type A (augmented) and type B (bizarre) reactions. Type A reactions are dose-dependent, predictable, and result from the pharmacological action of the drug. For instance, anticoagulants are known to induce bleeding in the patient through their direct mechanism of action. Type B reactions, however, are unpredictable, idiosyncratic, and result from genetic causes or immune responses. Type B reactions may lead to severe consequences, such as anaphylaxis or severe skin reactions that may not be directly related to the known pharmacological effects of the drugs. GPS must be familiar with these classifications since they dictate the process of clinical decision-making and the risk management involved in prescribing medications. The incidence of ADRs is very challenging in clinical practice, particularly in patient safety and the effectiveness of treatments. A study assessing ADRs in a tertiary care hospital documented that a high percentage of patients experienced adverse events, stressing the importance of monitoring and reporting (Adhikari et al., 2009). Specifically, 250 out of 1250 patients admitted during the course of the study exhibited adverse reactions, with a significant percentage (76.8%) being mild, while 66% were severe and required critical medical intervention. Moreover, the research found that a substantial percentage of ADRs were resultant from antimicrobial agents and medications that affect the central nervous system (CNS). These findings underline the significance of healthcare providers conducting keen ADR monitoring to provide patients with effective and safe care with minimal risk of medication complications. The integration of network pharmacology with personalized medicine further emphasizes the necessity for managing ADRs based on a more advanced understanding of drug interactions and patient-specific factors. Based on principles of network pharmacology, physicians can design individualized therapeutic regimens that consider not only the pharmacologic properties of drugs but also their likelihood of causing adverse effects based on individual patient profiles (Marsh et al., 2010). This approach facilitates the identification of safer pairs of therapies and reduces the risk of Type A and Type B reactions. Personalized medicine represents a paradigm shift in pharmacotherapy, calling for an interdisciplinary approach to rationalize drug development, enhance safety, and ultimately improve patient outcomes in everyday practice (Figure 4.11).

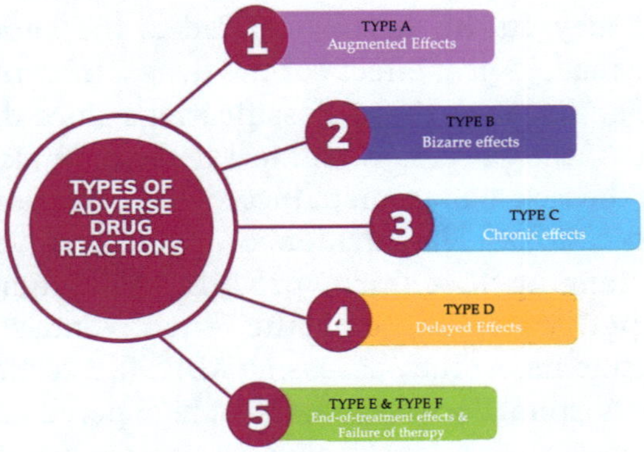

Figure 4.11. Adverse drug reaction types.

Source: https://lh5.googleusercontent.com/u_xvKgpYqMmEyFb4Oi0T_13-mz-keUHVyVxpwKCvos4GU2Z71I6FsddZ8v73as--86rzjEuYKCzKtAAYJtpQyF0PMZUhxIhLmKnAn9J2gK5zn8yoxvRoW1gW0Jnn_9s1R2LB4j_8gGR9Ue0R-w=s1600.

4.4.2. Importance of Monitoring Drug Interactions

Drug interaction monitoring is of significant importance in the practice of pharmacology, particularly in general practice. As an increasing number of healthcare providers prescribe an extended list of drugs to manage multifactorial diseases, the dangers of drug-drug interactions become a noteworthy concern. Drug interactions can lead to adverse effects, therapy failure, or even severe clinical implications. For example, two drugs might modify each other's metabolism, thereby enhancing toxicity or reducing effectiveness, which requires careful monitoring to ensure optimal patient safety and treatment benefit. Thus, implementing guidelines for evaluating patients' medication regimens can minimize such risks and improve overall therapeutic outcomes in accordance with best practices in drug therapy management. Also, patients tend not to report all medications they are taking, such as over-the-counter drugs and supplements, which makes it harder to monitor. Practitioners face challenges in taking comprehensive medication histories and identifying potential interactions that may not be apparent at first sight. EHRs and clinical decision support systems (CDSS) offer a solution to this problem today, as these technologies can prompt providers to examine potential interactions during the point of care. This proactive strategy enhances communication between healthcare providers and patients, enabling the detection of hazardous combinations and the delivery of safe and effective treatments based on patients' specific health profiles. In addition, continuing education of healthcare providers in pharmacology and drug interaction management is essential. Continuing professional development and training allow practitioners to remain abreast of the latest research and clinical guidelines regarding drug interactions. Understanding the pharmacokinetic and pharmacodynamic profiles of drugs can enable practitioners to assess risk appropriately, using strategies to monitor and adjust therapy accordingly. Considering the heterogeneity of the individual drug response and the vast array of determinants for drug interactions, including genetics and co-morbid disease, medication expertise is even more essential in guiding appropriate prescribing. This reinforces the contention that monitoring drug interactions is not an adjunct function of pharmacology but a central aspect critical to optimizing patient treatment within general practice, as highlighted in discussions at professional gatherings such as the 2017 conference. Biennial meeting (Bailey et al., 2018; Kitsiou et al., 2013) (Figure 4.12).

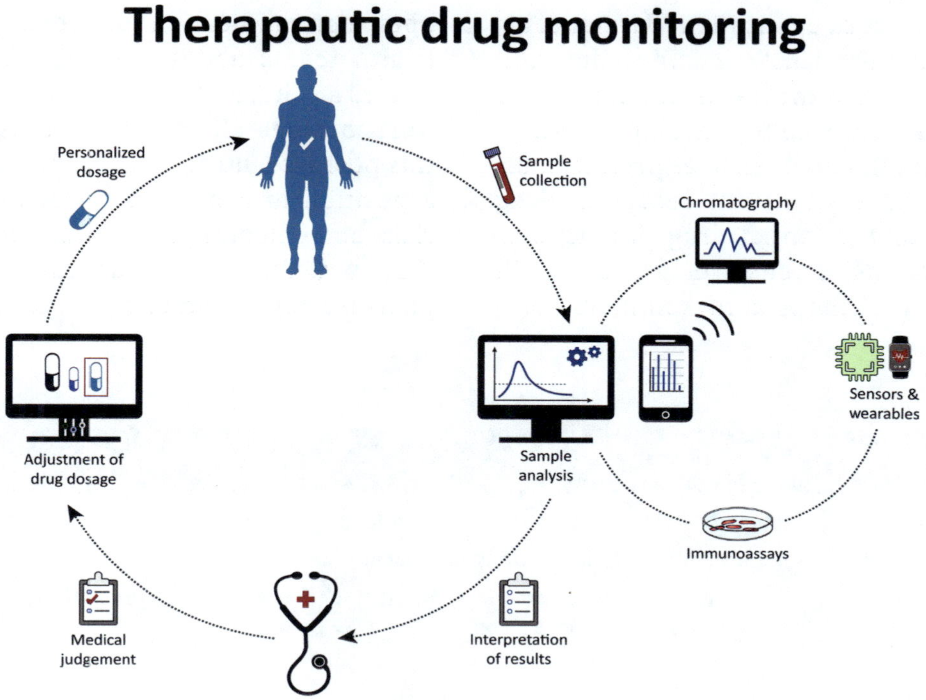

Figure 4.12. Therapeutic drug monitoring.

Source: https://www.cell.com/cms/10.1016/j.tibtech.2020.03.001/asset/f0fc0d11-5c01-4de5-ab0a-dcecc55259f6/main.assets/gr1_lrg.jpg.

4.4.3. Strategies for Minimizing Risks in Prescribing

Mitigating the dangers of drug prescriptions requires a strategy that considers the complex nature of patient-centered care. A viable approach is the performance of thorough medication reviews among, for example, older people, who are often at risk of adverse drug effects due to polypharmacy. Greater understanding of aging physiology and pharmacology can assist health professionals in selecting the appropriate drugs to prevent the onset of iatrogenic complications. Creating a uniform template, such as the revised Beers Criteria, provides primary care doctors with guidelines for identifying inappropriate medications in older populations. The process of systematic review guarantees that medications are not just safe but also weigh appropriate non-pharmacological interventions when available, ultimately improving the QoL of the patients and reducing health concerns related to unneeded medications (Bhanji et al., 2013). In addition to targeted medication review, CDSS are also a method for lowering prescribing risk. Such systems can maintain adherence to evidence-based clinical guidelines, like opioid treatment for chronic pain syndromes. By using computerized algorithms that integrate patient data from electronic medical records, CDSS can provide precise, patient-related advice at the time of consultation. The cyclic testing and design of CDSS ensure that they address standard prescribing rule uncertainties, thus enhancing the usability and clarity of recommendations. As a result, the tools not only improve the safety of opioid prescribing practices but also capitalize on expertise, thereby bridging the gap between clinical guidelines and primary care practice application (Farmer et al., 2010). Last but not least, ongoing education and training for healthcare professionals are necessary to ensure safe prescribing practices. Professional development enables professionals to stay updated with recent research, drug preparations, and potential drug interactions, thereby fostering a culture of safety in prescribing. Workshops and seminars with case studies can provide opportunities for peer-to-peer discussions of difficult prescribing situations, allowing professionals to learn from their collective experience. Besides, encouraging open communication between patients and health teams about the risks of medication fosters a culture where patients are encouraged to report side effects or concerns. By evolving this positive culture, health professionals are in a position to considerably reduce prescribing risks and enhance the therapeutic outcomes of their patients, thereby advancing an effective pharmacological practice in general medicine.

Test Your Knowledge

1. What are the different types of ADRs, and how do they vary in severity and mechanism?
2. Why is it important to monitor for drug interactions in clinical practice?
3. What are some common examples of drug interactions that can lead to serious adverse effects?

4.5. Patient Education and Medication Adherence

Learning Outcome

1. Understand the importance of educating patients about their medications
2. Describe techniques to improve medication adherence
3. Define the role of healthcare providers in supporting patients

Effective patient education is a central factor in enhancing drug compliance, a critical element of effective pharmacotherapy in primary care. Research indicates that patients who have a clear understanding of their drug regimen are more likely to adhere to prescribed therapy. Knowledge not only encompasses the nitty-gritty of when and how to take the drug but also the condition for which the drug is intended. When healthcare providers educate patients about potential side effects and desired outcomes, patients are likely to be more in charge of their own health. Such patient empowerment alleviates feelings of helplessness usually associated with chronic illnesses, promoting a healthier attitude towards medical interventions and adherence. The incorporation of personalized education strategies further expedites the process, allowing healthcare professionals to tailor their communications to the specific needs of unique patients, thereby increasing the effectiveness of educational interventions (Gasser et al., 2018). Moreover, the effectiveness of patient adherence interventions is directly proportional to how closely they align with the determinants of non-adherence. Evidence suggests that a single approach in all cases does not work; thus, healthcare professionals must identify and address patient-specific barriers to medication adherence. Existing evidence noted in the literature emphasizes aligning interventions with modifiable and unmodifiable determinants of medication adherence. This patient-specific approach provides support tailored to patients' individual conditions, with the highest chances of achieving adherence outcomes. By systematically categorizing such determinants and aligning them with appropriate educational interventions, clinicians can implement measures not only for educating but also for motivating patients to adhere to their medication regimens (Bart et al., 2016). This matching thus emphasizes the imperative for healthcare professionals to implement continuous monitoring and tailoring of adherence strategies. In conclusion, the connection between patient education and medication adherence in family practice is crucial for achieving optimal pharmacological treatment outcomes. Understanding the multifaceted nature of adherence challenges, healthcare providers must adopt a more holistic model of patient education. This involves establishing open communication, fostering patient involvement in their healthcare, and making the exchange of information a cooperative experience. Moreover, such initiatives must be supported by health systems via the planning of integral educational programs that equip patients with the skills to manage their medicines appropriately. Through such measures, general practice can manage the widespread barriers to adherence and establish a framework for ongoing patient engagement. Last but not least, enhancing medication adherence through targeted education interventions not only improves individual health outcomes but also reduces healthcare expenses associated with non-adherence, demonstrating the extensive impact of successful patient education (Gasser et al., 2018).

4.5.1. Importance of Educating Patients About Their Medications

Patient education regarding their medication is a vital component of pharmacological care in the primary setting. An informed patient will be more inclined to adhere to prescribed treatments, having an awareness of the reason for the medication as well as its potential side effects. Not only does this optimize the success of the treatment regimen, but it also minimizes the potential for drug errors. For instance, if patients understand the need for their medication at specific times or with specific foods, they can minimize the risk of side effects and hospitalization. As observed in similar literature, the gap in communication between hospital junior doctors and GPs regarding discharge medicine instructions highlights the importance of involving both patients and healthcare providers in adequate information (Bhattacharya et al., 2014). If patients are adequately informed, they become active partners in their care, leading to enhanced health outcomes. Moreover, the learning process must extend beyond the provision of step-by-step instructions on the administration of drugs. Patients need to understand the big picture of their drug treatment, including drug interactions with other drugs, and that they need to adhere to treatment for chronic conditions. Patient empowerment results from education, which enables them to recognize symptoms that need medical attention, therefore acting proactively rather than reactively. For example, when the medication administration skills of nursing students were evaluated, it was evident that structured assessments, such as objective structured clinical examinations (OSCE), can significantly enhance their confidence in medication administration (Hemingway et al., 2013). This indicates the need for educational models that incorporate patient involvement in their medication regimens, emphasizing that well-informed patients can better guide their healthcare trajectories. In addition, by creating a patient-educating culture within the general practice setting, a sustainable healthcare approach is fostered. Follow-up appointments can be utilized as opportunities to review medication planning and listen to patient questions or concerns. By creating an open and ongoing dialogue regarding medications, practitioners can assess patients' comprehension and compliance more adequately. This process not only reinforces the therapeutic relationship between health professionals and patients but also motivates patients to become more empowered in their own health. Finally, a partnership model for medication education strengthens physician-patient communication and enhances adherence, resulting in improved health outcomes for pharmacological care. As medication management dialogue continues to evolve, adopting a patient-centered model of education remains crucial to effective general practice (Figure 4.13).

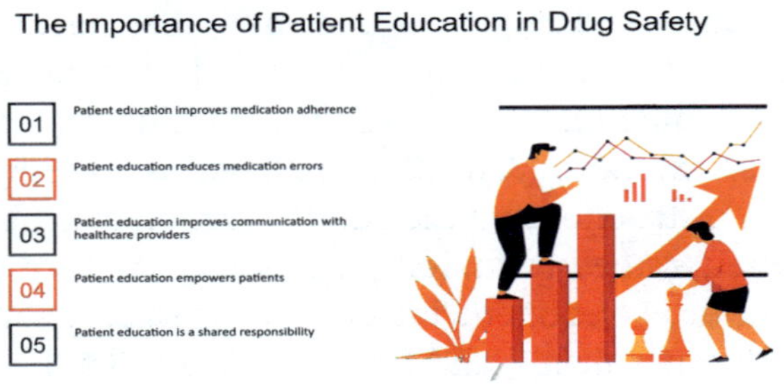

Figure 4.13. The importance of patient education in drug safety.

Source: https://fastercapital.co/i/The-Role-of-PPIPLA-in-Enhancing-Drug-Safety-and-Patient-Education--The-Importance-of-Patient-Education-in-Drug-Safety.webp.

4.5.2. Techniques to Improve Medication Adherence

Compliance with medication is highly significant in the effective pharmacologic therapy, but many patients are not able to stick to prescribed regimens consistently. One of the principal means of enhancing compliance is by educating patients on the importance of taking drugs as instructed, using concise, plain language. After patients are aware of the potential consequences of non-adherence, i.e., the aggravation of their disease or possible complications, they become more likely to take an active part in their treatment regimen. Furthermore, enhancing the level of trust between patients and healthcare professionals can create an environment where patients are willing to discuss their medication schedules. As noted by Cox et al. (2012), identification of a patient's need to take medicines, primarily for asymptomatic conditions such as glaucoma, is critical in enhancing the outcomes of adherence. Therefore, focused education can significantly impact patient self-management and adherence. The integration of technology in medication management is another efficient approach to enhancing adherence. Tools such as mobile apps and computerized reminders can assist patients by alerting them to drug timing and encouraging timely dosing. These technology-mediated interventions are beneficial for patients with chronic diseases who may be required to take complex medication regimens. Through reminders, patients can minimize the risk of missed doses because of forgetfulness. In addition, patient information collected through such platforms can also be utilized by healthcare professionals to assess patterns of adherence and establish likely barriers. As Boons et al. (2017) put it, the facilitation of patients with evidence-based methods, such as the identification of probable adherence barriers and proposing solutions, can enhance medication management. Not only does this ease compliance, but it also fosters patient involvement in their overall healthcare process. Multidisciplinary collaborative care approaches have also proven to be successful in optimizing medication adherence. These approaches promote communication among various healthcare professionals, including physicians, nurses, and pharmacists, who collectively devise interventions for overcoming medication management problems. For instance, pharmacists can play a vital role in advising patients on their medications, walking them through potential side effects and the importance of adherence. This comprehensive support can significantly contribute to developing patients' self-efficacy, thereby improving adherence rates in the long term. Shared decision-making strategies allow patients to be proactive concerning their treatment process and, therefore, more likely to be adherent. Establishing these collaborative environments is supported by evidence from Boons et al. (2017), facilitating the multidisciplinary strategy to ensure personalized approaches for adherence implementation (Figure 4.14).

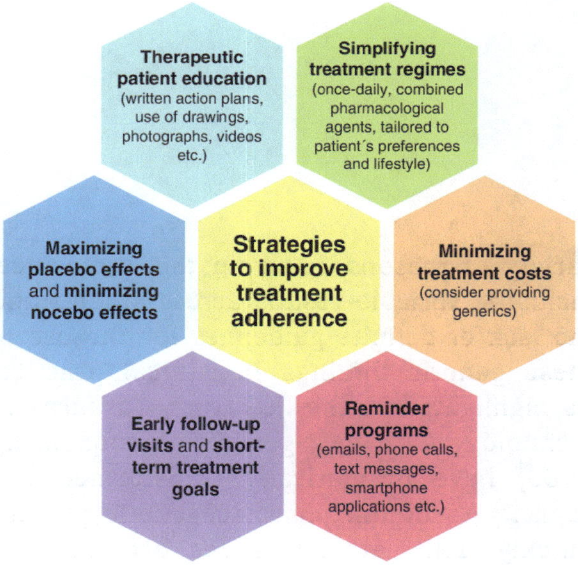

Figure 4.14. Strategies to improve treatment adherence.

Source: https://iimtu.edu.in/blog/wp-content/uploads/2023/07/Strategies-to-improve-treatment-adherence.png.

4.5.3. Role of Healthcare Providers in Supporting Patients

Healthcare professionals play a central role of leading the patient through multidimensional care that involves clinical, educational, and emotional components. Such care is particularly relevant in the context of pharmacology, since drug selection, their dosage, and control directly determine the patient's treatment outcome. Providers must keep pace with the evolving environment of drug approvals and treatments, finding a balance between spurring innovation in treatment and meeting safety requirements (Abbott et al., 2014). By communicating well with patients, providers are able to deliver individualized information on medication regimens, correct usage, and potential side effects, enhancing adherence and therapeutic efficacy. Also, education in patient engagement helps healthcare providers overcome potential barriers, such as health literacy or financial constraints, thus empowering patients throughout the course of care. As a matter of fact, beyond their role as providers of information, healthcare providers must actively participate in chronic disease management through a system of organized care delivery. This is achieved through the use of internal EHRs, which enhance continuity of care and enable improved monitoring of treatment outcomes (McCarthy et al., 2009). These systems would allow providers to monitor patients' response to drug therapies and change therapeutic strategies accordingly. Secondly, by using standardized care processes for chronic care management, the providers minimize the variation of care, which in the long term enhances patients' experience as well as outcome. Through these best practices, healthcare providers not only improve their patients' immediate health but also ensure the integration of pharmacologic therapies within the larger healthcare system. Finally, the emotional and psychological support by healthcare professionals also plays a vital role in fostering patient empowerment and resilience. Through establishing trust-based relationships, professionals can encourage patients to voice their opinions, pose questions, and take an active role in making their treatment choices. Through active engagement, patients become empowered to take control of their well-being, which can lead to better medication compliance (McCarthy et al., 2009). Moreover, since patients must cope with complex treatment regimens, professionals can serve as role models, guiding them through challenges and helping them further understand the role of pharmacology in their overall well-being. The interaction between these facilitative roles ensures compliance not only with therapy but also with establishing a more holistic perception of health, where drug interventions become part of a patient's own habits and needs without tension.

Test Your Knowledge

1. Why is patient education important in ensuring safe and effective medication use?
2. Which techniques or tools have been shown to improve medication adherence in patients?
3. What role do healthcare providers play in supporting patients to follow their prescribed medication regimens?

4.6. Ethical Considerations in Pharmacology

Learning Outcome

1. Understand informed consent and patient autonomy
2. Focus on issues of drug pricing and accessibility
3. Describe ethical dilemmas in prescribing practices

Ethics are at the forefront in pharmacology, particularly with the expanded horizon of personalized medicine. The advent of pharmacogenetics is a two-edged sword because it attempts to individualize drug therapy based on specific genetic profiles. As tremendous as the promise of enhanced efficacy and reduced adverse effects is, pharmacogenetics is not yet applied widely within clinical practice. A variety of reasons underpin this reluctance, including variable results across studies and the lack of definite guidelines for the use of these genetic findings in clinical practice. As highlighted in the literature, advances in technology with next-generation sequencing (NGS) have dramatically transformed our capacity to obtain pharmacogenetic profiles quickly. Still, ethical issues around data quality, interpretation, and confidentiality are overshadowing this. Resolution of these ethical dilemmas is fundamental in the proper adoption of individualized pharmacological therapy into mainstream practice (Paepe et al., 2013). Novel pharmacological intervention always raises ethical concerns and issues of informed consent and patient autonomy. Proper care should be taken to ensure that patients are fully informed about the outcomes of pharmacological treatment, especially in situations involving complex treatment regimens. Successful communication between healthcare professionals and patients plays a fundamental role in developing trust and establishing a culture of collaborative decision-making. Practitioners, therefore, need to tread a thin line: the urgent need for successful treatment against ethical demands to respect a patient's preferences and rights. Besides, with the evolving healthcare context placing increasing emphasis on population health and social determinants, as discussed in the emerging nursing curricula, medical practitioners and pharmacists must be equipped to explore how these broader determinants influence individual treatment choices and outcomes (Bouchaud et al., 2017). Equitable access to drugs is another significant ethical concern in relation to pharmacology. Health disparities often lead to unequal access to necessary pharmacologic therapy, highlighting differences between population groups. Healthcare practitioners and pharmacists must advocate for policies that ensure fair drug distribution, recognizing the impact of social determinants that can significantly affect patient compliance with pharmacologic therapy. This disquiet is not merely in the office of the single clinician but requires broader societal changes to eliminate barriers to access to medications. Effective measures might include outreach programs in the community or collaboration with policymakers to ensure that safety and efficacy are not undermined by cost or by socioeconomic status. Emphasizing access to equitable pharmacological therapy by healthcare practitioners can help move towards an equitable healthcare system while still ensuring ethical practice in the profession.

4.6.1. Informed Consent and Patient Autonomy

Informed consent is a cornerstone of ethical medical practice, particularly in pharmacology. Informed consent underscores the significance of patients' complete comprehension of their treatment options, including the risks and advantages of pharmacological intervention. In general practice, where physicians often balance the complexities of patient needs with the rules of medical practice, informed consent becomes paramount in upholding patient autonomy. By ensuring that patients are provided with adequate information, healthcare providers are honoring patients' rights to make informed decisions regarding treatment planning. This aligns with ethical standards, which expect patients not only to comprehend the information but also to make voluntary decisions without duress, thereby leading to their active involvement in their own healthcare. Patient autonomy is connected to informed consent and is a key consideration in general practice, particularly in ethical treatment. Patient-centered care has shifted the power dynamic in the clinician-patient relationship, prioritizing cooperation when making decisions. Professionals need to realize that autonomy means more than just consent; it encompasses a patient's values and preferences regarding the overall objective of their health. In practice, this translates to clear communication and articulation of how pharmacological interventions address individual patient circumstances. Building a trust relationship enables practitioners to have sensitive treatment discussions while taking into account the diverse cultural, personal, and social factors that motivate patient preference. In addition to enhancing compliance, this maintains an element of agency for patients to control their own health. The ethical dilemma of informed consent is directed towards the problem in achieving patient autonomy by medical professionals, especially among vulnerable populations such as children or mentally challenged individuals. The complexity of such situations demands both an appreciation of ethical principles and an awareness of the practicalities of clinical practice. To physicians and other healthcare providers, this means that there must exist a framework for balancing the need for patient autonomy with the need to make decisions in the best interests of the patient when he or she may not be able to make informed choices. As a result, ongoing discussions about ethics codes and practice become crucial for guiding practitioners on how to manage such dilemmas. In the face of the shifting healthcare landscape, clinicians must address such issues through continuous learning and self-reflection, ensuring that informed consent remains a dynamic process protecting patient rights and safety in pharmacology (Coleman et al., 2011; Montalto et al., 2014) (Figure 4.15).

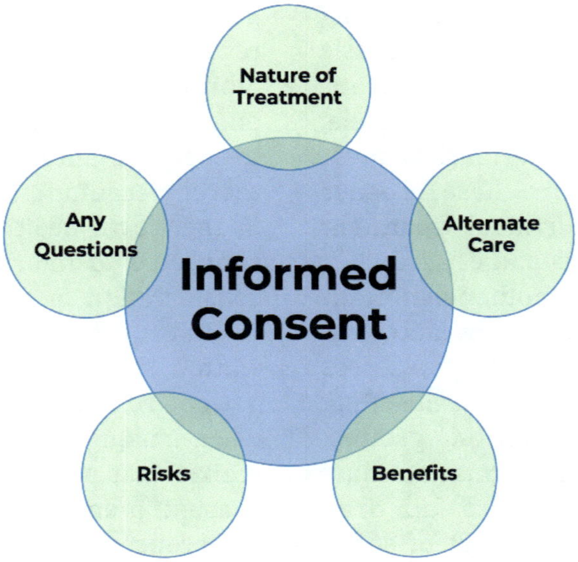

Figure 4.15. Informed consent.

Source: https://postgraddc.com/wp-content/uploads/2022/08/Informed-Consent.png.

4.6.2. Issues of Drug Pricing and Accessibility

The issues of drug availability and pricing are critical matters in the field of pharmacology, particularly in primary practice. The gap between medicine affordability and patient financial limitations has far-reaching implications for patient outcomes. In the majority of low- and middle-income countries (LMICs), antibiotic resistance is exacerbated by improper access to medicines of first essence, which are overly priced or unavailable. As identified by agencies like the WHO, over 50% of medications are inappropriately prescribed or dispensed, highlighting systemic frailties in healthcare infrastructure. Access to affordable drugs must be strengthened through policy overhauls to foster the effective management of common diseases. This not only necessitates regulatory intervention but also demands interagency collaboration among healthcare stakeholders to ensure drugs are both accessible and utilized as they should be. With the introduction of biologic therapeutic products, the landscape of drug therapy has evolved, and new challenges in pricing and accessibility have arisen. These products, based on living organisms and produced with state-of-the-art recombinant methods, tend to be associated with high production costs, resulting in prices that are too high for most patients. Although such therapies have the promise of transforming the control of disease, regulatory bodies must quickly develop guidelines to ensure the accessibility and responsible use of such drugs. There is a desperate need for more potent policies to facilitate fair access to biological agents, especially in low-resource settings. Without concerted efforts to make such treatments accessible, the transformative potential of biological drugs might be undone by the deep-seated inequalities in access to good-quality medical care. Because antibiotics are such a critical component of infection treatment, availability is most critical, particularly within the pediatric population, where infectious disease remains a leading cause of mortality. Programs like Make medicines child size by agencies like the WHO aim to address drug formulation and availability issues in children in LMICs. But more and more emphasis is being put on the misuse of antibiotics, which has the potential to lead to some very severe issues like antimicrobial resistance (AMR). To counter these risks, it is necessary to construct holistic strategies that improve access to rational prescribing habits and provide the required medicines. By fostering evidence-based clinical guidelines and utilizing correct drug formulations, healthcare systems can enhance treatment outcome amplifications and consequently reduce health inequities among vulnerable populations. Continued observation and concerted effort will be necessary to ensure that pharmacological advancement translates into increased access to care for all (Figure 4.16).

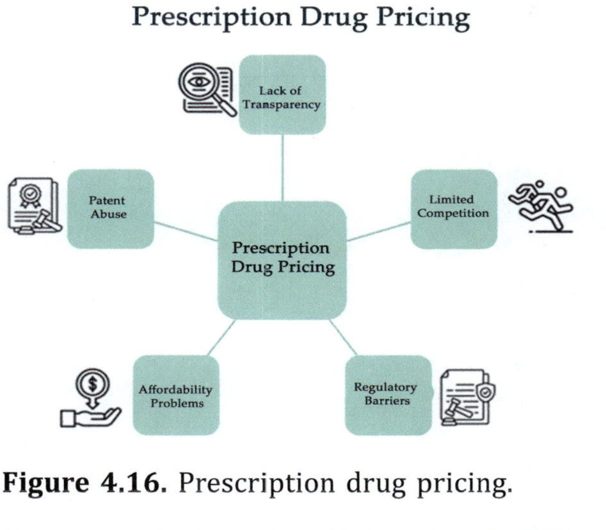

Figure 4.16. Prescription drug pricing.

Source: https://wallstreetmojo-files.s3.ap-south-1.amazonaws.com/2024/03/Prescription-Drug-Pricing.jpg.

4.6.3. Ethical Dilemmas in Prescribing Practices

Where pharmacology meets clinical practice, ethical issues often arise in the process of prescribing, particularly where patient autonomy and professional responsibility must be balanced. Practitioners weigh numerous parameters, including drug efficacy, side effects, and financial implications on patients' lifestyles. For instance, a change from being a student doctor to a foundation trainee places extraordinary responsibility on the decision-making process, which is further compounded by the quick-fix-oriented healthcare system and risk management. As a result, understanding that responsibility is not incremental but also contextual and fluid is key to unfolding these moral dilemmas (Zukas et al., 2013). This identification not only shapes the understanding of junior doctors' duties but also influences their prescribing choices, with patient care and safety ramifications resonating throughout their careers. Promoting compliance with medication regimes in patients is another area of ethical concern within prescribing practice. It is against this background that community pharmacists often take on a role, issuing patients emergency prescriptions when they are unable to receive their regular supply promptly. A study highlighted that emergency drugs are routinely dispensed out of practice hours, to older patients with chronic conditions in particular. While this is an agreeable practice ensuring care continuity, it at the same time raises issues on the adequacy of communication between GPs and pharmacists. When pharmacists respond to ad hoc medicine requests without reference to physicians, the terrain for ethical dilemmas in patient care becomes available, primarily concerning compliance and the level of medical management (Ashcroft et al., 2015). The solutions to such issues call for establishing formal communication channels between pharmacists and general practices to resolve dilemmas and improve patient outcomes. Furthermore, prescribing behavior is often determined by system influences, including the workload of providers and health policy, which may generate ethical challenges. GPs' pressures may, in some instances, result in hurried prescribing in lieu of thorough consideration of each patient's needs. These stressful environments increase the likelihood of unethical prescribing practices, hence threatening the health of patients and undermining the trust that underpins the doctor-patient relationship. It is understood that responsibility in healthcare environments is dynamic rather than constant, but variable based on the nature of the situation being presented, which can help doctors rethink their prescribing practice as responsibilities and risk management roles (Zukas et al., 2013). Given these nuances, formal consideration of ethical guidelines is necessary, asserting priority of both accountability and optimal patient care in the setting of general practice.

Test Your Knowledge

1. What is the importance of informed consent and patient autonomy in pharmacological treatment?
2. How do issues of drug pricing and accessibility impact ethical decision-making in pharmacology?
3. What are some common ethical dilemmas faced by healthcare providers when prescribing medications?

SUMMARY

In summary, the incorporation of pharmacology in general practice plays a vital role in maximizing patient care via evidence-based management of medications. Such broad knowledge allows medical practitioners to weigh the therapeutic benefits against the harms of pharmacologic interventions. The EBPs outlined in the paper highlight the importance of ongoing training and practice reforms towards enhanced clinical outcomes. Moreover, the use of formal frameworks, as demonstrated in studies on benefit-risk assessments, is an active intervention to protect patient safety and facilitate optimal exchange of essential information among actors in the healthcare network (James et al., 2015). This demonstrates the imperative to foster harmony in settings where pharmacological advancements can be seamlessly integrated into everyday practice. Furthermore, the new animal drug safety evaluation is a poignant reminder of pharmaceutical principles with relevance outside human pharmacology. The highly accurate preclinical experiments to determine efficacy and toxicity demonstrate that high standards are practiced in veterinary as well as in human pharmacology (Polova et al., 2018) These experiments ensure both safety and efficacy in addition to facilitating informed professional decisions. Because GPs are exposed to such a diverse range of drugs, identifying similarities through pharmacology remains an integral part of patient care, ultimately improving the therapy process. Ultimately, the integration of pharmacology and general practice is not merely an intellectual endeavor but a practical necessity that will drive future healthcare provision. As the practice of medicine continues to evolve, ongoing research and debate into pharmacological use will ensure that safety, efficacy, and patient-centered care remain the primary considerations. Findings from various studies support open communication and evidence-based clinical practice, enabling health professionals to adeptly navigate challenging pharmacological environments (James et al., 2015). In a continuously evolving field, embracing these principles is imperative to achieve optimal gains from pharmacological treatment with fewer associated risks, resulting in a safer and better healthcare system.

The integration of pharmacology within general practice indicates a multifaceted approach to patient care that seeks to maximize the benefits of drug treatment. Key themes include the necessity for practitioners to control pharmacological principles to maximize treatment benefits. This entails not only understanding and being familiar with the mechanisms of drug action but also staying up-to-date with the latest therapeutic developments and recommendations. The place is attributed to clinical trials and peer-reviewed evidence, such as that published by Clinical Pharmacology and Therapeutics, to emphasize the need for practitioners to critically evaluate new treatments to ensure the best are applied in general practice. By combining extensively screened pharmacological science with clinical experience, healthcare clinicians can tailor treatment regimens that address the individual needs of their patients and thereby enhance the quality of care administered across different settings (Terzic et al., 2017). In the instance of specific pharmacological interventions, anal fissure treatment describes the intricacies of general practice. The discussions regarding the application of pharmacological agents demonstrate the extent to which these therapies can improve the QoL of patients. The latest studies on rectal cream application, such as the favorable results of the combined composition No. 4 rectal cream, prove the potential of new drugs to cure chronic conditions. These findings offer invaluable information about the properties that such medications must possess, such as anti-inflammatory and analgesic effects, to facilitate healing. Therefore, clinical practice is informed by the emphasis on empirical evidence and drug assessment through systematic approaches to ensure that therapeutic interventions for patients are not only effective but also safe (Stakhorska et al., 2019). Finally, it is evident that the current debate on pharmacology in general practice positively contributes to improving patient outcomes and enhancing professional enlightenment. By gathering essential information from ongoing research and clinical practice, health professionals are better equipped to address the challenges of managing medications. New intervention therapy and traditional pharmacological approaches continue to evolve, further enhancing patient-centered care. These debates raise the critical question of ongoing education and training for professionals in managing the dynamic pharmacotherapy arena properly. As healthcare continues to evolve, having a strong foundation of pharmacological expertise will continue to be crucial in providing patients with complete and adequate care suited to their unique needs (Terzic et al., 2017).

KEY TERMS FROM THIS CHAPTER

- Adverse drug reactions (ADRs)
- Clinical decision support systems (CDSS)
- Drug-drug interactions
- Evidence-based pharmacology
- Health provision
- Healthcare professionals
- High-throughput screening practices
- Antibiotic resistance
- Drug action
- Drug-related side effects
- Health practitioners
- Healthcare clinicians
- Heterogeneous physiological responses
- Central nervous system (CNS)

CRITICAL THINKING QUESTIONS

1. **What does pharmacokinetics primarily study?**
   a. The effects of drugs on the body
   b. The absorption, distribution, metabolism, and excretion of drugs
   c. The ethical considerations in drug prescription
   d. The adverse effects of drugs
2. **Which term describes the relationship between drug concentration and its effect on the body?**
   a. Pharmacokinetics
   b. Therapeutic index
   c. Pharmacodynamics
   d. Bioavailability
3. **An example of a common adverse drug reaction is:**
   a. Weight gain after taking antipsychotics
   b. The therapeutic effect of an antibiotic
   c. The interaction between aspirin and warfarin causes bleeding
   d. Drug absorption in the stomach
4. **What is an essential component of patient education regarding medication adherence?**
   a. Explaining the drug's mechanism in detail
   b. Discussing the importance of completing the prescribed course
   c. Providing only written instructions
   d. Focusing on adverse drug reactions only
5. **Which ethical principle is most relevant when prescribing medications?**
   a. Autonomy
   b. Justice
   c. Confidentiality
   d. Non-maleficence

Short Answer Questions

1. How did early medicinal practices and herbal remedies contribute to the historical development of pharmacology?
2. What are the key differences between pharmacokinetics and pharmacodynamics, and why are both important in drug therapy?
3. What categories of medications are most commonly prescribed in general practice, and how do these medications address common health conditions?
4. Why is monitoring for adverse drug reactions and drug interactions critical in general practice, and what are some strategies to minimize these risks?
5. What role does patient education play in improving medication adherence, and what techniques can healthcare providers use to support patients?
6. How can ethical considerations, such as informed consent and patient autonomy, influence prescribing practices in general practice?

Answers to Critical Thinking Questions

1. (b) 2. (c) 3. (a) 4. (b) 5. (d)

REFERENCES

1. Lees, P., Pelligand, L., Whiting, M., Chambers, D., Toutain, P., & Whitehead, M. L. (2017). Comparison of veterinary drugs and veterinary homeopathy: part 1. *Veterinary Record, 181*(7), 170–176. https://doi.org/10.1136/vr.104278Abbott, R., & Ayres, I. (2014). Evidence and extrapolation: Mechanisms for regulating off-label uses of drugs and devices. https://core.ac.uk/download/62566275.pdf (accessed on 27th June 2025).
2. Abdelfatah, S., Abu-Darwish, M. S., Banerjee, M., Bhakta-Guha, D., et al. (2019). Biopiracy *versus* one-world medicine–From colonial relicts to global collaborative concepts. https://core.ac.uk/download/228178415.pdf (accessed on 27th June 2025).
3. Abdel-Rahman, S. M., Ahsman, M. J., Ambrose, P. G., Anderson, B. J., Anderson, G. D., Anderson, S. L., Andes, D., et al. (2014). Pharmacokinetic/pharmacodynamic modelling approaches in pediatric infectious diseases and immunology. https://core.ac.uk/download/29469548.pdf (accessed on 27th June 2025).
4. Abduljalil, K., Aghazadeh-Habashi, A., Aigrain, P., Aitman, T. J., Al Za'abi, M., Alegre, B., Alnaqeeb, M. A., et al. (2019). Current trends in drug metabolism and pharmacokinetics. https://core.ac.uk/download/286361678.pdf (accessed on 27th June 2025).
5. Abrahamsson, H., Abramiuk, M., Aitken, M., Ajram, L., Akers, J., Aldhouse-Green, S., Andrews-Hanna, J., et al. (2017). The odyssey of dental anxiety: From prehistory to the present. A narrative review. https://core.ac.uk/download/84923580.pdf (accessed on 27th June 2025).
6. Adhikari, P., Padmaja, U., & Pereira, P. (2009). A prospective analysis of adverse drug reactions in a South Indian hospital. https://core.ac.uk/download/pdf/87416.pdf (accessed on 27th June 2025).
7. Advisory Council on the Misuse of Drugs. (2011). *Consideration of the Novel Psychoactive Substances ('Legal Highs')*. https://core.ac.uk/download/1643031.pdf (accessed on 27th June 2025).
8. Ameer, B., & Weintraub, M. (2018). Pediatric obesity: Influence on drug dosing and therapeutics. https://core.ac.uk/download/155271623.pdf (accessed on 27th June 2025).
9. Antrobus, R., Bujar, M., Crisp, N., Dukes, G., Gouws, J., Gouws, J., Green Thompson, R., et al. (2018). The South African regulatory system: Past, present, and future. https://core.ac.uk/download/287581368.pdf (accessed on 27th June 2025).
10. Aramin, H., Crowe, S. E., Gupta, S., Park, J. S., et al. (2016). Review article: The global emergence of *Helicobacter pylori* antibiotic resistance. https://core.ac.uk/download/323064594.pdf (accessed on 27th June 2025).
11. Ashcroft, D. M., Gray, N. J., Mackridge, A. J., Mensah, N., et al. (2015). Emergency supply of prescription-only medicines to patients by community pharmacists: A mixed methods evaluation incorporating patient, pharmacist and GP perspectives. https://core.ac.uk/download/42138326.pdf (accessed on 27th June 2025).
12. Attard Montalto, S. (2014). Ethical principles in pediatric practice. https://core.ac.uk/download/46603075.pdf (accessed on 27th June 2025).
13. Bailey, J., Bon, C., Cox, S., Darwich, A. S., Dorey, J., Duwal, S., Ette, E. I., et al. (2018). Population variability in animal health: Influence on dose-exposure-response relationships. Part II: Modelling and simulation. https://core.ac.uk/download/159992803.pdf (accessed on 27th June 2025).

14. Bajorek, B., & Singh, S. (2014). Defining 'elderly' in clinical practice guidelines for pharmacotherapy. https://opus.lib.uts.edu.au/bitstream/10453/35163/1/Defining%20%27elderly%27%20in%20clinical%20practice%20guidelines%20for%20pharmacotherapy.pdf (accessed on 27th June 2025).

15. Banoo, S., Keyter, A., Salek, M. S. S., Walker, S. R., et al. (2019). The South African Medicines Control Council: Comparison of its registration process with Australia, Canada, Singapore, and Switzerland. https://core.ac.uk/download/287581585.pdf (accessed on 27th June 2025).

16. Barke, E., Coghill, D., & Cornforth, C. (2010). Stimulant drug effects on attention deficit/hyperactivity disorder: A review of the effects of age and sex of patients. https://core.ac.uk/download/55797029.pdf (accessed on 27th June 2025).

17. Barker, C. I., Irwin, A., Le Doare, K., Sharland, M., et al. (2015). Improving antibiotic prescribing for children in the resource-poor setting. https://core.ac.uk/download/29469533.pdf (accessed on 27th June 2025).

18. Bhanji, S., Qidwai, W., & Sabzwari, S. R. (2013). Polypharmacy in elderly: A cautious trail to tread. https://core.ac.uk/download/47258911.pdf (accessed on 27th June 2025).

19. Bhattacharya, D., Poland, F., Wright, D., Yemm, R., et al. (2014). What constitutes a high-quality discharge summary? A comparison between the views of secondary and primary care doctors. https://core.ac.uk/download/41989602.pdf (accessed on 27th June 2025).

20. Boons, C. C. L. M., Hugtenburg, J. G., Timmers, L., van den Bemt, B. J. F. M., et al. (2017). Supporting adherence to oral anticancer agents: Clinical practice and clues to improve care provided by physicians, nurse practitioners, nurses and pharmacists. https://core.ac.uk/download/84046723.pdf (accessed on 27th June 2025).

21. Boothroyd, D. (2011). *Pharmacology*. https://core.ac.uk/download/29175462.pdf (accessed on 27th June 2025).

22. Bouchaud, M., Brown, D., & Swan, B. A. (2017). Creating a new education paradigm to prepare nurses for the 21st century. https://core.ac.uk/download/129190945.pdf (accessed on 27th June 2025).

23. Boussery, K., Mehuys, E., Petrovic, M., Somers, A., et al. (2015). Older patients' prescriptions screening in the community pharmacy: Development of the Ghent Older People's Prescriptions Community Pharmacy Screening (GheOP3S) tool. https://core.ac.uk/download/55843875.pdf (accessed on 27th June 2025).

24. Cochetti, C. S. (2009). *Integrating 'Traditional' And 'Scientific' Medicine in Contemporary Cuba*. https://core.ac.uk/download/74352.pdf (accessed on 27th June 2025).

25. Coleman, D. L., & Rosoff, P. M. (2011). The case for legal regulation of physicians' off-label prescribing. https://core.ac.uk/download/62564977.pdf (accessed on 27th June 2025).

26. Cox, C. L. (2012). Adherence, compliance, persistence and concordance in the management of glaucoma, Part I. https://core.ac.uk/download/9983106.pdf (accessed on 27th June 2025).

27. De Paepe, A., & Vanakker, O. (2013). Pharmacogenomics in children: Advantages and challenges of next generation sequencing applications. https://core.ac.uk/download/55848729.pdf (accessed on 27th June 2025).

28. Diallo, G., Foguem, C., & Kamsu-Foguem, B. (2013). Conceptual graph-based knowledge representation for supporting reasoning in African traditional medicine. https://core.ac.uk/download/12044019.pdf (accessed on 27th June 2025).

29. Farmer, A. P., Garg, A. X., Kuehn, B. M., Vucic, B., Sintek, C. D., Wang, D., Clark, D. J., et al. (2010). Designing an automated clinical decision support system to match clinical practice guidelines for opioid therapy for chronic pain. https://core.ac.uk/download/pdf/8407473.pdf (accessed on 27th June 2025).

30. Fenech, A. G., & Grech, G. (2009). Biotech drugs: Biological therapeutic agents. https://core.ac.uk/download/46603869.pdf (accessed on 27th June 2025).

31. Forte, J. S. (2000). How safe are herbal products? https://core.ac.uk/download/46604508.pdf (accessed on 27th June 2025).

32. Gasser, M., Gutzwiller, F. S., Keininger, D. L., Price, D., et al. (2018). Factors associated with appropriate inhaler use in patients with COPD–Lessons from the REAL survey. https://core.ac.uk/download/152415582.pdf (accessed on 27th June 2025).

33. Giovagnoli, A., & Zagoraiou, M. (2025). *Simulated Clinical Trials: Some Design Issues*. https://core.ac.uk/download/pdf/6820410.pdf (accessed on 27th June 2025).

34. Griese-Mammen, N., Ihle, P., Krueger, K., Laufs, U., et al. (2019). Comparison of different strategies to measure medication adherence via claims data in patients with chronic heart failure. https://core.ac.uk/download/225124687.pdf (accessed on 27th June 2025).

35. Hanekom, S., Patman, S., Plani, N., van Aswegen, H., et al. (2017). Developing minimum clinical standards for physiotherapy in South African ICUs: A qualitative study. https://core.ac.uk/download/213606949.pdf (accessed on 27th June 2025).

36. Hemingway, S., McCann, T., Roberts, B., Stephenson, J., et al. (2013). Mental health and learning disability nursing students' perceptions of the usefulness of the objective structured clinical examination to assess their competence in medicine administration. https://core.ac.uk/download/20363416.pdf (accessed on 27th June 2025).

37. Hemingway, S., Mutsatsa, S., Newell, R., & Turner, J. (2014). Can student mental health nurses be prepared for medicines management? https://core.ac.uk/download/30731081.pdf (accessed on 27th June 2025).

38. Hunt, C. A., Kennedy, R. C., Kim, D. Y., et al. (2013). Agent-based modeling: A systematic assessment of use cases and requirements for enhancing pharmaceutical research and development productivity. https://core.ac.uk/download/323079387.pdf (accessed on 27th June 2025).

39. Kitsiou, A., Caforio, A. L. P., Porta-Sanchez, A., Vahanian, A., Iung, B., Carrera, C., Szymanski, C., et al. (2013). *ESC Core Curriculum for The General Cardiologist (2013)*. https://core.ac.uk/download/55756305.pdf (accessed on 27th June 2025).

40. Kraft, W. K., Mantravadi, S., & Ogdie, A. (2017). Tumor necrosis factor inhibitors in psoriatic arthritis. https://core.ac.uk/download/83049994.pdf (accessed on 27th June 2025).

41. Leong, J., Salek, S., & Walker, S. (2015). A practical approach to communicating benefit-risk decisions of medicines to stakeholders. https://core.ac.uk/download/287582324.pdf (accessed on 27th June 2025).

42. Marsh, A., Singer, D. R. J., Taylor, P. C., Watkins, C., et al. (2010). Personalized medicine: The impact on chemistry. https://core.ac.uk/download/45676.pdf (accessed on 27th June 2025).

43. McCarthy, D., & Mueller, K. (2009). *Marshfield Clinic: Health Information Technology Paves the Way for Population Health Management.* https://core.ac.uk/download/71352965.pdf (accessed on 27th June 2025).

44. Overy, C., & Tansey, E. M. (2014). *Migraine: Diagnosis, Treatment and Understanding c1960–2010.* https://core.ac.uk/download/30696936.pdf (accessed on 27th June 2025).

45. Polova, Z. (2018). Study of acute toxicity of a new veterinary drug for intramammary introduction. https://media.neliti.com/media/publications/297577-study-of-acute-toxicity-of-a-new-veterin-a8c4d87e.pdf (accessed on 27th June 2025).

46. Reynolds, L. A., & Tansey, E. M. (2008). *Clinical Pharmacology in the UK, c.1950–2000: Industry and Regulation.* https://core.ac.uk/download/30696180.pdf (accessed on 27th June 2025).

47. Roth, D., & Cuatrecasas, P. (2010). The distributed partnering model for drug discovery and development. https://core.ac.uk/download/71350819.pdf (accessed on 27th June 2025).

48. Schenk, K. (1959). *A Study to Determine If Facts About Drugs and Drug Therapy Can Be Learned as Effectively by A Patient-Centered Approach as By Classroom Presentation* (Master's thesis). https://open.bu.edu/bitstream/2144/21940/1/Schenk_Katharine_1959_web.pdf (accessed on 27th June 2025).

49. Siriwardena, A. N. (2006). The rise and rise of non-medical prescribing. https://core.ac.uk/download/52725.pdf (accessed on 27th June 2025).

50. Stakhorska, M., & Zaychenko, G. (2019). Experimental approval of the efficacy of the combined composition rectal cream new test-samples in the conditions of acute complicated anal fissure in rats https://core.ac.uk/download/322516330.pdf (accessed on 27th June 2025).

51. Terzic, A. M., & Waldman, S. A. (2017). Peer review certifies quality and innovation in *Clinical Pharmacology & Therapeutics.* https://core.ac.uk/download/129191658.pdf (accessed on 27th June 2025).

52. van den Bemt, B. J. F., Arnet, I., Hersberger, K. E., Nieuwlaat, R., & Allemann, S. S. (2016). Matching adherence interventions to patient determinants using the theoretical domains framework. https://core.ac.uk/download/95845988.pdf (accessed on 27th June 2025).

53. Zukas, M., Kilminster, S., & Fenwick, T. (2013). Responsibility matters: Putting illness back into the picture. https://core.ac.uk/download/16467837.pdf (accessed on 27th June 2025).

CARDIOVASCULAR SYSTEM: DISEASES, RISK FACTORS, DIAGNOSTIC APPROACHES, AND TREATMENT MODALITIES

5

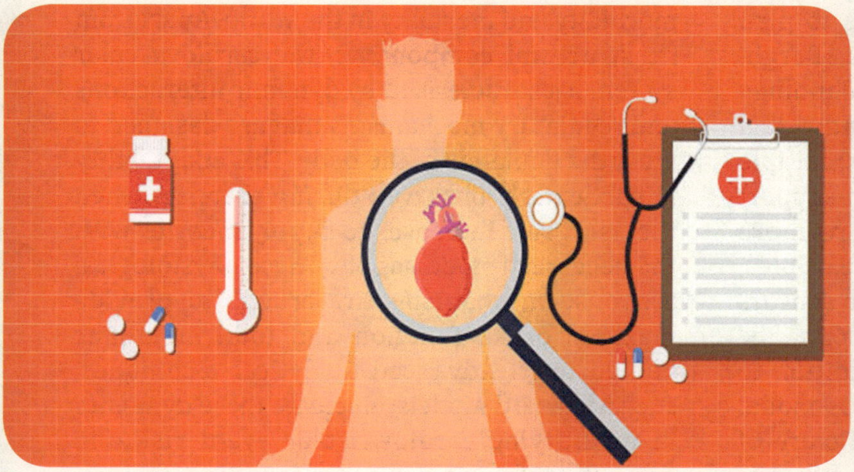

LEARNING OBJECTIVES

After studying this chapter, you will be able to:

1. Understand the anatomy of the cardiovascular system
2. Describe common cardiovascular diseases
3. Explain risk factors for cardiovascular disease
4. Discuss diagnostic approaches in general medicine
5. Define treatment modalities
6. Focus on effective preventive measures in addressing cardiovascular diseases

Introduction

The cardiovascular system is also the key to maintaining overall health because it transports oxygen and nutrients to tissues and removes metabolic waste products. This complexity necessitates a holistic approach in the practice of general medicine, where doctors must contend with many interrelated variables influencing cardiovascular health. Traditional interventions for treatment often focus on single symptoms or quantitative measures, such as blood pressure and cholesterol, and may well overlook the general context of a patient's way of life, genetics, and environmental factors. As cardiovascular illnesses are still among the leading causes of morbidity and mortality globally, there is an increasingly strong need to establish systemic solutions addressing not only the physiological but also the psychosocial aspects of patient care. Breakthroughs in tailored medicine will radically alter the overall therapeutic approach to CVD. Understanding that no two patients are alike, physicians must consider individual variables—genetic background and personal risk factors—in arriving at treatment decisions. Present reductionist models, which are prone to oversimplifying disease etiology, can lead to futile treatment, with patients never having proper management of their condition. Personalized medicine aims to individualize treatment based on each patient's characteristics, potentially maximizing adherence to treatment protocols and the treatment of CVDs. This revolution is underpinned by emerging systems biology tools and technical progress that facilitate more nuanced insight into personal health parameters, allowing clinicians to plan more optimal management strategies (Borghi et al., 2017). With the emerging technology that creates large volumes of data on individual patients, it is now feasible to integrate multiple types of health measures into a decision-support system, rendering cardiovascular care more informed in its decision-making. Wearables, social media usage, and several other sensors provide valuable information about patients' lifestyle and physical condition, in addition to past clinical measurements. This cross-modal analysis of data provides a holistic picture of cardiovascular health, enabling a more dynamic understanding of the overall well-being of the patients. Moreover, new approaches can estimate genetic traits, environmental exposures, and other factors that may influence cardiovascular risk, thereby improving the clinical context (Banister et al., 2018). Consequently, a general medicine approach that properly combines these varied streams of information can enhance diagnostic accuracy and personalized treatment, ultimately leading to improved patient outcomes for those suffering from CVD.

Definition of Cardiovascular System

The cardiovascular system plays a central role in ensuring homeostasis and general well-being within the human body. It comprises the heart, blood vessels, and blood, and they function together to distribute oxygen, nutrients, hormones, and other vital substances to tissues while allowing carbon dioxide and metabolic wastes to be removed. While the central pump is the heart, pumping blood through an arterial and venous system, the physiology of this system is much more intricate than simple transportation. The internal and external forces of physical exercise, nutrition, and genetics influence the physiological laws that regulate this system. Healthcare professionals need to understand the complexity of the cardiovascular system because it is the foundation of CVD diagnosis and management, one of the leading causes of morbidity and mortality in the world. Apart from its structural components, the cardiovascular system is characterized by dynamic interactions and regulatory mechanisms that are designed to meet the demands of the body. This adaptability is particularly observed during exercise, when the heart rate increases to supply muscles with the necessary blood supply. These physiological response mechanisms are crucial to provide maximal organ function and total metabolic homeostasis. Advanced analytical techniques, such as hazard models, elucidate these dynamics in quantifying cardiovascular event risk and correcting for possible confounding factors. These models incorporate time-to-event analysis and can potentially enhance our understanding of the complexity of cardiovascular well-being and disease progression, resulting in personalized prevention and therapeutic interventions (Abrahamowicz et al., 2020). Furthermore, recent advances in biomedical science highlight the application of physiological signals for evaluating cardiovascular well-being. Techniques such as the synchrosqueezing transform (SST) enable the study of oscillatory physiological signals, including those from pulse wave analysis. By analyzing such signs, researchers can acquire characteristics like the spectral pulse signature to more precisely describe hemodynamics. The application of such novel techniques to cardiovascular studies enhances the monitoring and diagnosis capabilities of CVDs. This multi-dimensional approach highlights the potential of incorporating advanced analytical models into the master medical strategy to address cardiovascular issues, ultimately leading to improved patient outcomes and a better understanding of cardiovascular health (Chang et al., 2016) (Figure 5.1).

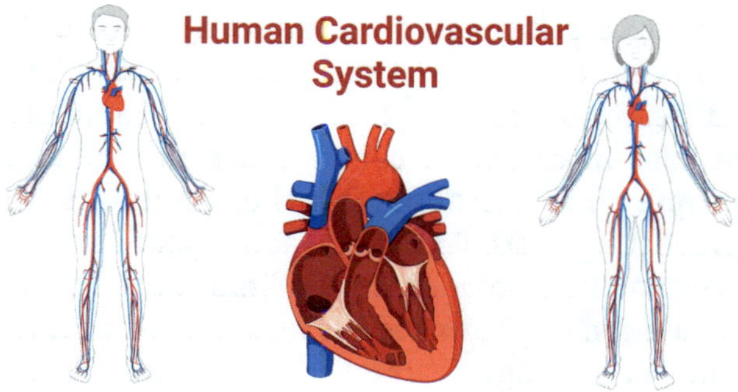

Figure 5.1. Illustration of human cardiovascular system.

Source: https://microbenotes.com/wp-content/uploads/2023/02/Human-Cardiovascular-System-1.jpg.

Importance of Cardiovascular Health

Cardiovascular health forms a critical component of overall well-being, significantly influencing morbidity and mortality on the global platform. The incidence of CVD keeps increasing, emphasizing the need for public health intervention and personal education regarding risk factors. Preventative strategies, such as lifestyle modifications involving diet and exercise, form the core of reducing CVD risk factors. Emphasizing regular check-ups and consultation with physicians can lead to early interventions that make it possible to control hypertension, diabetes, and cholesterol levels properly. Since the diseases have such a significant impact on populations, particularly in developing nations, interventions also need to address accessibility of therapies, not just prevention. Increased education and awareness programs might drive a culture of CVD prevention, eventually translating into better health outcomes and reduced healthcare spending in the long run. Social implications of CVD are particularly incisive, given its prevalence and demographic effects on various populations, with gender-based factors being considered in particular. In countries such as Saudi Arabia, for example, the rate of CHD has been increasing, with common risk factors following the same trend as found in Western nations. Smoking, physical inactivity, and obesity are key contributors to cardiovascular burden, which is further compounded by cultural practices that might make it challenging for the effective provision of health services to specific groups of individuals, like Saudi women. Improving cardiovascular health among such marginalized groups is in jeopardy if these differences are not addressed. There is an imperative need to address culturally distinct concerns for these populations, since varying awareness and availability of prevention result in increased morbidity and mortality among women and erode general public health measures. Therefore, one must understand and buffer such gender-specific variations to form targeted policies in the realm of health. Access to effective treatment and preventive drugs is another key factor in promoting cardiovascular health. Despite clear evidence of the link between CVDs and numerous health inequities, millions of individuals all over the world lack access to essential medicines and healthcare. The global emphasis on enhancing access to medicines, as part of the 2011. The UN political declaration on non-communicable diseases (NCDs) highlights the imperative of policy measures to close gaps in treatment. By adopting successful HIV treatment models, healthcare systems can integrate scalable, affordable, and fair approaches. Moreover, better procurements and more effective use of generic drugs will go a long way in enhancing treatment access, especially in LMICs. By focusing on systemic issues and implementing effective policies, we can make rapid strides in preventing and controlling CVDs, ultimately improving the health future of millions worldwide.

Overview of General Medicine's Role in Cardiovascular Care

General medicine plays a key role in cardiovascular management, particularly in the prevention and treatment of CVD. GPs serve as the first point of contact for patients, a factor that allows early detection of risk factors such as hypertension, hyperlipidemia, and diabetes. Because CVDs are mostly multifactorial, integrated intervention by general medicine clinicians allows comprehensive evaluation of the health status of a patient. In addition, their ability to coordinate referrals to the specialists allows that the patient receives overall treatment appropriate to his/her needs. World health systems are increasingly recognizing the importance of primary care in managing NCDs, with a special emphasis on cardiovascular health. For instance, maximizing the use of available budgets through efficient selection and procurement of drugs can enhance access to treatment for such conditions, reflecting the role of general medicine in driving better patient outcomes (Abdraimova et al., 2013). Additionally, compliance of patients with prescribed pharmacotherapy remains a significant problem in cardiovascular treatment, particularly for the condition of hypertension. Despite the effectiveness of antihypertensive medication, evidence exists that suggests that noncompliance with antihypertensive treatment can have undesirable health effects, putting patients at risk of cardiovascular complications. GPs, as they manage their patients' care, must make efforts to promote compliance, including shared decision-making during consultations. This allows for the incorporation of patients' beliefs and perceptions of their diseases, which can enhance their compliance with treatment regimens. By encouraging open communication and transparency about the requirement for compliance, general medicine cannot only improve patient outcomes on an individual basis but also participate in overall public health campaigns to reduce the prevalence of CVD (Banning et al., 2009). Furthermore, the role of general medicine in cardiovascular practice emphasizes the necessity to address health inequities, particularly in low- and middle-income nations. These populations often face access hurdles for basic drugs and CVD interventions. General medical physicians can advocate for policies that favor the equitable utilization of health commodities to facilitate proper interventions for their patients in preventing CVDs. This can be done by influencing policymakers to address the limitations in the regulation of pharmaceuticals and drug access. The knowledge gained through dominant models, such as those used for HIV care, can be tapped as effective templates to enhance the availability of CVD care. With concerted efforts aimed at prevention and control, general medicine can assume a critical role in changing cardiovascular health outcomes among diverse populations (Abdraimova et al., 2013).

5.1. Anatomy of the Cardiovascular System

Learning Outcome

1. Understand the structure of the heart
2. Describe major blood vessels and their functions
3. Explain circulatory pathways

The cardiovascular system, or the heart and blood vessels, is the basis on which adequate blood circulation in the human body is achieved. The heart functions as a two-pump system: the right pump handles pulmonary circulation, while the left pump manages systemic circulation. The composition of the heart involves atria and ventricles, both of which play vital roles in receiving and pumping blood out. The cardiac muscle, or the myocardium, is responsible for contraction, providing oxygenated blood to tissues and organs. In addition, the intricate network of arteries, veins, and capillaries constitutes the vascular system, facilitating the delivery of nutrients and waste at the cellular level. Appreciating such anatomical complexity is key to the diagnosis and management of CVD, with cardiovascular system diseases remaining the leading causes of morbidity and mortality globally, further driving the necessity for a comprehensive knowledge of cardiovascular anatomy in clinical medicine. Being more specific, the chambers of the heart are lined with specialized tissues that optimize efficiency and minimize turbulence in blood flow. The mitral and tricuspid valves between the atria and ventricles regulate unidirectional blood flow, preventing backflow during contraction. The aortic and pulmonary valves regulate blood egress from the heart into the aorta and pulmonary artery, respectively. The conduction system of the heart, including the sinoatrial node and the atrioventricular (AV) node, regulates the heartbeat through electrical impulses, which are crucial for maintaining appropriate heart rhythms. Abnormal operation in any of these components could lead to arrhythmias or HF, thus making it essential that anatomical knowledge be translated into clinical practice. Exposing medical practitioners to such information gives them the skills needed to diagnose and treat CVDs effectively. Moreover, the vascular elements of the cardiovascular system, which are arteries, veins, and capillaries, play a vital role in overall health. Arteries, with muscle-thick walls, can sustain high pressure to carry oxygen-rich blood from the heart to the peripheral tissues. Veins are equipped with valves that help return deoxygenated blood to the heart, particularly from the lower extremities. Capillaries, with a single layer of endothelium, are the primary sites for the exchange of gas and nutrients. As described in existing literature, such as the assessment of enhancing the role of PAs and NPs in cardiovascular diagnosis, understanding this anatomy is essential because the health-care setting is changing to address the heightened demand for cardiology procedures due to a workforce shortage (Moon et al., 2017). Hence, a solid understanding of the anatomy of cardiovascular systems is not just the foundation of general medicine but is also essential in developing comprehensive strategies to address cardiovascular health needs.

5.1.1. Structure of the Heart

The heart, a muscle organ essential for survival, is the core component of the cardiovascular system responsible for maintaining circulation within the body. Its operation is intricate with four chambers: the right and left atria, and the right and left ventricles. The atria receive blood from the lungs and body, and the ventricles pump blood to the systemic circulation and lungs, respectively. This coordinated flow of blood is made possible through valves, ensuring a one-way passage. The right atrium receives the deoxygenated blood through the superior and inferior vena cavae and is then pumped to the right ventricle, which forwards it to the lungs for oxygenation. It is essential to understand the heart's structure in order to know how CVD can disrupt these processes and lead to a decline in health and well-being, including its importance to the practice of general medicine (Link et al., 2008). It also has valves and chambers, but the muscular wall of the heart, or the myocardium, is essential to its functioning. Composed primarily of cardiac muscle fibers, the myocardium possesses unique characteristics that allow it to contract rhythmically and forcefully to circulate blood through the circulatory system. The muscular layer is not equal in thickness; the left ventricle's wall is thicker than the right ventricle's wall to accommodate the higher pressures of systemic circulation. The pericardium is a two-walled sac that envelops the myocardium, providing structural support and containing fluid that reduces friction between heartbeats. Perception of myocardial integrity and pathology, such as hypertrophy or ischemia, has an effect in diagnosing and treating CVD (Meirhaeghe et al.,

2011). In addition, the electrical conduction system of the heart plays a crucial role in rhythmic contractions. Sinoatrial (SA) node, or the natural pacemaker, initiates the electrical impulses that propagate through the atria, triggering them to contract. The impulses are relayed to the AV node, where there is a brief pause before messages are forwarded on to the ventricles via the His-Purkinje system. This precise timing ensures chambers contract synchronously, thereby optimizing blood flow. Abnormalities of this electrical system may lead to arrhythmias, making familiarity with the heart's conduction pathways particularly important in general medicine. Advances in therapy for such conditions, including ablation therapies and pacemaker therapy, demonstrate the complement of anatomical data to clinical practice (Link et al., 2008) (Figure 5.2).

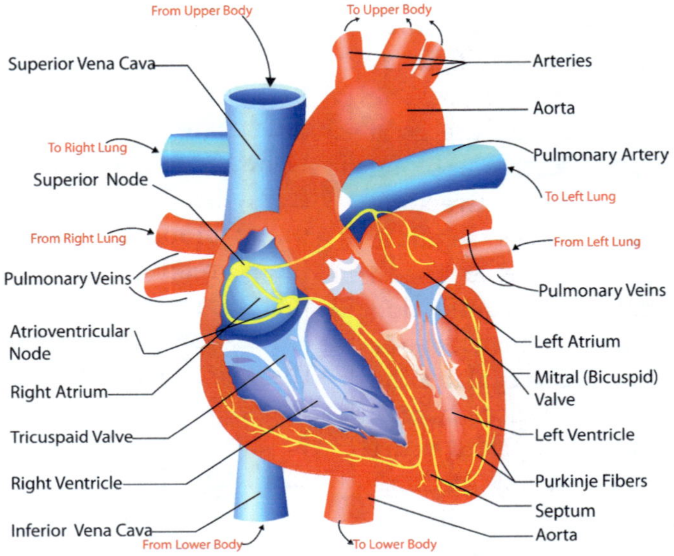

Figure 5.2. Heart structure.

Source: https://www.news-medical.net/image-handler/picture/2018/7/shutterstock_139537109.jpg.

5.1.2. Major Blood Vessels and Their Functions

The circulatory system in the human body highly depends on the large blood vessels, which serve as the tubes to transport the blood to and from the body. Arteries, veins, and capillaries all have distinct and essential functions to attain homeostasis. Arteries carry oxygenated blood from the heart to tissues, where it delivers essential nutrients and oxygen. The largest artery, the aorta, branches out into smaller arteries that supply all of the organs with an adequate amount of blood. Deoxygenated blood, however, is taken to the heart by veins and utilizes a one-way flow that prevents backflow through the use of valves. This intricate network of blood vessels helps control blood pressure and flow, both of which are critical for overall cardiovascular health. Capillaries, being the most minute of blood vessels, are the primary locations for oxygen, carbon dioxide, nutrients, and waste material exchange between blood and tissues. Gases and solutes can diffuse through thin walls for the efficient supply of nutrients and removal of wastes at the cellular level. The pattern of capillary beds follows the metabolic needs of the tissues and varies in density.

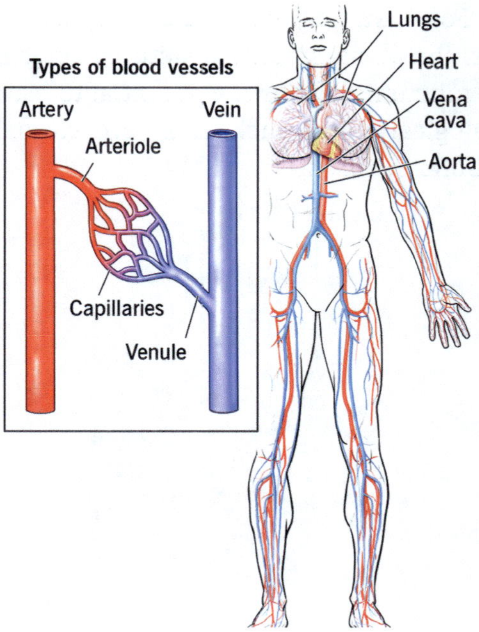

Figure 5.3. Blood vessels.

Source: https://my.clevelandclinic.org/-/scassets/images/org/health/articles/blood-vessels.

For instance, muscle tissue has a tight plexus of capillaries to support high metabolic demand, whereas other tissues may have a relatively loose network. Such dynamic flexibility emphasizes the importance of capillaries in the circulatory system and that they play a vital role in ensuring tissue homeostasis while enabling vital body functions. Cardiovascular technology advancements have initiated unprecedented advances in understanding and managing vascular health. Techniques such as real-time contouring of EKG displays and the measurement of blood pressure without invasive devices have revolutionized clinicians' ability to monitor vascular function non-invasively. Another approach to modeling blood flow dynamics applies highly sophisticated mathematical formulas to simulate blood flow in arterial circuits with high precision. According to recent evidence, these models provide predictions of physiological fluid flows, enhance diagnostics, and enable more individualized treatment regimens for vascular diseases. These developments not only increase our understanding of blood vessel function but also highlight the convergence of technology and clinical practice in advancing medical policy toward cardiovascular health (San et al., 2012; Schafer et al., 2025) (Figure 5.3).

5.1.3. Overview of the Circulatory Pathways

The circulatory circuits are the life-supporting pipelines of the cardiovascular system, required to maintain physiological equilibrium and organ function. Composed of two primary circuits—the systemic and pulmonary circuits—this intricate system presents an effective method of dispensing oxygenated blood to the body while simultaneously eliminating carbon dioxide and other metabolic waste. The systemic pathway begins with oxygenated blood being discharged from the left ventricle of the heart to the aorta, from which it branches out to small arteries and ultimately reaches capillaries. These are the places where blood and tissue exchange gases and nutrients, emphasizing the pathway's significance in sustaining cellular processes and overall metabolism. Furthermore, the circulation of deoxygenated blood begins in the venous system and moves to the right atrium, achieving a circular pattern. Such coordination forms one of the rudimentary principles of cardiovascular physiology and deserves continuous research in clinical sciences. The efficiency of the circulatory pathways is also reflected through the complex coordination of hormones such as natriuretic peptides (NPs), which form the cornerstone for regulating cardiovascular mechanisms. These peptides are directly involved in the regulation of blood pressure and in fluid balance, and are essential to both homeostasis and disease response (Figure 5.4).

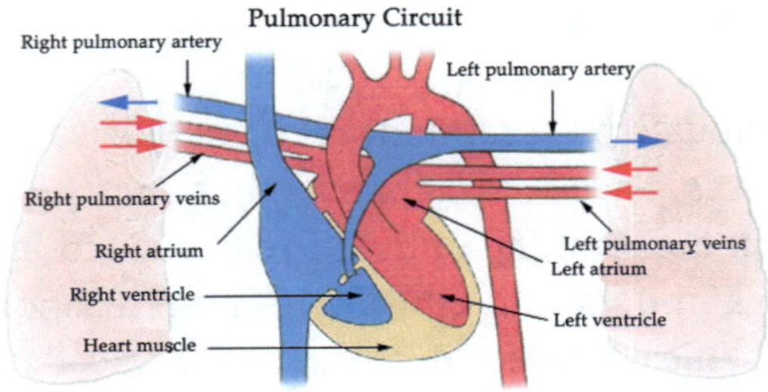

Figure 5.4. Pulmonary circuit.

Source: https://storymd.com/journal/jk7qlkqubm-circulatory-pathways/page/b5gzgh4l2kl-circulatory-pathways.

Dysregulation of NP signaling underlies a variety of cardiovascular conditions, including hypertension and HF, and thus underscores the importance of understanding their molecular mechanisms better. Increasing research has been devoted to exploring the therapeutic application of NPs, suggesting that targeting these molecules may represent new opportunities for intervention in numerous CVDs. This knowledge underlies modern medical treatment aimed at targeted and individualized therapy because it underlines the involvement of hormonal mechanisms in the overall picture of cardiovascular health, discussed in recent studies on the physiology and pathophysiology of the cardiovascular system (Rubattu et al., 2019). Circulatory mechanisms also exhibit dynamic effects from a variety of outside influences, including lifestyle determinants, environmental determinants, and genetic predisposition. Understanding the impact of these adipose tissues on the circulatory system is essential for the development of preventive strategies against CVD. For instance, epicardial adipose tissue deposition about cardiac structures determines heart function and has the potential to promote pathological states such as atherosclerosis or metabolic syndrome.

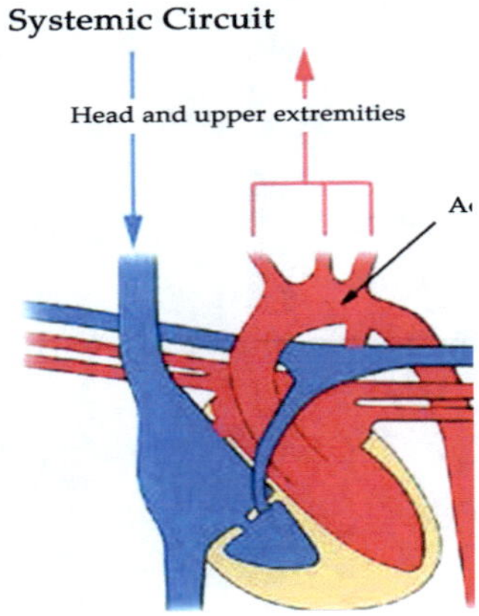

Figure 5.5. Systemic circuit.

Source: https://storymd.com/journal/jk7qlkqubm-circulatory-pathways/page/b5gzgh4l2kl-circulatory-pathways.

Development in imaging technology has enabled better studies of these adipose tissues, providing opportunities for new forms of interventions that can minimize their harmful effects. Also, as advocated in the ideologies of contemporary medicine, information from such research may promote the advancement of less harmful therapies that target root causes, which disquiet the delicate equilibrium of the cardiovascular system (Agra et al., 2017). Through insight into the complexities of these pathways, the path is set for more efficient general medicine approaches, endeavoring to optimize cardiovascular well-being (Figure 5.5).

Test Your Knowledge

1. What are the main structural components of the heart, and what roles do the atria and ventricles play in circulation?
2. Which are the major blood vessels connected to the heart, and what are their primary functions in blood circulation?

5.2. Common Cardiovascular Diseases

Learning Outcome

1. Describe coronary artery disease
2. Explain the causes of heart failure
3. Understand heart arrhythmia

Common CVDs constitute a range of disorders affecting the heart and blood vessels, with hypertension, coronary artery disease (CAD), and HF being particularly frequent. Hypertension, also known as the silent killer, typically does not have noticeable symptoms but can lead to severe complications, such as stroke and heart attack, if left untreated. Hypertension prevalence indicates the need for intensive screening and management procedures within the overall general medicine approach to CVD. Hypertension therapy is not only pharmacologically insufficient but must also consider the multifaceted nature of each patient's health status, lifestyle, and individual risk factors to mitigate associated cardiovascular risks (Borghi et al., 2017). CAD is another column of CVDs, which fundamentally results from plaque buildup in the coronary arteries and can result in myocardial ischemia. CAD has enormous implications and oftentimes results in angina and myocardial infarction. CAD patients typically present with a series of risk factors, including high cholesterol, smoking, and inactivity. General medicine adopts a comprehensive approach to treating CAD by promoting lifestyle changes alongside medical therapies that stabilize plaque formation and enhance endothelial function. Notably, gaining insight into the varied clinical manifestations of CAD enables practitioners to adopt individualized therapy, which maximizes patient outcomes in general. Due to the complex dynamics of CAD, a comprehensive plan involving education and drug compliance is of paramount importance to stem its effects on public health. CHF is a severe stage in CVD pathogenesis, with reduced capacity of the heart to pump blood. CHF tends to complicate earlier heart diseases and is most often caused by diseases such as hypertension and CAD. The global medicine approach to CHF management requires an interdisciplinary model merging symptom relief and quality-of-life medicines with lifestyle changes for fluid balance and nutrition modulation. Advances in personalized medicine offer promising opportunities in the management of CHF, putting patient-specific parameters at the forefront of developing effective management protocols. This tailored approach is essential because CHF presents differently in various populations, necessitating adaptable interventions that consider individual patient profiles to provide optimal care (Borghi et al., 2017). The evolution of more sophisticated treatment techniques for CVD highlights the importance of treating these common diseases by involving patients and using personalized therapies.

5.2.1. Coronary Artery Disease (CAD)

Coronary artery disease (CAD) is one of the most serious issues in the big picture of CVDs, which is characterized by narrowing or blockage of the coronary arteries due to the atherosclerotic process. Apart from resulting in reduced supply of blood to the heart muscle, CAD leads to serious complications such as myocardial infarction and HF. Despite advances in prevention and treatment over the past decades, CAD remains an epidemic cause of morbidity and mortality worldwide. The prevalence of risk factors such as hypertension, hyperlipidemia, and smoking speaks for targeted public health initiatives to reduce the overall burden of the disease. As described in the literature, broad dual approaches to the prevention of CVD are not well suited to individual patients and require an integrated, multifaceted strategy that considers both population-level and individual risk factors (Battistoni et al., 2015). The intricacies involved in managing CAD extend beyond routinely adjusting risk factors; they also require understanding the anatomical variations in coronary artery morphology, particularly when using interventions like stenting. Modern studies have reassured the need for recognizing and quantifying these morphological factors in a manner that can maximize treatment efficacy. For instance, accurate descriptions of bifurcation anatomies can facilitate determining the appropriate stenting technique both in the short and long run. These three-dimensional imaging-based computational models provide critical information about artery geometries and anatomy, enabling healthcare providers to incorporate more accurate treatment techniques for individual patients.

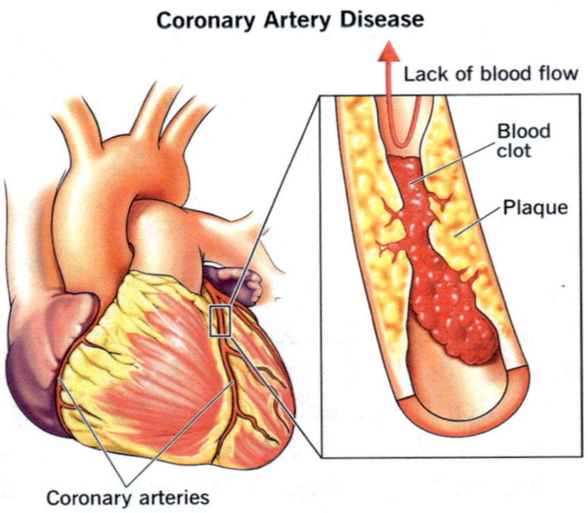

Figure 5.6. Coronary artery disease (CAD).

Source: https://my.clevelandclinic.org/-/scassets/images/org/health/articles/16898-coronary-artery-disease.

This data not only lends strength to intervention strategies but also lays the groundwork for future innovation in stent technology to improve results in the treatment of diseased arteries (Ellwein et al., 2016). The best way to counter the CAD burden is by implementing a multi-faceted strategy that addresses medical, lifestyle, and technological advances. Advanced risk stratification processes can be implemented by employing novel techniques that incorporate both conventional and novel risk factors so that high-risk patients receive early interventions. Public health interventions in the form of lifestyle modifications, such as dietary, exercise, and smoking cessation changes, are equally crucial for reducing the burden of CAD. Furthermore, more research on personalized medicine, particularly through newer imaging and computational modeling, can potentially simplify treatment approaches. With more convergence of these techniques, healthcare systems will become increasingly capable of preventing and managing CAD and ultimately improving outcomes and reducing the CVD socioeconomic burden (Battistoni et al., 2015) (Figure 5.6).

5.2.2. Heart Failure (HF)

Heart failure (HF) is a significant public health problem within the cardiovascular system, where the heart's inability to pump an adequate amount of blood to meet the body's requirements characterizes it. HF can be due to various etiologies, including ischemic heart disease, hypertension, and cardiomyopathy. The prevalence of HF is also significantly increasing, particularly due to the increase in the population of the elderly and the growing rates of obesity and diabetes. In addition, management of HF requires a comprehensive treatment process that involves lifestyle changes, drug therapy, and patient education. Multidisciplinary care teams that integrate various aspects of the disease help maximize treatment outcomes by addressing the physiological and psychosocial dimensions of the condition. Acknowledgment of such complexities is vital for healthcare practitioners interested in designing comprehensive strategies for HF management, ultimately to result in enhanced QoL in affected individuals. Diagnosis of HF involves an exacting consideration of the clinical presentation, results of physical examination, and several diagnostic tests. Dyspnea, fatigue, and edema are characteristic symptoms that need precise differentiation from other conditions that mimic HF. Diagnostic imaging, such as echocardiography, is at the core of cardiac function measurement and identification of intrinsic structural defects (Figure 5.7).

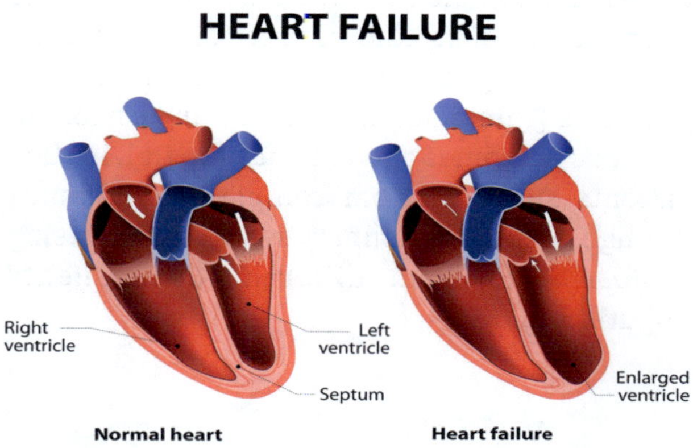

Figure 5.7. Heart failure (HF).

Source: https://continentalhospitals.com/uploads/mceu_22197202211699430774969.jpg.

Biomarkers like NPs also assist in confirming the diagnosis. Furthermore, practitioners must observe demographic factors that influence the presentation of the disease and treatment options. For instance, disparities in healthcare resources can hinder treatment compliance as well as outcomes, especially in rural areas or among minorities. All of these are determinable to enhance equal access to healthcare, leading to better health outcomes among all patients with HF. Management of HF is geared towards both pharmacologic and nonpharmacologic therapy. The merit of individualized management is emphasized. Medication-based therapies, such as ACE inhibitors, beta-blockers, and diuretics, alleviate symptoms and improve survival. Beyond pharmacotherapy is lifestyle change, including diet, exercise, and smoking cessation, for successful management. The social and cultural conditions of living among patients could also play a significant role in influencing treatment compliance. For example, in Australia, the socioeconomic status-health status relationship is reflected as disparities in access among rural populations, including Indigenous Australians (Clark et al., 2008). Likewise, in Saudi Arabia, culture-specific health concerns and gender differences impact care and secondary prevention strategies for CVD, necessitating culturally sensitive approaches to the management of HF (Clark et al., 2012) (Figure 5.8).

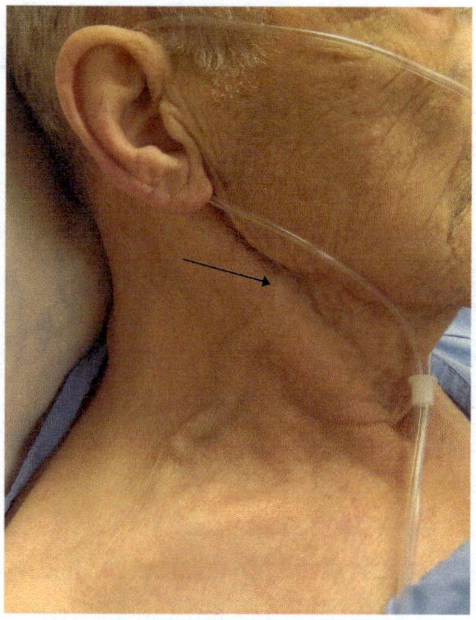

Figure 5.8. A man with congestive heart failure and marked jugular venous distension. An arrow marks the external jugular vein.

Source: https://upload.wikimedia.org/wikipedia/commons/thumb/4/4d/Elevated_JVP.JPG/800px-Elevated_JVP.JPG.

5.2.3. Arrhythmias

Arrhythmias, or irregular heart rhythms, are a significant clinical issue in the field of cardiovascular medicine. These disturbances in the normal rhythm of the heart can lead to tachycardia, bradycardia, or irregular rhythm, and cause a wide variety of clinical presentations ranging from palpitation and dizziness to more severe outcomes such as syncope or sudden cardiac arrest. The etiology of arrhythmias is multifactorial, usually involving a combination of intrinsic cardiac illness, environmental sources such as electrolyte abnormalities, and structural heart anomalies. Physicians must perform careful evaluation of patient history and appropriate diagnostic testing, such as electrocardiograms (ECGs) and electrophysiological studies, to adequately determine the etiology of the arrhythmia and formulate subsequent treatment plans accordingly. The management of arrhythmias must be both comprehensive and delicate, considering advances in medical technology and pharmacotherapy. Treatment can range broadly depending on the type and severity of the arrhythmia; it can be as simple as changes in lifestyle, pharmacological treatment using antiarrhythmic drugs, and more complex procedures such as catheter ablation or the placement of implantable cardioverter-defibrillators (ICDs). Furthermore, some populations, such as patients with congenital heart disease, have an increased risk for arrhythmias and need close monitoring and multidisciplinary care planning. Present evidence shows that patients with congenital heart disease are nearly twice as likely to have comorbidities, which further add complexity to the management of their arrhythmias, providing a strong impetus for an individualized treatment strategy (Agarwal et al., 2019). The relationship between comorbidities and arrhythmias profoundly impacts the clinical outcomes, such that the overall consideration of the patients' general health becomes essential. Most patients with arrhythmias also experience other CVDs or diseases that predispose them to complications. For instance, it is vital to understand the prevalence of comorbidities among patients with congenital heart disease because they are accompanied by unique challenges different from those in the rest of the population. They also have a higher incidence of both cardiovascular and noncardiovascular comorbidities, making them more complex to handle and requiring the interventions of healthcare professionals putting their hands together to mend such complicated problems (Kitsiou et al., 2013). It is possible to optimize outcomes and enhance the QoL in such patients suffering from complex arrhythmias through an interdisciplinary strategy comprising professionals from different departments (Figure 5.9).

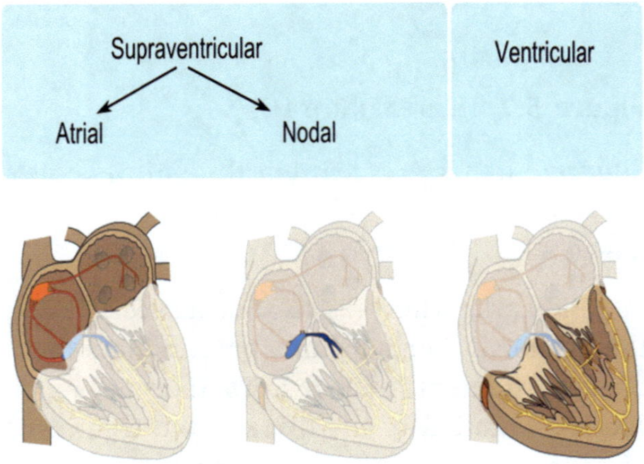

Figure 5.9. Broad classification of arrhythmias according to the region of the heart required to sustain the rhythm.

Source: https://upload.wikimedia.org/wikipedia/commons/7/77/De-Atrial_ventricular_%28CardioNetworks_ECGpedia%29.png.

Test Your Knowledge

1. What are the primary causes and symptoms of coronary artery disease?
2. What is heart failure, and how does it affect the function of the heart and circulation?
3. What are arrhythmias, and how can different types of arrhythmias impact heart function and patient health?

5.3. Risk Factors for Cardiovascular Disease

Learning Outcome

1. Describe lifestyle factors for cardiovascular disease
2. Understand the relationship between genetic predispositions and cardiovascular health
3. Explain comorbid conditions

Cardiovascular disease (CVD) remains one of the leading causes of morbidity and mortality globally, making it especially important to know of its multifactorial risk factors. Lifestyle determinants such as diet, exercise, and smoking play vital roles. Poor dietary habits, i.e., the consumption of high-fat and high-sugar foods, are significant risk factors for the development of obesity, hypertension, and dyslipidemia—all being pivotal predisposing conditions to CVD. In addition, sedentary behavior increases these risks, which emphasizes the importance of promoting exercise as a component of standard practice medicine. Identification of these lifestyle determinants allows clinicians to develop tailored interventions that will rectify lifestyles, hence restricting the incidence of CVD. It is a critical measure of prevention since early intervention of lifestyle factors will lead to improved outcomes and decreased healthcare expenditure on advanced CVDs. Another crucial factor in CVD risk is the comorbid illness, more specifically, the metabolic illnesses of diabetes and CKD. Not only do they raise the risk for CVD, but they also pose an additive challenge to clinical practitioners. Diabetic patients often have dysfunctional glucose metabolism that accelerates the development of atherosclerosis and magnifies the risk for cardiovascular events. Similarly, CKD is associated with hypertension as well as with electrolyte imbalance, adding further pressure to the cardiovascular system. A study conducted in primary care identified that healthcare providers often face constraints in effectively managing CKD, such as time, resources, and the availability of information on best practices (Abdel-Kader et al., 2019). Therefore, clinicians ought to be careful about such overlapping risk factors and prioritize management strategies that address cardiovascular status and coexisting comorbidities concurrently to optimize patient outcomes. Psychosocial factors have emerged as crucial predictors of CVD, thus giving rise to a complicated relationship between mental health and bodily status. Research has indicated that individuals with serious mental illness (SMI) are vulnerable to CVD due to numerous reasons, including the side effects of pharmacological therapy, which increase CVD risk (Braga et al., 2018). Mental illnesses such as depression and anxiety can result in lifestyle changes, such as weight gain and consumption of an unhealthy diet, further leading to cardiovascular events. To this, social determinants of health, such as access to healthcare and socioeconomic status, have an even higher level of influence when determining the health outcomes in these people. Therefore, mental healthcare has to be addressed holistically in primary care, and for this to occur, psychological and physical health considerations must be included in one overall approach to caring for the patient (Figure 5.10).

Cardiovascular risk factors

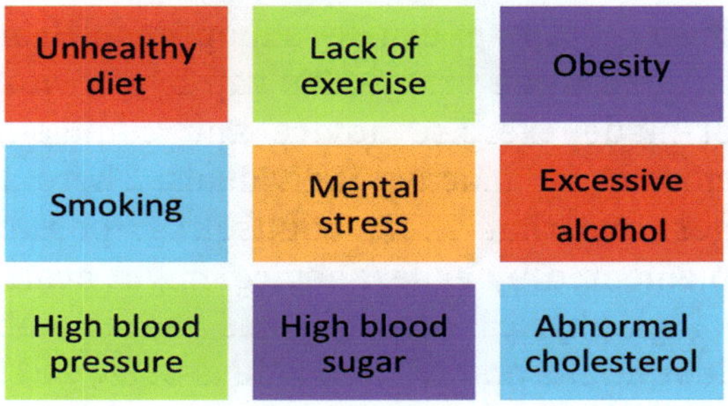

Figure 5.10. Cardiovascular risk factor.

Source: https://www.cardiacwellnessinstitute.com/heart-disease-treatment-prevention/wp-content/uploads/2019/12/Slide1.jpg.

5.3.1. Lifestyle Factors (Diet, Exercise, Smoking)

The relationship between cardiovascular health and lifestyle determinants is profound, particularly concerning different patterns of food, physical activity, and smoking. A diet rich in fruits, vegetables, whole grains, and low-fat protein is essential for cardiovascular health and the prevention of chronic diseases. Diets rich in saturated fats, trans fats, and salt cause atherosclerosis, hypertension, and ultimately cardiovascular issues. While single nutritional interventions yield minimal alterations in cholesterol, the evidence is inconsistent regarding their impact on morbidity and mortality, suggesting that nutritional management may not fully address cardiovascular needs. Despite this, nutritional improvement is paramount as it supports overall health efforts, indicating the need for long-term nutritional counseling and education in patient care, as noted in studies of lifestyle interventions. Also critical is the contribution made by physical exercise in cardiovascular well-being, as frequent physical exercise promotes beneficial metabolic shifts and decreases the obesity and high blood pressure. Not only does regular physical exercise contribute to maintaining weight, but it also improves vascular function and decreases inflammation. While the actions of exercise are well known, patient adherence to exercise therapy is usually suboptimal. Health practitioners can bridge this gap by providing tailor-made exercise advice and counseling specifically for inactive individuals. There are suggestions that short counseling, possibly supplemented by expert advice, might achieve very high physical activity gains, most notably in older adults and women (Aluas et al., 2019). Through such comprehensive approaches, practitioners can best ensure compliance with lifestyle changes that are crucial for cardiovascular wellness. Smoking cessation is also a leading lifestyle intervention in the model of general medicine in the management of the cardiovascular system, as smoking is a firmly entrenched risk factor for CVD. The evidence indicates that smoking cessation can lead to significant reductions in cardiovascular risk, although maintaining adherence to cessation strategies is challenging. General advice from health professionals has been shown to increase quit rates substantially among smokers, including those who are at higher risk of smoking-related illness. Incorporating various supportive interventions, such as counseling, smoking cessation therapy, and specially designed self-help materials, can also augment the likelihood of successful quitting (Aluas et al., 2019). The intersecting effects of smoking's adverse impacts on cardiovascular health underscore the importance of a combined approach that incorporates behavior modification into medical management, offering an all-encompassing method for optimizing patient outcomes in cardiovascular care (Aluas et al., 2019) (Figure 5.11).

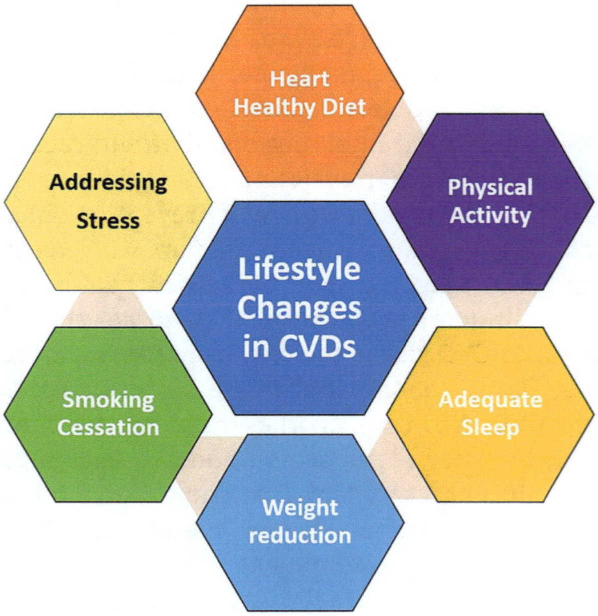

Figure 5.11. Lifestyle changes in CVDs.

Source: https://assets.cureus.com/uploads/figure/file/688742/article_river_49d74ce022d111ee9a792dbb7719cd14-Lifestyle.png.

5.3.2. Genetic Predispositions

The multifactorial relationship between cardiovascular wellness and hereditary susceptibilities has increasingly been recognized within the field of primary medicine. Hereditary factors contribute significantly to the etiology of most CVDs, including congenital heart defects (CHDs) and hypertension. The identification of specific genetic variants associated with these diseases enables health professionals to comprehend associated pathophysiological processes more accurately. As highlighted in the literature, CHDs are present in approximately 1% of live births and are a significant cause of mortality and morbidity in pediatrics. A comprehensive understanding of genetic susceptibilities allows for more personalized intervention and prevention strategies, thereby potentially improving patient outcomes. In addition, advances in genetic research allow one to shift from the traditional categorical diagnoses to more nuanced views of the genetic foundations, paving the way for innovative treatment protocols tailored to every patient. Perhaps the best example of advancement in this direction relates to the use of experimental systems in the study of genetic determinants of CVDs.

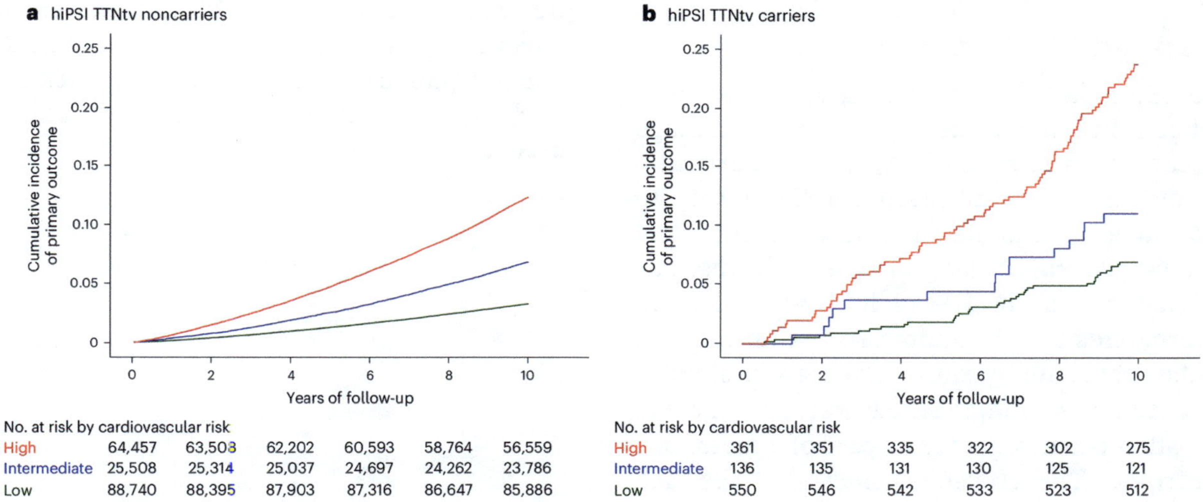

Figure 5.12. Impact of cardiovascular risk factors on genetic predisposition to heart disease.

Source: https://scx2.b-cdn.net/gfx/news/hires/2024/study-unveils-impact-o-1.jpg.

For instance, studies of coarctation of the aorta (CoA) employed new models to determine differential gene expression for this congenital condition. Scientists have isolated various factors of morbidity following repair using such models, including the involvement of genetic predispositions in impacting long-term health outcomes. By studying dysregulated pathways linked to CoA, particularly those involved in hypertension and cardiovascular dysfunction, a greater understanding is developed regarding how genetic influences interact with environmental and developmental forces. In doing so, this information not only provides guidance but also enables the development of targeted interventions designed to reduce the burden of CVD. Moreover, the potential to implement precision medicine in the treatment of CVD hinges upon unraveling the complexity of inherited susceptibility. Current literature emphasizes the necessity of intensive genetic stratification to inform clinical decisions, particularly in the management of intricate cardiovascular syndromes. The incorporation of phenotypic data with genetic and epigenetic information enables clinicians to gain a better integrated perception of individualized risk profiles. Systematic correlation of genomic sequencing and clinical assessment has the potential for identification of specific molecular pathways involved in CVD. Hence, the formulation of biobanks and patient cohorts for utilization in ongoing research will prove to be crucial in bringing to light the genetic etiology of CVDs. All these efforts are geared towards positioning cardiac care to advance toward a more personalized and streamlined model that safeguards against the long-term sequelae of genetic susceptibility on outcomes in patients (Figure 5.12).

5.3.3. Comorbid Conditions (Diabetes, Hypertension)

The existence of comorbidities, particularly diabetes and hypertension, is tough to manage in cardiovascular health, as it generally exacerbates the cardiovascular risks specific to heart disease. Diabetes mellitus, characterized by hyperglycemia, is a significant cardiovascular risk factor, mainly due to its involvement in atherogenesis and endothelial dysfunction. Studies consistently show that diabetics are at increased risk of high blood pressure, and the two often occur together as part of a metabolic syndrome. The crossover increases the risk of undesirable cardiovascular events such as heart attack and stroke, indicating the necessity of close monitoring and early treatment. Understanding the interdependence of these comorbid conditions can guide a more effective strategy in general medicine, aiming to address the multicomponent nature of cardiovascular well-being and reduce the overall disease burden. Hypertension, or high blood pressure, is a dominant risk factor that combines with synergistic cardiovascular effect from diabetes. The pathophysiologic mechanisms that underlie the association between hypertension and diabetes include chronic inflammation, increased vascular resistance, and autonomic dysfunction, all of which can eventually lead to organ damage. Hypertension is extremely prevalent in patients with diabetes, and most of them are not well-controlled in their blood pressure. Not only does this compounded diagnosis increase the risk of cardiovascular events, but it also complicates treatment. For instance, both disease conditions may require a multidimensional approach in the form of lifestyle change and pharmacological intervention that addresses both conditions simultaneously. Recognizing such complexities underscores the importance of an individualized management program within the framework of general medicine, ensuring that hypertension and diabetes are appropriately addressed and discussed to optimize outcomes. Moreover, the implications of comorbid diabetes and hypertension extend beyond individual health, reaching public health systems due to increased morbidity and expense of care for chronic disease.

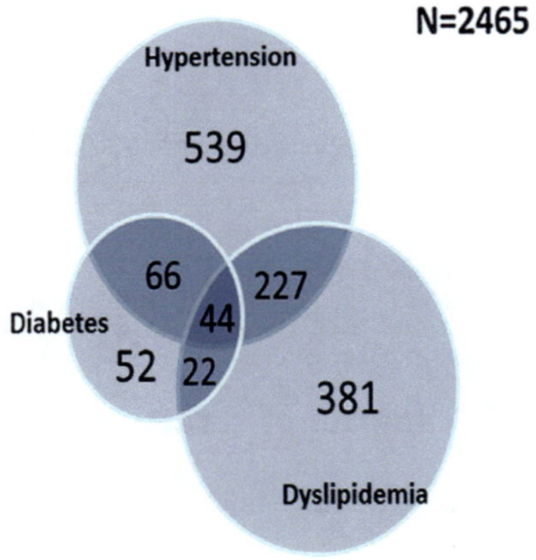

Figure 5.13. Comorbidities and overlap between diabetes, hypertension, and dyslipidemia.

Source: https://www.researchgate.net/profile/Jaya-Tripathy/publication/315948998/figure/fig1/AS:563823363215360@1511437373401/Co-morbidities-and-overlap-between-Diabetes-Hypertension-and-Dyslipidemia-India.png.

Evidence points to the fact that patients who are combating both diseases eventually experience much higher healthcare expenses and perhaps lower overall QoL. For instance, targeted interventions on specific chronic conditions can produce substantial quality improvements in diabetes care metrics, particularly when comorbid conditions like obesity and psychiatric disorders are present (Bolt et al., 2015). Interestingly, further, there are findings to suggest that mood disorders, including bipolar disorder, may be underdiagnosed in the context of diabetes-hypertension comorbidity, with treatment adherence and outcomes implications (Weeke et al., 2013). This under-recognition by the system highlights the need for healthcare professionals to adopt a holistic approach that acknowledges and addresses all aspects of a patient's health, ultimately leading to a more effective model for managing cardiovascular system-related illnesses (Figure 5.13).

Test Your Knowledge

1. How do lifestyle factors such as diet, physical activity, and smoking influence the risk of developing cardiovascular disease?
2. In what ways can genetic predispositions contribute to an individual's likelihood of developing cardiovascular conditions?
3. How do comorbid conditions like diabetes and hypertension increase the risk of cardiovascular disease, and why is managing these conditions important?

5.4. Diagnostic Approaches in General Medicine

Learning Outcome

1. Understand physical examination techniques in the cardiovascular approach
2. Discuss imaging studies in the assessment and management of cardiovascular health
3. Focus on laboratory tests (lipid profile and biomarkers)

The diagnostic techniques in general medicine have evolved significantly, especially in the cardiovascular system, where identification is critical and must be done in a timely and precise manner. Several techniques, including history-taking and physical examination, are steps that clinicians take toward diagnosing CVD. Advanced diagnostic equipment, such as ECGs, echocardiograms, and stress testing, refines the clinicians' capability further to quantify cardiovascular well-being. Such technologies play a pivotal role in revealing underlying conditions, such as hypertension and arrhythmias, that are not observable during first-ever encounters. Further, the use of patient-centered approaches allows for considering individual risk factors, thereby improving the efficacy of clinical decision-making for intervention and treatment plans. By making personalized medicine a priority, medical professionals are in a position to manage better the individuality of each patient's cardiovascular data, such that diagnostic procedures play an essential role in individualized treatments. Going beyond the traditional methods, biomarkers increasingly play an essential role in diagnostics for CVD. The use of NPs has taken center stage for their physiological and pathological relevance to cardiovascular function. NPs have a key function in cardiac performance and blood pressure regulation, with their levels serving as indicators of heart insufficiency or strain. Elevations in peptide levels may reflect underlying cardiac insufficiency or other CVD, warranting further investigation and immediate therapy. Furthermore, intensive analyses of the molecular mechanisms underlying NP actions enhance our understanding of their role in disease pathogenesis, thereby paving the way for improved diagnostic procedures and therapeutic management. The ongoing search for NP-targeted therapies is remapping treatment paradigms and emphasizes the necessity for constant innovation in diagnostic routines in general medicine. A critical aspect of enhancing diagnostic accuracy is addressing the multifactorial nature of diseases, such as hypertension. The widespread excessive dependency on a reductionist "trial-and-error" approach to treating hypertension leads to ignoring the patient-specific variations in physiological responses and produces less-than-ideal treatment outcomes. Recognizing the richness of complexity that exists in CVDs requires embracing an integrated, system-oriented diagnostic process wherein patient-specific factors assume prominence. With the implementation of personalized medicine, healthcare providers can tailor therapeutic regimens based on individualized genetic, environmental, and lifestyle factors affecting each patient. This is aimed not only at optimizing the therapeutic effect but also at avoiding possible complications, thus optimally addressing the increasing global burden of CVDs. Adoption of these new diagnostic tools and individualized treatment models is an arena with promise for augmenting the general medicine approach to managing cardiovascular health in contemporary healthcare settings.

5.4.1. Physical Examination Techniques

Physical examination skills within the cardiovascular approach are critical for clinicians to ascertain the status of the cardiovascular system. The assessment begins with an in-depth history and progresses to a methodical evaluation through observation, palpation, percussion, and auscultation. All these approaches have crucial information; for instance, observation allows clinicians to examine the contour, chest symmetry, as well as signs of distress, while palpation helps assess pulse strength and variation. Accurate auscultation of heart sounds should be done to identify abnormalities such as murmurs or gallops, which can indicate the presence of conditions. In particular, specific methods, such as the use of a stethoscope to identify heart rhythms, can lead to early identification of issues such as arrhythmias, critical to determine subsequent management.

The effectiveness of these examination techniques can influence patient outcomes in cardiovascular wellness and necessitates periodic reinforcement of these fundamental skills for practitioners. Standardized training in physical exam skills has been espoused in recent literature as critical, particularly with the increasing need for skilled practitioners due to the anticipated increase in CVD. Innovative education programs based on entrustable professional activities (EPA) may improve the competence of health providers, such as physician assistants (PAs) and nurse practitioners (NPs). A pilot curriculum for teaching echocardiography skills to PAs has been proposed to cover theoretical foundations as well as practical utilization through guided clinical practice. Through addressing knowledge gaps and augmenting practical skills, the curriculum intends to endow PAs with proficiency in conducting and interpreting echocardiography effectively. Developing the abilities of mid-level practitioners is essential because of the cardiology workforce shortage, as it can alleviate the workload from cardiologists and enhance the availability of high-quality cardiovascular care to patients (Moon et al., 2017). The incorporation of sophisticated physical examination methods into clinical practice can also affect diagnosis and treatment planning.

For instance, echocardiography, both in clinical technique and interpretive ability, allows an individual to comprehensively visualize cardiac structure and function. As the demand for echocardiography increases, it is necessary to integrate it into the skill acquisition routine of healthcare practitioners. Students enrolled in well-designed curricula can become competent in the use and interpretation of echocardiographic findings, thereby maximizing their capacity to treat cardiovascular disorders effectively. Standardization of such training not only increases individual expertise but also ensures consistency of quality in care provision across health facilities. As witnessed by current initiatives empowering ATs through specialty training, physical examination skills development will be key to the future of cardiovascular health (Kitsiou et al., 2013) (Figure 5.14).

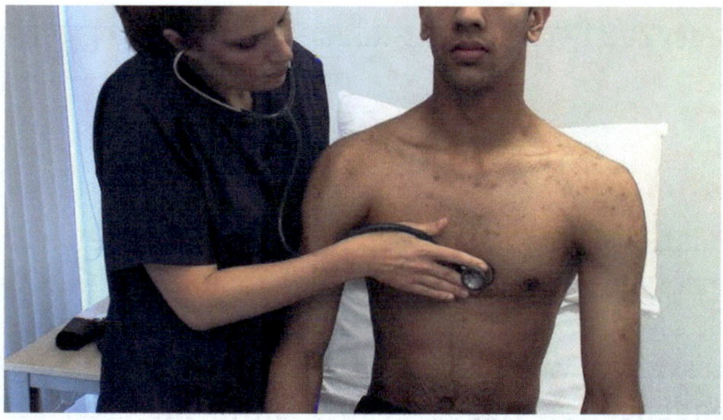

Figure 5.14. Cardiac physical examination.

Source: https://i.ytimg.com/vi/vreCONlSwZs/hq720.jpg?sqp=-oaymwEhCK4FEIIDSFryq4qpAxMIARUAAAAAGAElAADIQj0AgKJD&rs=AOn4CLBbnMEXfxKHMHo8kE-3idY2Akv9Ug.

5.4.2. Imaging Studies (ECG, Echocardiogram)

Imaging tests have a pivotal role to play in the assessment and management of cardiovascular status, with ECG and echocardiogram being the pillars of clinical application. An ECG provides excellent information about the electrical activity of the heart, which makes it possible to diagnose arrhythmias, ischemia, and other cardiac disorders. In athletes, for instance, a resting 12-lead ECG may detect genetic or structural heart diseases that may put a person at risk of sudden cardiac death (SCD). The growing refinement in ECG interpretation, based on increasing scientific data, has made it essential for clinicians to discern normal physiological adaptations in athletes from pathologically significant observations. This data is critical, as the incidence of SCD among this subgroup highlights the need for standard protocols for interpreting ECGs in the sports cardiology context (Aagaard et al., 2017). Echocardiography, another key imaging method, complements ECG by providing dynamic imaging of cardiac form and function. It enables measurement of left ventricle size and function, valvular integrity, and underlying structural abnormalities not discernible on an ECG alone. This non-invasive imaging technique plays a key role in the diagnosis of conditions such as HF, hypertrophic cardiomyopathy, and valvular heart diseases. Additionally, echocardiograms can aid clinical decision-making, particularly in acute presentations with chest pain. An examination of patients admitted with chest pain has demonstrated that echocardiographic evaluation in the acute environment can lead to earlier intervention, potentially lowering morbidity and mortality rates in the high-risk population. The integration of echocardiography into the standard cardiovascular assessment process is necessary to comprehend patient health fully (Camilleri et al., 2009). Both ECG and echocardiographic assessments, when integrated with the overall philosophy of general medicine for the cardiovascular system, enhance diagnosis and patient management. Depending on the type of CVDs, the application of these imaging tests allows clinicians to have a structured and risk-based assessment strategy. For patients, especially those admitted for acute chest pain, employing a combination of ECG and echocardiography can help in the successful detection of underlying causes, preventing unnecessary admissions, treatments, or complications. Continuous education and training of healthcare workers in modern imaging methods are essential to improve patient outcomes. As clinical practice continues to evolve, these imaging studies will continue to be an integral part of the overall management of cardiovascular patients, allowing for timely intervention and individualized treatment strategies that reflect current best practices in medicine (Figure 5.15).

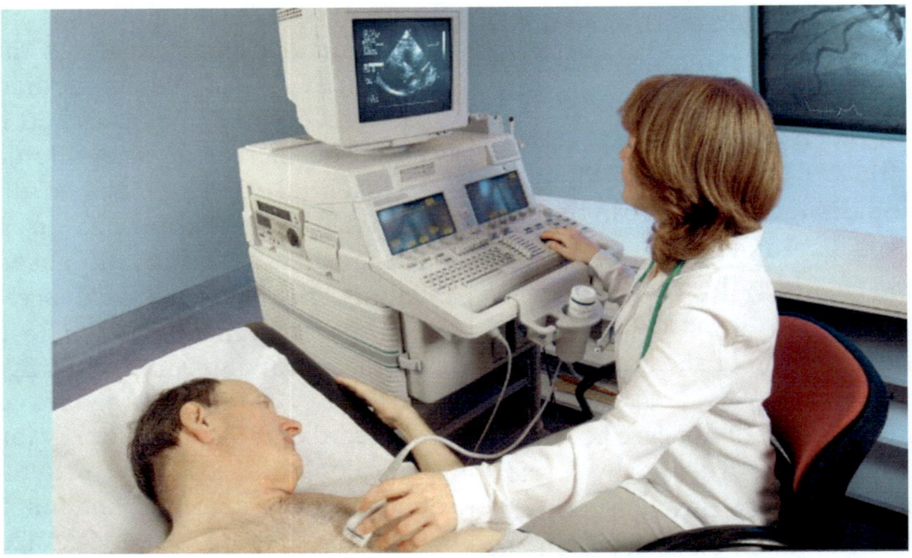

Figure 5.15. Patient undergoing echocardiogram testing which involves using an ultrasound machine to look at the structure and function of the heart.

Source: https://post.healthline.com/wp-content/uploads/2021/10/Patient-taking-a-echocardiogram-body2.jpg.

5.4.3. Laboratory Tests (Lipid Profile, Biomarkers)

Laboratory tests, in this case, lipid profiles and biomarkers, are equally significant in the general medicine approach to cardiovascular health. Lipid profiles measure the levels of cholesterol and triglycerides, which are critical in assessing the risk of contracting CVDs. Elevated levels of low-density lipoprotein (LDL) cholesterol and triglycerides, along with depressed levels of high-density lipoprotein (HDL) cholesterol, indicate a greater tendency for plaque deposition in the arteries, thereby increasing the risk of heart disease. This is the numerical analysis used to determine which lifestyle adjustments and medical therapies can lower cardiovascular risk. Furthermore, lipid profiles are priceless for monitoring the efficacy of drug therapies, enabling clinicians to adjust therapies in line with the patient's fluctuating lipid levels. Other than lipid profiles, biomarkers such as markers for oxidative stress reveal deeper aspects of cardiovascular health. Oxidative stress, which arises from a difference in the rate of production of reactive oxygen species (ROS) and antioxidant defense in the body, is a major contributor to cardiovascular pathologies. Biomarkers of oxidative damage to lipids, proteins, and DNA are increasingly being useful tools in the evaluation of cardiovascular risk. As highlighted in recent studies, a comprehensive oxidative stress index, which includes several markers, can enhance clinical assessment and individualize treatment protocols based on redox status estimations (Altieri et al., 2017). Incorporation of these biomarkers with traditional lipid profiles can help clinicians risk-stratify patients more accurately for cardiovascular events and guide interventions accordingly. Assessment of non-conventional biomarkers has gained acceptance in the setting of metabolic syndromes and their association with cardiovascular illness. For instance, studies have found serum vitamin E concentrations associated with liver disease such as simple steatosis (SS) and non-alcoholic steatohepatitis (NASH), which are also tied to increased cardiovascular risk (Angelico et al., 2015). Investigating biomarkers, particularly in groups with cardio-metabolic risk factors, is another aspect of understanding the complex nature of cardiovascular health. Thus, the constant evolution of laboratory diagnostic technologies paves the way for even more advanced techniques in overall medicine, enabling physicians to actively prevent CVDs through targeted therapy based on intensive biomarker examination (Figure 5.16).

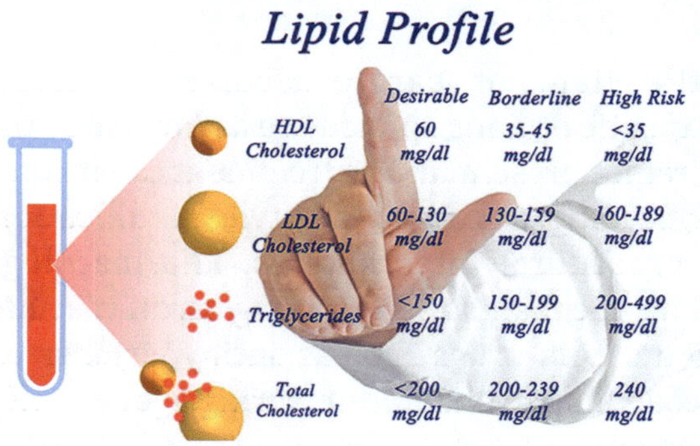

Figure 5.16. Lipid profile.

Source: https://pathkindwebsiteprod.blob.core.windows.net/websiteprod/uploads/blogs/2021-08/32.jpg.

Test Your Knowledge

1. What are some key physical examination techniques used to assess cardiovascular health, and what findings might indicate a problem?
2. How do imaging studies such as ECG and echocardiograms help in diagnosing cardiovascular conditions?
3. What information can laboratory tests like lipid profiles and cardiac biomarkers provide in the evaluation of cardiovascular disease risk or presence?

5.5. Treatment Modalities

Learning Outcome

1. Focus on pharmacological interventions in the management of cardiovascular diseases (CVD)
2. Describe lifestyle modification strategies
3. Understand surgical options (angioplasty, bypass surgery)

In the field of cardiovascular medicine, therapeutic options applied are as diverse as the syndromes presented. The treatment can include pharmacologic therapy, lifestyle modification, and procedural interventions. Pharmacology remains the mainstay in treating cardiovascular ailments with drugs such as antihypertensives, anticoagulants, and lipid-lowering agents. They are integral to the management of risk factors and symptom alleviation. Also, behavioral changes such as diet, exercise, and smoking cessation are necessary for the promotion of overall health and the prevention of cardiovascular risks. The synergism of these modalities has been shown to revolutionize patient outcomes, making them components of any treatment plan for cardiovascular disorders. In acute conditions, high-technology treatment modalities become indispensable for stabilizing and recovering the patient. For instance, in acute heart failure (AHF) presenting with severe respiratory compromise, non-invasive ventilation (NIV) is vital. NIV lowers the need for intubation and improves respiratory function primarily through modalities such as continuous positive airway pressure (CPAP) and pressure support ventilation. Both modalities have various benefits, with CPAP being more straightforward to employ for low-resource settings since it is simple to use. This adaptability highlights the importance of selecting the proper treatment modality based on clinical presentation and available resources, thereby allowing for early and effective treatment in the acute setting. In addition, new treatment modalities are continuously revolutionizing the field of cardiovascular therapy. New modalities such as high-flow nasal cannula therapy have been promising, particularly in patients with AHF and less severe respiratory failure. These newer techniques not only maximize oxygen delivery but also facilitate patient comfort and convenience. Also, constant advances in technology and science continue to expand the arsenal available to medical practitioners, allowing treatments to be maximized to address specific patient requirements. This dynamic character of cardiovascular treatment modalities serves as a reminder of the need to remain current with the latest advances, as they hold the promise of being translated into better health outcomes and QoL among patients living with CVDs.

5.5.1. Pharmacological Interventions

Pharmacological therapy is central to treating CVD and is administered in the form of these medications as foundational therapies for myriad conditions, including hypertension, HF, and ischemic heart disease. Antihypertensives, statins, and anticoagulants are administered daily to diminish risk factors and prevent adverse cardiovascular events. These drug treatments act through multiplex mechanisms, such as decreasing blood pressure, reducing cholesterol levels, or preventing the development of thrombi, and in combination, they provide improved patient outcomes. As an illustration, antihypertensive medications are typically used to treat hypertension , an established risk factor for cardiac disease. Effective management through pharmacotherapy not only improves symptoms but also affects the long-term prognosis of patients, highlighting the pivotal contribution that such treatments make to contemporary cardiovascular medicine. In addressing the wholeness of pharmacologic interventions, it is essential to recognize the significance of individualizing treatment approaches in response to individual variations. Heterogeneity of patient response to treatment could be a result of genetic predispositions, comorbid disease, or habit factors. Tailoring of medication regimens according to patient profiles optimizes therapeutic action and minimizes adverse effects, thus enhancing the treatment of CVD. Statins, for example, are commonly prescribed to lower cholesterol but with different efficacies in different population groups, validating the importance of a tailored therapy strategy. This model of personalized medicine not only enhances the EBP model but also improves the quality of care in CVD treatment, ultimately boosting patient compliance and outcomes.

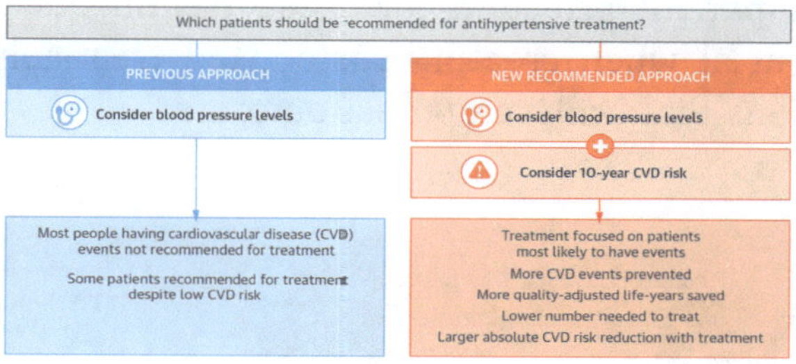

Figure 5.17. Cardiovascular risk and antihypertensive treatment.

Source: https://ars.els-cdn.com/content/image/1-s2.0-S0735109717367360-fx1.jpg.

In addition, the cardiovascular health of vulnerable populations is increasingly being considered within the realm of pharmacological therapy. For instance, those particular risk factors and the prevalence of CVD in women, particularly in culturally distinct environments like in Saudi Arabia, need to be addressed with gendered pharmacologic interventions. Recent studies indicate that traditional risk factors have different manifestations for women, leading to gendered epidemiological trends in the morbidity of heart disease. It is essential to understand these differentiations to develop effective treatment plans based on gender-based conditions in pharmacotherapy. As pharmacological therapies advance, health professionals must place greater emphasis on gender-responsive interventions to further develop care quality and outcomes for women, who have historically been accorded less consideration to their cardiovascular needs (Clark et al., 2012) (Figure 5.17).

5.5.2. Lifestyle Modification Strategies

Effective lifestyle change interventions are critical to the prevention and management of CVDs, particularly in high-risk groups. A coordinated approach to lifestyle changes centers on exercise, healthy diets, and the avoidance of smoking, all of which are established to favor cardiovascular protection. Community-based interventions, targeted toward special populations, such as African Americans in rural communities, have proven to be effective in reversing barriers resulting from physical and social environments. Evidence-based treatments (EBTs) used in a way congruent with community-based participatory research (CBPR) principles ensure that methods address local practice and culture. For instance, tailoring lifestyle interventions through community participation ensures better retention and engagement, ultimately resulting in a population better able to manage their cardiovascular risk factors (Bess et al., 2019). Changing patterns of AF treatment reinforce the importance of lifestyle intervention in disease recurrence prevention. Modern studies highlight that not only do lifestyle modifications neutralize risk factors, but they also enhance the efficacy of existing medical therapies. By promoting regular exercise, balanced diet, and weight management, patients can significantly reduce the frequency of AF attacks. The incorporation of lifestyle interventions in the overall context of cardiovascular management has increasingly gained recognition, highlighting the imperative of tailored approaches based on patient-specific profiles. As technology advances and clinical practices evolve, the ultimate enrichment of AF management remains, with its foundational basis in lifestyle change a reality that cannot be overemphasized, as it offers a forward-looking strategy for enhanced cardiovascular outcomes (Calkins et al., 2017). In our case, the long-term sustainability of the lifestyle transition relies on extended support systems within healthcare and community systems.

Education that emphasizes skill-building for health-oriented decision-making can empower individuals to make and maintain healthier lifestyle choices. Health professionals play a key role in facilitating this process, offering assistance and resources to persons who wish to transition their lifestyle. Collaborative interventions that align healthcare professionals, community agencies, and families establish a constructive environment for long-term change. Additionally, tracking the efficacy of such interventions through systematic measures can guide future improvements and optimizations of lifestyle modification efforts, keeping them current and effective in the fight against cardiovascular disorders (Bess et al., 2019).

5.5.3. Surgical Options (Angioplasty, Bypass Surgery)

Within the overall general medical schema of CVD, surgical treatments such as angioplasty and bypass grafting play pivotal roles in the treatment of CAD. Angioplasty, an invasive intervention, involves positioning a balloon catheter within the vessel to expand stenosed or blocked blood vessels, either with or without stent placement to maintain vascular patency.

This technique has gained popularity as it restores circulation quickly, inhibits symptoms, and reduces the risk of myocardial infarction. However, angioplasty, while successful with particular lesions and patient populations, does not address the underlying cause in multivessel disease, so alternative solutions such as bypass surgery need to be utilized for more complete treatment. On the other hand, coronary artery bypass grafting (CABG) provides a more extensive solution for individuals with extensive blockages or multiple arteries involved. CABG is a procedure in which a bypass is made around clogged coronary arteries using segments of healthy blood vessels obtained from the rest of the body. In addition to augmenting perfusion, CABG has been shown to also have survival benefits in the long term with complicated CAD. The decision between angioplasty and CABG frequently rests on considerations of coronary disease anatomy, clinical presentation, and patient preference. Attunement to the subtleties of patient selection for these treatments is crucial when creating customized treatment plans that achieve optimal outcomes.

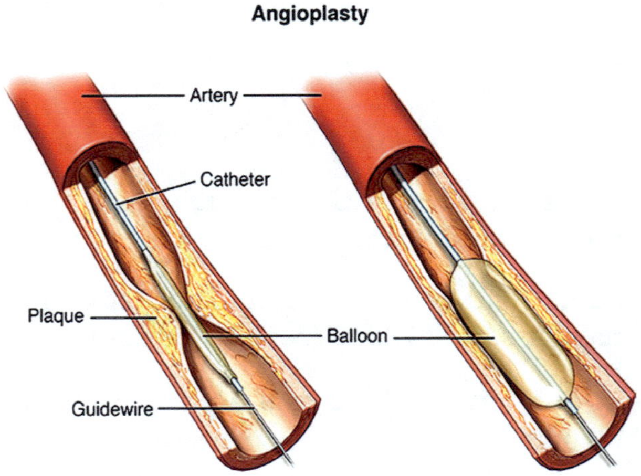

Figure 5.18. Angioplasty.

Source: https://www.hopkinsmedicine.org/-/media/images/health/2_-treatment/cardiovascular/coronary-artery-disease-treatment/pcardio20140402v0001.jpg.

Also, current thought encourages the use of outcome measurements in operations, noting especially the need for tracking cost-effectiveness and QoL following operations like angioplasty and CABG. These measurements enhance understanding of the impacts of these surgical options on healthcare systems, and the chosen approach is the ideal measure of patient-focused care. Through these dimensions, critically measured, healthcare workers can identify systems that not only adopt appropriate technologies but execute them effectively too. These are essential considerations in developing comprehensive treatment programs that not only respond to immediate health requirements but also lead to long-term sustainable outcomes for cardiovascular patients (Chandra et al., 2008) (Figure 5.18).

Test Your Knowledge

1. What are the common pharmacological interventions used in the treatment of cardiovascular diseases, and how do they work?
2. What are the main surgical options for treating cardiovascular disease, such as angioplasty and bypass surgery, and when are they typically indicated?

5.6. Preventive Measures

Learning Outcome

1. Explain the importance of regular health screenings
2. Focus on patient education and awareness in the management and prevention of cardiovascular disease (CVD)
3. Discuss community health initiatives

Good prophylaxis is vital in addressing CVDs, which are the most significant cause of death globally. It requires educating patients about risk factors such as hypertension, hyperlipidemia, diabetes, and lifestyle, including diet and physical activity. Moreover, screening in an orderly manner, coupled with early intervention, can contribute significantly to reducing the incidence of serious CVDs. In Croatia, despite a high incidence of such risk factors and an established public health system, there are significant barriers to the effectiveness of prevention measures. They relate to ineffectiveness and the lack of consistency in assigning responsibilities to actors, which complicates the application of prevention programs. Better coordination and definition of roles between public health agencies, clinicians, and community organizations are needed to support an integrated approach towards CVD prevention, as outlined in the findings of Andrić et al. (2009). Another crucial element of preventive practice is patient involvement in their own treatment, especially about medication adherence. Studies have shown that patients are likely to weigh the benefits of preventive therapies based on their perceived risk and outcomes. For example, research has established that a high percentage of the population, approximately 48%, would be prepared to take preventive medication if they believed it would prolong their lives or yield a substantial reduction in their overall risk of cardiovascular events (Albarqouni et al., 2017). To encourage compliance with preventive interventions, medical professionals must properly educate patients regarding the potential benefits and risks of drugs and modifications in lifestyle. This mandate addresses the essence of individualized care, where medical practitioners assess each patient's needs and preferences, thereby encouraging preventive strategies and supporting healthy lifestyles. Further, investigations on the social determinants of health play a crucial role in implementing effective prevention of CVD. Social determinants such as socioeconomic status, availability of medical treatment, and education play a significant role in influencing health outcomes. Disparities in social determinants could lead to unequal access to necessary preventive interventions and thus the prevalence of CVD. Interventions toward these social determinants must be prioritized to eradicate health inequities and equal access to education, screening for health, and focused interventions for all populations. By harmonizing public health policy with broader socio-economic policy, the health systems can strengthen their prevention against CVD. It is a cross-cutting strategy required to overcome current barriers and create an environment suitable for improved cardiovascular health, according to the suggestions provided by Andrić et al. (2009).

5.6.1. Importance of Regular Health Screenings

Regular health checks are of most significant value in the early detection and management of CVDs, involving a proactive healthcare strategy. The regular checks frequently include taking measurements of risk factors like blood pressure, cholesterol levels, and blood glucose levels. Identification of abnormalities from these parameters enables physicians to institute preventive care or early interventions that significantly avoid the development of serious complications such as heart attacks or strokes. In populations with high chronic disease prevalence, identification of risk factors through routine screenings is imperative. It is particularly touching to address systemic health disparity because, by identifying risk factors, effective mechanisms for improving public health outcomes are formed (N/A, 2006). Routine health screenings thus serve as a gateway to enhanced patient awareness and comprehensive management of cardiovascular health. In addition, incorporating school programs into routine health screenings can make them more effective. For instance, short interventions provided within the healthcare environment, such as counseling about lifestyle modification and disease prevention, can make patients active contributors to their own health. Evidence indicates that when patients are taught about the consequences of unmonitored conditions such as high blood pressure and cholesterol, they demonstrate higher levels of motivation in adopting healthy behaviors (Kopecky et al., 2016). Such information components not only increase individual health literacy but also influence community health by decreasing the overall burden of chronic cardiovascular illnesses. When healthcare systems prioritize frequent screenings and health education, they foster a culture of more engaged and educated patients, who are able to adopt radical lifestyle changes. In summary, the contribution of frequent health screenings to cardiovascular health cannot be overstated. Such screenings enable early detection of risk factors, provide a basis for patient education, and facilitate active disease management. As the U.S. population is getting older and is increasingly developing chronic illnesses, ensuring routine screenings is a top priority. Older adults, who often have more than one condition, highly appreciate being regularly checked and counseled on how to keep their cardiovascular system in check (Kopecky et al., 2016). By including routine health screenings as part of the overall medicine plan for the cardiovascular system, physicians can significantly improve patient outcomes and general QoL (Figure 5.19).

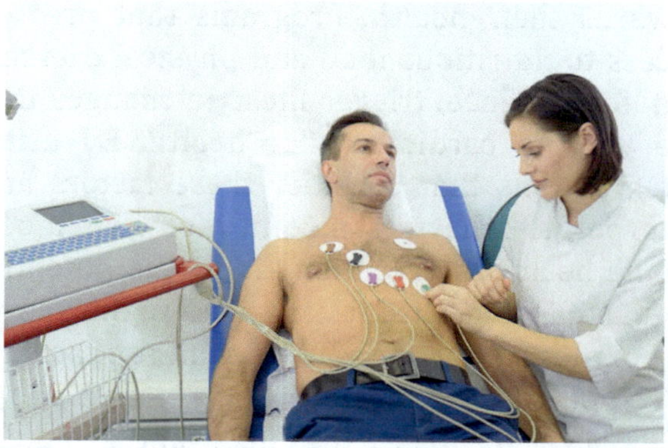

Figure 5.19. Health screenings in the early detection and management of cardiovascular diseases.

Source: https://manhattancardiology.com/wp-content/uploads/2022/12/heart-screening-services-new-york-city.jpg.

5.6.2. Patient Education and Awareness

Health education and patient awareness are the key to the prevention and control of CVD. An educated patient population is maximally involved in their healthcare, resulting in better health outcomes and adherence to treatment plans. Literature highlights the significance of mass education processes in addressing existing knowledge gaps among patients regarding CVD risk factors and their management. Interestingly, elderly patients usually exhibit a disoriented understanding of the significance of their prescribed medication for CVD prevention, indicating an imperative necessity for tailored education strategies. To be specific, results suggest that the majority of elderly patients do not discern the complexities of treatment decision-making, usually viewing it as unilateral rather than as a collaborative process with healthcare providers. Thus, raising awareness of the consequences of CVD medication and lifestyle habits can encourage proactive involvement in collaborative decision-making processes, thereby improving patient satisfaction and outcomes (Bonner et al., 2019). To further improve patient participation, healthcare practitioners must include targeted education methods for diverse patient populations, particularly underrepresented groups. Disparities in healthcare access and knowledge perpetuate uneven health outcomes, particularly in cardiovascular care in minority populations. A recent study revealed that while the majority of physicians recognized the importance of addressing minority health disparities through effective communication interventions, much remains to be done in the practical application of such interventions in practice environments. For instance, only 40–66% of physician respondents indicated employing strategies to enhance patient education and awareness among high-risk minority patients for CVD. This is in concordance with a primary barrier to the offering of equal healthcare, further emphasizing constant training and education of practitioners to make use of culturally sensitive learning tools and interventions capable of engaging various patient groups, further supporting the theory of a shared model of decision-making (Gadon et al., 2012). The integration of patient education programs within primary care settings is central to building an educated patient population capable of addressing their cardiovascular well-being. Such interventions are workshops, targeted consultation sessions, and available written information, all aimed at de-mystifying the control of cardiovascular health. For example, the application of a patient-centered model of communication can significantly enhance patients' understanding of their illness, treatment options, and strategies for lifestyle modification. Moreover, an environment in which patients are encouraged to express their preferences and concerns can lead to improved and more personalized care plans. By closing the four critical steps of shared decision-making in CVD prevention—awareness of choice, discussion of harms and benefits, investigation of preference, and informed decision-making—physicians can significantly enhance patient outcomes and adherence to therapeutic recommendations.

Making patients well-informed will eventually allow them to become active partners in their path to cardiovascular health, which results in better long-term outcomes (Bonner et al., 2019).

5.6.3. Community Health Initiatives

Community health programs are significant interventions in view of the rising cardiovascular health disorders among diverse populations. These programs are more likely to focus on preventive measures, education, and providing access to requisite health facilities, which are essential to reduce the prevalence of heart diseases. Community involvement-based programs can inform individuals about risk factors such as hypertension, diabetes, and obesity, which can be focal areas for cardiovascular disorders. As documented in healthcare reports, targeting outreach to high-risk groups like American Indians and Alaska Natives has been successful in closing gaps in care and improving overall health outcomes within these groups (Roubideaux, 2004). By developing health programs that carefully tailor interventions to the unique cultural needs of populations, healthcare providers can foster heightened awareness and adherence to preventive measures, ultimately reducing the burden of CVD. Successful community health programs also encompass an integrated response to resolving the social determinants of health that impact cardiovascular conditions. Socioeconomic status, educational attainment, access to healthy food, and safe environments are all factors that influence individuals' behaviors towards their health. Programs that provide access to nutritious food and physical exercise can, for instance, trigger lifestyle changes that are vital to cardiovascular health. By using interventions that consider these factors and incorporate behavioral modification techniques, public health interventions have the potential to make a significant impact. Furthermore, as explored in policy recommendations, developing committees to analyze and adopt EBPs can also enhance the effectiveness of these interventions in narrowing racial and ethnic disparities in care (Alexander et al., 2009). This combined approach ensures the identification and remediation of community-specific needs, promoting balanced health improvement across different populations. Additionally, coordination with neighborhood groups, schools, and health organizations plays important and vital role in amplifying the reach and impact of community health programs. Combined efforts can help share resources, coordinate educational workshops, and implement comprehensive health campaigns to educate the public on cardiovascular risk and prevention strategies. Engaging stakeholders in co-designing and implementing such programs not only fosters trust in the community but also guarantees participation. Involving residents and leaders from various sectors, programs can be readily embraced and sustained in the long run. This engagement reinforces the process of building a culture of health at the community level, where cardiovascular health becomes the shared agenda. It therefore establishes a permanent legacy of health empowerment and protection against heart disease.

Test Your Knowledge

1. Why are regular health screenings (e.g., blood pressure, cholesterol, glucose levels) important in the early detection and prevention of cardiovascular diseases?
2. How does patient education and awareness contribute to the prevention and better management of cardiovascular risk factors?
3. What role do community health initiatives play in promoting heart-healthy behaviors and reducing the incidence of cardiovascular diseases at a population level?

SUMMARY

The synopsis of a comprehensive review of the general medicine treatment model for the cardiovascular system highlights the necessity of understanding cardiovascular health through a holistic approach. Noting the prevalence of CVD as one of the leading causes of morbidity and mortality, health professionals must integrate an integrative model founded on prevention, early detection, and individualized treatment measures. Health professionals' ability to interpret a wide range of clinical information, ranging from lipid profiles and blood pressure levels to new epidemiological data, determines the improvement of patient outcomes. For instance, recent studies have shown that statin treatment not only reduces cholesterol but may also reduce the risk of community-acquired pneumonia (CAP), suggesting synergistic effects of cardiovascular medication and their viability in prolonged health-related environments (Khan et al., 2013). In addition, advancements in diagnostic devices and therapeutic techniques have created the potential for increased clinical control of cardiovascular conditions. Understanding the intricate interactions among the different risk factors—lifestyle choice, hypertension, and diabetes—has allowed clinicians to design more focused and effective interventions. Public education programs aimed at cardiovascular wellness are imperative for prevention. Informing the populace about the importance of lifestyle modifications, such as diet and exercise, will enable communities to foster a heart health-oriented culture. Additionally, the incorporation of genetic and molecular research into the practice of clinical care will likely transform cardiovascular medicine in the future, with increasingly targeted therapies that can lead to better patient outcomes and reduced rates of occurrence of heart disease. Finally, the necessity for ongoing research and continued updating of clinical guidelines cannot be overstressed. The continually evolving nature of medical science necessitates that practices must be updated constantly in line with new evidence. For instance, in the case of bibliometric studies, the accuracy of journal classification systems is of overriding significance to enable the sharing of excellent clinical practice and studies (Waltman et al., 2016). With the continuous evolution of the medical field, health practitioners must stay current with recent advancements and exemplary practices to ensure they deliver services aligned with modern standards. In brief, an effective and progressive strategy for cardiovascular health, combining research progress, education, and clinical practice, will eventually result in better patient care and public health.

In cardiology, it is crucial to understand the relationship between disease outcomes, treatment complications, and patient-reported outcomes (PRO) when designing effective management approaches. One of the key advancements in this field has been the creation of standardized outcome measures, specifically for conditions such as AF. As emphasized by recent stories, the International Consortium for Health Outcomes Measurement (ICHOM) established a comprehensive set of standards by engaging a wide variety of health professionals and patient representatives. Through a Delphi exercise suited to the nature of the question, these stakeholders identified key outcomes that reflect both the long-term consequences of the disease and those of its treatment, thereby highlighting the importance of a patient-centered definition of quality of care within the cardiovascular system. This convergence signals a key move toward value-based healthcare, underpinning the delivery of care through open benchmarks and driving continuous innovation in cardiovascular management (Arbelo et al., 2020). In addition, the inclusion of demographic and clinical risk adjusters contributes to the robustness of such measures of outcome. The findings derived for the treatment of CVD extend beyond clinical signs themselves; they include an array of patient-specific factors like comorbidities, cognition, and lifestyle determinants like smoking and exercise. These allow for a more nuanced appreciation of cardiac health influenced by diverse factors. The focus of ICHOM efforts on the application of standardized formats, such as ICD codes, facilitates the standard use of such measures across various healthcare settings. This effort not only supports clinicians in monitoring and improving chronic AF care but also enriches the available clinical research data, thus enabling healthcare systems to make informed decisions to improve patient outcomes on a broader scale (Arbelo et al., 2020). With structured outcomes, addressing psychosocial determinants is now commonly recognized as a critical component of the comprehensive management of CVDs. The quality of well-being among patients is often tied to the efficacy of their emotional resilience and coping against stress. A study with police officers in Santa Clara County indicated how HeartMath training provided practical skills to manage stress, hence evidencing positive effects of emotional self-care on health. The findings showed that significant reductions in physiological and psychological stress responses, which are core to cardiovascular well-being, were achieved. Significantly, the study highlighted improved interpersonal relationships and communication, suggesting emotional well-being directly correlates with physical well-being outcomes. This confluence of mental well-being and cardiovascular medicine indicates the necessity of a multidisciplinary approach in daily medicine, aligning with the general aims of advancing patient-centered care practices in cardiovascular systems.

KEY TERMS FROM THIS CHAPTER

- Angioplasty
- Antihypertensive treatment
- Arrhythmias
- Cardiovascular care
- Cardiovascular medicine
- Cardioverter-defibrillators (ICDs)
- Circulatory system
- Anticoagulants
- Antihypertensives
- Blood glucose levels
- Cardiovascular disease (CVD)
- Cardiovascular system
- Cholesterol levels
- Congenital heart defects (CHDs)

CRITICAL THINKING QUESTIONS

1. **Which of the following blood vessels carries oxygenated blood from the lungs to the heart?**
   a. Pulmonary artery
   b. Pulmonary vein
   c. Aorta
   d. Superior vena cava
2. **Which condition is characterized by a blockage of blood flow to the heart muscle?**
   a. Stroke
   b. Myocardial infarction
   c. Hypertension
   d. Atrial fibrillation
3. **Which of the following is a modifiable risk factor for cardiovascular disease?**
   a. Family history
   b. Age
   c. Smoking
   d. Gender
4. **Which diagnostic test is commonly used to evaluate the electrical activity of the heart?**
   a. MRI
   b. Chest X-ray
   c. Electrocardiogram (ECG/EKG)
   d. Echocardiogram
5. **Which of the following interventions is most effective in the primary prevention of cardiovascular disease?**
   a. Coronary artery bypass graft (CABG)
   b. Beta-blockers
   c. Angioplasty
   d. Lifestyle modification (e.g., diet, exercise, smoking cessation)

Short Answer Questions

1. What are the major anatomical components of the cardiovascular system, and what roles do the heart, arteries, veins, and capillaries play in circulation?
2. Describe the pathophysiology, common symptoms, and management options for three major cardiovascular diseases: coronary artery disease, heart failure, and arrhythmias.
3. What lifestyle and behavioral factors significantly increase the risk of developing cardiovascular disease, and how can these risks be reduced?
4. How do genetic predispositions and comorbid conditions like hypertension and diabetes contribute to cardiovascular disease development?
5. What physical examination techniques and diagnostic tools (e.g., ECG, echocardiogram, blood tests) are commonly used to assess cardiovascular health in general practice?
6. What pharmacological treatments are commonly used in managing cardiovascular conditions, and how do they help in improving heart function or preventing complications?

Answers to Critical Thinking Questions

1. (b) 2. (b) 3. (c) 4. (c) 5. (d)

REFERENCES

1. Drezner, J. A., Sharma, S., Baggish, A., Papadakis, M., Wilson, M. G., Prutkin, J. M., La Gerche, A., Ackerman, M. J., Borjesson, M., Salerno, J. C., Asif, I. M., Owens, D. S., Chung, E. H., Emery, M. S., Froelicher, V. F., Heidbuchel, H., Adamuz, C., Asplund, C. A., Cohen, G., . . . Corrado, D. (2017). International criteria for electrocardiographic interpretation in athletes: Consensus statement. *British Journal of Sports Medicine, 51*(9), 704–731. https://doi.org/10.1136/bjsports-2016-097331Abdel-Kader, K., Agrawal, V., Cavanaugh, K., Choi, M. J., et al. (2019). Primary care physicians' perceptions of barriers and facilitators to management of chronic kidney disease: A mixed methods study. https://core.ac.uk/download/323073389.pdf (accessed on 27th June 2025).
2. Abdraimova, A., Alleyne, G., Atun, R., Barrington, W., Bigdeli, M., Cameron, A., Cameron, D., et al. (2013). Promotion of access to essential medicines for non-communicable diseases: Practical implications of the UN political declaration. https://core.ac.uk/download/pdf/10674416.pdf (accessed on 27th June 2025).
3. Abrahamowicz, M., Andersen, P. K., Cook, R. J., Joly, P., et al. (2020). Analysis of time-to-event for observational studies: Guidance to the use of intensity models. http://arxiv.org/abs/2005.13271 (accessed on 27th June 2025).
4. Agarwal, A., Broberg, C. S., Dudley, R. A., Foster, E., et al. (2019). Age- and lesion-related comorbidity burden among US adults with congenital heart disease: A population-based study. https://core.ac.uk/download/323079618.pdf (accessed on 27th June 2025).
5. Agra, A., Alexander, J., Alexopoulos, D., Arora, V., et al. (2017). Investigating interactions between epicardial adipose tissue and cardiac myocytes: What can we learn from different approaches? https://core.ac.uk/download/82983603.pdf (accessed on 27th June 2025).
6. Albarqouni, L., Doust, J., & Glasziou, P. (2017). Patient preferences for cardiovascular preventive medication: A systematic review. https://core.ac.uk/download/196605102.pdf (accessed on 27th June 2025).
7. Altieri, F., Marrocco, I., & Peluso, I. (2017). Measurement and clinical significance of biomarkers of oxidative stress in humans. https://core.ac.uk/download/127587179.pdf (accessed on 27th June 2025).
8. Aluas, M., Bordea, R. I., Budin, C. E., Ciumarnean, L., et al. (2019). Therapeutic alternatives with CPAP in obstructive sleep apnea. https://core.ac.uk/download/232440313.pdf (accessed on 27th June 2025).
9. Andrić, A., Džakula, A., Juriša, A., Polašek, O., et al. (2009). Cardiovascular diseases, risk factors and barriers in their prevention in Croatia [Kardiovaskularne bolesti, rizični faktori i zapreke za prevenciju u Hrvatskoj]. https://core.ac.uk/download/11699660.pdf (accessed on 27th June 2025).
10. Angelico, F., Baratta, F., Bucci, T., Cangemi, R., et al. (2015). Similar reduction of cholesterol-adjusted Vitamin E serum levels in simple steatosis and non-alcoholic steatohepatitis. https://core.ac.uk/download/54525153.pdf (accessed on 27th June 2025).
11. Arbelo, E., Banerjee, A., Bollmann, A., Caffrey-Armstrong, J., et al. (2020). Development of an international standard set of outcome measures for patients with atrial fibrillation: A report of the International Consortium for Health Outcomes Measurement (ICHOM) atrial fibrillation working group. https://core.ac.uk/download/286716298.pdf (accessed on 27th June 2025).

12. Banister, E. W., Coyle, E. F., Dorsey, R., Collins, F., Goff, D. C., Maier, T., Pärkkä, J., et al. (2018). Cross-modal health state estimation. http://arxiv.org/abs/1808.06462 (accessed on 27th June 2025).

13. Banning, M. (2009). Medication taking behavior and hypertension: A review of the literature. https://core.ac.uk/download/335817.pdf (accessed on 27th June 2025).

14. Battistoni, A., Mastromarino, V., & Volpe, M. (2015). Integrated preclinical cardiovascular prevention: A new paradigm to face growing challenges of cardiovascular disease. https://core.ac.uk/download/54519397.pdf (accessed on 27th June 2025).

15. Belch, J., Boc, V., et al. (2019). *ESVM Guideline on Peripheral Arterial Disease*. https://core.ac.uk/download/286715349.pdf (accessed on 27th June 2025).

16. Bess, K. D., Cene, C. W., Corbie-Smith, G., Dave, G., et al. (2019). Adaptation of an evidence-based cardiovascular health intervention for rural African Americans in the Southeast. https://core.ac.uk/download/286537358.pdf (accessed on 27th June 2025).

17. Bolt, D. M., Fink, J., Greenlee, R. T., Magnan, S., et al. (2015). The relationship of individual comorbid chronic conditions to diabetes care quality. https://core.ac.uk/download/323070914.pdf (accessed on 27th June 2025).

18. Bonner, C., Doust, J., Jansen, J., McCaffery, K., et al. (2019). Shared decision-making about cardiovascular disease medication in older people: A qualitative study of patient experiences in general practice. https://core.ac.uk/download/222450519.pdf (accessed on 27th June 2025).

19. Borghi, C., Grassi, G., Rosei, E. A., Savoia, C., et al. (2017). Personalized medicine—A modern approach for the diagnosis and management of hypertension. https://core.ac.uk/download/96884785.pdf (accessed on 27th June 2025).

20. Bozdag, S., Eddinger, T. J., Kersten, J. R., LaDisa, J. F., et al. (2015). Gene expression in experimental aortic coarctation and repair: Candidate genes for therapeutic intervention? https://core.ac.uk/download/213083552.pdf (accessed on 27th June 2025).

21. Braga, O. G. (2018). Antipsychotic drug use: Managing cardiometabolic and cost effects. https://core.ac.uk/download/212899184.pdf (accessed on 27th June 2025).

22. Bueno, H., Christ, M., Cowie, M., Cullen, L., et al. (2017). Indications and practical approach to non-invasive ventilation in acute heart failure. https://core.ac.uk/download/144473095.pdf (accessed on 27th June 2025).

23. Calkins, H., Cleland, J. G. F., Heist, E. K., Kowey, P. R., et al. (2017). The burden of proof: The current state of atrial fibrillation prevention and treatment trials. https://core.ac.uk/download/80696856.pdf (accessed on 27th June 2025).

24. Camilleri, R., Camilleri, R., & Gerada, E. (2009). A clinical practice audit of management and outcomes of patients presenting with chest pain to the Medical Admissions Unit. https://core.ac.uk/download/46602238.pdf (accessed on 27th June 2025).

25. Chandra, A., Fisher, E. S., & Skinner, J. S. (2008). *Outcomes Assessment and Healthcare Reform*. https://core.ac.uk/download/71346829.pdf (accessed on 27th June 2025).

26. Chang, H. H., Tsai, T. H., Wang, C. L., Wu, C. Y., et al. (2016). Modeling the pulse signal by wave-shape function and analyzing by synchro squeezing transform. http://arxiv.org/abs/1507.05943 (accessed on 27th June 2025).

27. Clark, R., Davidson, P., Driscoll, A., Newton, P., et al. (2008). Heart failure nursing in Australia: Challenges, strengths, and opportunities. https://core.ac.uk/download/10904833.pdf (accessed on 27th June 2025).

28. Clark, R., Rawas, H., Windsor, C., Yates, K., et al. (2012). Cultural challenges to secondary prevention: Implications for Saudi women. https://core.ac.uk/download/10909715.pdf (accessed on 27th June 2025).

29. Delles, C., Dominiczak, A., & Padmanabhan, S. (2017). Genomics and precision medicine for clinicians and scientists in hypertension. https://core.ac.uk/download/77601341.pdf (accessed on 27th June 2025).

30. Ellwein, L. M., Foley, D., LaDisa, J. F., et al. (2016). Image-based quantification of 3D morphology for bifurcations in the left coronary artery: Application to stent design. https://core.ac.uk/download/213075193.pdf (accessed on 27th June 2025).

31. Gadon, M., Klein, J. W., Schubiner, L. O., Wynia, M. K., et al. (2012). Physicians' experiences and opinions regarding strategies to improve care for minority patients. https://digitalscholarship.unlv.edu/cgi/viewcontent.cgi?article=1094&context=jhdrp (accessed on 27th June 2025).

32. Green, A. R., Betancourt, J. R., & King, R. R. (2009). *Improving Quality and Achieving Equity: A Guide for Hospital Leaders*. https://core.ac.uk/download/71352207.pdf (accessed on 27th June 2025).

33. Hillsdon, M., Summerbell, C., & Thorogood, M. (2006). Changing behavior. https://core.ac.uk/download/46332.pdf (accessed on 27th June 2025).

34. Khan, A. R., Bin Abdulhak, A. A., Waterer, G. W., Kung, H. C., Tleyjeh, I. M., Peters, J. L., Higgins, J. P., et al. (2013). The role of statins in prevention and treatment of community acquired pneumonia: A systematic review and meta-analysis. https://core.ac.uk/download/19937734.pdf (accessed on 27th June 2025).

35. Kitsiou, A., Caforio, A. L. P., Porta-Sanchez, A., Vahanian, A., Iung, B., Carrera, C., Szymanski, C., et al. (2013). *ESC core curriculum for the general cardiologist (2013)*. https://core.ac.uk/download/55756305.pdf (accessed on 27th June 2025).

36. Kopecky, E. G. (2016). *Waiting Room Health Promotion for Older Adults in Rural Primary Care* (Doctoral dissertation). https://core.ac.uk/download/51067936.pdf (accessed on 27th June 2025).

37. Link, B., Morroni, C., Myer, L., Susser, E., et al. (2008). Social epidemiology. https://core.ac.uk/download/1670083.pdf (accessed on 27th June 2025).

38. Meirhaeghe, A., Ropero, A. B., Tabak, A. G., Meirhaeghe, A., Voight, B. F., Newton-Cheh, C., Sengenes, C., et al. (2011). Mendelian randomization study of B-type natriuretic peptide and type 2 diabetes: Evidence of causal association from population studies. https://core.ac.uk/download/1437139.pdf (accessed on 27th June 2025).

39. Moon, S. (2017). Echocardiography curriculum development for physician assistants using entrustable professional activities. https://core.ac.uk/download/215924737.pdf (accessed on 27th June 2025).

40. N/A. (2006). *Creating Community Environments That Promote Comprehensive Health and Wellness*. https://core.ac.uk/download/71350530.pdf (accessed on 27th June 2025).

41. Reemtsen, B., Finn, J. P., Alejos, J., Touma, M., Halnon, N., Nelson, S. F., et al. (2017). A path to implement precision child health cardiovascular medicine. https://core.ac.uk/download/323077346.pdf (accessed on 27th June 2025).

42. Roubideaux, Y. (2004). A review of the quality of healthcare for American Indians and Alaska Natives. https://core.ac.uk/download/71354480.pdf (accessed on 27th June 2025).

43. Rubattu, S., & Volpe, M. (2019). Natriuretic peptides in the cardiovascular system: Multifaceted roles in physiology, pathology and therapeutics. https://core.ac.uk/download/231746948.pdf (accessed on 27th June 2025).

44. San, O., & Staples, A. E. (2012). An improved model for reduced-order physiological fluid flows. http://arxiv.org/abs/1212.0188 (accessed on 27th June 2025).

45. Schafer, G. (2025). A case study of technology transfer: Cardiology. https://core.ac.uk/download/pdf/42897756.pdf (accessed on 27th June 2025).

46. Tomasino, D., Sundram, J., Atkinson, M., & McCraty, R. (1999). Impact of the Heart Math self-management skills program on physiological and psychological stress in police officers. https://core.ac.uk/download/71342457.pdf (accessed on 27th June 2025).

47. Waltman, L., & Wang, Q. (2016). Large-scale analysis of the accuracy of the journal classification systems of Web of Science and Scopus. http://arxiv.org/abs/1511.00735 (accessed on 27th June 2025).

48. Weeke, A., Ferrari, A. J., Mitchell, A. J., Felker, B., Ya-Mei, B., Guthrie, B., Astrup, C., et al. (2013). Multimorbidity in bipolar disorder and under-treatment of cardiovascular disease: A cross-sectional study. https://core.ac.uk/download/16458216.pdf (accessed on 27th June 2025).

RESPIRATORY SYSTEM: COMMON RESPIRATORY DISORDERS, DIAGNOSTIC TOOLS, AND PHARMACOLOGICAL TREATMENTS

6

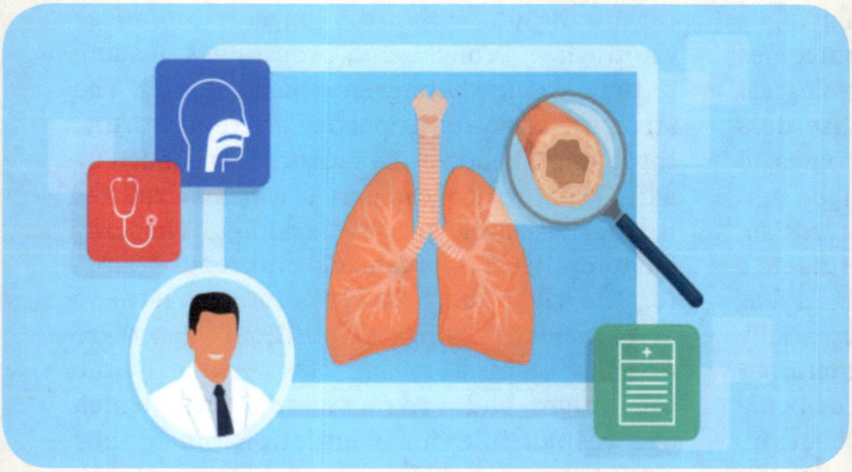

LEARNING OBJECTIVES

After studying this chapter, you will be able to:

1. Understand the physiology of breathing
2. Describe common respiratory disorders
3. Discuss diagnostic tools in respiratory medicine
4. Focus on pharmacological treatments
5. Define non-pharmacological interventions
6. Deal with preventive measures and public health

Introduction

The respiratory system is the main pathway for gas exchange, facilitating the movement of oxygen into the body and carbon dioxide out of the body. It is made up of main structures such as lungs, trachea, bronchi, and alveoli, and it works through coordinated physiological processes to meet the metabolic requirements of the organism. Lungs' lobes provide a high surface area that increases oxygen intake. The anatomical structures are significant in maintaining cellular respiration, the process by which cells receive their energy. Furthermore, the interaction of the circulatory and respiratory systems ensures the provision of oxygenated blood to the body, depicting the interdependence of the body systems and the significance of respiratory activity in ensuring homeostasis. In addition to its fundamental function of gas exchange, the respiratory system has several ancillary functions that highlight its significance in general medicine. One such function is thermoregulation, as the introduction of air into the body can control the body's temperature. Moreover, the respiratory system acts as a line of defense for the organism against invading pathogens and harmful substances from the exterior, using structures like cilia and mucus to catch and destroy foreign material. This defense mechanism demonstrates how shifts in respiratory well-being can lead to significant consequences, such as increased susceptibility to infection and chronic illness. Ethnic differentials in occupational health, as supported by studies, express how certain demographic groups are more likely to experience higher rates of limiting long-term illness, thereby having a direct impact on respiratory health outcomes (Clay et al., 2004). Lastly, the psychological aspects that go along with respiratory disorders are significant, particularly when it comes to public health and emergency management. The emergence of threats from bioterrorism attacks and pandemic infectious disease outbreaks can potentially lead to rigorous fear and anxiety among the population, potentially causing exacerbation of the current respiratory illnesses or even the new syndrome of being over-wary and susceptible to fearful behaviors (Bracha et al., 2006). The overlap of physical and psychological health demands a combined model of respiratory medicine that goes beyond mere physiological management to include psychological assessments and interventions. By recognizing the multidimensionality of respiratory health, healthcare professionals can attempt to develop more comprehensive care strategies that address not only physical symptoms but also patients' psychological well-being.

Overview of Respiratory Anatomy

Understanding the anatomy of the respiratory system is key to comprehending its total function and role in human physiology. The respiratory system consists primarily of the upper and lower respiratory tracts that, together, facilitate the exchange of gases. The upper tract includes the nasal cavity, pharynx, and larynx and plays a vital role in filtering, warming, and humidifying air before inhalation. This separation is responsible for protecting the lower respiratory pathways and optimizing the amount of air that reaches the lungs. Joined to these passages are the various cartilages and muscles surrounding the larynx, which aid in phonation and indirectly enhance communication and interaction in society, further contributing to the respiratory system's multifaceted nature. Transitioning to the lower respiratory tract, this section is tasked with the critical exchange of oxygen and carbon dioxide within the lungs. It comprises the trachea, bronchi, and bronchioles, leading to the alveoli, where gas exchange occurs. The structure of alveoli is particularly noteworthy; these small, balloon-like sacs are surrounded by a dense network of capillaries, which maximizes the surface area for gas exchange. The lung anatomy itself is organized into lobes—three for the right lung and two for the left—to accommodate the heart's position. Then there are the respiratory muscles, primarily the diaphragm and intercostal muscles, which are responsible for ventilation since they alter thoracic pressure during breathing. All these anatomical features are necessary to comprehend how various respiratory diseases may be halting normal function. Furthermore, anatomical and environmental variations can influence the effectiveness of the respiratory system. Syndromes such as Brachycephalic Obstructive Airway Syndrome, in particular, may be found in certain breeds of dogs, where anatomy plays a part in keeping the respiratory system healthy. The syndromes develop due to morphological changes that, although aesthetically pleasing, can lead to serious health issues. This resonates with the broader idea that human respiratory anatomy can also exhibit variance that predisposes patients to respiratory disease, such as asthma or obstructive sleep apnea (OSA). Hence, it is now of utmost significance that medical professionals consider anatomical variance when diagnosing and managing respiratory illnesses, ensuring their approach is holistic and personalized. Modifying treatments based on anatomical considerations can best enhance therapy outcomes, illustrating the intricate relationship between structure and function in respiratory health (Reiter et al., 2015) (Figure 6.1).

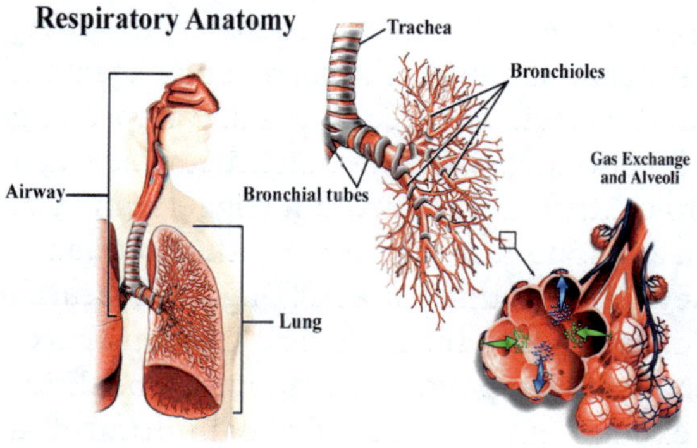

Figure 6.1. Respiratory anatomy.

Source: https://www.nhlbi.nih.gov/sites/default/files/inline-images/How%20Lungs%20Work%20Illustration_edited.jpg.

Importance of Respiratory Health

The importance of respiratory health is underscored by its central position in overall health and its effect on other functions within the body. The respiratory system is critical in gas exchange, introducing oxygen into the bloodstream and eliminating carbon dioxide produced as a byproduct of metabolism. Such processes are the foundation for physical condition and mental processes because an insufficient supply of oxygen will leave brain performance and overall energy levels depleted. The function of the lungs is also directly related to QoL since compromised lung function can limit physical exercise and lead to an inactive lifestyle. These are not just limitations in physical function but also tend to enhance emotional and mental health conditions to create a cycle that is difficult to break. Therefore, emphasizing thoughtful respiratory care is necessary, as it allows for healthier living and facilitates increased activity in daily life tasks. Progress towards retaining respiratory health must transcend individual actions to include broader policy efforts and community health initiatives. Local governments and health agencies play significant roles in developing guidelines to mitigate environmental poisons that are harmful to lung function and respiratory well-being. Both air quality monitoring and smoking cessation programs are staple components of public health policy plans for enhanced respiratory health. As hypothesized by contemporary research on AMR and its implications for health systems, specific policies are required to address the complexities of respiratory-related illnesses at both national and regional levels (Aarestrup et al., 2015).

Through such concerted effort, in addition to addressing acute respiratory infections, preventive measures that protect vulnerable populations are targeted, enhancing community health resilience in general. Other than policy interventions at the systemic level, promotion of exercise is a critical component of lung health preservation, particularly in the elderly. With the aging population, the risk of respiratory complications increases accordingly, necessitating the development of interventions that foster long-term exercise. Lifestyle intervention programs have been proven to improve lung capacity and general fitness significantly. Interventions tailored to older adults to enhance physical activity can lead to favorable respiratory outcomes through enhanced aerobic function and reduced dyspnea during exercise (N/A, 2001). By establishing environments that favor regular exercise and supporting the provision of educational materials, healthcare providers may facilitate patients to take an active role in managing respiratory health. Therefore, the combination of community organization with personal commitment creates a whole-system solution for the management of respiratory health in various populations.

Common Respiratory Diseases

Acute respiratory diseases are a public health problem that presents in patients from multiple populations. Among these diseases, pneumonia is of special interest due to its frequency and severity. The disease is often precipitated by various pathogens, such as bacteria, viruses, and fungi, which induce inflammation of the lung tissue. For instance, bacterial pneumonia may often result as a secondary effect of viral infections that compromise the respiratory defenses, making the host immunocompromised and predisposed to secondary infections. Accurate identification of the offending organisms is significant since it immediately determines appropriate antibiotic therapy and supportive care. Proper management of pneumonia is further reliant on an understanding of such underlying mechanisms, and therefore, the importance of rigorous clinical evaluation and research into respiratory disease pathogenesis is paramount, ultimately determining patient outcomes (Dear et al., 2020). COPD is yet another prevalent respiratory condition, which is characterized by chronic respiratory symptoms and airflow limitation due to abnormal lung responses to inhaled noxious gases or particles. The primary risk factor for COPD is tobacco smoke, but environmental and occupational exposure to toxic substances also contributes significantly to its causation. The patient may present with progressive respiratory symptoms such as dyspnea, chronic cough, and sputum production, significantly affecting QoL. COPD treatment is typically a combination of pharmacologic interventions, pulmonary rehabilitation (PR), and lifestyle modification to relieve symptoms and prevent exacerbations. Public interventions aimed at smoking cessation and environmental improvement are essential in stemming the rising incidence of COPD and leaving healthier respiratory systems for future generations (Agache et al., 2016). Asthma, a common respiratory disorder, primarily occurs in children but can extend into adulthood. It is characterized by long-term inflammation of the airways, leading to recurring wheezing, chest tightness, breathlessness, and coughing. Asthma inducers are varied, including allergens, viral infections, and environmental toxins, requiring individualized treatment regimens. Prevention and control with inhaled corticosteroids (ICS) and bronchodilators are the current management aimed at relieving acute attacks and improving daily functioning. Crucially, patient education on how to control asthma, prevent triggers, and use action plans is key in reducing the frequency and severity of asthma attacks. Ongoing research continues to probe the biological mechanisms of asthma to develop novel therapeutic modalities and expand knowledge of the multifaceted disease (Dear et al., 2020).

6.1. Physiology of Breathing

Learning Outcome

1. Understand the mechanisms of inhalation and exhalation
2. Describe the gas exchange process in the alveoli
3. Focus on the regulation of breathing by the nervous system

The physiology of breathing consists of several complex processes necessary for maintaining homeostasis and transferring gases within the body. The mechanics of breathing essentially involve the synergistic contraction of the diaphragm, intercostal muscles, and accessory muscles to create a pressure gradient that allows air to flow into and out of the lungs. As the person inhales, the diaphragm relaxes and descends, and the intercostal muscles push the rib cage upward, increasing the volume of the thoracic cavity and lowering intrapulmonary pressure. Negative pressure pulls air into the lungs, with oxygen being exchanged for carbon dioxide over the alveolar membranes. Understanding the physiological mechanism is relevant when dealing with conditions such as respiratory distress and COPD. They have a tendency to confuse the normal mechanics of breathing, secondarily affecting tissue oxygen delivery. The interaction of respiration with emotional status also affects breathing physiology. Emotions can dramatically influence autonomic functions and respiratory rates, with unpleasant emotions typically leading to inappropriate respiratory rates and volumes. Current controversy in the literature suggests that interventions such as meditation and controlled breathing can reverse the adverse effects of stress and anxiety on respiratory physiology. By changing breathing patterns, these practices can induce positive feedback in the autonomic nervous system, inducing relaxation and making possible greater gas exchange in the lungs. This overlap of respiratory physiology and emotional health mirrors the need for an integrated understanding of the body's systems and their interconnected nature, particularly in the treatment of psychological and physiological ailments that are dependent upon successful respiratory function (Barnes et al., 2015). In light of the changing landscape of medical interventions and the integration of old practices, including Qigong, with new methods, promising improvements in respiratory health lie ahead. Qigong places a focus on breath control and being mindful of one's body, which could regulate breathing patterns and enhance lung function naturally. By applying machine learning to the analysis of Qigong breathing signatures, researchers aim to link specific breathing rhythms to various pathologies and offer personalized healthcare strategies that combine Eastern holistic principles with Western scientific accuracy. This new approach not only acknowledges the body's physiological function of respiration but also leverages technology to enhance therapy benefits. It may open the door to developing a vitality score index (VSI) that can predict the outcomes of lifestyle choices and medical interventions on individuals. These interdisciplinary strategies hold promise to revolutionize the general medicine of the respiratory system by providing individually tailored treatments based on a systematic understanding of physiology and patient health (Dethlefs et al., 2019).

6.1.1. Mechanisms of Inhalation and Exhalation

Inhalation and exhalation are fundamental processes inherent in the functioning of the respiratory system. Inspiration or inhalation occurs when the diaphragm becomes relaxed and descends, simultaneously widening the thoracic cavity. This creates negative pressure relative to atmospheric pressure, and air enters the lungs. Intercostal muscles also get involved in lifting the ribcage, further enhancing the expansion of the thoracic cavity. This is crucial for maintaining adequate ventilation, which allows the exchange of gases needed for cellular respiration. For this step, it is critical to the composition of air entering the lungs because it can influence subsequent biochemical reactions. These include trace gas quantification in exhaled breath, which reflects ongoing metabolic processes, as outlined in recent studies on respiratory diagnostics (Amann et al., 2010). Expiration, or exhalation, is a passive process for regular breathing, where the intercostal and diaphragm muscles relax, making the thoracic cavity smaller. As the volume decreases, the pressure within the lungs increases, pushing air out through the conducting airways. Negative pressure mechanics exist for both inhalation and exhalation, but there are physiological nuances that ensure adequate gas exchange. Interestingly, exhalation efficiency can be influenced by numerous determinants, including patterns of breathing as well as the presence of some pathologies. For instance, diseases such as asthma have been shown to alter airflow and contribute to respiratory symptoms that impact both inhalation and exhalation. Understanding the mechanism of airflow limitation during expiration is also essential in the management of occupational asthma, which requires early detection and proper treatment strategies to prevent long-term respiratory morbidity (Axon et al., 2000). The intricate process of inhalation and exhalation not only allows external respiration but also plays a vital role in homeostasis and the regulation of metabolism. For example, concentrations of substances like nitric oxide and volatile organic compounds in exhaled breath can be a significant determinant of the metabolic condition and respiratory health of an individual. Quantification of these substances to the accurate decimal place can inform clinical practice, especially in respiratory diagnosis. Breath compound variability has been shown to be primarily a function of airway gas exchange, rather than systemic concentration alteration, highlighting the importance of understanding how exhalation and inhalation work. It may ultimately provide the foundation for new diagnostic methods and therapeutic strategies in respiratory medicine, thereby improving patient care and outcomes (Amann et al., 2010) (Figure 6.2).

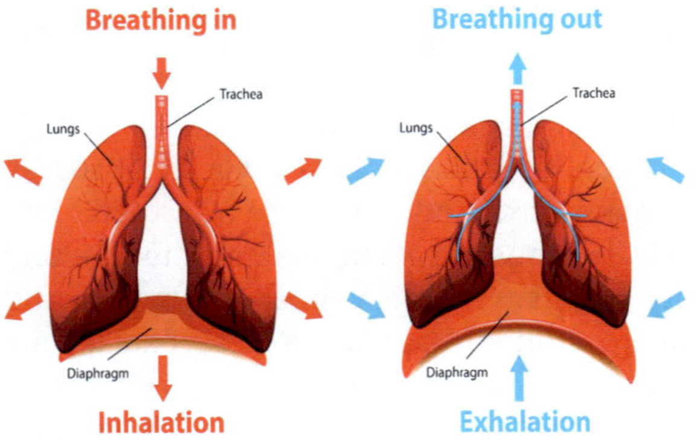

Figure 6.2. Inhalation and exhalation mechanisms.

Source: https://media.geeksforgeeks.org/wp-content/uploads/20220613110834/processbreathingexplained130855066.webp.

6.1.2. Gas Exchange Process in the Alveoli

The alveolar gas exchange is an essential part of respiratory physiology in which oxygen and carbon dioxide are exchanged from air to blood or vice versa. Alveoli are tiny air sacs at the terminus of bronchioles, covered by a single layer of epithelial cells, and possess a large surface area, allowing efficient gas exchange. Oxygen, which is in the air breathed in, diffuses through the alveolar membrane into the pulmonary capillaries, in which it combines with hemoglobin in the red blood cells. On the other hand, carbon dioxide, a byproduct of metabolism, diffuses from the blood into the alveoli to be exhaled. This process relies on the differences in partial pressures, with gases diffusing from areas of higher to lower concentration so that oxygen exchange and carbon dioxide removal are effectively maintained (Amann et al., 2010). The process of gas exchange in the alveoli is multifaceted and includes various physiological mechanisms that enhance the efficiency of respiration. Alveolar ventilation, or the air delivered to alveoli and participating in gas exchange, is regulated by both rate of breathing and tidal volume. In a normal subject, with perfect coordination between the two, a healthy person would have the maximum amount of fresh air entering and the minimum amount of stale air retained. Additionally, the presence of pulmonary surfactant, a lipoprotein complex secreted by type II alveolar cells, reduces surface tension, preventing collapse of the alveoli and facilitating lung compliance. This biophysical property is important during shallow breathing or pathological states, supporting the alveoli's function as not merely passive gas-exchange structures, but as active participants in respiratory health (Amann et al., 2010). Furthermore, the maintenance of the delicate balance of gases within the alveoli and their interaction with systemic circulation underlines the importance of understanding this process in the clinical context. Alterations in gas concentrations may reflect associated metabolic or pulmonary pathology. For instance, quantification of exhaled nitric oxide and other trace molecules can be applied as diagnostic markers, revealing the presence of respiratory inflammation or disease state. Development of standardized protocols for such measurements, as exemplified by professional association guidelines, is required for the advancement of respiratory medicine. As research into lung repair and regeneration nuances continues, the functional characteristics of alveoli will remain pivotal in therapeutic innovations to enhance gas exchange and pulmonary function in general (Basil et al., 2020) (Figure 6.3).

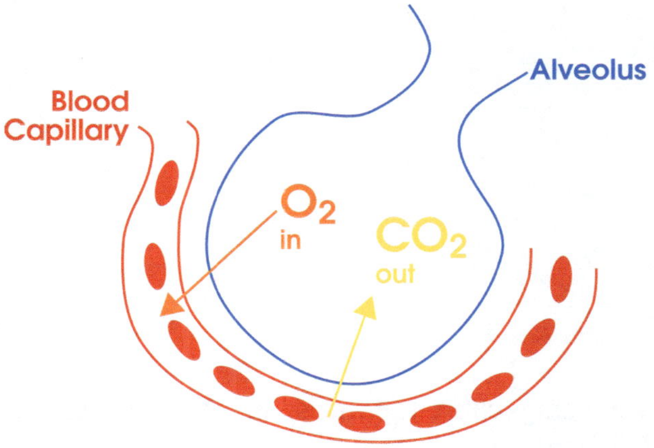

Figure 6.3. Gas exchange in humans. Oxygen and carbon dioxide switch places between a capillary (part of the bloodstream) and an alveolus (an air sac in the lungs).

Source: https://upload.wikimedia.org/wikipedia/commons/thumb/c/c4/Gas_exchange_in_the_aveolus_simple_%28en%29.svg/1024px-Gas_exchange_in_the_aveolus_simple_%28en%29.svg.png.

6.1.3. Regulation of Breathing by the Nervous System

Control of breathing by the nervous system is a very complex process and is primarily undertaken by the brainstem respiratory centers, which are the medulla oblongata and the pons. These brain regions are provided with sensory input from the body regarding the status of the respiratory needs of the body, and combine this information to adjust the rate and depth of breathing accordingly. For instance, carotid and aortic arch chemoreceptors detect rises in the level of carbon dioxide and oxygen in the blood. When there is an increase in carbon dioxide, it induces an increase in respiratory rate and volume to eliminate excess carbon dioxide and ensure adequate oxygenation. This intricate feedback mechanism reflects the key function of the nervous system in maintaining homeostasis in the respiratory system, thus the importance of neural control in the respiratory process.

Furthermore, the interaction between emotions and breathing rhythms confirms the nervous system's stronger role in the regulation of respiration. Anxiety and stress can trigger the sympathetic division of the autonomic nervous system, inducing shallow, rapid breathing, which can augment the feelings of panic and distress. Recent evidence exists that mindfulness therapies, such as meditation and controlled breathing patterns, are capable of triggering parasympathetic responses that control feelings and improve respiratory status (Barnes et al., 2015).

By controlling their breathing patterns, individuals can reverse the detrimental effects of stress, suggesting that incorporating breathing exercises in therapeutic settings promises an integrated solution to healing stress disorders. Such findings highlight the relevance of exploring the interaction between the nervous system and respiration in mental health. In addition, advances in technology have led to greater insight into the control of breathing and its quantification. Photoplethysmography-based non-invasive wearable sensors provide data on various physiological parameters, including respiration rate, without the burdensome weights of traditional methods like polysomnography (Combertaldi et al., 2018). The equipment provides ongoing observation of respiratory movements in real life, enabling researchers to explore the nuances with which the nervous system regulates breathing in different states, like sleep or mixed emotions. With the development of the ability to diagnose and interpret sleep-borne illnesses, understanding the control of respiration in terms of physiological and psychological health becomes increasingly important. The integration of technology into this field not only enhances clinical diagnosis but also opens up avenues for creating new treatments that have the potential to improve overall respiratory health.

Test Your Knowledge

1. What are the key mechanisms involved in inhalation and exhalation?
2. How does gas exchange occur in the alveoli, and what role do oxygen and carbon dioxide gradients play in this process?
3. How is breathing regulated by the nervous system?

6.2. Common Respiratory Disorders

Learning Outcome

1. Understand the causes and symptoms asthma
2. Describe chronic obstructive pulmonary disease (COPD)
3. Explain the types and treatment options of pneumonia

The spectrum of usual respiratory illness encompasses a variety of conditions that can significantly impair pulmonary function and general health. Asthma, characterized by chronic airway inflammation and hyperresponsiveness, is a common, age-independent disorder. Its pathogenesis involves environmental triggers and genetic predisposition, resulting in episodic wheezing, chest tightness, and breathlessness. Optimal management typically consists of the combination of pharmacotherapeutic measures, including ICS and bronchodilators, and adjustment of lifestyle to prevent exposure to established precipitants. Educational interventions aimed at improving patient awareness and adherence to treatment further enhance control of this chronic disease, ultimately leading to improved QoL and prevention of exacerbation. The correct answer is E. The second primary respiratory disease is OSA, a condition characterized by recurring upper airway obstruction during sleep, resulting in nocturnal disturbances and hypoxia. OSA has wide-reaching consequences since it is also associated with a myriad of complications, from CVD to metabolic diseases. The gold standard for the treatment of moderate to severe OSA is CPAP therapy, whose clinical effectiveness depends on variable patient compliance. With the exclusion of CPAP, other modalities such as lifestyle modification, surgery, and oral appliances address individual patient needs. Lastly, OSA pathology heterogeneity necessitates an individualized treatment strategy, considering personalized treatment regimens to optimally maximize patient outcomes (Aluas et al., 2019). COPD is also a prevalent condition that is so challenging in respiratory medicine, primarily owing to prolonged exposure to harmful particulates or gases, most commonly as a result of tobacco smoking. This progressive and chronic disease is characterized by airflow limitation and by chronic respiratory symptoms, including sputum production and chronic cough. The pathophysiology of COPD lies in the complex interaction between inflammatory and remodeling processes and airway and alveolar destruction. The treatment of COPD typically involves both pharmacological therapies, such as steroids and bronchodilators, and non-pharmacological interventions, including smoking cessation programs and PR. Continuous attempts to introduce prevention and early diagnosis into people's knowledge are crucial since early treatment significantly improves patient prognoses and QoL (Akyol et al., 2019).

6.2.1. Asthma: Causes and Symptoms

Asthma, a chronic inflammatory airway disease, is marked by augmented sensitization to a variety of environmental stimuli. The pathogenesis of asthma is multifactorial, involving genetic predisposition, environmental triggers, and lifestyle. Genetic factors are the major determinants, with individuals having a positive family history for asthma or allergy having a greater susceptibility. Further, environmental exposures such as pollen, dust mites, mold, pet dander, and cigarette smoke can trigger symptoms. Further, air pollution, particularly in urban areas, has also emerged as a significant driving force behind the upsurge of asthma. Data from various studies have spotlighted the relationship between outdoor air pollution and the prevalence of asthma, particularly among vulnerable groups who may not have access to adequate healthcare or measures to avoid it (American Lung Association, 2001). Identification of these etiologies is an essential step in developing particular interventions to regulate and reduce the incidence of asthma. Presentation of asthma can be very unpredictable across individuals and also over time, thereby being challenging for diagnosis and management. Common presentations include wheezing, cough, shortness of breath, and chest tightness, particularly at night or in the early morning hours. Various factors like physical activity, cold air, and respiratory tract infection can induce these presentations. Additionally, the severity of symptoms can vary with changes in the environment or exposure to triggers, causing acute asthma episodes. A critical part of disease control is identifying these symptoms in time and how they correlate with underlying causes. Successful control of asthma often requires implementing a tailored action plan that includes drug therapy, lifestyle changes, and education on identifying precipitating factors. This integrated approach could significantly improve the QoL for individuals suffering from asthma and minimize the frequency of exacerbations. Through a study of asthma's relationship with environmental disparities, the uneven effect of this disease on particular communities is evident. Urban populations, particularly low-socioeconomic-status and ethnic minority groups, are more likely to have higher levels of air pollution, thereby leading to a higher incidence of asthma. These disparities have their roots in structural factors, including inadequate housing, limited access to healthcare, and limited means of pollution control (American Lung Association, 2001). Policy intervention aimed at decreasing asthma's impact on high-risk groups can address these disparities. Promotion of cleaner environments and targeted public health interventions are the first steps toward reducing asthma's effects on high-risk populations. The interface of environmental justice and respiratory health highlights the importance of ongoing research into the health effects of the environment, further improving our practice of managing and preventing asthma (Figure 6.4).

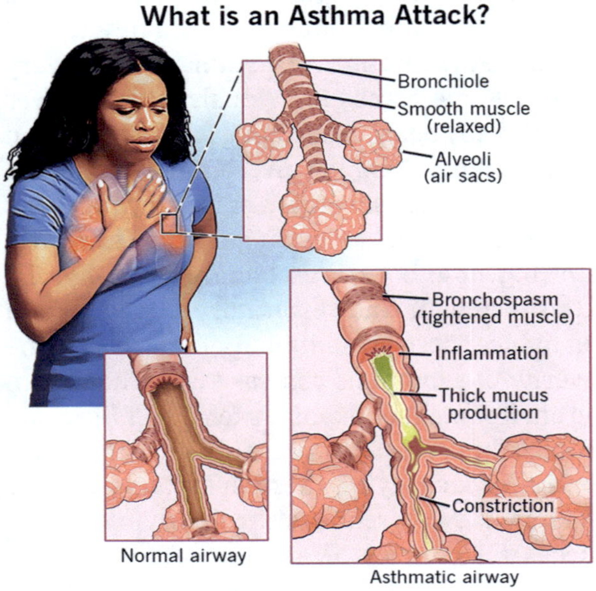

Figure 6.4. Asthma.

Source: https://my.clevelandclinic.org/-/scassets/images/org/health/articles/6424-asthma.

6.2.2. Chronic Obstructive Pulmonary Disease (COPD)

Chronic obstructive pulmonary disease (COPD) is a permanent lung disease characterized by airflow constriction and breathing difficulty. Primarily caused by long-term exposure to harmful substances such as tobacco smoke and outdoor air pollution, COPD is a significant health expense worldwide. The disease is characterized by chronic cough, sputum, and dyspnea on exertion, which significantly impacts patients' QoL. As the respiratory status deteriorates in the patient, acute exacerbations are more prone to occur, and ongoing medical management and intervention become necessary. Understanding COPD pathophysiology plays a central role in the successful management of regimens, both pharmacologic and non-pharmacologic, for alleviating symptoms and enhancing patient comfort. Therapeutic modalities of COPD management commonly include the use of bronchodilators, corticosteroids, and PR. These are designed to relieve symptoms, improve lung function, and enhance physical tolerance. One such recent study aimed at the significance of dyspnea management strategies employed by patients with COPD, including the subjects' liking for therapeutic practices like bronchodilator therapy and breathing postures, like leaning forward (Matchim et al., 2014).

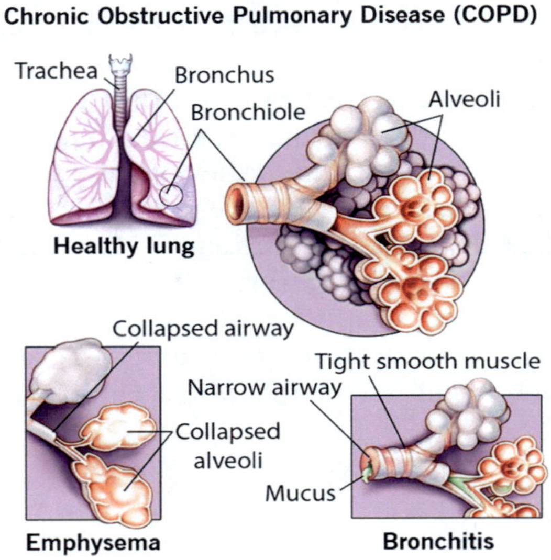

Figure 6.5. Chronic obstructive pulmonary disease (COPD).

Source: https://my.clevelandclinic.org/-/scassets/images/org/health/articles/8709-copd.jpg.

The finding that most patients find bronchodilators somewhat beneficial highlights the importance of educating patients about proper medication practices and the necessity of adhering to treatment protocols. Besides, effective management also relies on understanding the specific patient's experience with dyspnea, allowing tailored strategies to be incorporated alongside routine medical treatments. In addition to pharmacologic therapy, lifestyle modification is very crucial for the care of COPD. Smoking cessation is the gold standard, with tobacco being the most prevalent cause of the disease. Regular exercise and proper physical activity tailored to the patient's ability can also increase lung function and overall health. Self-management skills, including patient education, equip patients with the knowledge to better manage their condition. Instructing COPD patients on their disease and including symptom management skills can significantly improve QoL (Amaducci et al., 2018). The development of ongoing treatment modalities and a full understanding of problems confronting patients contribute to the advancement of care strategies, ultimately leading to better health outcomes in this high-risk group (Figure 6.5).

6.2.3. Pneumonia: Types and Treatment Options

Pneumonia is a severe respiratory illness characterized by inflammation of lung tissue, most often caused by infectious pathogens such as bacteria, viruses, and fungi. Pneumonia had traditionally been classified into distinct syndromes like CAP, hospital-acquired pneumonia (HAP), and immunocompromised pneumonia, among others. Each has specific etiologic reasons and clinical manifestations. For instance, Streptococcus pneumoniae is a common etiologic pathogen of CAP, whereas HAP is more likely associated with drug-resistant pathogens such as Pseudomonas aeruginosa. Identification of such differences remains an essential criterion for guiding appropriate treatment regimens based on the type of pneumonia and specific patient considerations. Proper and timely identification of the type of pneumonia is a key prognostic factor and a necessary prerequisite for therapeutic interventions, ultimately maximizing outcomes in respiratory therapy. It's therapy also relies on its etiology, the pathogenic infecting agent, and the patient's clinical status. Antibiotic therapy remains the cornerstone of treatment for bacterial pneumonia, and antibiotic choice relies on local resistance patterns and patient-specific factors such as age and allergy. Therapy in uncomplicated CAP, for example, is typically attained with outpatient therapy by macrolides or doxycycline, while complications may require hospitalization with intravenous antibiotics. In addition, antiviral drugs are also utilized for viral pneumonia, particularly when influenza viruses cause it. Also essential in the treatment regimen is supportive care, including hydration, supplementary oxygenation, and respiratory therapy, to ensure adequate ventilation and oxygenation of the patient.

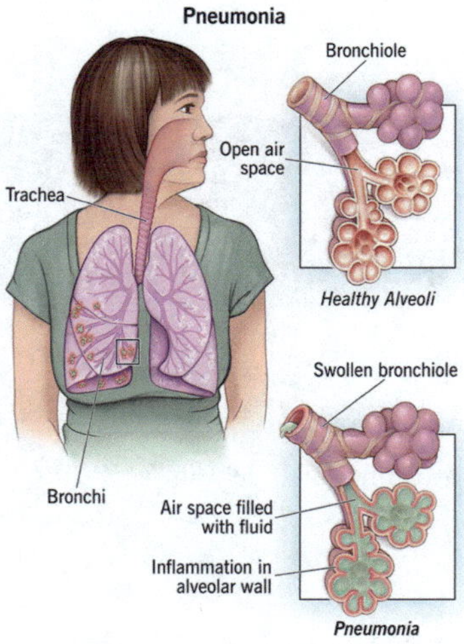

Figure 6.6. Pneumonia.

Source: https://my.clevelandclinic.org/-/scassets/images/org/health/articles/4471-pneumonia-01.

This multi-pronged strategy ensures effective management of pneumonia and protects against complications. Prevention is also an essential key to managing pneumonia's public health significance. Immunization remains a viable method, especially for vulnerable populations like the elderly or those with chronic illnesses, to reduce the incidence of *Streptococcus pneumoniae* and *Haemophilus influenzae* bacterial pneumonia. Moreover, adopting lifestyle changes, such as quitting smoking and implementing proper hygiene practices, can significantly minimize the risk of acquiring pneumonia. These prophylactic measures are essential, particularly in the background of ongoing research that connects respiratory illnesses to more general medical issues. The need to treat infections such as periodontal disease has been emphasized through research demonstrating a connection between systemic disease and respiratory problems. Therefore, an integrated pneumonia care approach, including prevention, treatment, and patient education, is essential for improving respiratory health outcomes among populations with various disparities (Bandeeri et al., 2004; Weissenfluh et al., 2019) (Figure 6.6).

Test Your Knowledge

1. What are the common causes and symptoms of asthma, and how is the condition typically managed in general practice?
2. What is Chronic Obstructive Pulmonary Disease (COPD), and how does it differ from other respiratory conditions in terms of progression and treatment?
3. What are the different types of pneumonia, and what are the standard treatment options for each type?

6.3. Diagnostic Tools in Respiratory Medicine

Learning Outcome

1. Describe pulmonary function tests
2. Understand imaging techniques
3. Define bronchoscopy and its applications

In respiratory medicine, the diagnostic armamentarium plays a vital role in diagnosing, observing, and treating various pulmonary diseases. Imaging procedures such as chest X-ray and CT scans play a key role in visualizing the morphology of the lung and identifying abnormalities, including tumors, infections, or COPD. These imaging modalities provide clinicians with precise information about the respiratory system's morphology, which can significantly impact treatment. In addition, advancements in imaging technology, including high-resolution CT, have enhanced early ILD diagnosis, enabling prompt intervention and better patient outcomes. It is vital to incorporate these imaging modalities within the clinic, as they provide a non-invasive evaluation of the respiratory system, complementing other diagnostic methods necessary for overall patient care. Other than imaging, spirometry remains one of the most sought-after diagnostic means of ascertaining lung function. This sensitive pulmonary function test measures several parameters, such as forced expiratory volume (FEV1) and forced vital capacity (FVC), allowing practitioners to characterize the degree of airway restriction or obstruction. Spirometry is particularly valuable in asthma and COPD diagnosis since it provides measurable values that guide treatment protocols and monitor disease progression. The simplicity and convenience of this test make it suitable for mass screening, particularly among at-risk populations. Accuracy, on the other hand, depends on proper technique and the use of standard reference points, highlighting the need for consistent training and adherence to protocols among health providers. The application of spirometric data in clinical evaluation enhances our understanding of respiratory status and guides therapeutic interventions toward improved patient management. The recent advances in diagnostic techniques, especially for tuberculosis (TB), reflect the ongoing advancement in respiratory medicine. Despite its status as one of the global infectious diseases, TB diagnosis has long been handicapped by the lack of rapid, point-of-care tests. Current gold-standard techniques for active pulmonary TB diagnosis are typically laboratory-based assays that delay therapy. The gaps still prevail, underscored by the critical need for improved access and accuracy in diagnostic instruments to effectively control TB. New diagnostic tests for latent infection and drug-resistant type identification have been established, but the path towards a point-of-care test for all is still elusive. The gaps need to be filled as rapid case detection relies on progress in diagnosis technology, political will, and sufficient funding to facilitate sustainable health interventions. Accordingly, ongoing R&D of TB diagnostics offers a significant promise towards enhancing global respiratory wellness (Harari et al., 2012; Blakey et al., 2017).

6.3.1. Pulmonary Function Tests (PFTs)

Pulmonary function tests (PFTs) are a critical part of respiratory health evaluation, providing helpful information on lung function and lung capacity. PFTs consist of a range of methods, from spirometry to lung volume measurement and gas diffusion, each yielding varying information about the respiratory system. Spirometry, the most common PFT, quantitates the volume and rate of air a patient can exhale and thus determines potential obstructive or restrictive airway patterns. The results of such tests are essential for the diagnosis of conditions such as asthma, COPD, and pulmonary fibrosis. Furthermore, PFTs are found to be very valuable in determining disease progression and treatment efficacy, allowing physicians to appropriately adjust therapeutic interventions. In addition to their application in diagnostics, PFTs are utilized significantly in preoperative care and occupational medicine. In preoperative assessment, especially for operations involving anesthesia, PFTs help determine whether a patient's pulmonary function can withstand procedural stresses. Preoperative evaluation is critical in the case of patients with existing lung disease since compromised respiratory function can create substantially increased perioperative risk. Similarly, in occupational health practice, PFTs assist in diagnosing respiratory conditions at work, and appropriate interventions are implemented to prevent complications. Standardization becomes imperative to achieve reliability and consistency in practice, as has been the case with efforts to develop recommendations for cardiopulmonary exercise testing in chronic lung disease (Aguilaniu et al., 2019). On top of this, the interpretation of pulmonary function test results will need several factors, including patient age, existing medical condition, and environmental considerations, to be factored in. Variations in age, gender, height, and ethnicity will all result in differences in lung capacity and function, necessitating population-specific predictive values. This calls for accurate calibration of PFT equipment against known standards and normal data to effectively label results as either normal or abnormal. Of special interest is the continued evolution of pulmonary function testing technology and respiratory physiology research, to further sharpen the diagnostic precision and clinical utility of such tests. Such innovations will increasingly guide the holistic management of respiratory disorders and shape the direction of future investigative approaches in respiratory health (Singanayagam et al., 2015) (Figure 6.7).

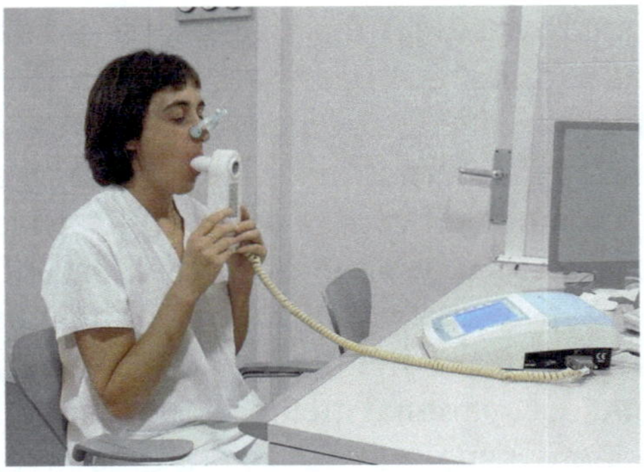

Figure 6.7. Spirometry.

Source: https://upload.wikimedia.org/wikipedia/commons/thumb/2/27/DoingSpirometry.JPG/800px-DoingSpirometry.JPG.

6.3.2. Imaging Techniques: X-rays and CT Scans

Application of imaging technologies such as X-rays and CT scans is now a necessity in the diagnosis and management of respiratory system illnesses. X-rays are a simple imaging technique useful for visualizing thoracic structures and providing information on conditions such as pneumonia, pleural effusion, and lung tumors. Though relatively quick and cheap, interpretation needs an experienced eye to identify obvious pathologies. However, their disadvantage is that when more complex cases arise, they demand advanced imaging tools like CT scans. CT scans, with their ability to produce cross-sectional images at high resolution, are particularly beneficial in diagnosing complicated lung and respiratory disorders like ILD and pulmonary embolism. Together, these imaging modalities enhance clinicians' diagnostic acumen and allow for more targeted treatment protocols and ultimately improved patient outcomes in respiratory medicine. The incorporation of imaging modalities into the clinical setting is not without controversy, especially when the risks from radiation exposure are taken into account. While X-rays have been available for more than a century, their dependence on ionizing radiation calls for a careful weighing of the risk/benefit ratio in every imaging decision. Literature nowadays stresses the need for a worldwide approach to radiation risks, particularly in instances of repeated imaging examinations performed on individuals with chronic respiratory disease (Donya et al., 2014). Doctors must weigh the diagnostic advantages against potential long-term effects, such as increased cancer risk. This act of balancing is required to reap the maximum benefits for patients from technological advancements in imaging while minimizing their exposure to harmful radiation. Well-defined guidelines and judicious utilization of these imaging modalities are, therefore, extremely crucial in the field of general medicine for the respiratory system. With advancing technology, investigations are being carried out to maximize best practices for their use in clinical settings. Interestingly, studies have documented varying frequencies of ailments such as cocaine abuse among patients with acute respiratory presentation, and these can be explained by imaging modalities (Bandeeri et al., 2004). This serves to emphasize the importance of context in understanding imaging findings, especially where atypical presentations render diagnosis problematic. Further, the advancements in imaging technology, e.g., the implementation of low-dose CT scans, hold the promise of reduced exposure to radiation while enhancing diagnostic ability. As the medical community focuses on improving patient outcomes and safety, education on the use of imaging modalities in respiratory medicine continues to gain significance. The convergence of clinical knowledge, technological innovation, and patient care provides an evolving platform for establishing diagnostic services across general medicine for the respiratory system.

6.3.3. Bronchoscopy and Its Applications

Bronchoscopy is a critical diagnostic and therapeutic tool in general medicine that provides for the direct visual examination of the air passages and lungs. Using a bronchoscope, doctors can enter the passages of the bronchi to detect pathologic conditions like infection, tumors, or inflammatory disease. This process not only facilitates diagnosis but also allows for targeted interventions, including biopsy, drainage of secretions, or the direct administration of medications into the target zone. With increased indications of bronchoscopy, it remains a fast-evolving method in respiratory medicine. The utilization of more advanced imaging technologies during bronchoscopy enhances its diagnostic capability, thereby maximizing patient benefits and treatment algorithms. Apart from its application in diagnosis, bronchoscopy also plays a significant role in the treatment of chronic respiratory conditions, for example, cystic fibrosis. In this genetic condition, the airways of victims are blocked by thick mucus, resulting in frequent infection and ultimately lung failure. Through bronchoscopy, it is possible to remove such mucus, improving symptoms and lung function. Recent findings indicate the efficacy of bronchoscopy in combination with gene therapy as a new drug treatment, particularly for patients participating in clinical trials to assess new CFTR gene treatments. These advances establish bronchoscopy as an active instrument not just for the diagnosis of respiratory states but also as part of new therapeutic regimens (Alton et al., 2016). Further, the therapeutic application of bronchoscopies has been significantly improved with the incorporation of novel technologies such as autofluorescence imaging (AFI). By using this method, the detection and viewing of precancerous lesions and airway structures in real time are enhanced, resulting in more precise interventions. Autofluorescence bronchoscopic techniques are becoming more widespread outside traditional applications after showing promise in other clinical domains, including dermatology and surgery (Aigner et al., 2020). The increased interest in newer imaging modalities reflects a further commitment to enhancing clinical effectiveness in respiratory disease. While bronchoscopy continues to utilize the most recent technology, its use in the integrated management of respiratory disease will assuredly be supplemented, eventually resulting in improving patient care in numerous different ways (Figure 6.8).

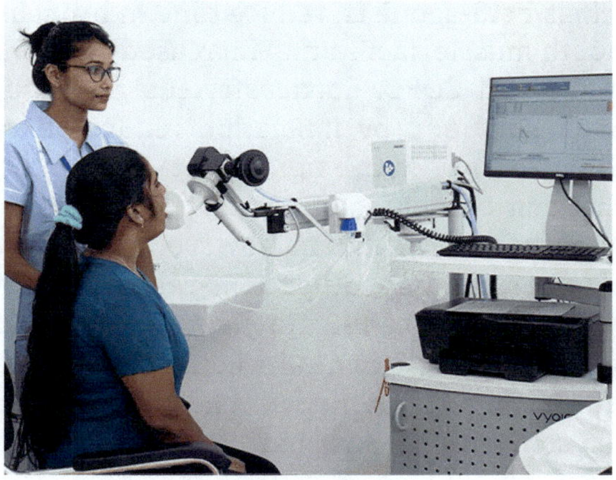

Figure 6.8. Bronchoscopy test.

Source: https://www.apexhospitals.com/_next/image?url=https%3A%2F%2Fbed.apexhospitals.com%2Fuploads%2Fbronchoscopy_ebfe11c0ed.png&w=1200&q=75.

Test Your Knowledge

1. What are pulmonary function tests, and how do they help in diagnosing and monitoring respiratory diseases?
2. How are imaging techniques such as chest X-rays and CT scans used in evaluating respiratory conditions?
3. What is bronchoscopy, and in what clinical situations is it typically used?

6.4. Pharmacological Treatments

Learning Outcome

1. Describe bronchodilators and their mechanisms
2. Understand corticosteroids for inflammation control
3. Discuss antibiotics for bacterial infections

The therapy of respiratory diseases is generally pharmacological and tailored to reduce symptoms while optimizing patients' QoL. Common agents include bronchodilators, corticosteroids, and anticholinergics, acting on various aspects of respiration. Bronchodilators, such as beta-agonists, reduce tone in bronchial smooth muscle, facilitating increased airflow in asthma and COPD. Corticosteroids given both systemically and by inhalation reduce airway inflammation with significant therapeutic benefit in chronic inflammatory diseases. The success of such treatment, however, necessitates an understanding of patient-related factors that may influence PK and pharmacodynamics, highlighting the essential role of personalized medicine in respiratory pharmacotherapy. Apart from conventional pharmacologic management, increasing evidence demands that there is an integration wherein the conventional drugs are complemented by alternative therapy, particularly in managing stress and anxiety related to respiratory disease. There is evidence that meditation and some breathing exercises can be employed as complementary additions to drug treatment. These practices address both the physical and emotional dimensions of respiratory function by achieving homeostasis and reducing sympathetic predominance of the autonomic nervous system. Early results confirm such measures in reversing the adverse effects of stress on respiratory function, so they are to be considered as a first-line or adjunct therapy in patients with accompanying anxiety or emotional disorder along with their respiratory illness, as stated in recent articles (Barnes et al., 2015). Added to this is the dynamic nature of pharmacological management in respiratory medicine, particularly with reference to the pharmaceuticalization and medicalization of disorders like insomnia, which is also a disorder characterized by comorbidity with chronic respiratory disease. The intersection, therefore, is proper management of insomnia for improved patient outcomes. The research indicates that the majority of medical management is actually practiced in general practice communities. Yet, an excessive overreliance on pharmaceutical interventions also calls their effectiveness and appropriateness into question (Coveney et al., 2019). As the field develops, it will be essential to understand the complexities of pharmaceutical interventions in treating insomnia related to respiratory illness. This understanding will help design interdisciplinary treatment options that promote overall patient wellness and minimize the side effects of long-term medication.

6.4.1. Bronchodilators and Their Mechanisms

The role of bronchodilators in the treatment of respiratory diseases is pivotal, particularly in diseases with airway constriction such as asthma and COPD. The medications function primarily by inducing relaxation of the bronchial smooth muscles, which leads to widening of the airway and enhanced airflow to the lungs. Bronchodilators are short-acting and long-acting drugs, which find their specific place in various clinical scenarios. Short-acting beta-agonists, for instance, provide immediate relief and are indispensable in acute situations. Still, long-acting formulations are typically administered in chronic conditions to enhance overall lung capacity and decrease exacerbations. It is thus imperative to understand the PK and dynamics of bronchodilators to achieve maximum patient benefit in respiratory medicine. Evaluation of the effectiveness of bronchodilators entails an extensive review of their mechanisms, which demonstrates that there is a multifaceted strategy towards alleviating respiratory distress. These drugs mainly work by stimulating beta-adrenergic receptors in bronchial smooth muscle, which triggers a cascade of intracellular changes culminating in smooth muscle relaxation. Certain bronchodilators also possess anti-inflammatory effects, influencing the respiratory disease pathophysiology beyond merely relaxing muscles. Therapeutic application of bronchodilators, however, is not without complexity. Studies have found that the efficacy of these medications can be influenced by individual patient factors, including the severity of illness and comorbidities.

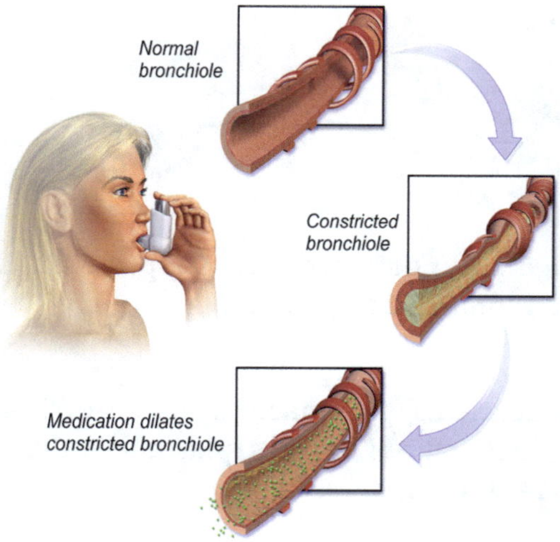

Figure 6.9. Bronchodilators.

Source: https://upload.wikimedia.org/wikipedia/commons/e/e3/Bronchodilators.png.

These clinically useful attributes need to be known by healthcare professionals who want to give tailored and effective treatment to patients suffering from respiratory ailments (Fernandes et al., 2015). Despite the well-established efficacy of bronchodilator therapy, current research and debate target maximizing their utilization, with a special emphasis on combination with other treatments such as corticosteroids. Clinical trials have identified that the combination of bronchodilators with corticosteroids can provide superior clinical results in patients with severe bronchial inflammation, such as those suffering from bronchiolitis. The literature demands well-designed clinical trials to demarcate primary areas of concern, including the definition of disease and appropriate selection of outcomes in evaluating the efficacy of treatment (Fromer et al., 2014). This critical methodology message highlights the need for a research initiative in this field to ensure that therapeutic treatment protocols for bronchodilators are not only evidence-based but also harmonizable with current clinical practice, thereby efficiently treating respiratory illnesses (Figure 6.9).

6.4.2. Corticosteroids for Inflammation Control

Corticosteroids have become the focal point in respiratory disease treatment, particularly due to their potent anti-inflammatory effect. The synthetic drugs imitate the effect of hormones produced by the adrenal glands and target the immune system to inhibit its activity, thus treating conditions with inappropriate inflammation. For asthma and COPD, corticosteroids have been demonstrated to effectively reduce airway inflammation, alleviating symptoms such as wheezing, breathlessness, and cough. Beyond relieving symptoms, studies have shown that corticosteroids improve lung function and overall health in patients suffering from COPD and asthma. The inclusion of corticosteroids in treatment regimens is generally determined by clinical information, further solidifying their status as a keystone within respiratory medicine (Blakey et al., 2017). While effective, corticosteroids do possess potential side effects, thus their application becomes an issue of cautious consideration. Prolonged use of systemic corticosteroids can lead to conditions such as osteoporosis, hyperglycemia, and increased susceptibility to infection. To offset these dangers, clinicians typically prescribe ICS, which direct the drug to the lungs, lowering systemic absorption and accompanying side effects. ICS have been highly effective in managing asthma, as they reduce inflammation in the area of action without the far-reaching systemic side effects associated with oral or injectable drugs. Because of their favorable profile, ICS were approved as first-line therapy for persistent asthma, and the evidence indicates that the early treatment may block disease progression and reduce the frequency of exacerbations (McKay et al., 2011). Moreover, corticosteroids are also administered in conjunction with other therapeutic agents with the purpose of amplifying their effect and dealing with the multifactorial nature of respiratory diseases (Figure 6.10).

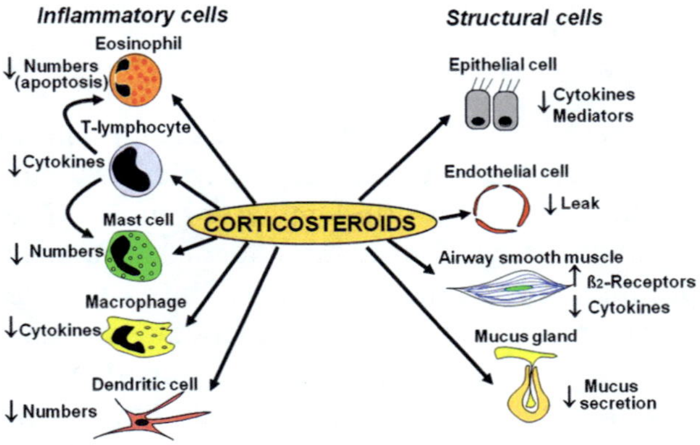

Figure 6.10. Cellular effect of corticosteroids.

Source: https://www.mdpi.com/pharmaceuticals/pharmaceuticals-03-00514/article_deploy/html/images/pharmaceuticals-03-00514-g001.png.

For instance, the association of ICS with long-acting beta-agonists (LABAs) has been demonstrated in clinical trials and provides synergistic advantages that improve overall airway control and patient outcomes. The dual strategy allows for both the reduction of inflammation and bronchodilation, which addresses multifaceted aspects of respiratory pathophysiology. The importance of individualized therapy cannot be overstated, as patient response to corticosteroids is potentially very heterogeneous. Monitoring and adjusting treatment plans based on patient-specific considerations are essential to attain the optimal therapeutic outcomes and enhance management strategies for respiratory diseases effectively (Blakey et al., 2017) (Figure 6.11).

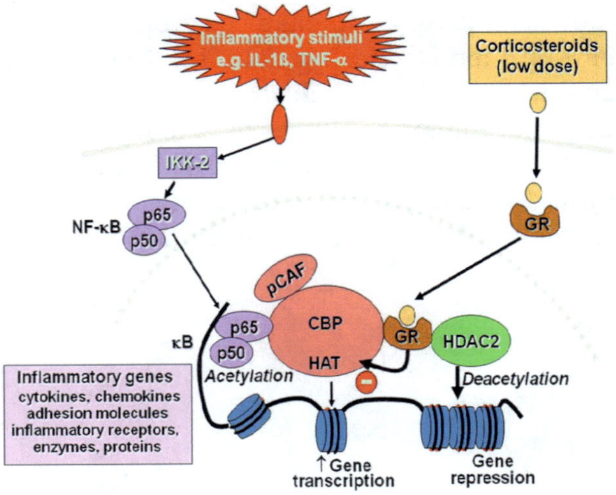

Figure 6.11. Corticosteroid suppression of activated inflammatory genes.

Source: https://www.mdpi.com/pharmaceuticals/pharmaceuticals-03-00514/article_deploy/html/images/pharmaceuticals-03-00514-g004.png.

6.4.3. Antibiotics for Bacterial Infections

Antibiotic therapy for respiratory system infections is an important aspect of general practice. Antibiotics are employed against bacterial pathogens that can lead to infections such as pneumonia, bronchitis, and exacerbations of COPD. The choice of the antibiotic is typically made based on presumptive or isolated bacterial species, as well as the patient's history and risk factors, most notably age and comorbidities. Here, the issue of antibiotic resistance is crucial because misuse can contribute to the growing threat from resistant organisms, thereby complicating treatment. Effective management involves not just employing the appropriate antibiotic, but also employing strategies which delay resistance development and optimize patient benefits, given the evolving nature of bacterial infections. Elderly patients particularly present particular challenges in the control of respiratory bacterial infections. With advancing age, immune function is compromised and increased susceptibility to chronic diseases, which in turn raises the risk of developing COPD and chronic bronchitis exacerbations. In such patients, the most frequently occurring organisms during acute exacerbations are typically infectious agents such as *Haemophilus influenzae* and *Streptococcus pneumoniae*, as well as more resistant organisms like *Pseudomonas aeruginosa*. Current risk-stratified antibiotic therapy guidelines emphasize the importance of tailoring therapy to the risk of exposure to resistant organisms, particularly in older patients with chronic respiratory disease or increased disease expression (Albertson et al., 2010). The selection of appropriate antibiotics has a significant impact on both morbidity and mortality in such patients. Besides, the application of combined antimicrobial stewardship programs is essential to enhance the effectiveness of antibiotics in the management of respiratory infections. The purpose of these programs is to monitor and evaluate antibiotic prescribing habits to reduce unnecessary prescriptions that are likely drivers of AMR. Various policy strategies, such as encouraging responsible use, good surveillance, and infection control practices, may prevent the problem of resistance in different healthcare environments (Aarestrup et al., 2015). By promoting intersectoral collaboration across the healthcare continuum — human, animal, and environmental health sectors—as underscored by the One Health approach, policymakers can create customized solutions that proactively confront the issues of antibiotic use in respiratory diseases. This multifaceted endeavor is central to the guarantee of antibiotics as an effective tool in the war against bacterial infections, resulting in both patient health and public health sustainability.

Test Your Knowledge

1. What are bronchodilators, and how do they work to relieve symptoms in respiratory conditions such as asthma and COPD?
2. How do corticosteroids help control inflammation in respiratory diseases, and what are some common routes of administration?
3. When are antibiotics indicated in respiratory conditions, and why is it important to distinguish bacterial infections from viral ones before prescribing?

6.5. Non-Pharmacological Interventions

Learning Outcome

1. Understand the importance of pulmonary rehabilitation
2. Explain the role of oxygen therapy
3. Focus on lifestyle modifications for respiratory health

The management of respiratory diseases, particularly chronic ones such as asthma, now incorporates the use of non-pharmacological interventions coupled with conventional pharmacotherapy. Interventions typically entail lifestyle modification, psychological counseling, and educational interventions aimed at improving patient outcomes. A good example is smoking cessation, a critical non-pharmacological intervention that can significantly improve lung function and reduce exacerbation rates in COPD patients. Furthermore, the application of PR programs has been shown to enhance exercise capacity and QoL in chronic respiratory disease patients. The interventions not only allow patients to become more actively engaged in disease management but also increase treatment compliance with pharmacologic regimens. By focusing on integrated patient care, healthcare practitioners can promote a more holistic intervention for respiratory well-being that addresses not only the physiological condition of chronic disease but also the psychological dimensions (Singanayagam et al., 2015). Coupled with lifestyle modification, psychological interventions are key factors in integrative management of respiratory disorders. These treatments address the psychological comorbidities that are often present in asthma patients, including anxiety and depression, and they are responsible for exacerbating respiratory symptoms and drug noncompliance. Although there is varying evidence regarding the efficacy of psychological treatments, some studies have found that cognitive-behavioral therapy helps improve self-management skills and subsequently asthma control. Significantly, the inclusion of these psychological treatments helps to decrease the emotional burden of chronic illness. Evidence for such therapies, while not yet conclusive, is indicative of the advantages they can bring to those with challenges in asthma control (Brewin et al., 2015). As demand for integrated care grows, the importance of non-pharmacological interventions in clinical practice also increases. Education interventions also assume particular significance in the non-pharmacological treatment of respiratory disease. Interventions to develop patient awareness of their condition can significantly empower patients to adopt self-management behaviors. Education of patients regarding asthma triggers, inhaler use, and action plans can enhance symptom control and reduce acute exacerbations. Moreover, group education classes can provide social support, allowing patients to learn from one another and develop strategies for managing their conditions. As adjuncts to medication, these educational interventions are critical to enhancing overall patient engagement and compliance. With the complex nature of respiratory illnesses, incorporating educational elements into treatment regimens can be vital in promoting a more cooperative partnership between patients and healthcare professionals, culminating in enhanced long-term patient outcomes (Singanayagam et al., 2015).

6.5.1. Importance of Pulmonary Rehabilitation

Pulmonary rehabilitation (PR) plays a significant role in the restoration of the QoL among patients with chronic respiratory disorders, including COPD and ILDs. The treatment is multidisciplinary and involves exercise training, education, and psychological support, which combine to improve the overall physical and emotional state of the patient. Clinical studies have indicated that patients who participate in PR exhibit significant decreases in dyspnea, increased physical ability, and improved health-related QoL. Importantly, the exercises within PR programs are individually selected to increase respiratory muscle strength, consequently improving lung function and allowing patients to manage their disease better. This structured process is critical because it enables patients to become more of an active partner in their own healthcare, engendering a sense of empowerment that can become a driver of better treatment compliance and lifestyle intervention. Furthermore, PR addresses not only the physical components of chronic respiratory disease but also the psychological and social barriers with which patients may struggle. The inclusion of educational and counseling components in PR allows patients to better understand the disease and manage symptoms to avoid flare-ups. Feeling supported within a group setting, patients indicate decreased loneliness and anxiety, for improved mental health status. Existing recommendations emphasize including mental health considerations in respiratory treatment, as psychological well-being significantly affects patients' ability to attend rehabilitation therapy and adhere to treatment protocols (Pelliccia et al., 2020). Thus, based on this multidisciplinary practice, PR becomes a cornerstone of chronic respiratory disease management, addressing various patient needs. Finally, the worth of PR is not merely in patient gain, but also in its significance for healthcare systems. Through enhanced disease control and potentially fewer, less intense acute exacerbations, PR can lead to reduced hospital admissions and healthcare costs in the long term. Such cost-saving interventions are valuable in light of the increasing prevalence of chronic respiratory diseases worldwide. Evidence shows that proper implementation and dissemination of PR programs can extend to have a broad impact on public health benefits, reducing healthcare system burdens while improving overall patient well-being (Alexander et al., 2022). This two-pronged benefit—enhancement of patient QoL and reduction in healthcare utilization—highlights the pivotal contribution of PR as an integral part of the respiratory care continuum, warranting ongoing investment and emphasis in everyday medicine practice for respiratory care (Figure 6.12).

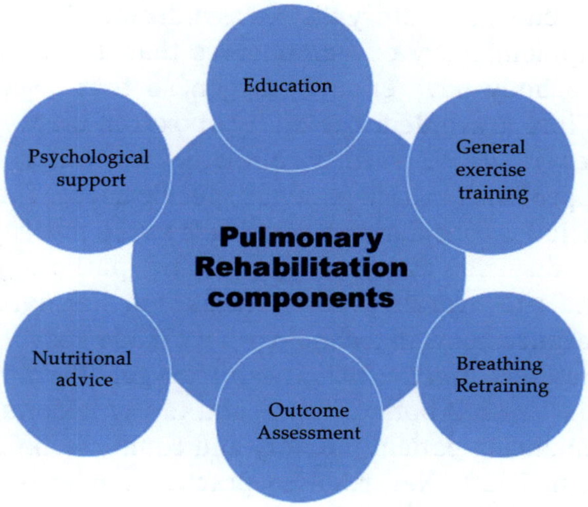

Figure 6.12. Components of pulmonary rehabilitation.

Source: https://www.cardiacwellnessinstitute.com/heart-disease-treatment-prevention/wp-content/uploads/2017/10/pulmonary-rehabilitation-pptx-6-638.jpg.

6.5.2. Role of Oxygen Therapy

Oxygen therapy is a crucial component in the management of numerous respiratory illnesses, particularly those with impaired gas exchange, such as COPD and OSA. Through the provision of supplemental oxygen, medical providers can decrease hypoxemia and heighten the concentration of oxygen saturation among patients, ultimately improving overall respiratory function and QoL. In OSA, oxygen therapy is typically used as an adjunct to primary treatments like CPAP therapy to correct nocturnal oxygen deficits caused by periodic airflow obstruction. Notably, the efficacy of such treatment modalities is largely dependent on patient compliance and individualized treatment regimens since non-compliance will compromise the therapeutic benefits of adjunct therapy like oxygen supplementation (Aluas et al., 2019). The application of oxygen therapy extends beyond COPD and OSA to include a variety of clinical situations where hypoxia is a significant threat. For instance, in pneumonia or acute respiratory distress syndrome (ARDS), supplementary oxygen ensures that tissues in the body have enough oxygen so that organ failure is avoided. The utility of oxygen therapy lies in its versatility, allowing for tailored approaches to each patient's specific needs. This includes considering factors such as the severity of disease, the underlying lung pathology, and the overall patient status. Furthermore, advancements in technology have made delivery methods more efficient, and oxygen therapy can be used both at home and in the hospital, enhancing patient mobility and comfort (Akyol et al., 2019). Nevertheless, practical application of oxygen therapy is not without challenges, primarily with respect to the risk of long-term exposure to adverse effects. Some comorbid patients can experience oxygen toxicity or carbon dioxide retention complications if the oxygen levels are not checked and regulated with proper management. These complications highlight the importance of frequent clinical checks and the implementation of evidence-based guidelines for directing oxygen therapy initiation and titration. In addition, professionals must be keen on patient education so that patients know why they should adhere to oxygen orders. As the dynamics of respiratory care continue to evolve, there must be ongoing research to adapt oxygen therapy protocols for maximum optimization and to study their long-term impact on outcomes in the overall practice of medicine for the respiratory system (Aluas et al., 2019) (Figure 6.13).

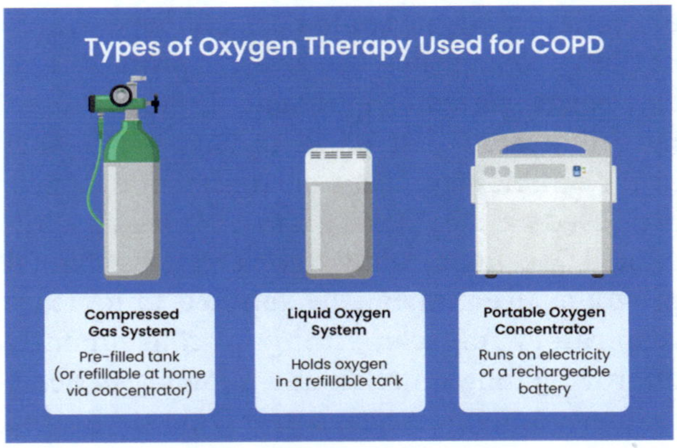

Figure 6.13. Types of oxygen therapy used for COPD.

Source: https://images.ctfassets.net/yixw23k2v6vo/1UnMz71uOxnaku2MBD5uUW/4f7601bd58b8cb83cfb1660b68652104/large-GettyImages-1766510692_-2042805249-copd-oxygen-therapy.jpg.

6.5.3. Lifestyle Modifications for Respiratory Health

Lifestyle interventions play an important role in maximizing respiratory health and avoiding the risk of respiratory disorders. The single optimal intervention is to quit smoking; since it has been unequivocally established that tobacco smoke induces lung cancer and COPD, which are two of the most significant causes of chronic respiratory morbidity. Smokers who quit can significantly improve their lung function and overall health, with a decreased risk of many respiratory outcomes. In addition, physical exercise develops lung volume and respiratory muscle strength. Physical training also improves the body's overall cardiovascular health, which is intrinsically linked with effective respiratory functioning. By means of such a life change, individuals can enhance their QoL and decrease the risk of respiratory diseases, thus emphasizing the importance of active health management in respiratory medicine. Nutritional intake is another critical part of lifestyle modifications for respiratory well-being. A proper diet that includes plenty of fruits, green leafy vegetables, and whole grains can strengthen the immune system, thereby reducing the risk of respiratory infection. Foods that are high in antioxidants, such as berries and green leafy vegetables, may combat oxidative stress in the lungs and improve respiratory function. Furthermore, omega-3 fatty acids found in fish and flaxseed have been found to possess anti-inflammatory properties, which can reduce inflammation in the airways. Conversely, overconsumption of processed food and foods with trans fats or added sugar can cause respiratory distress and worsen conditions.

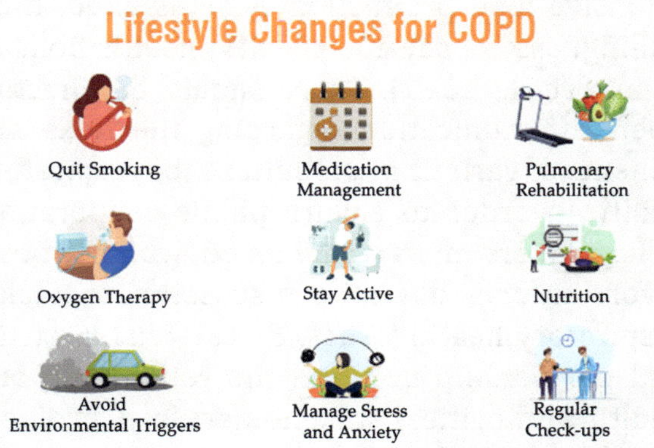

Figure 6.14. Lifestyle changes for COPD.

Source: https://www.yashodahospitals.com/wp-content/uploads/Living-with-COPD3.jpg.

A healthy diet, in that sense, not only ensures overall wellness but also directly ensures respiratory wellness through its anti-inflammatory and immune-boosting properties. Finally, managing stress and environmental problems is part of lifestyle modifications that improve respiratory health. Reducing exposure to allergens, irritants, and pollutants—such as secondhand tobacco smoke and environmental toxins—is important for improving lung function and reducing the incidence of respiratory disease. Using air purifiers and ventilation at home to minimize airborne pollutants is advisable. Moreover, stress-free activities such as yoga, meditation, or deep-breathing exercises can enhance lung volume and psychiatric well-being. It is also known that stress has been shown to have damaging effects on physical health, including exacerbating respiratory diseases. By incorporating these lifestyle modifications and focusing on both environmental and psychological well-being, patients can adopt a holistic strategy to promote robust respiratory function and overall health, illustrating the interconnectedness of many lifestyle components in respiratory medicine (Figure 6.14).

Test Your Knowledge

1. What is pulmonary rehabilitation, and why is it essential in the management of chronic respiratory diseases?
2. How does oxygen therapy benefit patients with respiratory conditions, and what are the indications for its use?
3. Which lifestyle modifications can help improve respiratory health and reduce the progression of respiratory diseases?

6.6. Preventive Measures and Public Health

Learning Outcome

1. Understand vaccination against respiratory infections
2. Describe smoking cessation programs
3. Focus on air quality and its impact on respiratory health

Preventive best practices in public health can significantly help stem respiratory disease, especially given the burgeoning pressures on healthcare systems. These include promoting vaccination programs, awareness campaigns for air quality, and lifestyle education on healthful choices. Influenza and pneumococcal disease vaccination has been shown to reduce morbidity and mortality rates substantially in those at risk, such as the elderly and those with chronic illness. Additionally, public health interventions intended to lower tobacco use and educate the population on the hazards of secondhand smoke have been important in lessening the incidence of chronic respiratory ailments. Encouraging active health behaviors and enlisting community support through prevention activities can consolidate a robust public health model focused on preserving respiratory health and advancing overall well-being. Public health and the integration of healthcare services are essential in framing an integrated response to the prevention of respiratory disease. Historically, public health agencies have endured chronic underfunding and relative neglect compared to healthcare systems, limiting their capacities. Shifting attention towards building stronger public health infrastructures can enhance health by prioritizing prevention over treatment. Strategies will have to encompass the formulation of policies that improve environmental health, improve access to clean air, and adopt policies for reducing harmful pollutants. By encouraging an integrated system that ensures both public health education and healthcare accessibility, communities can better alleviate respiratory health inequalities, resulting in a more harmonized health environment for everyone. Moving towards such dual approaches will ensure that measures receive proper attention and support, leading to better respiratory health throughout the nation in the long run (Gostin et al., 2011). Additionally, the public's contribution towards preventive healthcare measures cannot be discounted. There is evidence that indicates how public opinion for interventions can influence the effectiveness of health plans. For instance, public concerns about food animal welfare and intensive food production systems affect their willingness to pay for specific health policies (Clark et al., 2019). There should be effective open communication regarding the risks and benefits of various interventions for respiratory health in order to ensure public cooperation. Policymakers must create an environment that favors informed public discussion to tackle respiratory health issues. By establishing trust and partnership between the community and health authorities, stakeholders can promote healthier lifestyles and create compliance with preventive practices. Ultimately, increased public involvement and trust in health programs will create a better foundation for long-term respiratory health in populations.

6.6.1. Vaccination Against Respiratory Infections

The complexity of respiratory infections necessitates a robust public health reaction, with vaccination taking center stage as a key protective option. Vaccination generates immunity against common causes of respiratory infections, drastically decreasing the incidence and severity of conditions like influenza and TB, which pose major health threats worldwide. The persisting problems with traditional vaccines, including the BCG vaccine used against TB, highlight an urgent need for innovation in vaccine strategies. The understanding that Mycobacterium tuberculosis infects the human body via inhalation highlights the potential of mucosally delivered vaccines, which may offer more protection by provoking a targeted immune response at the level of the respiratory tract. Accordingly, the development of vaccines targeting respiratory infections is pivotal in achieving public health outcomes to overcome these diseases (Barclay et al., 2019). The disparities in perception and knowledge between laymen regarding the prevention of respiratory infection also underscore the necessity for education and advocacy in improving the immunization coverage. A study of three European countries reported that the population confuses the common cold with influenza, leading to a generalized prevention strategy that does not target the specific benefits of the influenza vaccine. The majority of the respondents were negative in their attitudes towards the flu vaccine, viewing it as largely beneficial only to individuals with risk factors. Such a misunderstanding discourages its general acceptance as a preventive measure among the general population. To meet this challenge, primary care physicians must actively encourage patients to be vigilant about vaccination as a key determinant of prevention, dispel widespread myths, and reinforce preventive health behaviors that can substantially reduce the reservoir of respiratory infections (Divjak et al., 2019). Given the ongoing respiratory infection issues and public health concerns with vaccination, maximizing immunization efforts remains a priority. Development of novel delivery systems, i.e., aerosolized vaccines, is a promising direction in the prevention of TB, able to produce a more effective immune response in the mucosal tissue of the respiratory system. Parallel to that, integration of vaccination programs into routine healthcare may improve acceptance and coverage rates, in particular in the time of emerging infectious diseases. Promoting equitable access to vaccines and addressing the socio-economic barriers to vaccination coverage are key components of an all-out public health campaign. Giving priority to vaccination against respiratory infections ultimately reinforces individual health and contributes to population immunity, thereby reducing the overall burden of disease in populations (Barclay et al., 2019; Divjak et al., 2019) (Figure 6.15).

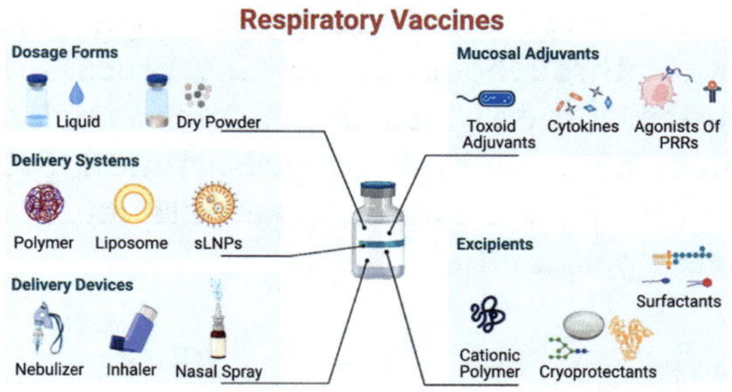

Figure 6.15. Respiratory vaccines.

Source: https://ars.els-cdn.com/content/image/1-s2.0-S016836592300113X-ga1.jpg.

6.6.2. Smoking Cessation Programs

Smoking cessation programs are necessary in controlling the respiratory disease epidemic caused by tobacco use. Smoking cessation programs are measures that enable people to quit smoking, which is linked to numerous respiratory diseases, including COPD and lung cancer. Using a combination of evidence-based interventions such as behavioral therapy, drug interventions, and educational resources, programs of cessation provide tailored support that meets the unique needs of smokers. The comprehensive program of such interventions complements anti-smoking campaigns in reducing the incidence of smoking, thereby improving respiratory health among the community at large. Furthermore, smoking cessation has been proven to lead to significant improvement in the lungs. As such, these programs are an essential part of preventing further respiratory complications and enhancing the QoL in individuals who have quit smoking. The effectiveness of smoking cessation programs is generally measured by their ability to suppress withdrawal symptoms and tobacco cravings, thereby promoting long-term behavior modification. Current research highlights the importance of personalized approaches since individuals respond in varying degrees to various cessation strategies. Treatments involving counseling and guidance from physicians have greater success rates and suggest applying social support throughout the quitting process. For severe conditions, medications such as nicotine replacement therapy or prescription drugs are part of the treatment to ensure maximum success possibilities.

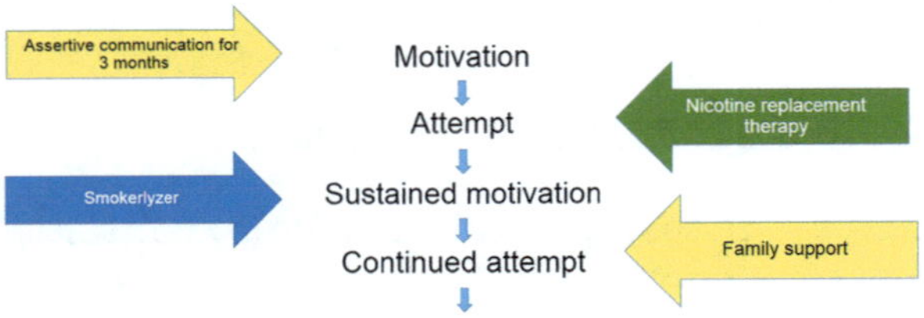

Figure 6.16. Conceptual model of newly devised smoking cessation service.

Source: https://www.researchgate.net/publication/331292976/figure/fig1/AS:729307727028226@1550891920860/Conceptual-model-of-newly-devised-smoking-cessation-service.png.

Specifically, maintaining follow-up and continued care is central to long-term success rates for cessation. This underscores the need for ongoing research to establish the most effective combination of strategies employed in smoking cessation programs targeting diverse populations. Further, the broader importance of smoking cessation programs extends beyond individual-level health effects to include significant public health impacts. Reduced smoking prevalence through such programs can lead to reduced healthcare costs from smoking-induced ailments, thereby benefiting society at large. Further, successful programs for smoking cessation reduce health inequalities, particularly among high-risk groups who may have higher smoking and concomitant respiratory disease incidence. For instance, smoking prevention among Indigenous communities has been linked to improved overall health outcomes, including infant mortality and a reduction in respiratory diseases, as documented in the literature. Thus, investment in effective smoking cessation programming increases individual health and increases the health of populations and communities, and creates a ripple effect in public health improvement (Figure 6.16).

6.6.3. Air Quality and Its Impact on Respiratory Health

Air quality is a critical determinant of respiratory health and the incidence and severity of respiratory disease. Urban environments tend to expose individuals to a cocktail of pollution, including particulate matter, nitrogen dioxide, and sulfur dioxide, significantly elevating the risk for respiratory diseases such as asthma and COPD. Vulnerable groups, including racial or ethnic minorities and low-income individuals, are likely to have a disproportionate share of these health risks because they are exposed more frequently to pollution in the urban environment. As indicated by findings of the American Lung Association, legislation has been enacted one after another to promote environmental status; even with this, disparities still prevail in exposure to pollution and point to a need for targeted intervention strategies that consider the unique challenges of marginalized populations (American Lung Association, 2001). Second, indoor air quality remains an essential domain of respiratory health, particularly in developing countries where a majority of residences utilize biomass fuels for heating and cooking. These solid fuels, upon combustion, emit indoor air pollutants, which have been linked to a wide range of respiratory diseases. Studies have revealed that nearly 3 billion individuals globally are affected by indoor air pollution and have proved through evidence that it has a causal relationship with high morbidity and mortality from respiratory diseases. This background emphasizes the critical need for public health interventions to reduce exposure to indoor air pollution through improved energy systems and ventilation, as well as community health education concerning the effect of such pollutants on well-being (Ezzati et al., 2025). Reducing the challenge of air quality on respiratory diseases calls for an integrated approach to public health and policy. Interventions must be grounded in rigorous scientific research that delineates the populations at risk and the type of pollutants to which they are exposed. Additionally, an interdisciplinary approach that takes inputs from environmental science, toxicology, and social sciences can come up with innovative solutions to the multifaceted issues of air quality and respiratory health. By prioritizing environmental ecological justice programs, policymakers can work towards creating healthier environments for all communities, especially those most exposed to air pollution. A comprehensive and well-informed approach must be used to reverse the respiratory health implications of air quality issues identified in both urban and indoor environments (American Lung Association, 2001; Ezzati et al., 2025).

Test Your Knowledge

1. How do vaccinations help prevent respiratory infections, and which vaccines are commonly recommended?
2. Why is smoking cessation critical in preventing respiratory diseases, and what strategies support individuals in quitting smoking?

SUMMARY

Synthesis of literature in general medicine of the respiratory system highlights the complex interplay between various forms of treatment and their effectiveness against respiratory diseases. Self-medication and complementary therapy, particularly for conditions like asthma and COPD, are concerns of interest and concern as reflected through existing literature. This setting is also complicated by heterogeneity in quality of studies, sample, and treatment interventions, all of which challenge the evidence base informing alternative treatments. Therefore, self-medication must be handled with care, as there is room for adverse health effects through ineffective or inappropriate treatments, and it is thus crucial to conduct further research and standardized guidelines to inform practitioners and patients (Kilgore et al., 2010). Moreover, the need for extensive research extends beyond mere effectiveness to encompass broader health aspects of respiratory disease. As noted in organic animal production discourse, research quality becomes central to our understanding of health implications. The ongoing release of data on various health implications complicates the urgent need for peer-reviewed literature to guide assertions about alternative treatments, such as herbal medicine. Such gaps in evidence erode the process of clinical decision making since practitioners must balance embracing conventional therapies with the potential benefits and risks of alternative interventions (Eijck et al., 2003). Thus, there is a need for a multidisciplinary approach to manage the complexities and deliver optimal patient care. In short, with the emerging field of respiratory system medicine, knowledge of contemporary and emerging therapies is essential for both patients and health practitioners. The integration of mainstream and complementary treatment modalities calls for a critical examination of evidence to inform practice. With the future of respiratory care constantly expanding, future research must be aimed at robust clinical trials and systematic reviews that address the shortcomings of the current evidence. By prioritizing methodological rigor, the medical profession can enhance the quality of care and address the complex needs of patients with respiratory diseases, ultimately improving health outcomes and patient satisfaction in this critically vital branch of medicine.

The management of respiratory system disorders involves a sophisticated understanding of the various therapeutic techniques employed in contemporary medicine. Emphysema, among the foremost problems, has a critical effect on public health, particularly in regions like South Africa. An increase in the number of emphysema cases with limited therapies triggers the exploration of new treatments such as endoscopic lung volume reduction (ELVR). This method offers a tantalizing alternative to traditional surgery, hoping to restore lung function with fewer associated risks and costs. These requirements have been defined by the South African Thoracic Society, and experts were convened to discuss the application of ELVR in the local context, with special regard to the key role of patient selection to optimize results. This focused treatment falls within a broader movement in general medicine towards treatments that are specific to the patient, such that the therapeutic benefit justifies the intrinsic costs and sophistication of elaborate medical intervention (Allwood et al., 2015). In addition to technological advances in the treatment of respiratory diseases, the self-medication process in cases of upper respiratory tract infections and chronic illnesses like asthma and COPD is noteworthy. Self-medication prevalence reveals a shift in the behavior of patients, where they increasingly seek over-the-counter treatment, both herbal and conventional, without consulting a professional. While the trend proves patients' willingness to master their health, it raises concerns regarding the efficacy and safety of such interventions. A. A review of the available evidence suggests that although some herbal therapies have potential, the quality of studies for their application is generally low. This the need for more robust clinical trials to validate the evidence surrounding these treatments, establishing a culture whereby patients can make evidence-informed choices as opposed to informed choices (Kilgore et al., 2010). The importance of blending traditional and innovative modalities of treatment in respiratory medicine cannot be overstated. The interface between advancements in procedural techniques and self-medication necessitates a re-definition of how healthcare practitioners engage with patients. Adequate training on the appropriate forms of treatment, for example, the risks and benefits of self-medication, is crucial in creating healthier safety practices. Also, the clinicians are urged to discuss and consider all the possible therapeutic alternatives with their patients, both traditional and new. Through shared decision-making, healthcare providers can facilitate patient adherence to prescribed therapy and realize enhanced overall health outcomes. Ultimately, therefore, an unprejudiced approach that respects patient choice but rests on evidence will result in more effective management of respiratory illness across general medicine (Kilgore et al., 2010).

KEY TERMS FROM THIS CHAPTER

- Aerobic function
- Autonomic nervous system
- CFTR gene treatments
- Diaphragm
- Environmental variations
- Hospital-acquired pneumonia (HAP)
- Imaging modalities
- Airflow constriction
- Breathing rhythms
- Corticosteroids
- Environmental considerations
- Gas exchange
- ILD diagnosis
- Inflammatory disease

CRITICAL THINKING QUESTIONS

1. **Which of the following muscles is primarily responsible for inspiration during normal, quiet breathing?**
   a. Internal intercostal muscles
   b. External intercostal muscles
   c. Diaphragm
   d. Abdominal muscles
2. **In chronic obstructive pulmonary disease (COPD), which of the following is a common physiological change?**
   a. Increased lung compliance and airway obstruction
   b. Decreased lung compliance and airway obstruction
   c. Increased lung compliance and airway dilation
   d. Decreased lung compliance and airway dilation
3. **Which diagnostic tool is considered the gold standard for assessing lung volumes and airflow limitation?**
   a. Chest X-ray
   b. Spirometry
   c. Arterial blood gas analysis
   d. Pulse oximetry
4. **Which of the following pharmacological agents is commonly used as a bronchodilator in asthma management?**
   a. Beta-2 adrenergic agonists
   b. Corticosteroids
   c. Antibiotics
   d. Antihistamines
5. **Which of the following non-pharmacological interventions is most effective in preventing respiratory infections at a community level?**
   a. Regular use of inhalers
   b. Chest physiotherapy
   c. Annual pulmonary function testing
   d. Smoking cessation programs

Short Answer Questions

1. What are the main physiological mechanisms involved in inhalation and exhalation, and how do the lungs facilitate efficient gas exchange?
2. Describe the causes, symptoms, and management strategies for common respiratory disorders such as asthma, COPD, and pneumonia.
3. What diagnostic tools are used in respiratory medicine, and how do pulmonary function tests, imaging techniques, and bronchoscopy contribute to diagnosis?
4. How do bronchodilators and corticosteroids work pharmacologically to treat respiratory conditions?
5. When are antibiotics indicated in respiratory disease management, and why is it essential to distinguish bacterial from viral infections?

Answers to Critical Thinking Questions

1. (c) 2. (a) 3. (b) 4. (b) 5. (d)

REFERENCES

1. Dar, O. A., Hasan, R., Schlundt, J., Harbarth, S., Caleo, G., Dar, F. K., Littmann, J., Rweyemamu, M., Buckley, E. J., Shahid, M., Kock, R., Li, H. L., Giha, H., Khan, M., So, A. D., Bindayna, K. M., Kessel, A., Pedersen, H. B., Permanand, G., . . . Heymann, D. L. (2015b). Exploring the evidence base for national and regional policy interventions to combat resistance. *The Lancet, 387*(10015), 285–295. https://doi.org/10.1016/s0140-6736(15)00520-6Agache, I., Bachert, C., Bedbrook, A., Bergmann, K. C., et al. (2016). *ARIA 2016: Care Pathways Implementing Emerging Technologies for Predictive Medicine in Rhinitis and Asthma Across the Life Cycle.* https://core.ac.uk/download/77614616.pdf (accessed on 27th June 2025).
2. Aguilaniu, B., Armstrong, D., Kampouras, A., Beaver, D., Bell, J., Borg, B., Boyce, M., et al. (2019). ERS statement on standardization of cardiopulmonary exercise testing in chronic lung diseases. https://core.ac.uk/download/286027730.pdf (accessed on 27th June 2025).
3. Aigner, F., Pratschke, J., Schumann, T., Stockmann, M., et al. (2020). Recent advances and the potential for clinical use of autofluorescence detection of extra-ophthalmic tissues. https://core.ac.uk/download/323257980.pdf (accessed on 27th June 2025).
4. Akyol, M. U., Alden, T. D., Amartino, H., Ashworth, J., et al. (2019). Recommendations for the management of MPS VI: Systematic evidence- and consensus-based guidance. https://core.ac.uk/download/323074857.pdf (accessed on 27th June 2025).
5. Albertson, T. E., Chan, A. L., & Louie, S. (2010). The diagnosis and treatment of elderly patients with acute exacerbation of chronic obstructive pulmonary disease and chronic bronchitis. https://core.ac.uk/download/323070598.pdf (accessed on 27th June 2025).
6. Allwood, B. W., Bruwer, W. W., Dheda, K., Herth, F., et al. (2015). Recommendations for the use of endoscopic lung volume reduction in South Africa: Role in the treatment of emphysema. https://core.ac.uk/download/77019684.pdf (accessed on 27th June 2025).
7. Alton, E. W. F. W., Armstrong, D. K., Ashby, D., Bayfield, K., et al. (2016). A randomized, double-blind, placebo-controlled trial of repeated nebulization of non-viral cystic fibrosis transmembrane conductance regulator (CFTR) gene therapy in patients with cystic fibrosis. https://core.ac.uk/download/154748380.pdf (accessed on 27th June 2025).
8. Aluas, M., Bordea, R. I., Budin, C. E., Ciumarnean, D., et al. (2019). Therapeutic alternatives with CPAP in obstructive sleep apnea. https://core.ac.uk/download/232440313.pdf (accessed on 27th June 2025).
9. Amaducci, S., Bacci, E., Baldacci, S., Bartoli, M., et al. (2018). Inhalation therapy in the next decade: Determinants of adherence to treatment in asthma and COPD. https://core.ac.uk/download/152415584.pdf (accessed on 27th June 2025).
10. Amann, A., Lumb, A. B., Schrikker, A. C., Mörk, A. K., Amann, A., et al. (2010). A mathematical model for breath gas analysis of volatile organic compounds with special emphasis on acetone. http://arxiv.org/abs/1003.4475 (accessed on 27th June 2025).
11. American Lung Association. (2001). *Urban Air Pollution and Health Inequities: A Workshop Report.* https://core.ac.uk/download/323074325.pdf (accessed on 27th June 2025).
12. Axon, E. J., Balmes, J. R., Frew, A., Gannon, P. F., Balmes, J. R., Jajosky, R. A., et al. (2000). Occupational asthma: A review. https://core.ac.uk/download/323081929.pdf (accessed on 27th June 2025).

13. Bandeeri, N., Henry, J. A., Meredith, C., Treacy, C., et al. (2004). The prevalence of cocaine-associated chest pain in a London hospital. https://core.ac.uk/download/5230488.pdf (accessed on 27th June 2025).
14. Barclay, W. R., Stylianou, E., McShane, H., Paul, M. J., Reljic, R., Resende Co, T., Rodriguez, A., et al. (2019). Mucosal delivery of tuberculosis vaccines: A review of current approaches and challenges. https://core.ac.uk/download/286270868.pdf (accessed on 27th June 2025).
15. Barnes, V. A., Crawford, M. W., Harden, K., Ravinder, S., et al. (2015). Self-regulation of breathing as a primary treatment for anxiety. https://core.ac.uk/download/131210063.pdf (accessed on 27th June 2025).
16. Basil, M. C., Chapman, H. A., Engler, A. E., Guo, M., et al. (2020). The cellular and physiological basis for lung repair and regeneration: Past, present, and future. https://core.ac.uk/download/305124289.pdf (accessed on 27th June 2025).
17. Blakey, J., Chisholm, A., Kocks, J. W. H., Lisspers, K., et al. (2017). Use of electronic medical records and biomarkers to manage risk and resource efficiencies. https://core.ac.uk/download/80686081.pdf (accessed on 27th June 2025).
18. Bracha, H. S., & Burkle, F. M., Jr. (2006). Utility of fear severity and individual resilience scoring as a surge capacity, triage management tool during large-scale, bio-event disasters. https://core.ac.uk/download/pdf/86672.pdf (accessed on 27th June 2025).
19. Brewin, A., Morice, A., Khan, A. U., Alexander, B. A., Nickel, C., Put, C., et al. (2015). Psychological interventions in asthma. https://core.ac.uk/download/30611340.pdf (accessed on 27th June 2025).
20. Clark, B., Frewer, L. J., Jones, P., Kyriazakis, I., et al. (2019). Consumer attitudes towards production diseases in intensive production systems. https://core.ac.uk/download/187087240.pdf (accessed on 27th June 2025).
21. Clay, D., Davies, R., Elias, P., Gumber, A., et al. (2004). *Review of the Occupational Health and Safety of Britain's Ethnic Minorities*. https://core.ac.uk/download/105299.pdf (accessed on 27th June 2025).
22. Combertaldi, S., Dammeier, F., Delgado-Gonzalo, R., Kübler, D., et al. (2018). Respiratory and cardiac monitoring at night using a wrist wearable optical system. http://arxiv.org/abs/1710.11026 (accessed on 27th June 2025).
23. Coveney, C., Gabe, J., & Williams, S. J. (2019). Medicalization, pharmaceuticalisation or both? Exploring the medical management of sleeplessness as insomnia. https://core.ac.uk/download/160278437.pdf (accessed on 27th June 2025).
24. Dear, J. D. (2020). Bacterial pneumonia in dogs and cats: An update. https://core.ac.uk/download/286361309.pdf (accessed on 27th June 2025).
25. Dethlefs, B. A., Lee, K. L., Li, S. C., Loudon, D., et al. (2019). Breathing signature as vitality score index created by exercises of Qigong: Implications of artificial intelligence tools used in traditional Chinese medicine. https://core.ac.uk/download/323075335.pdf (accessed on 27th June 2025).
26. Divjak, A. C., Hoffmann, K., Mayrhuber, E. A. S., Peersman, W., et al. (2019). Laypersons' perception of common cold and influenza prevention: A qualitative study in Austria, Belgium and Croatia. https://core.ac.uk/download/237011876.pdf (accessed on 27th June 2025).

27. Donya, M., ElGuindy, A., Firmin, D., Radford, M., et al. (2014). Radiation in medicine: Origins, risks and aspirations. https://core.ac.uk/download/77008838.pdf (accessed on 27th June 2025).

28. Eijck, I., Groot, M., Kasteel, D., Kijlstra, A., et al. (2003). Analysis of black holes in our knowledge concerning animal health in the organic food production chain. https://core.ac.uk/download/10919416.pdf (accessed on 27th June 2025).

29. Ekström, T. J., Nordfors, L., Shiels, P. G., Stenvinkel, P., et al. (2017). Current epigenetic aspects the clinical kidney researcher should embrace. https://core.ac.uk/download/84340482.pdf (accessed on 27th June 2025).

30. Ezzati, M., & Kammen, D. (2025). The health impacts of exposure to indoor air pollution from solid fuels in developing countries: Knowledge, gaps, and data needs. https://core.ac.uk/download/pdf/9308128.pdf (accessed on 27th June 2025).

31. Fernandes, R. M. R. M. C. (2015). *Interventions and Outcomes in Bronchiolitis Clinical Trials.* https://core.ac.uk/download/32336113.pdf (accessed on 27th June 2025).

32. Fromer, L., Kaplan, A., Price, D., Román-Rodríguez, M., et al. (2014). Is there a rationale and role for long-acting anticholinergic bronchodilators in asthma? https://core.ac.uk/download/25497566.pdf (accessed on 27th June 2025).

33. Gostin, L. O., Hardcastle, L. E., Jacobson, P. D., Record, K. L., et al. (2011). Restoring health to health reform: Integrating medicine and public health to advance the population's well-being. https://core.ac.uk/download/70374138.pdf (accessed on 27th June 2025).

34. Harari, A., Zumla, A., Armand, M., Axelsson-Robertson, R., Banada, P., Marais, B., Betsou, F., et al. (2012). Tuberculosis diagnostics and biomarkers: Needs, challenges, recent advances, and opportunities. https://core.ac.uk/download/9839032.pdf (accessed on 27th June 2025).

35. Kilgore, D., & Najm, W. (2010). Common respiratory diseases. https://core.ac.uk/download/323075715.pdf (accessed on 27th June 2025).

36. Lyon, A. R., López-Fernández, T., Couch, L. S., Asteggiano, R., Aznar, M. C., Bergler-Klein, J., Boriani, G., et al. (2022). *2022 ESC Guidelines on Cardio-Oncology Developed in Collaboration with the European Hematology Association (EHA), the European Society for Therapeutic Radiology and Oncology (ESTRO) and the International Cardio-Oncology Society (IC-OS). European Heart Journal, 43,* 4229–4361. https://doi.org/10.1093/eurheartj/ehac244 (accessed on 27th June 2025).

37. Matchim, Y., Parveen, S., & Thaniwattananon, P. (2014). Dyspnea experience and dyspnea management in patients with chronic obstructive pulmonary disease in Bangladesh. https://media.neliti.com/media/publications/155883-EN-dyspnea-experience-and-dyspnea-managemen.pdf (accessed on 27th June 2025).

38. McKay, A., Zeki, A. A., Greening, A. P., Joukhadar, C., McSharry, C., Weir, C. J., et al. (2011). Effects of short-term treatment with atorvastatin in smokers with asthma–A randomized controlled trial. https://core.ac.uk/download/110369.pdf (accessed on 27th June 2025).

39. N/A. (2001). *National Blueprint: Increasing Physical Activity Among Adults age 50 and Older.* https://core.ac.uk/download/71346800.pdf (accessed on 27th June 2025).

40. N/A. (2025). *Aerospace Medicine and Biology: A Continuing Bibliography with Indexes, Supplement 129, June 1974.* https://core.ac.uk/download/pdf/42893564.pdf (accessed on 27th June 2025).

41. N/A. (2025). *Timing Impact Assessment for COAG Closing the Gap Targets: Child Mortality.* https://core.ac.uk/download/pdf/30674535.pdf (accessed on 27th June 2025).

42. Pelliccia, A., Sharma, S., Gati, S., Bäck, M., Börjesson, M., Caselli, S., Collet, J. P., et al. (2020). *2020* ESC guidelines on sports cardiology and exercise in patients with cardiovascular disease. *European Heart Journal, 42*, 17–96. https://doi.org/10.1093/eurheartj/ehaa605 (accessed on 27th June 2025).

43. Reiter, A., Yucel, A., Drake, A. G., Hendricks, A., Noller, C., Ambrósio, C. E., Knecht, C. D., et al. (2015). Impact of facial conformation on canine health: Brachycephalic obstructive airway syndrome. https://core.ac.uk/download/36778815.pdf (accessed on 27th June 2025).

44. Singanayagam, A., Crockett, A. J., Ries, A. L., Yohannes, A. M., Fletcher, C., Bucknall, C. E., Fletcher, C. M., et al. (2015). Four patients with a history of acute exacerbations of COPD: Implementing the CHEST/Canadian Thoracic Society guidelines for preventing exacerbations. https://core.ac.uk/download/30697683.pdf (accessed on 27th June 2025).

45. Weissenfluh, N. G. (2019). *Periodontitis and the Elderly: An Overview of The Disease and Its Impact on An Aging Population.* https://core.ac.uk/download/213463617.pdf (accessed on 27th June 2025).

GASTROINTESTINAL SYSTEM: DISORDERS, DIAGNOSTIC APPROACHES, AND TREATMENTS

7

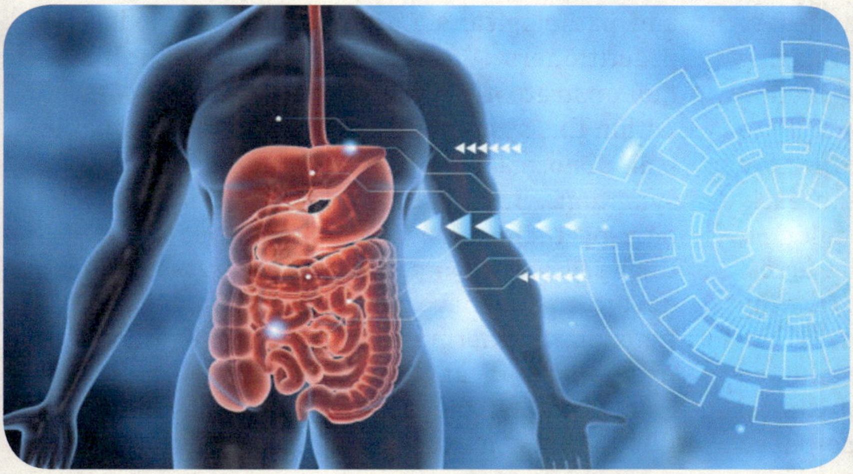

LEARNING OBJECTIVES

After studying this chapter, you will be able to:

1. Understand the anatomy of the gastrointestinal system
2. Describe common gastrointestinal disorders
3. Discuss diagnostic approaches in general medicine
4. Define treatment modalities
5. Focus on preventive measures for maintenance of the gastrointestinal (GI) system
6. Deal with emerging trends in gastrointestinal medicine

Introduction

Gastrointestinal (GI) function is an essential component of human health, fulfilling the vital role of digestion, absorption, and expulsion. A thorough comprehension of basic principles of general medicine in the GI system is essential for clinicians and healthcare providers who wish to diagnose and manage disorders that have the potential to impact QoL. The complexity of the GI tract, with organs such as the esophagus, stomach, intestines, and liver, requires a multidisciplinary approach that integrates disparate diagnostic and therapeutic modalities. The opening chapter will provide an overview of contemporary practices and advances in GI medicine, illustrating how integrating extensive knowledge can lead to better patient outcomes. Central to the evolution of GI medicine is the development and dissemination of clinical guidelines that guide practitioners in the use of diagnostic instruments. Notably, the founding of the gastrointestinal ultrasound (GIUS) task force by the European Federation of Societies for Ultrasound in Medicine and Biology in 2014 was a milestone. This initiative aimed to promote the clinical use of GIUS by establishing standardized practice guidelines for practitioners. The purpose of the task forces was not only to deliver best practices but, more importantly, to enhance awareness regarding diagnostic imaging in the GI system. Central to these projects is also standardization of the methods of examination and interpretation of sonoanatomical structures, which ultimately aids in enhancing the accuracy of diagnoses in GI disease (Calabrese et al., 2016). As medical technology continues to evolve, integration of state-of-the-art imaging modalities stands to serve an essential function in further advancing the entire strategy to the GI system. The emphasis on non-invasive techniques such as GIUS facilitates the early detection and intervention of GI pathologies, which are a prime determinant for the arrest of disease progression. An understanding of the complexities of these procedures and normal physiological characteristics evaluated by ultrasonography forms the basis of clinical practice. The task forces' evidence-based strategy addresses a broader trend in medicine towards evidence-led policy that maximizes treatment efficacy and patient safety. The following sections will therefore examine the various dimensions of GI disease, diagnostic innovation, and the resulting implications for treatment within the general medicine strategy (Calabrese et al., 2016).

Definition of the Gastrointestinal System

The digestive system, or GI system, is an intricate chain of organs that digest and absorb nutrient components from food. The system has numerous structures including the mouth, esophagus, stomach, intestines, liver, pancreas, and gallbladder. There is a function for each structure, which is to break down the food into nutrients for absorption into the blood system. The process of digestion is not just a mechanical and chemical breakdown, but also involves coordination by the nervous and hormonal systems to regulate digestive processes. The use of hormonal interactions, particularly with significant intestinal hormones, is important for attaining optimal digestion and understanding GI pathologies. Abnormalities in this system may lead to disease, such as irritable bowel syndrome (IBS) and IBD, that involve complex symptomatology requiring advanced general medicine treatment and management. An awareness of the GI system's physiological and pathological states is relevant to medical practitioners. Conditions like IBS and IBD demonstrate the way in which dysfunction within this system can cause severe abdominal pain, abnormal bowel habits, and other disabling symptoms. Both diseases are characterized not only by their physical symptoms but also by their psychic accompaniments, as stress is well-documented to have a deep impact on digestive function. Furthermore, symptomatology tends to manifest in an oscillatory fashion, which would suggest the possible role of hormonal fluctuations, most notably progesterone, to worsen symptoms. Recent studies suggest that investigating these hormonal interactions may unveil new therapeutic possibilities, allowing clinicians to treat the underlying dysfunctions rather than merely palliating symptoms. Such a holistic focus validates the intricacy of GI health within the overall scope of general medicine. An effective general medicine strategy for managing GI disease should incorporate interdisciplinary collaboration, emphasizing the need to cross clinical and basic sciences. Conceptual surgery, as defined in academic environments, shows a pattern where clinicians and basic scientists come together to formulate an integrated treatment paradigm for the issues faced in the GI tract. This is made possible by collaborative innovation in decision-making and enhancing treatment effect through assimilated knowledge and approaches. For instance, the use of decision trees and algorithms allows medical professionals to discuss patient symptoms in an organized fashion and modify treatment regimens—a fundamental aspect to manage GI disorders correctly. By closing the gap between clinical practice and empirical research, the method of general medicine not only improves diagnostic and curative outcomes but also helps achieve a better understanding of the GI system as the epicenter of total health (Figure 7.1).

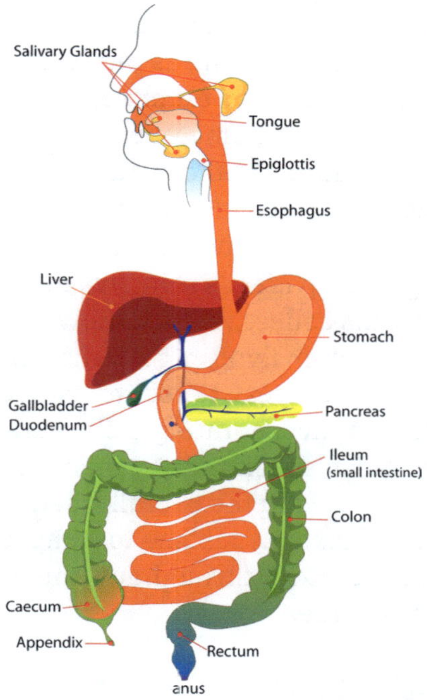

Figure 7.1. Illustration of digestive system.

Source: https://upload.wikimedia.org/wikipedia/commons/thumb/8/81/Digestive_system_simplified.svg/800px-Digestive_system_simplified.svg.png.

Importance of Gastrointestinal Health

The relevance of GI health cannot be stressed strongly enough, as it is a basis of overall well-being. The GI tract not only serves to break down food to absorb nutrients but also has immune function and homeostasis. A healthy GI tract serves to digest food into essential vitamins and minerals that the body employs to maintain crucial processes. Furthermore, the gut microbiota, with its complex community of bacteria, governs numerous areas of health, including metabolic regulation and inflammation. Malfunctions in the complex system may lead to a variety of disorders ranging from harmless indigestion to serious conditions like IBD or IBS. Therefore, it is essential to comprehend and maximize GI health in general medicine because it ultimately comes full circle with overall health outcome and QoL. Teaching about and marketing GI wellness are central parts of prevention medicine. With obesity, diabetes, and other diseases of lifestyle on the rise at epidemic proportions, GI wellness is directly connected with the prevention of these diseases. Increased awareness of food choices that offer gut benefits may be key to enhancing public health. For instance, adding prebiotics and probiotics to your food can help create a balanced microbiome that reduces the risk of GI disease and enhances immunity. Furthermore, healthcare professionals, including direct support professionals (DSPs), are increasingly involved with medication that supports GI health, as noted by more recent studies. Continuous education and appropriate training of DSPs on the importance of GI drug management significantly enhance competence levels and instill prudent practices in patient care (Auberry et al., 2017). Such programs highlight the multifaceted nature involved in enhancing GI health within a broader medical setting. Also, the consequences of impaired GI health do not affect physical health alone; they can also impact mental and emotional well-being. Much of the research suggests a direct linkage between gut health and mental health, referred to as the gut-brain axis. Dysfunction of gut flora is responsible for exacerbating conditions like anxiety and depression, which highlights the point that a system-based approach to medicine must consider GI health as a significant factor. In managing these issues, the general trend in medicine is the application of personalized management practices that include dietary adjustments, consistent physical exercise, and psychological guidance. Training through understanding the physiology of the GI system and its effects can make patients active participants in their own health care. Therefore, well-being in the GI system is more than a clinician's concern; it is a larger field of health that underscores the necessity of holistic processes in general medicine (Jang et al., 2019).

Overview of General Medicine's Role in Gastrointestinal Care

General medicine is also central to the care of the GI system through a holistic approach to diagnosing and managing various disorders of the GI tract. General medicine involves not only the evaluation of symptoms but also the complexity arising from interactions among the body's different systems, which often make GI diagnoses difficult. For instance, symptoms such as IBS or IBD require a thorough evaluation that includes a detailed patient history and physical examination, and appropriate laboratory and imaging studies. GPs should be cautious when identifying abnormal presentations, as these can indicate underlying pathologies that may require referral to a gastroenterologist. Thus, a balanced understanding of general medicine enables practitioners to effectively navigate the ambiguity of GI diseases, emphasizing a harmonized model of care that fosters patient-centered practice management. Beyond diagnosis and management, general medicine is also crucial in preventive care in GI health. Preventive measures commonly involve educating patients on food choices, lifestyle modifications, and compliance with regular screening tests, such as colonoscopies, which are critical in detecting colorectal cancer at an early stage. Practitioners are also duty-bound to encourage immunization against hepatitis viruses where applicable and counsel patients against excessive alcohol consumption and smoking, both of which have degrading effects on the functioning of the GI system. Furthermore, there is more being understood about gut microbiota's impact on general well-being, such as dysbiosis, which may lead to a variety of GI upset. By highlighting these preventive measures, general medicine further cemented its role in not only curing what ails us now but also in ensuring long-term GI health. The interfaculty cooperation between general medicine and gastroenterology is crucial in optimizing patient outcomes from GI tract care. The combined practice allows GPs to bridge the gap between primary care and specialist intervention, establishing a more responsive continuum of care. For example, when facing , complex cases of GI nematodes, generalists can call upon parasitology information and perform specialized management procedures, such as client-oriented selective treatment regimens according to the patient's status, as the literature indicates. This collective know-how accelerates clinical decision-making, particularly in treating conditions with resistance to conventional therapies. By incorporating information from other medical specialties, general medicine plays a major role in the overall treatment of GI conditions, ultimately leading to comprehensive and effective care throughout the patient's treatment course.

7.1. Anatomy of the Gastrointestinal System

Learning Outcome

1. Understand the structure and function of the digestive tract
2. Describe accessory organs and their roles
3. Discuss the interaction between different components of the system

The GI anatomy consists of extremely highly coordinated system of organs responsible for the digestion of food, the absorption of nutrients, and the expulsion of waste. Starting from the oral cavity, which includes the tongue, teeth, and salivary glands, the process continues to the pharynx and then to the esophagus, eventually reaching the stomach. All components of the GI tract play a vital role in both mechanical and chemical digestion. The stomach, for instance, uses hydrochloric acid and digestive enzymes to digest food, converting it into a semi-liquid form known as chyme. This intricate process illustrates how structures within the anatomy interact to facilitate digestion and highlights the importance of understanding these components when applying any general medical method to GI health. Following the stomach, chyme flows into the small intestine, which consists of three parts: the duodenum, jejunum, and ileum. The small intestine is primarily utilized for nutrient absorption, facilitated by its high surface area due to the presence of villi and microvilli. The specialization also emphasizes the small intestine in the study of nutrient deficiency and malabsorption syndromes. Following the absorption of nutrients, residual waste product enters the large intestine, which includes the cecum, colon, rectum, and anus. The primary functions of the large intestines include the absorption of water and fermentation of indigestible material, showing the key roles of each segment of the GI tract in maintaining homeostasis and overall wellness. The incorporation of sophisticated imaging techniques, such as GIUS, better elucidates GI anatomy and pathology. The establishment of the GIUS task force by the European Federation of Societies for Ultrasound in Medicine and Biology indicates the necessity for standardized examination protocols. Existing guidelines suggest including GIUS to illustrate normal anatomical details and physiological activity, facilitating the diagnosis of various GI diseases. This equipment not only facilitates real-time imaging but also allows precise estimates of pathologies using non-invasive methods. As suggested during deliberations within the pharmacology community, integrating sophisticated technology with anatomical data is imperative for enhancing the efficiency of clinical assessments and treatment plans in the realm of GI health (Calabrese et al., 2016; Bailey et al., 2018).

7.1.1. Structure and Function of the Digestive Tract

The very specialized digestive system is used to digest food, absorb nutrients, and remove waste products. Structured hierarchically, the digestive system consists of regions that have specific functions. The process begins in the oral cavity, where mechanical digestion occurs through chewing, and enzymes in saliva start degrading carbohydrates. As food travels down the esophagus, rhythmic muscular contractions known as peristalsis propel it along. This is required to push the food into the stomach, where gastric juice continues chemical digestion. The rhythmic contractions of the stomach ultimately blend the food into a chyme-like semi-fluid mixture, preparing it for future nutrient absorption. From the stomach, chyme flows on to the small intestine, an organ crucial for complex digestion and nutrient absorption. The small intestine, consisting of the duodenum, jejunum, and ileum, functions through both enzymatic processes and specialized structural mechanisms. Villi and microvilli offer greater surface area, optimizing absorption efficiency to a large degree. Pancreatic enzymes and liver bile function in conjunction within the duodenum to emulsify fat, break down protein, and metabolize carbohydrates. Interestingly, the synergy between hormonal activation and intestinal motility also plays a crucial role in regulating digestion, so that alterations can influence the rate of absorption and motility. These characteristics not only facilitate proper digestion but also highlight the complexity of GI interactions. These interactions may be responsible for explaining conditions like IBS, where fluctuating symptoms arise due to hormonal regulation of digestive processes. This understanding could lead to potential new therapeutic modalities (Linson et al., 2013). The final segments of the digestive system, the large intestine and rectum, are primarily responsible for water absorption and waste formation. The large intestine, including the cecum, colon, and rectum, is primarily responsible for solidifying indigestible food material. It is in this compartment that the gut flora break down leftover nutrients, further contributing to the absorption process and producing vital vitamins like vitamin K. The absence of some digestive processes, as seen in gastrointestinal stromal tumors (GISTs), can significantly impact nutrient absorption and overall digestive function (Georgescu et al., 2016). GISTs, though rare, can destroy the GI tract's structural integrity through obstructing or bleeding. The structure-function relationship within the digestive system highlights the importance of maintaining GI health, as imbalances in this system can lead to various medical ailments that affect general health (Figure 7.2).

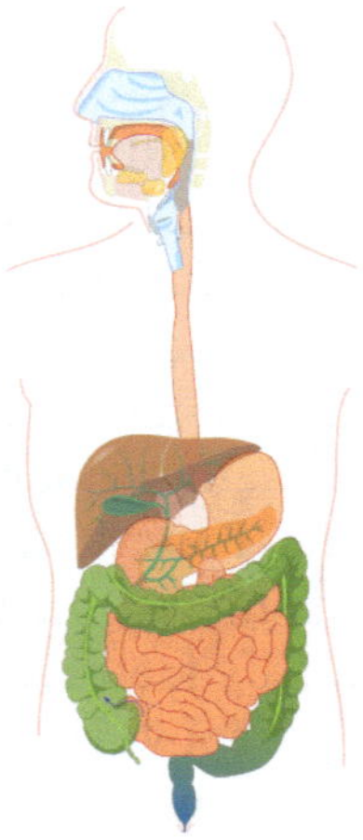

Figure 7.2. Diagram of the gastrointestinal tract in the average human.

Source: https://upload.wikimedia.org/wikipedia/commons/thumb/e/ed/Digestive_system_without_labels.svg/250px-Digestive_system_without_labels.svg.png.

7.1.2. Accessory Organs and Their Roles

Accessory organs play a critical role in the overall function of the GI tract because they are responsible for a large percentage of digestion and metabolism. Some of these accessory organs include the liver, pancreas, and gallbladder, which are not part of the digestive tract itself but play a key role in processing food and maintaining metabolic homeostasis. The liver, for instance, is tasked with bile production, which is required for emulsification and the absorption of fat. In addition, the liver plays a vital role in storing nutrients and detoxifying, cleaning blood from the GI tract before it is circulated to the rest of the body. This multifunctional organ is the quintessential example of the integrated functioning of the GI system because each essential structure contributes to a system that works together to enhance overall health and well-being. The pancreas is also an exocrine and endocrine organ, emphasizing its role in the GI system. As an exocrine, the pancreas releases digestive enzymes, such as amylase and lipase, into the small intestine to aid in carbohydrate and fat digestion. The pancreas also releases bicarbonate to neutralize stomach acid, creating an ideal pH for enzyme activity. Its endocrine function is, in contrast, primarily the regulation of blood sugar levels through the release of hormones like insulin and glucagon. This adaptability points to the pancreas's significant function not only in digestion but in maintaining overall metabolic balance within the body. Any disorganization of this organ could have substantial health repercussions, including diabetes or pancreatitis, pointing to its significant role in GI health. The gallbladder, often overshadowed by larger accessory organs, similarly plays a critical function in the digestive process. It is a reservoir for bile secreted by the liver, ejecting it as needed to facilitate fat digestion during meals. The timing and release of bile are accurate; however, a malfunctioning gallbladder may lead to issues such as gallstones, which can occlude bile flow and cause significant pain. Further, gallbladder function and the nature of one's diet could influence different health outcomes. For example, an excessively fat diet may lead to increased bile production, making dietary management imperative for maintaining gallbladder health. The relationship between the gallbladder and other accessory organs, and how they function together, contributes to the complexity of the GI tract and the need for a holistic approach in medical assessment of digestive health (Estrine et al., 2006; Darlington et al., 2017) (Figure 7.3).

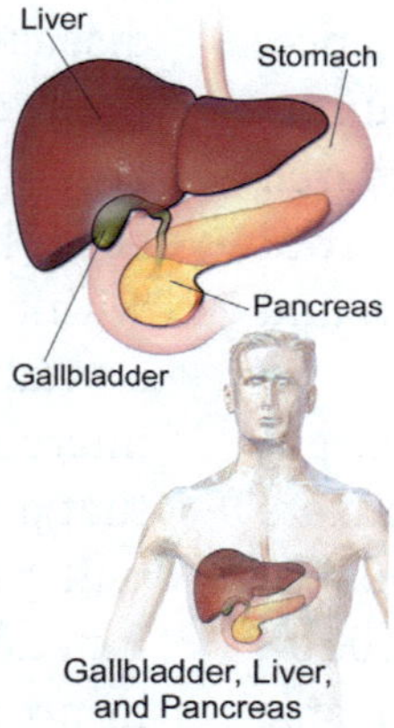

Figure 7.3. The liver, gallbladder, and pancreas are the major accessory organs of digestion.

Source: https://humanbiology.pressbooks.tru.ca/wp-content/uploads/sites/6/2019/06/Blausen_0428_Gallbladder-Liver-Pancreas_Location-1-512x1024.png.

7.1.3. Interaction Between Different Components of the System

It is critical to comprehend the relationship between most components of the gut system to have a practical approach to overall medicine. The gut is not only a conduit for waste and food but also assists in homeostasis by its complex relationships with the microbiota.

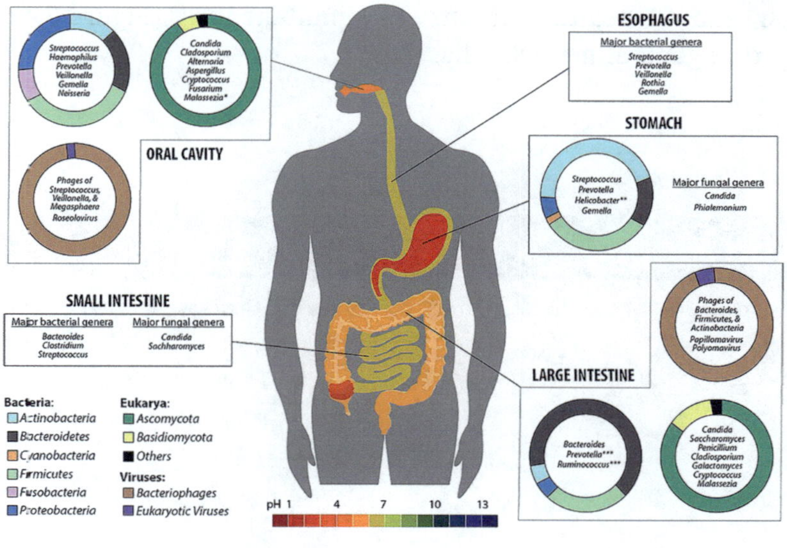

Figure 7.4. Diagram of human microbiota depicted in various regions of the gastrointestinal tract.

Source: https://upload.wikimedia.org/wikipedia/commons/thumb/5/52/Microbiome.jpg/1024px-Microbiome.jpg.

The microbiota, being present within the lumen of the GI tract, thrive in this intricate environment, maintaining a state called Eubiosis, where human hosts and microbes all benefit from each other. Destruction of this balance, however, may lead to Dysbiosis, profoundly impacting health outcomes. Recent research highlights such disruptions as probable root causes for IBDs, among others, to evolve and advance. It is, thus, essential to develop an understanding of the interaction between gut health and microbial health in order to formulate good practices for treatment of various GI diseases, as suggested by Andrada et al. (2020). Further, the interrelationship between chronic stress and GI health reflects the interactive nature of the system. Chronic stress is now well understood to initiate GI diseases through dysregulation and inflammation of gut flora. Major regulators of the body's stress response, specifically neuropeptides of the corticotropin-releasing hormone (CRH) family, have been found to modulate inflammatory pathways that predispose to diseases like colorectal cancer. This highlights the interrelatedness of psychological stress, inflammation, and GI health, with its layers of complexity that general medicine has to confront. By taking these interrelations into account, practitioners are better positioned to individualize treatment plans to not only treat the physiological presentations of GI diseases but also the psychosocial aspects of their continuation, as suggested by Baritaki et al. (2019). Lastly, the inclusion of nutrition complicates the dynamics of interaction within the GI system even further. Diet plays a vital role in determining the makeup of the microbiota and, by inference, GI health. Diets that promote the presence of beneficial bacteria will promote Eubiosis and increase immune function and absorption of nutrients. Diets high in processed foods and sugars will, conversely, induce Dysbiosis, leading to inflammation and GI disease. The discussion between diet, microbiota, and GI function is an example of the body's systems-based nature. Thus, a general medicine strategy needs to be multifaceted in nature with dietary management in addition to encouraging microbial health. This can ultimately lead to more effective interventions and prevention in GI disease management, confirming the necessity for considering different system components simultaneously (Figure 7.4).

Test Your Knowledge

1. What are the main structures of the digestive tract, and what are their primary functions in the digestive process?
2. Which organs are considered accessory organs of the digestive system?

7.2. Common Gastrointestinal Disorders

Learning Outcome

1. Understand gastroesophageal reflux disease (GERD) and irritable bowel syndrome (IBS)
2. Describe symptoms and diagnostic criteria
3. Explain the impact of gastrointestinal disorders on quality of life

The aforementioned high incidence of common GI disorders, including IBD and IBS, demands a good understanding of their pathophysiology as well as their potential interventions. The illnesses encompass numerous disabling symptoms like bloating, diarrhea, constipation, and abdominal pain, which differ in frequency and severity. Recent research suggests that hormonal etiologies, particularly the interplay of intestinal hormones and sex hormones like estrogen and progesterone, may account for the variable profile of symptoms in these diseases. To illustrate, alterations in levels of progesterone have been associated with worsening IBS-like symptomatology and have implied that such types of hormonal profiles may represent a novel therapeutic target for treatment of IBS and IBD. This approach can unlock the doors for more effective therapies that address the underlying cause rather than just treating symptoms, thereby highlighting the importance of integrated care in GI disorders (Linson et al., 2013). Despite the established pharmacological therapy for common GI disorders, there is growing interest in complementary and alternative medicine (CAM) therapies that patients will seek out. Such interventions could range from dietary alterations to herbal treatments and acupuncture. While patients can identify some advantages related to CAM therapy, the scientific evidence for their efficacy is generally incompatible. Healthcare practitioners must be careful and conduct informed conversations with patients regarding the safety and effectiveness of such alternative treatments. This entails a precise evaluation of evidence at hand and the hazards involved with untested treatment. Through the facilitation of an open conversation, medical professionals are better able to help their patients make well-informed decisions, balancing the desire for alternative treatments with the requirement of EBP (Ghosh et al., 2010). An understanding of the psychosocial aspects of GI disease is also central to the overall treatment plan. These conditions also frequently involve not just physical symptoms, but considerable psychological distress, which can worsen the severity of GI symptoms. IBS patients, for example, will often present with co-morbid depression and anxiety, setting up a complex interplay that can preclude effective management. Recognizing the importance of addressing these psychological factors is key to the provision of whole-person care. Cognitive-behavioral therapy, mindfulness training, and stress management are used in treatment plans to enhance patients' QoL. Adding psychological support to the entire treatment plan enhances patient outcomes and satisfaction, highlighting the need to address GI disorders within a multidisciplinary model that treats both psychological and physical conditions (Linson et al., 2013).

7.2.1. Overview of Prevalent Conditions (e.g., GERD, IBS)

GERD and IBS are among the most common GI conditions with a tremendous influence on the QoL of millions of individuals. GERD is the retrograde movement of gastric contents into the esophagus, producing symptoms of heartburn, regurgitation, and dysphagia. Chronic acid reflux can result in esophagitis, strictures, or Barrett's esophagus, an esophageal cancer precursor. Conversely, IBS is a functional GI disorder characterized by abdominal discomfort, bloating, and alteration in bowel habits. The disease is not associated with any identifiable organic etiology, which makes its diagnosis and management more difficult. Contemporary practice aims at symptom control and lifestyle adjustment, placing high importance on the need for an integrated approach to address both the psychological and physical aspects of these diseases. The link between gut disease and mental well-being emphasizes the complexity of conditions like IBS. Part of the new evidence is that stress, anxiety, and depression all exacerbate gut symptoms, implying a two-way relationship between gut function and mental state (Figure 7.5).

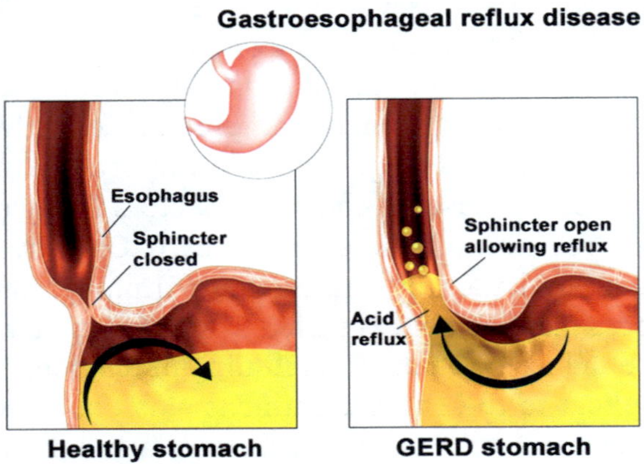

Figure 7.5. Gastroesophageal reflux disease (GERD).

Source: https://livgastro.in/wp-content/uploads/2023/01/Gastroesophageal-Reflux-Disease-feature.png.

For instance, patients with IBD are significantly anxious and depressed, particularly when the disease is acute. The prevalence of these psychiatric disorders among IBD patients is staggering; studies have shown anxiety and depression scores to be significantly higher in these patients compared to healthy controls, as emphasized by the importance of interventional care approaches inclusive of physical and mental disease management in gastroenterology (Graff et al., 2016). Such evidence points towards the importance of psychological comorbidity screening in the management of chronic GI disease. Lifestyle and dietary habits play central roles in both the prevention and management of GI disorders, such as IBS and GERD. The majority of the patients employ herbal drugs as adjunct therapy to conventional treatments, primarily due to perceived enhanced tolerability compared to pharmaceutical drugs (Mohiuddin et al., 2019). In fact, over 80% of the global population utilizes conventional medicine for various diseases, indicating a strong preference for incorporating holistic practices within it. Factors such as a well-balanced and fiber-enriched diet, moderate physical exercise, and stress-relief techniques can have significant impacts on the gastrointestinal system. Further, health professionals are encouraged to educate patients on the importance of maintaining their best bowel habits and recognizing precipitating factors that may exacerbate their symptoms. Finally, these strategies can be a fuller program of learning to recognize and manage common GI diseases (Figure 7.6).

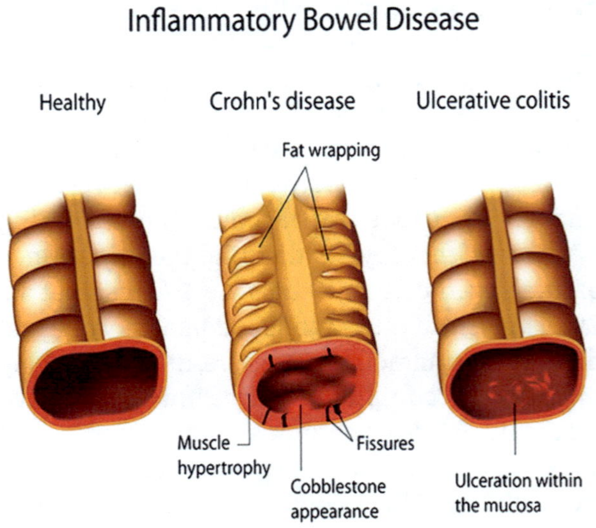

Figure 7.6. Illustration of inflammatory bowel disease (IBD).

Source: https://www.ibdrelief.com/uploads/files/ibd1_gallery_image_924_131.jpg.

7.2.2. Symptoms and Diagnostic Criteria

In GI disease, there needs to be a thorough understanding of symptoms and diagnostic features to act appropriately. The typical presentation in terms of abdominal pain, bloating, constipation, and diarrhea is characteristic of conditions such as IBS and IBD. The sporadic pattern of the changeable symptoms renders diagnosis a more challenging task. In recognizing the contributions of hormonal influences, such as those involving progesterone, there is an explanation for the varying symptom patterns and, therefore, improved diagnostic accuracy. This emphasizes the necessity not only to be aware of symptoms but also to appreciate the mechanisms thereof as possible pathways for targeted therapies and ultimately enhanced patient care (Linson et al., 2013). Diagnostic criteria are necessary to separate various GI conditions so that they can be treated with proper care at the appropriate time. Criteria such as the Rome IV criteria for functional GI disorders help clinicians categorize symptoms, standardizing the diagnostic process. This facilitates segregation between IBS and IBD, both of which have similar symptoms but are treated differently. In addition, comprehensive patient histories and symptom tracking can assist clinicians in refining diagnostic assessments, allowing for tailored treatment protocols that address the individualized needs of the patient and account for the multifactorial nature of GI disturbance (Marzorati et al., 2017). Breakthrough research into the gut microbiome has also broadened the diagnostic lens, demonstrating that alterations in microbial populations can significantly influence GI symptoms. For instance, studies that recognize the impact of prebiotic interventions, such as EpiCor fermentate, exhibit positive outcomes regarding symptom relief, for example, bloating and constipation. Such findings recognize the pivotal role of gut microbiota in symptomology as well as the significance of integrating microbiome analysis into routine diagnostic testing. In summary, a comprehensive understanding of symptoms, their diagnostic criteria, and the communication between the gut microbiome and nonsymptomatic conditions not only enhances diagnostic accuracy but also offers new dimensions for treatments in general medicine (Marzorati et al., 2017) (Figure 7.7).

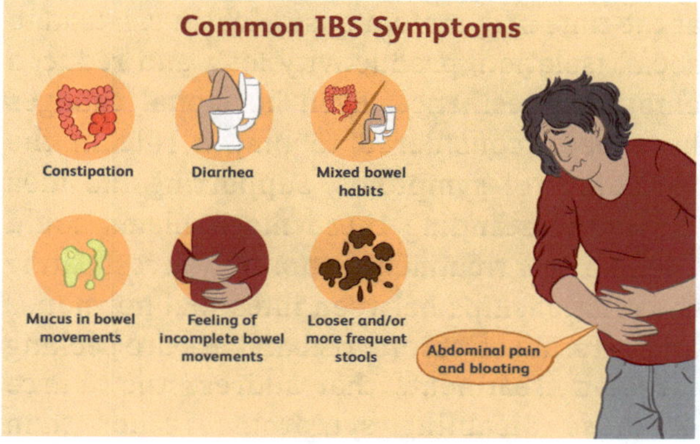

Figure 7.7. Common irritable bowel syndrome (IBS) symptoms.

Source: https://www.verywellhealth.com/thmb/dsJMWjLTkxrCzRhMeJkuL5LUegE=/1500x0/filters:no_upscale():max_bytes(150000):strip_icc()/ibs-pain-locations-1945305-5c04ab7ec9e77c0001dbe853.png.

7.2.3. Impact on Quality of Life

The quality-of-life effect of GI diseases is widespread and multifaceted, commonly resulting in significant physical discomfort and emotional distress. The patients with conditions like constipation or IBS usually have severe symptoms like bloating and pain in the abdomen that interfere with normal functioning. Not only do these symptoms undermine physical health, but they also contribute to a feeling of heightened anxiety and stress, establishing a vicious cycle that worsens the condition. Most importantly, it has been shown that successful management of these symptoms by novel interventions, such as EpiCor fermentate, improves quality-of-life scores. The modulation of the gut microbiome's composition as a mechanism for symptom relief is central to understanding how targeted interventions can alleviate discomfort and enhance patient well-being (Marzorati et al., 2017). Moreover, the psychological importance of GI symptoms cannot be overstated, particularly in the case of disorders such as IBD and the episodic course of IBS. Patients are more likely to feel uncertain at the time of symptom onset, which can lead to social isolation, productivity loss, and reduced emotional resilience. Even hormonal changes have been considered to play a role in the variability of symptoms, supporting the idea that understanding these mechanisms could open up new treatment options. By investigating the relationships between intestinal hormones and external stressors, researchers are seeking targeted treatments that address the source of these disabling symptoms rather than just alleviating the symptoms themselves (Linson et al., 2013). Successful management programs must, therefore, consider both the physiological and psychological implications of such disorders if they are indeed to enhance the QoL for their sufferers. Ultimately, a style of general medicine emphasizing the overall GI system must aim to incorporate symptom control and enhancement of QoL for patients as its paramount goal. This involves an interdisciplinary, team-oriented approach that not only emphasizes the essential need for new treatments but also assures the support of patients as they address their emotional and psychological concerns. As the body of evidence for the gut-brain axis continues to expand, it will increasingly become necessary to tackle how improved GI health can manifest as increased overall mental well-being and life satisfaction. With such comprehensive knowledge, healthcare professionals can develop highly individualized treatment plans that address both the medicinal and affective requirements of their patients, ultimately leading to a dramatically enhanced QoL (Marzorati et al., 2017).

Test Your Knowledge

1. What are some of the most prevalent gastrointestinal disorders (such as GERD, IBS, and peptic ulcers), and what are their key characteristics?
2. What are the common symptoms and diagnostic criteria used to identify disorders like GERD and IBS in clinical practice?
3. How can gastrointestinal disorders affect a patient's quality of life, and what factors contribute to the chronic nature of some conditions?

7.3. Diagnostic Approaches in General Medicine

Learning Outcome

1. Describe physical examination techniques
2. Understand laboratory tests and imaging studies
3. Explain endoscopic procedures and their significance

In the field of general medicine, diagnosis is at the core of giving an appropriate assessment of GI illnesses. In most cases, diagnosis combines clinical evaluation, imaging techniques, and patient history to present an insightful image of the primary cause. Diagnosis can begin with a GP with a comprehensive physical examination and taking a detailed medical history concerning GI symptoms. While traditional techniques such as colonoscopy and endoscopy remain essential, studies indicate that healthcare determinants outside of the clinical domain also contribute significantly to diagnostic efficiency. To wit, open-access models and high-volume centers have been reported to have higher detection rates for significant lesions, suggesting that the organizational structure of healthcare can enhance patient outcomes and diagnostic yield in general (Holly et al., 2025). Hence, integrating these systemic insights into practice can render the process of diagnosis finer-tuned, both qualitatively and quantitatively. Another critical component on the diagnostic side of GI medicine is the role of evolving technology. New imaging technologies, such as MRI and CT, provide images with high resolution that may uncover GI disorders that go undetected by any other technique. These new technologies allow for early diagnosis of serious diseases like cancers and inflammatory diseases. Growing evidence is stressing the importance of maximizing the use of these advanced methods to achieve a balance between cost-effectiveness and patient safety. For instance, the development of targeted imaging modalities may help pinpoint the exact locations of disease to achieve optimal diagnostic yield and therapeutic planning. Hence, a blending of state-of-the-art imaging and traditional methods facilitates enhanced understanding of GI health, along with delivery of personalized treatment protocols sensitive to the requirements of the patients. In addition to such diagnostic modalities, effective management and monitoring of GI infections is also vital. Since resistant GI nematodes present some intrinsic hurdles, diagnosis and therapeutic protocols must also respond to these obstacles. Traditional reliance on broad-spectrum anthelmintic drugs is increasingly being undermined by the development of drug resistance, leading to re-evaluation of strategies. Targeted selective therapy, as used in literature, targets selective recognition of individual affected hosts and their treatment with caution, enhancing therapeutic effect and restricting resistance potential (Borges et al., 2011). This paradigm shift not only highlights the need for new paradigms of control but also the need to include diagnostic techniques that account for the GI issues of the present. By accurate diagnosis and judicious management, healthcare providers can optimize patient outcomes and maintain the integrity of GI medicine.

7.3.1. Physical Examination Techniques

The physical examination techniques used to evaluate the GI system are crucial for precise diagnosis and effective patient management. One simple process begins with a comprehensive history-taking, wherein practitioners obtain signs of abdominal pain, change in bowel habits, or weight loss. Next, the hands-on examination typically involves inspection, palpation, percussion, and auscultation of the abdomen. Examination detects surface irregularities, while palpation aids in detecting tenderness, masses, or enlargement of organs. Percussion can detect air-containing structures or fluid retention, and auscultation detects bowel sounds and related vascular bruits, suggesting underlying conditions. Since these techniques are prone to the variability of anatomy and physiology among individuals, systematically employing them helps construct an integrated clinical picture. Apart from conventional examination techniques, technologies such as GIUS have further changed the physical examination scene. The use of GIUS in clinical practice has been stressed by the European Federation of Societies for Ultrasound in Medicine and Biology, as it is a non-invasive method to visualize GI structures in real-time. Techniques recommended by both professional societies and expert task forces provide clinicians with the ability to gather requisite diagnostic information in a timely and accurate fashion. Using GIUS, clinicians are increasingly able to assess normal sonoanatomical features and pathology, supplementing standard examination protocols. Including this data not only enhances diagnostic capability but also promotes more individualized and specific management plans, which are critical to outcomes in GI health. In addition, the role of education within the process of learning physical examination skills cannot be overstated. Health providers must be formally trained in both traditional techniques and emerging imaging technologies to offer complete disease assessment. Continuing education provides practitioners exposure to current guidelines and standardized guidelines, enhancing their knowledge of the physical examination in the context of the GI system. Enhanced skills translate into better diagnostic accuracy, which eventually affects treatment protocols and improves patient outcomes. Although the specialty progresses with the invention of new diagnostic modalities, adherence to acceptable guidelines, such as those of the GIUS task force, remains essential in integrating new procedures into everyday practice. This combination of broad education and specialist application of testing techniques actually supports the overall strategy towards the GI tract in general medicine (Figure 7.8).

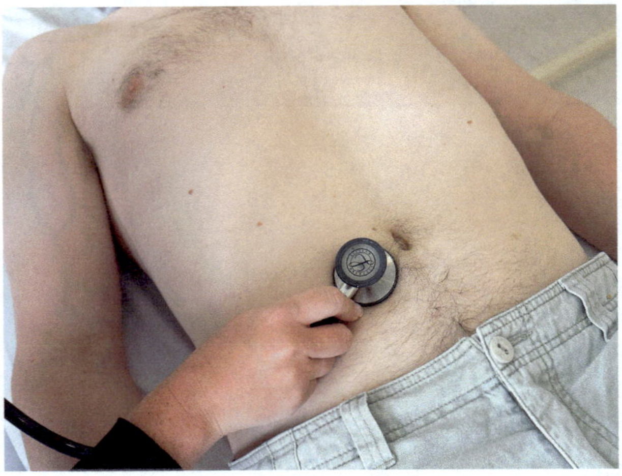

Figure 7.8. Auscultation for bowel sound.

Source: https://cdn.prod.website-files.com/6011a994ad210082aa98b668/60635d7383c39385d70895be_auscultation-for-bowel-sound.jpeg.

7.3.2. Laboratory Tests and Imaging Studies

Laboratory tests and imaging procedures are part of the general medicine approach to diagnosing GI disorders. The diagnostic procedures help providers ascertain the functionality and integrity of the GI tract and guide treatment. Laboratory tests, for instance, such as CBCs, liver function tests, and stool tests, provide critical information about underlying conditions. For instance, a rise in liver enzymes would refer to hepatobiliary disorders, and the presence of blood in stool may reflect GI bleeding, for which further investigations would be required. Thus, timely and accurate laboratory investigation not only helps to establish a diagnosis but also to assess the effectiveness of ongoing treatment regimens. Imaging studies supplement the diagnostic process by offering positive visual evidence of suspected GI disorders. Techniques such as ultrasound, CT, and MRI allow structural deficiencies, e.g., tumors, strictures, or inflammation, to be visualized. These methods excel in offering non-invasive examinations, which are crucial in cases where the application of traditional investigative methodologies is risky. An example is a CT scan that can specifically reveal how extensive IBD is or highlight lesions that are ideal for surgical intervention. Therefore, imaging has a vital role as it not only confirms laboratory findings but, in most instances, dictates management. Coordination between laboratory evaluation and imaging studies is integral in creating a global clinical picture of a patient's GI condition. Coordination of these diagnostic tools provides a better understanding of the disease to enable personalized treatment plans unique to the patient. As new technologies emerge and are developed, the efficiency and accuracy of these tests improve, and so do patient outcomes. The use of information from laboratory and imaging solutions requires physicians to remain vigilant in their diagnostic approach. These tools are not only used to confirm suspicions but also to detect unsuspected findings that might impact overall management plans (N/A, 2006, 2007).

7.3.3. Endoscopic Procedures and Their Significance

Endoscopic procedures have revolutionized the diagnosis and treatment of GI diseases, offering many more advantages than traditional surgery. The minimally invasive procedures allow physicians to explore the inside of the GI tract through the assistance of an endoscope, a medical instrument designed for this purpose. Upper endoscopy, colonoscopy, and endoscopic retrograde cholangiopancreatography (ERCP) are a few of the procedures that entail real-time imaging in addition to the harvesting of biopsies. Direct visualization of pathologic conditions, such as ulcers, tumors, and inflammatory disorders, enhances diagnostic sensitivity and aids in treatment planning. Furthermore, endoscopic techniques are more likely to yield shorter recovery times, fewer complications, and reduced postoperative pain, making them preferable to patients and physicians. Endoscopy has a role beyond diagnosis; it is a most valuable therapeutic tool. Techniques such as endoscopic mucosal resection (EMR) and endoscopic suturing facilitate the removal of neoplastic lesions with fewer invasive methods. This method offers treatment for conditions such as Barrett's esophagus and early cancers, thereby improving patient outcomes and QoL. These procedures usually adhere to principles of patient-centered care focused on minimally invasive methods, leading to safety and efficacy first and foremost.

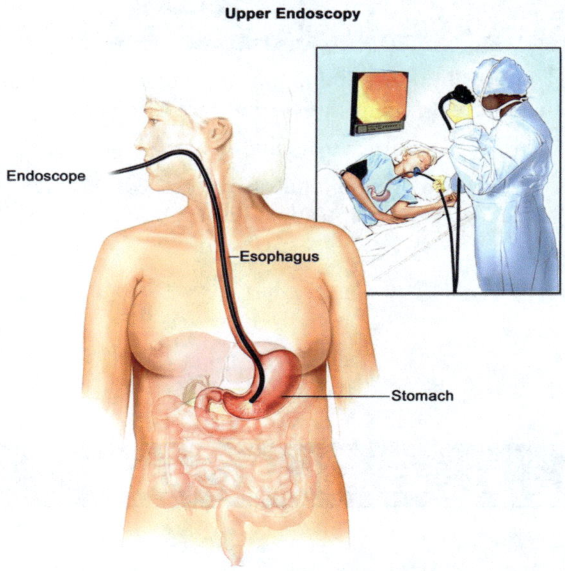

Figure 7.9. Upper endoscopy.

Source: https://www.niddk.nih.gov/-/media/Images/Health-Information/Digestive-Diseases/upper-endoscopy_715x756.jpg?h=756&w=715&hash=F2A2AE37DFB9B4F0AF2F7DF6BD35D1CD.

Additionally, the possibility of being performed in an outpatient setting further establishes its position in current gastroenterology practice, enhancing access and ease for patients. Recent advances in imaging technology, such as the integration of multidetector computed tomography (MDCT), have improved the precision of endoscopic intervention. For instance, the measurement of hiatal surface area (HSA) with MDCT allows patient-specific treatment planning in hiatal hernias, tailoring interventions to individual anatomies. As reported by recent literature, these advancements result in crucial preoperative information with a high correlation to endoscopic and patient outcomes (Boru et al., 2017). With these developments, medical practitioners can make informed choices regarding the management of GI disease, further emphasizing the importance of endoscopic procedures in contemporary clinical practice. As the prevalence of GI disease continues to rise, ongoing development and refinement of endoscopic methods will be pivotal to this growing healthcare burden (Figure 7.9).

Test Your Knowledge

1. What physical examination techniques are commonly used to assess gastrointestinal health, and what abnormal findings might indicate GI disorders?
2. Which laboratory tests and imaging studies are helpful in diagnosing GI conditions?
3. What is the role of endoscopic procedures such as upper GI endoscopy and colonoscopy in diagnosing and managing gastrointestinal disorders?

7.4. Treatment Modalities

Learning Outcome

1. Discuss about pharmacological interventions in managing gastrointestinal disorders
2. Understand dietary modifications and lifestyle changes
3. Focus on surgical options in the management of gastrointestinal conditions

The treatment modalities for the diseases of the gut have evolved significantly, blending pharmacologic and non-pharmacologic interventions to improve outcomes for the patient. Medications such as antacids, proton pump inhibitors, and other medications that target the gut microbiota are the accepted treatments for as disparate a range of conditions as GERD through to IBS. However, the response to therapy in patients varies, making a personalized approach based on the underlying pathophysiology critical. The use of patient-specific parameters, including genetic predisposition and psychosocial issues, is increasingly crucial. Such a comprehensive analysis enables targeted therapy, thereby maximizing the likelihood of successful treatment of GI disease and encouraging compliance with regimens. Concurrent to drug therapy, modification of lifestyle continues to play a significant role in GI disease treatment. Dietary change, increased physical activity, and stress management techniques can significantly alleviate symptoms and promote general GI health. For instance, dietary alteration in IBS patients has been correlated with symptomatic improvement since food intolerance may exacerbate the disease. Also, the incorporation of mindfulness and cognitive behavioral therapy (CBT) has been found to aid in the control of the psychosomatic component of GI illnesses. These drug-free methods augment present medical treatment, evoking a holistic healing environment that acknowledges the complex interconnection between mind and body within gut health. Current technical advances and imaging have further enhanced insight and treatment of GI illness. Techniques such as functional MRI (fMRI) allow investigation of the brain-gut axis, elucidating the neurological substrate for GI symptoms as well as their psychological counterparts. Not only do these imaging procedures diagnose distinct neural signatures for dysfunctions, but they also open the door to novel therapeutic approaches that integrate cognitive and behavioral strategies with biologic treatments. As the interactions between the gut microbiome and CNS are increasingly elucidated, tailor-made treatment protocols consisting of nutrition therapy, psychological counseling, and novel pharmacotherapy can yield improved outcomes in patients. Interdisciplinary collaboration will be crucial in realizing the most significant potential of these modalities, advancing the specialty to more effective, individualized care of gastroenterology patients (N/A, 2006; Aziz et al., 2019).

7.4.1. Pharmacological Interventions

In general medicine, pharmacologic intervention plays a central role in the management of GI disorders. Pharmacologic treatments are employed to alleviate symptomatology and restore the pathophysiology of various illnesses such as IBS, IBD, and peptic ulcer. Antispasmodics and laxatives, for instance, are widely applied to manage IBS-associated pain and constipation. Additionally, drugs such as proton pump inhibitors and H_2-receptor antagonists effectively inhibit gastric acid secretion and are thus used in conditions of excessive acidity. The selection of pharmacological agents typically demands a multifactorial approach that considers not only the specific GI symptoms but also the patients' general status and any comorbidities they may be experiencing. Thus, it is required to be well-versed in the pharmacodynamics and PK of these agents so that the therapeutic outcomes can be optimized. Despite the efficacy of pharmacological interventions, there is a challenge in their implementation, particularly in identifying and tailoring them to comorbid conditions. Patients with GI manifestations, for instance, may present with co-morbid mental disorders, e.g., late-life depression (LLD), which complicates their diagnosis and management. LLD typically presents with somatic symptoms, and thus patients present for GI complaints rather than their mood disorders. This overlap necessitates greater vigilance from family physicians to effectively screen and manage both conditions. With the utilization of screening tools along with tailored pharmacotherapy, practitioners can formulate a more comprehensive and effective treatment plan for both GI complaints and co-morbid mood disorders. Such dual management is crucial in optimizing patient outcomes as well as their QoL. New research also points to the necessity of systematic knowledge of pharmacologic therapy and its overall implications. The latest technology in neuroimaging has uncovered intricate interconnectivity between the brain, gut, and microbiome and significantly altered the treatment of GI disease. Brain signatures of conditions like IBS have been associated with chronic pain syndromes, and this shows that psychological and neurological factors play a significant role in these conditions. Therefore, drug treatments could not only to address GI disorders directly but also consider their neurobiological counterparts. Such cross-disciplinary approaches promise new regimes of treatment by integrating pharmacology with neuroscience and psychology, eventually enriching the overall medical ethos towards the gut (Declercq et al., 2018; Aziz et al., 2019) (Figure 7.10).

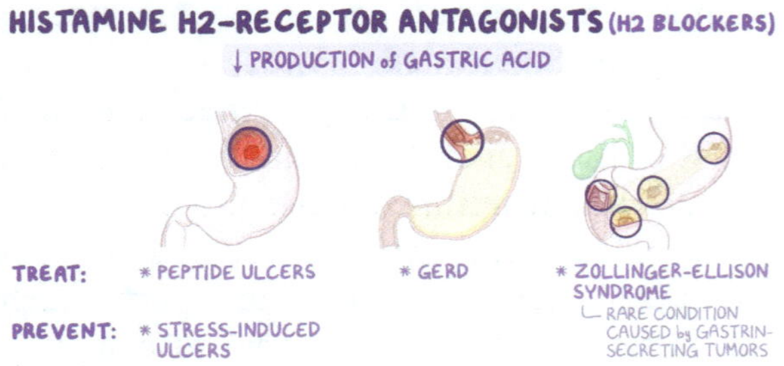

Figure 7.10. Histamine H_2-receptor antagonists.

Source: https://d16qt3wv6xm098.cloudfront.net/x8U1WHRIQbeiZe8QASYBlhclSgmVuZIt/_.jpg.

7.4.2. Dietary Modifications and Lifestyle Changes

Dietary modifications form the cornerstone of the treatment of GI disorders, particularly for constipation. Increasing fiber intake is a simple method that allows for normal bowel function and enhances colonic transit, thereby alleviating symptoms. A good diet involving fruits, vegetables, beans and legumes, and whole grains not only provides the necessary fiber but also essential nutrients that are accountable for overall intestinal well-being. Secondly, proper hydration is also to be integrated since water softens the stool and enhances GI motility. These dietary interventions have been observed to possess significant potential for improving the QoL for patients suffering from GI disorders, as they are a general medicine approach aimed at delivering both preventive and lifestyle interventions in treatment. Besides dietary change, lifestyle adjustments are also crucial to the resolution of GI disorders. Regular exercise has been shown to activate bowel movements and can alleviate symptoms of constipation. Regular moderate physical exercise aids normal metabolism and enhances circulation, which is essential for digestive health. Also, maintaining regularity in eating and bathroom usage helps the body get accustomed to the routine, thereby promoting healthier GI tracts. A diet with inclusion of recommendations for these lifestyle modifications, along with nutrition counseling, can have a cumulative effect, both on the symptoms and on the underlying causes related to digestive well-being. The synergistic effect of dietary and lifestyle modifications is enhanced by research highlighting their combined influence on conditions like constipation in individuals with Parkinson's disease (PD). Both lifestyle guidance and abdominal massage were believed to alleviate symptoms of constipation, suggesting that treatment of the condition from a variety of angles significantly enhances patient outcomes. Those who experimented with different changes to their behavior reported improved QoL, pointing to the importance of individualized interventions that are grounded in personal experience. As Aitchison et al. (2016) elucidate, while dietary habits form part of GI management, concurrent confluence of lifestyle adjustment can lead to improved symptom alleviation and total health. Such synergy with best practices, as demonstrated by Gardiner et al. (2016), is based on the provision of comprehensive measures in general medicine to approach GI dysfunction holistically.

7.4.3. Surgical Options and When They Are Indicated

It is essential to be familiar with the surgical procedures in GI disorders in order to optimize patient management. Surgical treatment is indicated in most GI conditions, particularly those not responsive to standard treatment. For instance, patients with complicated diverticular disease predominantly require surgical treatment when complications arise involving perforation and recurrent diverticulitis. In such a case, resection of the involved segment of the colon is a life-saving procedure. The decision to operate should be taken after careful consideration of the patient's overall health status and co-morbidities, as the outcome of the surgery might be severely compromised by these conditions. Significantly, when conservative care fails, the transition to surgical procedures usually can reverse QoL and eliminate the painful symptomatology associated with chronic GI disease. Additional study into surgical procedures finds their central role for curing multifaceted conditions like bowel obstruction or far-advanced cancer. In bowel obstruction, for example, an operation may be warranted to remove the obstruction when the blockage is not relieved by rest and medications. In patients with colorectal cancer, too, resection is typically a central component of the treatment. Italian Society of Colorectal Surgery (SICCR) emphasizes the importance of evidence-based guidelines to inform such decisions so that optimal utilization of surgical options as well as safety is ensured (Annibale et al., 2015). The surgeons must be vigilant in assessing the mode and timing of intervention because early or premature surgeries can lead to increased morbidity and undermine overall patient outcomes. Secondly, postoperative and long-term management of surgery is significant because complications may arise that require further intervention. Risks involved should be made clear to the surgical candidate, for example, infection, anastomotic leaks, and reoperation, particularly for advanced diseases of the GI tract. For extreme constipation, where surgical intervention in the form of colectomy might be an option, patients' bowel function must be assessed thoroughly and less invasive intervention held back at first (Gardiner et al., 2016). Ultimately, surgical intervention taken for GI disease must form part of a holistic, multidisciplinary management strategy that not only prioritizes immediate clinical needs but also provides long-term health through management and care (Figure 7.11).

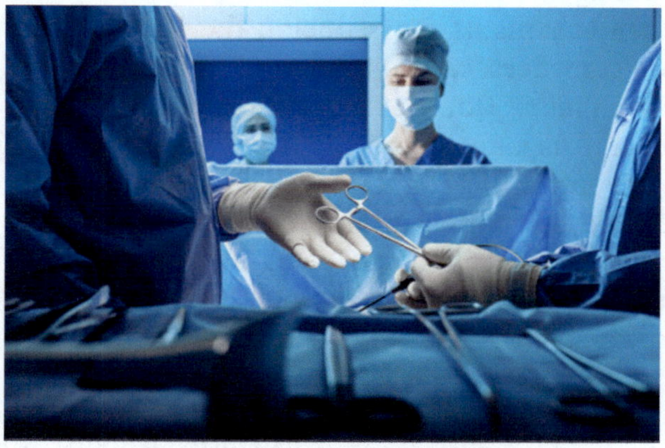

Figure 7.11. Surgical gastroenterology.

Source: https://prakashhospitalgn.com/wp-content/uploads/2024/09/Surgical-Gastroenterology.png.

Test Your Knowledge

1. What pharmacological interventions are commonly used to treat gastrointestinal disorders such as GERD, IBS, and IBD, and how do they work?
2. How can dietary modifications and lifestyle changes help manage or alleviate symptoms of common GI conditions?

7.5. Preventive Measures

Learning Outcome

1. Explain the importance of regular screenings
2. Understand the role of patient education in prevention
3. Describe lifestyle factors that promote gastrointestinal health

Preventive measures are highly critical in the management of GI overall health. Adherence to mechanisms for reducing the likelihood of GI disorders can minimize morbidity as well as enhance QoL. Patient education for dietary choice is one of the most critical aspects of prevention. Encouraging an eating pattern of high dietary fiber intake, fruits, and vegetables has been proven to lower significantly the risk of disease such as colorectal cancer and diverticulitis.

Additionally, altering behavior with regard to regular exercise and a healthy weight can be a factor for GI well-being. These efforts, along with routine screening regimens in high-risk groups, embody a proactive approach to preventive healthcare in managing GI disorders, ultimately fostering a culture of wellness rather than disease response. Pharmacologic treatment also constitutes a valuable addition to the arsenal of preventive measures in GI health. Co-prescription of gastroprotective drugs, especially in patients on NSAIDs, is significant due to the enhanced risk of GI complications with these medications.

Evidence indicates that awareness among healthcare providers of the necessity of gastroprotective cover has increased, yet adherence to prescribed dosage is inconsistent (Bilušić et al., 2006). Gastroprotective therapy must be administered to at-risk patients of NSAID-induced gastric ulcer. Implementation of evidence-based guidelines for these drugs can improve therapy results, reduce healthcare costs, and improve patient compliance with therapy regimens. Furthermore, an understanding of how prevention and nutrition are linked is essential. Probiotics, prebiotics, and other supplements have gained attention for their ability to enhance gut microbiota health, and hence perhaps treat numerous GI diseases. Much more research needs to be done, though, in order to make conclusive recommendations about using them. While phytotherapy and homeopathic drugs are routinely prescribed as natural treatments, their actual value in gastroprotection is largely unproven (Eijck et al., 2003). Therefore, it is an integrated plan founded on dietary management, proper medical advice, and lifestyle changes that can crack the code to maintaining a healthier GI system, actually decreasing the incidence of disease, and improving overall health.

7.5.1. Importance of Regular Screenings

Regular screening is essential for early diagnosis and prevention of GI diseases, with a significantly positive effect on patient outcomes. Colorectal cancer, which ranks as one of the leading causes of cancer death in the United States, is usually not symptomatic in its early stages, so regular screenings are essential. The fact that many colorectal cancers grow slowly is additional evidence supporting earlier detection through screening. Literature has proven that regular screening can lead to a decline in morbidity and mortality of these cancers.

However, despite being of utmost importance, the level of screening remains alarmingly low, which reveals a stark deficiency in preventive services. As noted in literature, an increase in awareness and education regarding such screenings is essential for maximizing patient compliance and lives being saved (Hardcorn et al., 2022). Educational interventions targeting patients' understanding of GI screening, such as colonoscopies and fecal occult blood testing, are critical in closing the gaps in screening rates. Literature suggests that patient-focused educational messages can improve awareness and knowledge of colorectal cancer, prevention, and hence active health control. In one recent project, those patients exposed to educational brochures demonstrated a considerable increase in awareness about colorectal cancer and screening techniques. Although the project's intervention had little influence on actual screening rates, it did demonstrate a substantial increase in awareness, thereby establishing a foundation for ongoing educational interventions. This case illustrates the effect of effective communication and the sharing of specific information in empowering individuals to take charge of their health by prioritizing routine screenings (Green et al., 2024).

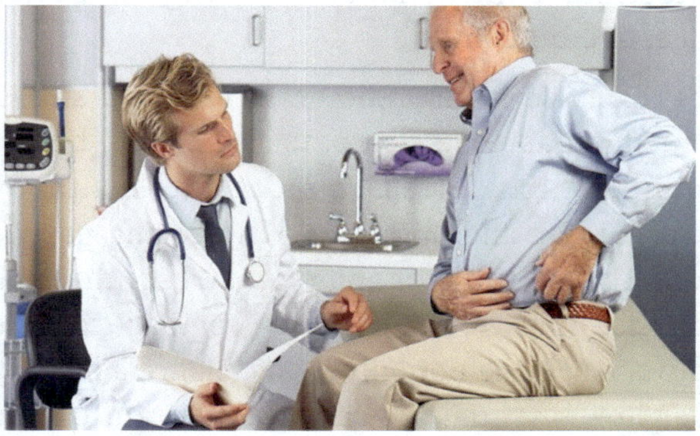

Figure 7.12. Screening for gastrointestinal disease.

Source: https://careplusvn.com/Uploads/t/tu/tu-van-kham-sang-loc-benh-duong-tieu-hoa-3_0003295_710.jpeg.

Additionally, the interaction between demographic traits and adherence to screening recommendations emphasizes the importance of routine screenings. Research has established that traits like age, socioeconomic status, and social support affect an individual's likelihood of enrolling in screening programs. By focusing only on education for specific populations, healthcare providers may enhance the acceptability and availability of screening to different populations. Recognizing that marital status and economic situation may determine health conduct can lead to the development of empowering interventions intended to eliminate these disparities. By aligning screening outreach programs with the unique needs of various demographic groups, the health system can maximize participation rates, resulting in early-stage diagnosis and better health outcomes for GI diseases (Green et al., 2024) (Figure 7.12).

7.5.2. Role of Patient Education in Prevention

Patient education is key to the prevention of GI diseases through empowering individuals with facts to make healthy choices. Proper knowledge of GI status risk factors helps the patient become aware of early signs of distress and seek timely healthcare. Being proactive in preventing morbidity related to IBD and GERD can significantly contribute to the management of these conditions.

Through the practice of awareness culture, medical practitioners can empower patients with the skills required to maintain digestive health. As noted, somatic complaints are common among patients, where they overlook symptoms related to such psychological conditions as LLD (Declercq et al., 2018). Thus, patient education regarding the interactions between GI health and psychological factors is essential for extensive preventive care. Also, patient education is provided to some habits that reverse unwanted side effects of prevalent treatments for GI illnesses. For instance, systemic corticosteroids are responsible for causing complications such as hyperglycemia and dyspepsia if not monitored correctly. Patient education about these potential side effects will enable them to take preventive measures, such as paying close attention to diet and bringing any abnormal symptoms to the attention of their healthcare professionals. In the instance of research on corticosteroid-induced hyperglycemia management, there was very poor adherence to guidelines, indicating improved patient education policies were in order (Fsadni et al., 2015).

By enabling physicians to enhance patients' knowledge about their therapy and associated risks, guideline adherence results, eventually translating to improved health outcomes and QoL. In addition, the description of the multi-dimensional function of patient education in prevention encompasses promoting lifestyle modifications that support GI well-being.

Dietary changes, physical activity, and stress management are some methods by which the risk for GI disease can be reduced to a great extent. Surveys show that patients who are well-educated about their illness and understand the lifestyle changes needed for prevention tend to lead healthier lives. This is especially applicable in the case of chronic diseases, where patients need to take charge of managing their health. As illustrated through research on corticosteroid management, if patients are well educated, their active participation can improve treatment efficacy and reduce complications (Fsadni et al., 2015). Ultimately, prioritizing patient education in practice not only informs individuals but also fosters an interactive healthcare environment that centers preventive care as the cornerstone of GI health treatment.

7.5.3. Lifestyle Factors That Promote Gastrointestinal Health

A worldwide awareness of GI well-being recognizes the key position of lifestyle within the body. Diet is a priority among the elements of lifestyle, as it is vital for maintaining a healthy GI tract. Diets rich in fiber from fruits, vegetables, and whole grains promote healthy bowel function and prevent constipation, which is one of the most common GI disorders. In addition, probiotics in fermented food items, like yogurt and kefir, are beneficial to gut microbiota, enhancing digestion. Meanwhile, water also plays an equally vital role; proper intake of water is essential to facilitate digestion, nutrition, and absorption. By prioritizing such nutrition, individuals can ensure the health of their GI system and reduce the risk of more serious digestive ailments, thereby complementing a general medicine approach of prevention and multi-faceted treatment. Regular exercise is also a critical factor that affects the health of the GI system.

Regular exercise raises the level of GI motility so that digestion occurs in a timely fashion, and one is less likely to develop conditions like constipation and GERD. Research shows that even moderate exercise can induce intestinal contractions, resulting in better digestive outcomes.

Exercise is also known to ward off stress, which tends to exacerbate GI-related health complications. Stress affects gut health by altering gut microbiota and increasing gastric sensitivity; thus, managing stress through exercise is two-fold. Bringing regular exercise into the routine not only helps ensure a healthy weight—essential for easing the strain on the gastric system—but also contributes to an overall feeling of well-being, which is important in a holistic strategy for GI health.

Mental status and emotional health strongly intersect with GI function, highlighting the significance of psychological factors in GI well-being. Stress, depression, and anxiety are chronic illnesses that can lead to alterations in gut motility and intestinal permeability and exacerbate IBS and IBD. Stress-reduction techniques such as meditation, yoga, and adequate sleep can improve mental wellness as well as GI health. As rightly stated in one study, it is of utmost importance to understand the close link between the brain and the gut, revealing that the brain guides responses that in turn influence GI function. Psychological treatment should be considered part of a broader medical approach, integrating psychological therapy with GI health to create a holistic and effective model of mental health treatment for patients (Estrine et al., 2006; N/A, 2014).

Test Your Knowledge

1. Why are regular screenings important in the early detection and prevention of gastrointestinal disease?
2. How does patient education contribute to the prevention of GI disorders, and what key information should be included in educational efforts?

7.6. Emerging Trends in Gastrointestinal Medicine

Learning Outcome

1. Discuss about advances in technology and diagnostics
2. Focus on research on gut microbiome and its implications
3. Deal with innovations in treatment approaches

The gastro medicine landscape is significantly changing due to the impetus provided by technological advancements and a better understanding of gut microbiome dynamics. The role of human gut microbiota in disease and human health has never been at the forefront of research to this extent, driving scientists to explore how shifts in microbiome may influence GI diseases such as IBD and IBS. Recent research has indicated that personalized microbiome therapeutics, such as probiotics and fecal microbiota transplantation, are regarded as promising strategies for preserving and restoring GI well-being. This trend towards customization highlights the importance of a personalized approach in managing GI diseases, enabling improved patient outcomes through more focused therapy plans based on unique microbial profiles. Apart from microbiome research, the intersection of AI and machine learning with gastroenterology is revolutionizing diagnostic and treatment work. AI systems are being designed to better analyze medical imaging and pathology reports, allowing for conditions like colorectal cancer to be diagnosed earlier. Machine learning algorithms can also predict patient outcomes from clinical information, allowing clinicians to create customized treatment plans. This technological advancement plays a central role in revolutionizing the precision of GI medicine, making interventions not just timely but also effective. With the health environment continuing to evolve, the implementation of AI in clinical practice could have a profound impact on the management of GI disease, revolutionizing patient care and improving health outcomes. Another trend within GI medicine of note is the increasing recognition of the psychosomatic aspects of GI illness. Psychological comorbidities such as depression and anxiety are present in the majority of chronic GI patients, which aggravate their symptoms as well as interfere with recovery. Recent research emphasizes bidirectional communication between the brain and gut and underscores the necessity of an interdisciplinary treatment approach that incorporates psychological management and standard medical treatments. The inclusion of mental health management in the care of GI disease not only cares for the whole patient but also significantly increases his or her QoL. By acknowledging the influence of psychological factors on physical well-being, gastroenterologists can adopt a more holistic therapeutic approach, leading to better patient cooperation and adherence to treatment strategies.

7.6.1. Advances in Technology and Diagnostics

The advancement in technology has significantly influenced the field of GI diagnostics, providing new avenues for enhancing patient care. One of them includes the use of point-of-care ultrasound (POCUS), a technology that offers real-time imaging and assessment of GI disease at the bedside. Recent literature has highlighted the potential of teleultrasound technologies such as FaceTime and Google Glass, with which experienced clinicians can remotely teach inexperienced practitioners how to perform essential ultrasound exams. This capability not only increases the availability of diagnostic equipment in emergency settings but also enhances the skills of less experienced medical personnel. By applying these technologies, healthcare providers can facilitate early assessment of cardiac, pulmonary, and abdominal illness, leading to accelerated clinical decision-making and potentially better patient outcomes (Austin et al., 2019). In addition to improvements in ultrasound technology, developments in colon capsule endoscopy (CCE) represent a significant advancement in non-invasive GI diagnosis. The technology allows for efficient colon investigation without the discomfort and invasiveness associated with traditional colonoscopy. A recent multicenter study demonstrated that the second-generation CCE system effectively maintained cleansing efficacy equivalent to that of standard preparation regimens without compromising overall procedure completion rate. Patients treated with the new regimen were more likely to complete the examination successfully, demonstrating that patient compliance is a factor in diagnostic accuracy. Also, despite some side effects of the new regimen, they were mostly minor and did not cause any serious issues. This is a significant leap for the treatment of colorectal screening (Burch et al., 2017). The synergy caused by these technological advancements boosts the overall medical approach towards GI disease by emphasizing rapid diagnosis and improved patient experience. Techniques like POCUS and CCE reflect the emphasis on more patient-focused care and efficient utilization of resources.

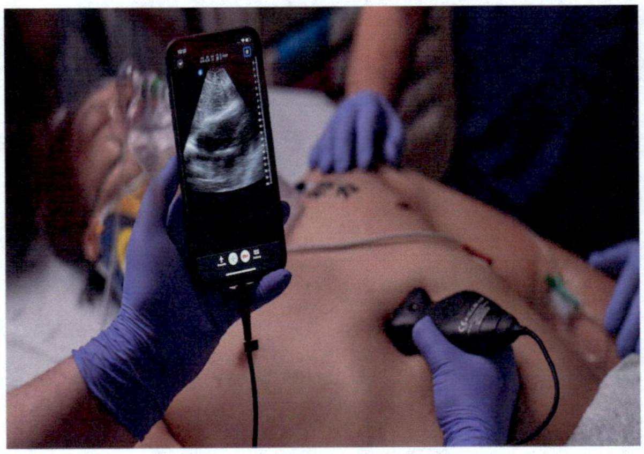

Figure 7.13. Point-of-care ultrasound (POCUS).

Source: https://aiumthescan.blog/wp-content/uploads/2023/05/POCUS.jpg.

As these technologies develop further, their integration into routine practice will become a reality, and clinicians will have even greater abilities for early diagnosis and intervention of GI disease. The combination of real-time imaging and non-invasive diagnostics has the capacity to minimize significantly the duration of hospital stays, decrease medical spending, and ultimately enhance patient health outcomes. Ongoing innovations and research in this field assure that the level of care in GI medicine will continue to increase, ensuring that healthcare providers are given the most effective diagnostic tools available today (Figure 7.13).

7.6.2. Research on Gut Microbiome and Its Implications

The evolving landscape of biomedical science increasingly highlights the gut microbiota as a key to unraveling human health and disease. This intricate community of trillions of microbes residing in the intestines not only engages in digestion but also modulates the immune system, metabolizes, and protects against infection. Central to this hypothesis is the distinction between eubiosis, the symbiotic condition of microbes, and dysbiosis, which describes imbalance and has been linked with disease states. More recent studies have led us to consider that disturbances in the gut microbiome can result in disease processes such as IBD, and the suggestion is that a precisely balanced microbiome may be a therapeutic modality (Andrada et al., 2020). Thus, a study of the uses of microbiome research might uncover new approaches in clinical practice, bridging the divide between basic science and actual applications in GI medicine. The Human Microbiome Project is a fine example of an integral project in understanding the complexity of microbiota and their interaction with human physiology. By sequencing the genomes of different microbial populations, scientists anticipate gaining a better understanding of the functional roles these microorganisms play within the human body. This effort transcends traditional views of the human genome as a disconnected blueprint, but instead suggests that humans are superorganisms where microbial genomes are intertwined irretrievably within human genes (Huss et al., 2009). This change not only reshapes our understanding of disease and health but also disrupts treatment models, prompting a transition toward personalized medicine that addresses microbial health as well.

In that regard, the integration of microbiome research within the broader paradigm of medicine is a comprehensive model for the management of GI disease with potential for better outcomes through the application of targeted therapies. As the dialogue regarding the gut microbiome grows, scientists are beginning to find the potential for association between microbiota composition and a vast range of health issues beyond the GI system. Current evidence shows that changes in the microbiome can influence metabolic disorders, autoimmune disease, and psychiatric illness through inflammation-mediated mechanisms and gut-brain interaction. The implications of the research call for a multidisciplinary framework incorporating microbiome examination into diagnostic and treatment plans. With developments such as probiotic treatment and dietary modification gaining increasing visibility, an enhanced understanding of the microbiome's role will redefine preventive strategies and therapeutic options for GI and systemic illnesses in equal proportion. Ongoing investigation in this field is crucial to optimize patient care and unveil the therapeutic potential of the gut microbiome in general medicine (Figure 7.14).

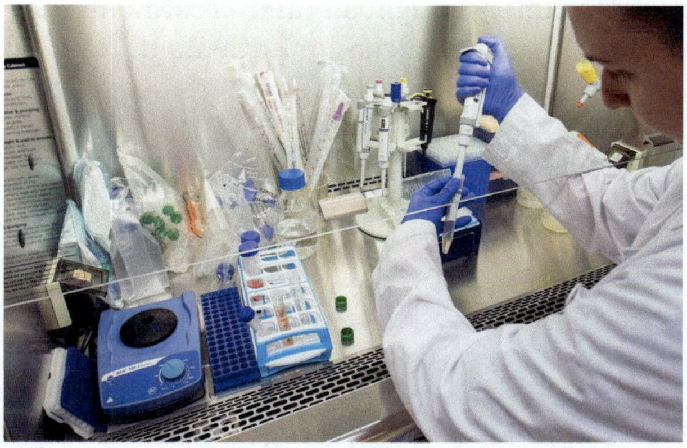

Figure 7.14. Gut microbiome research.

Source: https://lsmu.lt/wp-content/uploads/Mikrobiomo-tyrimuose-%E2%80%93-Lietuvos-mokslininku-proverzis.jpg.

7.6.3. Innovations in Treatment Approaches

In the past couple of years, treatment of the GI system has radically shifted with significant developments that not only patients but also improve care efficiency. One notable innovation is the employment of minimally invasive surgical techniques, such as laparoscopic surgery, which reduces recovery time and minimizes postoperative complications. By enabling surgeons to perform operations with minor cuts, these techniques allow quicker recovery and reduced hospital stays of the patients, and consequently lower costs of healthcare. Further, these technologies enhance patient satisfaction because patients experience less pain and scarring compared to open surgery. With the ongoing advancement of these technologies by the health community, there are bright prospects for improved treatment outcomes, underscoring the effectiveness of visionary interventions in gastroenterological medicine. Another critical innovation is the application of telemedicine in gastroenterology that has transformed access to healthcare for patients. Telehealth platforms enable patients to consult with experts remotely, avoiding geographical boundaries that typically restrict timely diagnosis and treatment. The technology is beneficial for patients in rural or disadvantaged communities where specialized care might be limited. Additionally, online consultation can accelerate the management of chronic GI disease by allowing for real-time observation and updating of treatment plans without having to consult the patient in the clinic. By integrating telehealth into the general medicine paradigm, healthcare workers can enhance patient involvement and adherence to treatment protocols, thereby improving overall GI health outcomes. Top-of-the-line facilities, such as ambulatory surgery centers and specialty clinics, have emerged as a significant innovation in the field of GI treatment. These centers are meant to provide some gastroenterological therapy less expensively and efficiently than standard full-service hospitals. By concentrating skills and equipment, specialty facilities can provide high-quality care while maintaining low patient waiting times. Their impact should also be evaluated on regular general hospitals, as the opening of such options would affect the scope of services delivered within larger health systems. While some studies indicate limited competitive advantages for these specialty centers, a well-balanced strategy is necessary to ensure that everyone receives complete GI care. Monitoring the development and performance of such centers is thus crucial since it highlights the changing trends in healthcare delivery in the GI market (N/A, 2007; Annemans et al., 2013).

Test Your Knowledge

1. What recent advances in technology and diagnostics are improving the detection and management of gastrointestinal disorders?
2. How is current research on the gut microbiome shaping our understanding of gastrointestinal health and its connection to systemic diseases?

SUMMARY

The general medical response to the GI system reflects the complexity of diagnosing and managing a broad spectrum of GI diseases. Even though the shared symptoms at times lead to straightforward clinical assessments, the variety of potential causes necessitates a wide knowledge of the systems' interaction, including immunologic reactions and environmental issues. New insight into diseases such as systemic sclerosis (SSc) and its impact on GI motility demonstrates the imperative need for ongoing research and multidisciplinary management. Special attention should be dedicated to knowing new therapeutic targets developed from novel pathophysiologic mechanisms, as suggested by the literature (Abraham et al., 2017). This ongoing research will allow more effective and tailored treatment approaches that will significantly improve patient outcomes. In addition, as the health effects of organic livestock production are gradually improving, it is clear that the nexus between diet, immune status, and gut health remains unexplored territory. The challenges inherent in organic animal husbandry, such as susceptibility to disease and the efficacy of immune modulation by alternative treatments, require serious investigation. The argument that animals produced organically possess inherently improved health is yet to be tested, and further research must be conducted to create concrete associations between production practices and health outcomes (Abraham et al., 2017). These determinations bear significant implications not only for the well-being of animals but also for human health, particularly with the continued expansion of knowledge regarding zoonotic diseases. A holistic approach must consider not only organic methods of agriculture but also international eating patterns correlated with GI health in human animals. Finally, the research of GI health in human and animal populations indicates an urgent need for integrative studies aimed at filling gaps in knowledge. Current trends indicate a sobering prevalence of GI disease in all demographic groups, demonstrating the need for education and early treatment. Designing prevention strategies capable of interrupting both environmental causes and genetic susceptibility may enhance the health prognosis for those affected. In particular, exploring the roles of dietary consumption and the potential role of phytotherapeutics is a notable development in treatment strategy that deserves more research (Eijck et al., 2003). By creating a setting for research among varied disciplines, more efficient and integrated solutions to GI health may emerge, for the benefit of clinicians and patients.

In assessing a general medicine course related to the GI tract, it is imperative to recognize pivotal factors that influence diagnosis and treatment. A key constituent is the understanding of the symbiotic relationship between GI health and gut microbiome. Current research emphasizes the role of microbial balance in cases of constipation and GI discomfort. For instance, a pilot study demonstrated how EpiCor fermentate, a prebiotic, was advantageous in modulating gut microbiota, leading to considerable symptom relief among participants with constipation. This emphasizes the importance of studying microbiome-directed treatments as part of a comprehensive treatment regimen, demonstrating how dietary interventions and microbial modulation may offer meaningful solutions to GI disease, particularly for patients with chronic bowel dysfunction symptoms (Marzorati et al., 2017). The contribution of patient education and lifestyle modification cannot be overemphasized either in the management of GI disease. Educating patients to see the connection between diet, stress, and intestinal health can be the key to symptom control. According to the research, gains in constipation-related QoL and reduced perceived stress levels can be achieved through specific interventions. Specifically, emphasizing the impact of particular prebiotics and dietary fiber on bowel consistency and frequency can lead to improved therapy.

As patients become engaged in self-management practice, they can integrate evidence-based recommendations with their experiences, leading to greater satisfaction from their treatment and improved overall health outcomes (Eskeland et al., 2025). Lastly, the role of healthcare systems in facilitating effective GI management is equally applicable. Current models are shown to exhibit discontinuity in service provision, particularly in rural settings where health promoters lack the skills and resources needed to make a meaningful impact on patient care. Experience shows that despite some excellent community health workers, the failures in the system remain significant barriers to optimum health service delivery. Learning from differences between government and nongovernment programs promises to align standard practice protocols, ensuring interventions are not only available but also effective for individuals suffering from GI disease. The implications emphasize the importance of an integrated approach that combines medical know-how, patient empowerment, and system reform to achieve optimal health benefits from GI treatment (Eskeland et al., 2025).

KEY TERMS FROM THIS CHAPTER

Abdominal pain
Accessory organs
Autoimmune disease
Broad-spectrum anthelmintic drugs
Colon capsule endoscopy (CCE)
Colorectal cancer
Conventional examination techniques
Corticosteroid management
Corticotropin-releasing hormone (CRH)
Diagnostic innovation
Dietary choice
Dietary modifications
Digestive enzymes
Direct support professionals (DSPs)

CRITICAL THINKING QUESTIONS

1. **Which condition is characterized by inflammation of the lining of the colon and rectum and often presents with bloody diarrhea?**
   a. Peptic ulcer disease
   b. Crohn's disease
   c. Ulcerative colitis
   d. Irritable bowel syndrome (IBS)
2. **Which of the following is the gold standard diagnostic tool for detecting colorectal cancer?**
   a. Abdominal ultrasound
   b. Stool occult blood test
   c. CT scan
   d. Colonoscopy
3. **The liver receives blood from the gastrointestinal tract via the:**
   a. Hepatic artery
   b. Portal vein
   c. Splenic vein
   d. Inferior vena cava
4. **Which of the following technologies is enhancing early detection of GI cancers?**
   a. Telemedicine
   b. Capsule endoscopy
   c. Manual rectal exam
   d. Nutritional counseling
5. **Fecal microbiota transplantation is an emerging treatment for:**
   a. GERD
   b. Pancreatitis
   c. Cirrhosis
   d. *C. difficile* infection

Short answer Questions

1. Describe the main anatomical structures of the gastrointestinal tract, from ingestion to defecation. What are the primary functions of each section?
2. What are the common causes, clinical manifestations, and potential complications of gastroesophageal reflux disease (GERD)?
3. What are the key diagnostic tools and procedures used to evaluate gastrointestinal disorders, and how do they differ in their applications (e.g., endoscopy vs. imaging vs. laboratory tests)?
4. Outline the pharmacological and non-pharmacological treatment options for irritable bowel syndrome (IBS).
5. What lifestyle and dietary changes are recommended to prevent common gastrointestinal conditions such as peptic ulcers, diverticulosis, and colorectal cancer?
6. What are some current or emerging technologies and treatments in GI medicine, and how are they changing clinical practice?

Answers to Critical Thinking Questions

1. (c)　2. (d)　3. (b)　4. (b)　5. (c)

REFERENCES

1. Migliori, G. B., Dheda, K., Centis, R., Mwaba, P., Bates, M., O'Grady, J., Hoelscher, M., & Zumla, A. (2010b). Review of multidrug-resistant and extensively drug-resistant TB: global perspectives with a focus on sub-Saharan Africa. *Tropical Medicine & International Health*, *15*(9), 1052–1066. https://doi.org/10.1111/j.1365-3156.2010.02581.x
2. Abraham, D. J., Assandri, R., Assassi, S., Auluck, P., Bacher, P., Baron, M., Baron, M., et al. (2017). Review article: Pathogenesis and clinical manifestations of gastrointestinal involvement in systemic sclerosis. https://core.ac.uk/download/83049880.pdf (accessed on 27th June 2025).
3. Aitchison, P., Cunnington, A., Dickinson, L., Hagen, S., et al. (2016). Abdominal massage for the relief of constipation in people with Parkinson's: A qualitative study. https://core.ac.uk/download/293881817.pdf (accessed on 27th June 2025).
4. Ameer, B., Weintraub, H., et al. (2018). Pediatric obesity: Influence on drug dosing and therapeutics. https://core.ac.uk/download/155271623.pdf (accessed on 27th June 2025).
5. Andrada, D., Sergiu, I., Micu, I., Manea, M. E., Marilena, D., et al. (2020). Microbiota: The missing link in the etiology of inflammatory bowel disease. https://core.ac.uk/download/304672907.pdf (accessed on 27th June 2025).
6. Annemans, L., De Regge, M., Duyck, P., Gemmel, P., et al. (2013). Physician-owned specialized facilities: Focused factories or destructive competition? A systematic review. https://core.ac.uk/download/55777137.pdf (accessed on 27th June 2025).
7. Annibale, B., Bellini, D., Binda, G. A., Cuomo, R., et al. (2015). Practice parameters for the treatment of colonic diverticular disease: Italian Society of Colon and Rectal Surgery (SICCR) guidelines. https://core.ac.uk/download/54522076.pdf (accessed on 27th June 2025).
8. Auberry, K., Shaver, C., & Wills, K. (2017). Improving medication practices for persons with intellectual and developmental disability: Educating direct support staff using simulation, debriefing, and reflection. https://core.ac.uk/download/189104549.pdf (accessed on 27th June 2025).
9. Austin, B., Davis, W., Le, D. Q., Ma, D., et al. (2019). Feasibility evaluation of commercially available video conferencing devices to technically direct untrained nonmedical personnel to perform a rapid trauma ultrasound examination. https://core.ac.uk/download/323310769.pdf (accessed on 27th June 2025).
10. Aziz, Q., Borsook, D., Elsenbruch, S., Kilpatrick, L. A., et al. (2019). Role of brain imaging in disorders of brain-gut interaction: A Rome Working Team Report. https://core.ac.uk/download/323078713.pdf (accessed on 27th June 2025).
11. Bailey, B., Cox, D., Darwich, A., Dorey, G., Duwal, S., Ette, E., et al. (2018). Population variability in animal health: Influence on dose-exposure-response relationships: Part II: Modelling and simulation. https://core.ac.uk/download/159992803.pdf (accessed on 27th June 2025).
12. Baritaki, S., Chatzaki, E., de Bree, E., Pothoulakis, C., et al. (2019). Chronic stress, inflammation, and colon cancer: A CRH system-driven molecular crosstalk. https://core.ac.uk/download/323076588.pdf (accessed on 27th June 2025).
13. Bilounga Ndongo, C., Etoundi Mballa, G. A., Hyder, A. A., Juillard, C., et al. (2010). Patterns of injury and violence in Yaoundé, Cameroon: An analysis of hospital data. https://core.ac.uk/download/323075033.pdf (accessed on 27th June 2025).

14. Bilušić, M., Erdeljić, V., Francetić, I., Huić, M., et al. (2006). Use of gastroprotective agents in recommended doses in hospitalized patients receiving NSAIDs: A drug utilization study. https://core.ac.uk/download/11699264.pdf (accessed on 27th June 2025).

15. Borges, F. A., Chagas, A. C. S., Fortes, F. S., Geldhof, P., et al. (2011). Challenges of nematode control in ruminants: Focus on Latin America. https://core.ac.uk/download/55744143.pdf (accessed on 27th June 2025).

16. Boru, E. C., Guida, A., Iossa, A., Rengo, C., et al. (2017). *25th International Congress of the European Association for Endoscopic Surgery (EAES) Frankfurt, Germany, 14–17 June 2017: Oral Presentations*. https://core.ac.uk/download/141696623.pdf (accessed on 27th June 2025).

17. Burch, W. C., Jr., Kashyap, P. K., Kastenberg, D., et al. (2017). Multicenter, randomized study to optimize bowel for colon capsule endoscopy. https://core.ac.uk/download/155271589.pdf (accessed on 27th June 2025).

18. Calabrese, E., Dietrich, C. F., Dirks, K., Gilja, P., et al. (2016). *EFSUMB Recommendations and Guidelines for Gastrointestinal Ultrasound–Part 1: Examination Techniques and Normal Findings (Long version)*. https://core.ac.uk/download/74321241.pdf (accessed on 27th June 2025).

19. Calabrese, E., Dietrich, C. F., Dirks, K., Gilja, P., et al. (2016). *EFSUMB Recommendations and Guidelines for Gastrointestinal Ultrasound–Part 1: Examination Techniques and Normal Findings (Short Version)*. https://core.ac.uk/download/74321243.pdf (accessed on 27th June 2025).

20. Darlington, L. G., & Stone, T. W. (2017). Microbial carcinogenic toxins and dietary anti-cancer protectants. https://core.ac.uk/download/80696830.pdf (accessed on 27th June 2025).

21. Declercq, T., Lemey, L., Petrovic, M., Tandt, H., et al. (2018). Late-life depression: Issues for the general practitioner. https://core.ac.uk/download/154408401.pdf (accessed on 27th June 2025).

22. Eijck, I., Groot, M., Kasteel, D., Kijlstra, A., et al. (2003). Analysis of black holes in our knowledge concerning animal health in the organic food production chain. https://core.ac.uk/download/10919416.pdf (accessed on 27th June 2025).

23. Eskeland, G. S., Lewis, M., & Traa-Valerezo, X. (2025). Challenging El Salvador's rural healthcare strategy. https://core.ac.uk/download/pdf/6616034.pdf (accessed on 27th June 2025).

24. Estrine, J., & DeLisle, L. (2006). Stress: Putting the brain back into medicine. https://core.ac.uk/download/71356692.pdf (accessed on 27th June 2025).

25. Fsadni, C. J. (2015). A study on the management of corticosteroid side effects in cancer patients. https://core.ac.uk/download/46603767.pdf (accessed on 27th June 2025).

26. Gardiner, A., & Hilton, A. (2016). Managing constipation in adults with co-morbidities. https://core.ac.uk/download/151161237.pdf (accessed on 27th June 2025).

27. Georgescu, L. C., Pătraşcu, T., Tobă, M. E., Ungureanu, A., et al. (2016). Gastrointestinal stromal tumor (GIST) of the Treitz's angle–A very rare cause of high bowel obstruction. https://core.ac.uk/download/144552989.pdf (accessed on 27th June 2025).

28. Ghosh, S., Koch, M., Rao, A. N., Suresh Kumar, P., et al. (2010). Do alternative therapies have a role in autism? https://core.ac.uk/download/pdf/87427.pdf (accessed on 27th June 2025).

29. Graff, L., Keefer, L., Knowles, S., Mikocka-Walus, A., et al. (2016). Controversies revisited: A systematic review of the comorbidity of depression and anxiety with inflammatory bowel diseases. https://core.ac.uk/download/42618534.pdf (accessed on 27th June 2025).

30. Green, S. (2024). Factors associated with digestive system cancer screening in Texas. https://core.ac.uk/download/621723249.pdf (accessed on 27th June 2025).

31. Holly, A., Burnand, B., Froehlich, F., Gonvers, J. J., Vader, J. P., Lamiraud, K., Juillerat, P., et al. (2025). The effect of non-medical factors on variations in the performance of colonoscopy among different healthcare settings. https://core.ac.uk/download/pdf/6617669.pdf (accessed on 27th June 2025).

32. Huss, J. E., & Juengst, E. T. (2009). From metagenomics to the metagenome: Conceptual change and the rhetoric of translational genomic research. https://core.ac.uk/download/237182407.pdf (accessed on 27th June 2025).

33. Jang, E. Y. (2019). A background of the opioid epidemic and its relationship to the Medicaid expansion. https://core.ac.uk/download/213463816.pdf (accessed on 27th June 2025).

34. Linson, E. A. (2013). *The Interplay Between Hormones and Irritable Bowel Disease.* https://open.bu.edu/bitstream/2144/12149/6/Linson_Elyse_2013_nosig_nocv.pdf (accessed on 27th June 2025).

35. Lorenz, W., & Rothmund, M. (1989). Theoretical surgery: A new specialty in operative medicine. https://core.ac.uk/download/11550720.pdf (accessed on 27th June 2025).

36. Marzorati, M., Pinheiro, I., Possemiers, S., Robinson, T., et al. (2017). A yeast fermentation improves gastrointestinal discomfort and constipation by modulation of the gut microbiome: Results from a randomized double-blind placebo-controlled pilot trial. https://core.ac.uk/download/147044915.pdf (accessed on 27th June 2025).

37. Mohiuddin, A. K. (2019). Alternative treatments of minor GI ailments. https://core.ac.uk/download/327073474.pdf (accessed on 27th June 2025).

38. N/A. (2006). *Focal Spot, Spring 2006.* https://core.ac.uk/download/129069350.pdf (accessed on 27th June 2025).

39. N/A. (2006). *Focal Spot, Winter 2005/2006.* https://core.ac.uk/download/129069348.pdf (accessed on 27th June 2025).

40. N/A. (2014). *Research Advances: January 2014.* https://core.ac.uk/download/75777581.pdf (accessed on 27th June 2025).

41. Pittman Hardcorn, B. (2022). Effects of tailored colorectal cancer patient education on colorectal cancer screening rates in an urban Kentucky clinic. https://core.ac.uk/download/519802123.pdf (accessed on 27th June 2025).

ENDOCRINE AND METABOLIC DISORDERS

8

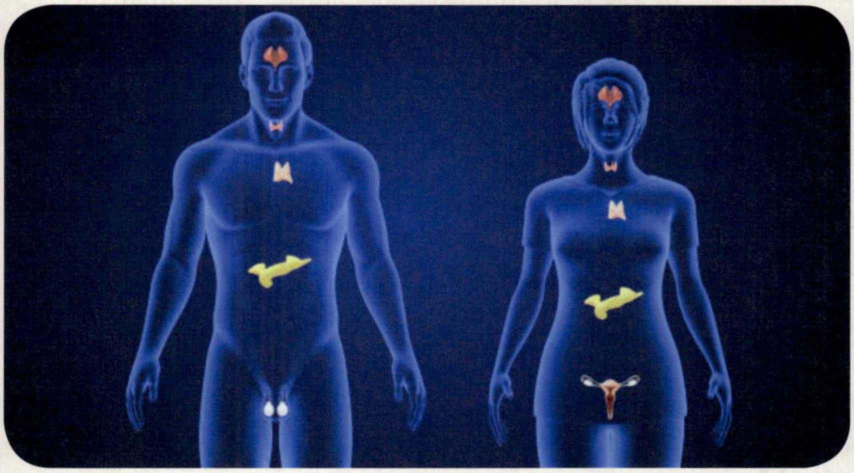

LEARNING OBJECTIVES

After studying this chapter, you will be able to:

1. Discuss the anatomy and physiology of the endocrine system
2. Understand common endocrine and metabolic disorders
3. Describe diagnostic approaches in managing endocrine and metabolic disorders
4. Deal with treatment modalities for managing endocrine and metabolic disorders
5. Focus on emerging research and future directions

Introduction

The area of general medicine involved with metabolic and endocrine disorders plays an extremely significant role in clarifying the complex physiological processes that regulate human health. Endocrine diseases, ranging from conditions of hormone synthesis and regulation, can lead to severe health complications. Metabolic diseases, on the other hand, encompass all types of metabolic balance disturbances of the organism, most often defined by genetic, environmental, and life factors. The interface of the two disciplines suggests that an integral method for diagnosis and therapy is necessary, as endocrine and metabolic derangements can worsen one another. An understanding of their interaction is required in order to develop effective, successful clinical approaches to the therapy of diseases such as diabetes, obesity, and thyroid disease. Lastly, understanding and appreciating these complexities lead to improved patient outcomes through directed interventions that consider endocrine and metabolic wellness as a multidimensional concept. In the last 10 years, there has been an increasing interest in obesity as a disease with significant effects on endocrine function and metabolic regulation. The prevalence of obesity has increased globally, with children and youth disproportionately affected, with severe obesity being a significant and important health problem. It not only causally contributes to many metabolic disorders like type 2 diabetes and CVDs but also presents special therapeutic and management challenges. More recent data indicate that the pathophysiology of obesity is more intricate than has been realized in the past, and this has implications for its treatment approach. For instance, Ameer et al. (2018) note that the effectiveness of treatment interventions is typically short-term, thus the importance of preventive interventions and a comprehensive approach that includes behavioral therapy, diet, and exercise. Obesity, therefore, calls for an interdisciplinary response that acknowledges both its hormonal and metabolic consequences. Furthermore, endocrine disorders such as anorexia nervosa (AN) demonstrate the critical impact that psychiatric disorders may have on metabolic well-being and endocrine function. AN, in particular among young females, illustrates how extreme caloric restriction can lead to profound hormonal derangements and reproductive dysfunction. The disorder is distinguished by underlying endocrine adaptations, which complicate the patients' health condition, resulting in long-term consequences that may affect fertility and pregnancy. According to Ciobanu et al. (2020), these endocrine function disruptions, while reversible, require a delicate understanding of the interconnectedness between endocrine regulation and mental health. Therefore, such disorders ought to be treated holistically, taking into account not only nutritional deficiency but also psychological determinants. This emphasizes the importance of interdisciplinary collaboration to address complex cases with both metabolic and endocrinological implications, ultimately improving patient care under the broad umbrella of general medicine.

Definition of Endocrine Disorders

Endocrine disorders represent a diverse group of ailments resulting from disturbances in the endocrine system, i.e., those glands that produce hormones required for various functions of the body. The hormones released by such glands are messengers that direct organs and tissues to perform specific functions and achieve homeostasis in the body. Both excessive production and lack of production of these hormones can lead to grave medical conditions. For instance, illnesses such as diabetes mellitus are the outcome of disturbed insulin regulation, and illness conditions such as hyperthyroidism and hypothyroidism result from thyroid hormone disturbances. This intricate interaction of hormones illustrates the pivotal role of the endocrine system in overall metabolic health. It highlights the importance of studying endocrine diseases to avert their extensive impact on patients' health. One of the most striking features of endocrine disorders is their multifactorial etiology, which can involve genetic, environmental, and lifestyle factors. Familial hypercholesterolemia is an inherited disorder that could be due to genetic susceptibilities creating faulty genes for producing excessive levels of cholesterol and increased cardiovascular risk. Environmental factors, e.g., exposure to endocrine-disrupting substances, could interfere with hormone function to create conditions for diabetes and obesity. Lifestyle itself contributes largely to endocrine health, as testified by the prevalence of type 2 diabetes, which has a strong link with sedentary lifestyle and obesity. This facet requires clinicians to adopt a holistic view when diagnosing and treating endocrine disorders, focusing instead on the unique case of the individual patient. Understanding the implications of endocrine disease goes beyond immediate clinical relevance; they affect patients' lives in the long term, particularly when attached to endocrine-condition-related conditions like obesity and AN. For example, people with AN may experience severe endocrine disturbances that lead to amenorrhea and infertility as a result of hypothalamic-pituitary-ovarian axis dysfunction. Along with the potential recovery, leftover endocrine consequences can impact maternal health and fertility during pregnancy (Ciobanu et al., 2020). Similarly, obesity has been characterized not only as a state of over-weight but also as a complex chronic disease of energy homeostasis with significant ramifications for metabolic well-being (Ameer et al., 2018). Therefore, a holistic understanding of such disorders is required for holistic healthcare, necessitating the use of individualized interventions that correspond to the complex nature of endocrine and metabolic disorders.

Overview of Metabolic Disorders

Metabolic diseases are a broad range of conditions that disrupt the body's normal metabolic processes, which have an effect on how the body utilizes energy from food. The diseases typically come from either genetic or acquired etiologies that weaken the efficiency of the metabolic pathways. The diseases include diabetes mellitus, obesity, and dietary deficiencies, and all play a significant role in increasing morbidity and mortality rates worldwide. Diabetes, particularly type 2, has reached epidemic proportions and is directly related to physical inactivity and obesity. The resulting metabolic dysfunction, resulting in many systemic complications, merely adds to the complexity of management and treatment. The prevalence of the disorders highlights the need for robust public health measures of prevention and early intervention. Among several metabolic disorders, AN is a complex interaction of psychological and physiological factors. AN is mainly reported in young women, and it leads to extreme caloric restriction, creating extreme nutritional deficits and endocrine disruption. As noted, the disorder evokes extreme endocrine adaptations, which lead to functional amenorrhea and influence reproductive health through its effect on the hypothalamic-pituitary-ovarian axis. Even though the acute effects can be reversed with treatment, the long-term implications significantly affect women's fertility and pregnancy outcomes, thus requiring a clear depiction of the clinical impact of AN. The seriousness with which AN has been examined in the context of metabolic disorders makes it imperative to have an integrated strategy involving psychiatric and nutritional management to achieve optimal recovery and reduce the negative consequences on health (Ciobanu et al., 2020). Obesity is a disease, chronic in nature, of multifactorial etiology based on an imbalance of energy and metabolic mechanism dysregulation. It presently affects a high percentage of the global population, particularly children and adolescents in the United States, where the rates are alarming. Obesity shows a myriad of health impacts. These include hypertension, type 2 diabetes, and cardiovascular illness, which occur in an obesity-grade dependent fashion. The nature of the disease obesity requires a shift in outlook from a simple accumulation of fat; it requires a thorough comprehension of its pathophysiology. Moreover, treatment, particularly for severe obesity, could prove challenging and necessitate a combination of behavioral measures and possibly pharmacologic management. Thus, ensuring a tailored strategy not only for weight management but also considering associated comorbidities is essential in achieving better health outcomes (Ameer et al., 2018).

Importance of Understanding These Conditions

It is crucial to understand the complexities of endocrine and metabolic disorders to provide successful diagnosis and treatment. These disorders, typically characterized by a wide range of symptoms involving hormonal imbalances and metabolic dysfunctions, directly affect the QoL in millions of individuals. A proper understanding of the disorders helps physicians devise intervention strategies for patient-specific needs. Integrative management with lifestyle modification, medication therapy, and patient education is essential for coping with such multifactorial conditions. The severe ramifications of untreated endocrine diseases, such as thyroid disease and diabetes, may lead to serious health outcomes, emphasizing the need for awareness and preventive actions. Hence, describing the pathophysiological mechanisms of these diseases enhances clinical practice and produces an educated patient population, ultimately maximizing overall healthcare efficiency. Beyond the direct health problems mentioned above, knowledge of endocrine and metabolic diseases also has a bearing on public health initiatives. These diseases have a multifactorial etiology, with genetic, environmental, and lifestyle contributions. Insight into how these factors interrelate facilitates more effective public health prevention and education programs. For instance, a focus on the role of obesity in the pathogenesis of type 2 diabetes underscores the importance of large-scale education programs that address diet and physical exercise. Other chronic conditions like hypertension and hyperlipidemia, which are often comorbid conditions with metabolic disorders, can result in staggering healthcare costs. By increasing public awareness of such diseases, health systems can consequently reduce disease burden, resulting in healthier populations and reduced economic burdens related to the management of chronic disease. It is such knowledge of these diseases that provides a foundation for promoting preventive health behaviors on the individual and population levels. One of the most critical components of this knowledge is an understanding of the interlinkage of chronic inflammation and disorders of multiple endocrine organs, such as diabetes and metabolic syndrome. The mechanisms by which hypoxia and inflammation are entwined can have a strongly influential impact on treatment and outcome in the patient. Chronic hypoxia, as defined in certain endocrine and metabolic diseases, may induce inflammatory processes that cause tissue damage and dysfunction. Such an interactive pathophysiologic process can exacerbate underlying disease, begetting a sequence of additional complications necessitating an integrated approach to therapy. For example, chronic hypoxia may provoke exaggerated inflammation that can result in diseases such as cardiovascular complications or neuropathy, the common occurrence of which is found in diabetic patients. Greater insight into these associations enhances the ability of health professionals to design tailored therapies that consider not only short-term symptoms but also the underlying disease mechanisms, thus refining patient management strategies in endocrinology and metabolism (Estrine et al., 2003; Carnevale et al., 2015).

8.1. Anatomy and Physiology of the Endocrine System

Learning Outcome

1. Describe major glands and their functions
2. Understand hormonal regulation and feedback mechanisms
3. Focus on the interaction between the endocrine and metabolic systems

The endocrine system is essential to the regulation of homeostasis by releasing hormones as chemical messengers to regulate various functions of the body. This intricate network includes glands such as the hypothalamus, pituitary, thyroid, adrenal, pancreas, and gonads, each secreting unique hormones that regulate metabolism, growth, reproduction, and stress. The homeostatic reactions involving such hormones are essential for the body's capacity to respond to internal and external alterations. For instance, the thyroid gland regulates the metabolic rates, and the adrenal glands initiate the fight-or-flight response through the secretion of cortisol and adrenaline, showcasing the system's wide-ranging role in physiological control and overall well-being (Sarmidi et al., 2012). Knowledge of the anatomical arrangement of the endocrine system is also required to understand its physiological functions. Each gland is in a strategically favorable position for it to communicate effectively with target organs and tissues. The pituitary gland, or the master gland, is located under the brain's hypothalamus and provides the system with the ability to communicate between the nervous system and the endocrine system.

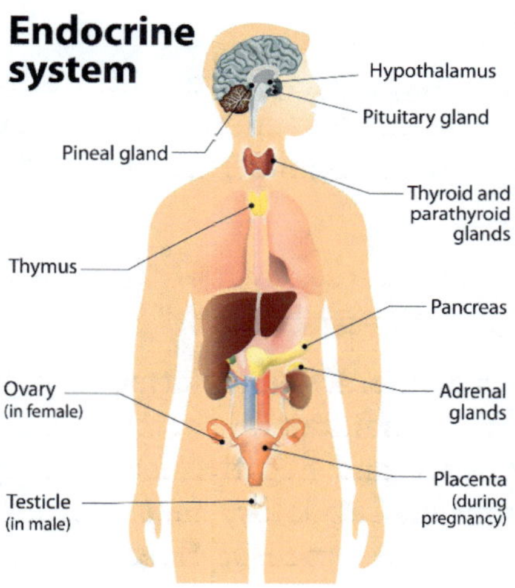

Figure 8.1. Endocrine system.

Source: https://www.inovifertility.com/wp-content/uploads/2024/11/Endocrine-System-scaled-1.jpeg.

This placement enables the pituitary to release hormones that stimulate other glands, creating complex feedback loops vital for regulating various body processes. Moreover, the rich vascular supply to glandular tissues enables quick hormone transportation throughout the body via the blood circulation, emphasizing the endocrine system's rapid capability to respond to physiological demand and stressors (Gardiner et al., 2016). Furthermore, the interaction between metabolism and the endocrine system contributes to good health and the preventionof metabolic disorders. Such hormones include insulin from the pancreas, which increases glucose absorption, and glucagon, which causes the release of glucose. Disruptions in hormone release or receptor sensitivity can lead to metabolic illnesses such as diabetes mellitus, highlighting the need for an interrelated approach to studying anatomy and physiology to address clinical issues. In the clinical context, the recognition of this interdependence allows clinicians to devise effective measures in managing endocrine disorder, thereby enhancing better patient outcomes and QoL (Sarmidi et al., 2012) (Figure 8.1).

8.1.1. Major Glands and Their Functions

The human endocrine system is made up of various major glands, each with vital functions to control various physiological processes. Among these glands, the pituitary gland, commonly known as the master gland, plays a crucial role based on its control over other glands and multiple hormonal pathways. Situated at the base of the brain, it releases essential hormones like growth hormone and prolactin, which are necessary for growth and reproductive functions, respectively. Furthermore, the pituitary gland's conversation with the hypothalamus illustrates the intricate feedback systems regulating hormone secretion, emphasizing its central role in endocrine regulation. This profound orchestration is used to show the necessity of homeostasis. Aberrations in pituitary function lead to disease states like acromegaly or hyperprolactinemia, illustrating the fine balance needed for normal physiological function and the vulnerability to metabolic derangements when imbalances occur. The thyroid gland, another large gland, has a significant influence on metabolic processes through the secretion of thyroid hormones, especially thyroxine (T4) and triiodothyronine (T3). Located in the anterior portion of the neck, the thyroid gland affects energy metabolism, psychosocial maturation, and heat control. Hyperthyroidism, or overactive thyroid, may lead to weight loss, anxiety, and an elevated heart rate, whereas hypothyroidism results in weakness, weight gain, and depression.

The essential role of the thyroid in energy expenditure is also linked to other metabolic diseases, where its function can have a direct impact on overall health. Thus, the understanding of the functioning of the thyroid and its hormone production is required in the diagnosis and management of all endocrine and metabolic diseases that result in systemic effects on health (Estrine et al., 2006). Except for the thyroid and pituitary glands, the adrenal glands are responsible for controlling how the body reacts to stress, as well as serving as metabolism regulators. Situated at the top of the kidneys, the glands have two distinct regions: the cortex and the medulla.

The adrenal cortex produces steroid hormones like cortisol, which control responses to stress, influence metabolism, and inhibit inflammation. In contrast, the adrenal medulla secretes adrenaline and norepinephrine, key players in the mechanism of fight or flight. This redundancy of the role of the adrenal glands serves to emphasize their role in acute stress response as well as in chronic metabolic regulation. Adrenal dysregulation, for example, that seen in Cushing's syndrome and Addison's disease, affects an individual's sense of well-being and metabolism, and therefore addresses the interconnectedness of endocrine functions and their implications for overall medicine (Donaldson et al., 2025) (Figure 8.2).

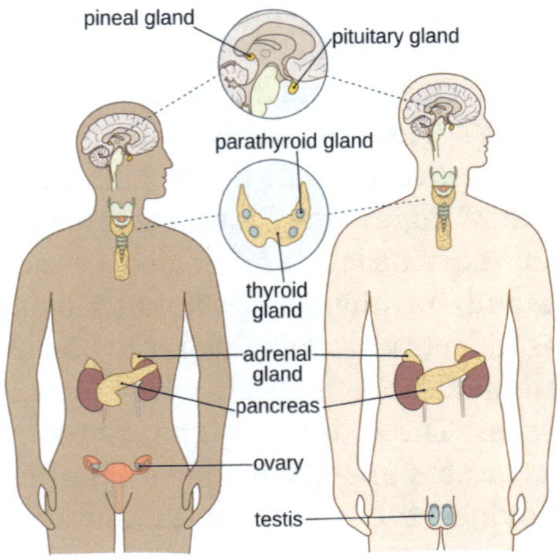

Figure 8.2. Main glands of the human endocrine system.

Source: https://upload.wikimedia.org/wikipedia/commons/thumb/7/78/Endocrine_English.svg/800px-Endocrine_English.svg.png.

8.1.2. Hormonal Regulation and Feedback Mechanisms

The delicate interaction of hormonal regulation is crucial to maintaining homeostasis in the body. Positive and negative feedback systems are significant regulatory mechanisms within the regulatory process. Negative feedback is significant in its role to reduce hormone oscillations and enable the body to stabilize its internal environment in response to deviations. For instance, the hypothalamic-pituitary-adrenal (HPA) axis describes this process: the secretion of cortisol by the adrenal glands inhibits the secretion of CRH and adrenocorticotropic hormone (ACTH), thereby controlling stress reactions. This self-regulation shows how endocrine imbalance results in a variety of disorders, underscoring the important role such feedback mechanisms play in general medicine, and indeed in endocrine and metabolic disease. In addition to negative feedback, positive feedback systems are also essential in the regulation of hormones, but on a minimal basis.

The mechanism reinforces certain physiological responses and is shown to be crucial when an immediate response is required. A classic example is the luteinizing hormone (LH) surge that occurs during ovulation, triggered by heightened estrogen levels. Such mechanisms are critical in order to achieve the hormonal changes needed in processes like reproduction. Health professionals need to comprehend these dynamics, particularly when managing reproductive health issues or metabolic disorders influenced by such cycles of hormones.

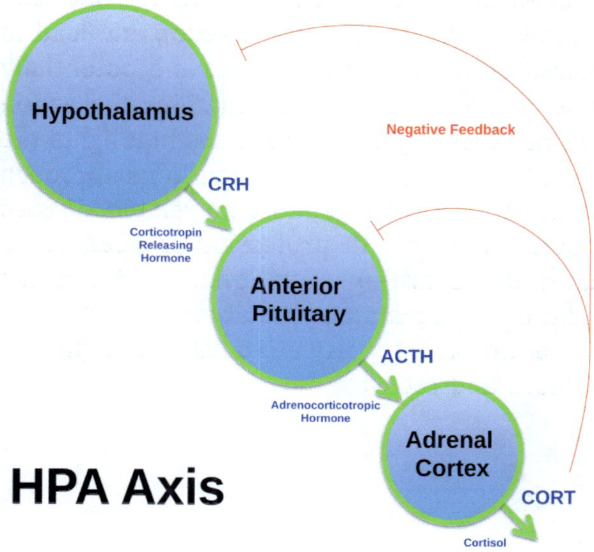

Figure 8.3. Schematic of the HPA axis (CRH: corticotropin-releasing hormone; and ACTH: adrenocorticotropic hormone).

Source: https://upload.wikimedia.org/wikipedia/commons/thumb/e/ee/HPA_Axis_Diagram_%28Brian_M_Sweis_2012%29.svg/800px-HPA_Axis_Diagram_%28Brian_M_Sweis_2012%29.svg.png.

Hormonal dysregulation resulting from breakdowns in the feedback mechanisms can have lasting consequences, like complications from endocrine diseases, thus the importance of these mechanisms in clinical practice. Further investigations have broadened our understanding of hormonal regulation, particularly in relation to circadian rhythms and their role in endocrine homeostasis. Molecular mechanisms behind biological clocks, and their connection to hormonal and metabolic processes, are increasingly becoming clear. Dysregulation of circadian rhythms has important implications for health, which can lead to endocrine diseases such as insulin resistance or disrupted reproductive function. The incorporation of circadian rhythms into the model of hormonal feedback mechanisms introduces a new vision for how hormone patterns play a part in overall well-being. Moreover, interventions on these interactions can provide new directions for the treatment of endocrine and metabolic disorders, further strengthening the need for research in this area to persist. In this field, developments may lead to more effective therapeutic strategies aimed at re-establishing balance to such intricate systems (Bruscalupi et al., 2017) (Figure 8.3).

8.1.3. Interaction Between the Endocrine and Metabolic Systems

There must be coordination of the endocrine and metabolic systems to maintain homeostasis and regulate various body functions. The endocrine system, through the use of hormones, transmits messages to multiple tissues to coordinate metabolic processes like glucose metabolism, lipid storage, and protein synthesis. For instance, insulin released from the pancreas plays a central role in the uptake of glucose by cells and consequently modulates energy availability and metabolic activity. On the other hand, metabolic alterations can feed back on endocrine function, as increased fatty acid availability is thought to lead to insulin resistance with its ensuing aberrant blood glucose control. This multidirectional interaction is a testament to the requirement for knowledge of both systems in the context of metabolic disease, such as diabetes and obesity. Therefore, physicians should be aware of how endocrine as well as metabolic derangements can worsen metabolic dysfunction reciprocally and vice versa, ultimately affecting patient care plans. In addition, the interactive correlation of metabolic syndrome with psychological factors highlights the multidimensionality of health. Increasing evidence indicates that metabolic syndrome is connected with depressive disorders and implies a bidirectional interaction between metabolic and mental health. Specifically, components of metabolic syndrome, such as elevated triglycerides and high blood pressure, have been linked to increased rates of depression, particularly in the pediatric population, where psychosocial problems may enhance metabolic risk. Conversely, anxiety has also been implicated in influencing metabolic syndrome, likely by means of stress- and inflammation-mediated mechanisms. The presence of such a twofold relationship dictates that the treatment of patients with endocrine and metabolic disorders should include a psychological evaluation besides routine metabolic management strategies. Awareness of such connections can lead to improved treatment and well-being among the concerned patients (Michael et al., 2017). Finally, diet influences the interaction between the endocrine and metabolic systems, complicating this interaction. For instance, the role of dietary fiber has been viewed in the context of pancreatic well-being and its overall importance in controlling metabolism. High-fiber diets have revealed protective roles in acute pancreatitis, with mechanisms likely present that maintain the integrity of the gut barrier and reduce systemic inflammation (Badiali et al., 2019). However, in patients with exocrine pancreatic insufficiency, fiber can inhibit pancreatic enzyme function and lead to increased fecal excretion of fat and potentially worsen metabolic derangement. This dual action of fiber and metabolic processes highlights the need for an individualized nutritional approach in the treatment of endocrine-related disease states. Thus, health professionals need to be cautious regarding nutritional factors when treating endocrine and metabolic disorders, as these interactions play a crucial role in patient welfare and recovery.

Test Your Knowledge

1. Name the major endocrine glands in the human body and briefly describe the primary hormone each gland secretes.
2. How do hormones secreted by the adrenal glands affect the body's metabolism and stress response?

8.2. Common Endocrine Disorders

Learning Outcome

1. Explain diabetes mellitus
2. Describe thyroid disorders
3. Define adrenal insufficiency

Endocrine homeostasis is preserved by the control of hormones, which is extremely crucial. Among the various disorders affecting this intricate system, common endocrine diseases such as diabetes mellitus, hyperthyroidism, and hyperparathyroidism have a significant impact on public health. Diabetes mellitus, a disorder that indicates either insulin resistance or disturbed insulin secretion, affects millions of individuals all over the world and results in severe complications such as CVD, neuropathy, and nephropathy. The widespread prevalence of this disorder highlights the importance of effective management and patient counseling to avoid associated risks. As the population ages, the impact of diabetes is likely to increase, thereby adding to the health system's load. It is now more imperative than ever that healthcare professionals recognize symptoms early and provide the appropriate lifestyle treatments and medication. Hyperthyroidism is another prevalent endocrine disorder caused by excess production of thyroid hormones, leading to a condition of hypermetabolism. Hyperthyroidism is often associated with weight loss, palpitations, and anxiety, significantly impairing QoL. Graves' disease is the most common cause, an autoimmune condition responsible for excess thyroid hormone activity. Treatment consists of effective antithyroid drugs, radioactive iodine, and surgery, depending on the severity of the disease and the patient's condition. Notably, there is a link between enhanced all-cause mortality in hyperthyroidism, particularly in elderly patients. This is caused, in part, by underlying diseases that the condition of hyperthyroidism may worsen. Continuation of monitoring and individualized treatment regimens is required to prevent complications and maximize patient outcomes. Finally, primary hyperparathyroidism (PHPT) is a severe endocrine disease, most prevalent in elderly adults, where it is generally detected incidentally on a routine blood test. PHPT is characterized by an increased parathyroid hormone level, causing increased blood calcium levels, which could lead to complications in the form of osteoporosis, nephrolithiasis, and potentially CVD. Evidence is also present for the possibility of a functional correlation between chronic hyperparathyroidism and elevated cortisol levels, both of which enhance the chances of comorbidities in such patients. Complications related to parathyroid surgery, such as transient thyrotoxicosis, further complicate the clinical presentation of these patients. Therefore, appropriate management—especially in older frail patients—is required to optimize recovery and outcomes of health, emphasizing the necessity for specialist-guided approaches in managing PHPT as well as its associated disorders (Armanini et al., 2015). Sleep disturbances resulting from hormonal imbalance may further exacerbate illnesses. Insomnia, particularly in older adults, can be induced by endocrine diseases, thereby creating a cycle of sickness that must be treated holistically (Estrine et al., 2003).

8.2.1. Diabetes Mellitus

The complexity of Diabetes Mellitus transcends its metabolic counterparts, with involvement of intertwinement with other mental conditions such as bipolar disorder. Type 2 diabetes has also been reported to be detrimental to psychiatric illness, particularly the outcome of bipolar disorder, when not well controlled. This relationship demonstrates a significant point of convergence between metabolic and neuropsychiatric disorders that need to be addressed through an interdisciplinary treatment regimen. Individuals diagnosed with both conditions often exhibit a higher severity of bipolar symptoms, which may contribute to neurodegenerative complications. These findings indicate the presence of overlapping clinical pathophysiology, suggesting that effective management of diabetes could also enhance the overall mental health outcomes for affected patients. As a result, collaboration between psychiatric and general medical practitioners is required to address the multi-faceted requirements of such individuals, pointing towards the need for integrated healthcare interventions in addressing co-occurring disorders (Ball et al., 2018).

Moreover, the treatment of Diabetes Mellitus is under transformation with the growing applications of newer surgical interventions. Recent surgical methods, like ileal interposition, have shown promise in providing noteworthy glycemic control, even for non-obese individuals. This process includes the repositioning of a section of the ileum to more effectively stimulate L cells, thereby facilitating the production of GLP-1 hormone. Improved L cell stimulation can augment glucose metabolism and assist in controlling diabetes symptoms. While the short-term results of these operations are promising, more research needs to be carried out to assess their long-term efficacy and histological effects on gut tissue.

As our understanding of the metabolic control role of the GI system develops, such surgeries may represent a welcome addition to the therapeutic repertoire against Diabetes Mellitus, engendering an integrative approach to treatment (Hirata et al., 2011). In this context, patient education and lifestyle modification should become the highest priority as adjuvant factors in the management of Diabetes Mellitus (Figure 8.4).

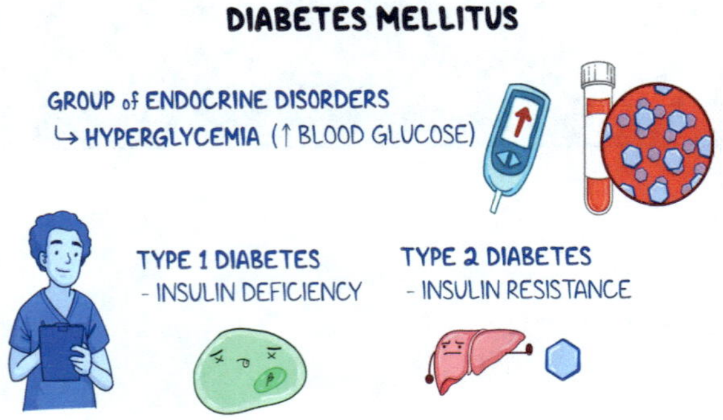

Figure 8.4. Diabetes mellitus.

Source: https://www.osmosis.org/_next/image?url=https%3A%2F%2Fd16qt3wv6xm098.cloudfront.net%2FrYDmLEhXTIa31kql5T6ImjTiQeesycwM%2F_.jpg&w=3840&q=75.

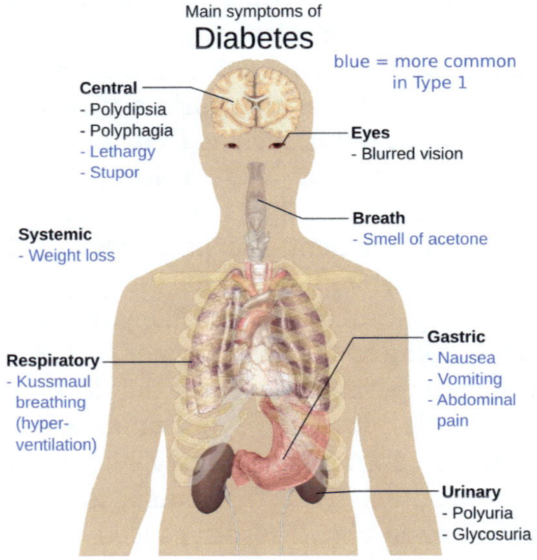

Figure 8.5. Overview of the most significant symptoms of diabetes.

Source: https://upload.wikimedia.org/wikipedia/commons/thumb/0/01/Main_symptoms_of_diabetes.svg/800px-Main_symptoms_of_diabetes.svg.png.

Treatment of this chronic illness includes a holistic practice of dietary adjustments, physical activity, and adherence to prescribed medical treatment. Effective patient education makes patients active partners in their health by helping them understand how their behavior affects blood glucose levels and overall wellness. Besides enhancing glycemic control, lifestyle changes also improve the QoL for patients. With healthcare professionals advocating holistic models of care, it is crucial to include metabolic and psychosocial considerations. In the long run, a holistic approach can significantly reduce the prevalence of Diabetes Mellitus and help appreciate its relevance in the framework of endocrine and metabolic disorders.

8.2.2. Thyroid Disorders

Thyroid disorders comprise a range of disorders that influence the production and regulation of hormones by the thyroid gland, considerably impacting the body's metabolic processes. The most common thyroid disorders are hypothyroidism and hyperthyroidism. Hypothyroidism, which is characterized by decreased hormone production, may appear in the form of fatigue, weight gain, and depression. In contrast, hyperthyroidism, which is marked by excessive levels of hormones, may lead to weight loss, increased heart rate, and anxiety. These imbalances disrupt metabolic homeostasis and affect body functions at the cellular and systemic levels. It is important to understand the biochemical mechanisms of thyroid hormone synthesis and activity to prevent these pathologies and improve patient management. As medical technology improves, the integration of nutritional therapies that support thyroid function has become increasingly important, hence bridging the knowledge gap between endocrinology and nutrition (Sarmidi et al., 2012). The diagnosis of thyroid diseases is often the integration of clinical assessment and laboratory testing. Thyroid-stimulating hormone (TSH) levels are usually measured by doctors as a screening test, with abnormal results necessitating further investigation of free thyroxine (FT4) and triiodothyronine (FT3) levels. While examination of hormone levels is valuable, it is also essential to consider the patient's clinical presentation, history, and risk factors. Increasing evidence suggests the significance of mitochondrial function in thyroid well-being and hormone production. Mitochondria have paramount functions in energy metabolism and steroid hormone biosynthesis, highlighting that mitochondrial dysfunction can be a causative component of thyroid disease (Achermann et al., 2017). Such complex interaction between the endocrine system and mitochondrial health highlights the significance of extensive clinical evaluations that incorporate both hormonal and metabolic assessment in thyroid dysfunction patients.

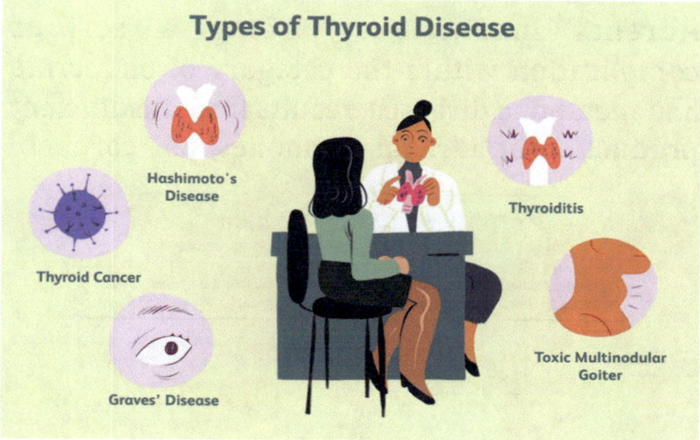

Figure 8.6. Types of thyroid diseases.

Source: https://www.researchgate.net/publication/365649056/figure/fig2/AS:11431281098902079@1669132341755/types-of-thyroid-diseases.png.

Treatment of thyroid diseases is a multi-dimensional process, and in many cases requires hormone replacement therapy or antithyroid drugs based on the type of disease. In patients diagnosed with hypothyroidism, the most common course of treatment involves levothyroxine, which is given to normalize the level of thyroid hormone and associated symptoms. On the other hand, hyperthyroidism is treated with antithyroid drugs, radioactive iodine, or surgery, depending on the severity of the disease and individual patient factors.

In addition, incorporation of lifestyle changes, such as exercise and diet, can improve treatment outcomes by maximizing metabolic health. Evidence suggests that food decisions have a significant influence on thyroid function and can be beneficial in symptom management (Sarmidi et al., 2012). As thyroid pathology continues to evolve, clinical manifestations continue to explore the interaction of thyroid function, metabolic regulation, and mitochondrial activity to formulate new therapeutic modalities and improve patient QoL (Figure 8.6).

8.2.3. Adrenal Insufficiency

Adrenal insufficiency, being a serious complication within the category of endocrine and metabolic diseases, results from insufficient production of adrenal hormones, i.e., cortisol.

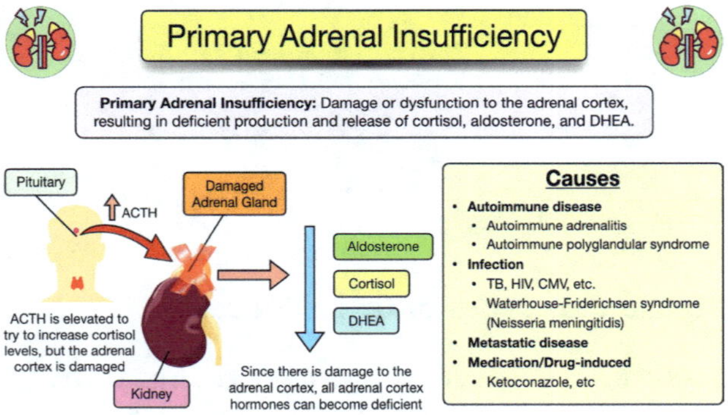

Figure 8.7. Primary adrenal insufficiency.

Source: https://images.squarespace-cdn.com/content/v1/5e48489da899cd09424943db/50ad45d6-9822-4596-8bcd-d453c01fd446/primary-adrenal-insufficiency-addisons-disease-causes.jpeg.

The disorder may present in two forms: primary adrenal insufficiency, or Addison's disease, and secondary adrenal insufficiency due to insufficient production of ACTH. In either subtype, the consequent hormone deficiency can cause a variety of metabolic disturbances such as hypoglycemia, disturbances in electrolyte levels, and impaired stress response. The systemic manifestations of adrenal insufficiency are significant, insofar as it is associated with increased morbidity and mortality due to cardiovascular, metabolic, and infectious disorders. It is essential to elucidate the pathophysiologic mechanisms of adrenal insufficiency in order to create ideal therapeutic strategies and to improve patient outcomes in the global population afflicted by this disorder (Figure 8.7).

Adrenal insufficiency care is disproportionately reliant on glucocorticoid replacement therapy; however, the complexity of treatment presents real challenges. It has been determined through studies that over-replacement of glucocorticoids—especially dosing and timing—most probably exacerbates coexisting metabolic disorders, including insulin resistance and dyslipidemia (Gianfrilli et al., 2018). Such complications are more difficult when adrenal insufficiency is accompanied by other deficiencies of the endocrine system, cumulatively having an unfavorable effect on overall health. Thus, treatment practices by healthcare providers are designed to tailor the application of new glucocorticoid regimens to align more closely with the body's own cortisol rhythms. Accurate patient education regarding medication adherence, stress-induced dose changes, and potential complications is of critical need in optimizing treatment outcomes while preventing acute adrenal crises from occurring. Acute adrenal crises are an emergent state of adrenal insufficiency requiring immediate medical care. Marked by profound hypotension, change in mental status, and electrolyte imbalance, adrenal crises occur unexpectedly, especially in the context of physiological stress like illness or surgery (Falhammar et al., 2017). The incidence ranges from 5 to 10 adrenal crises per 100 patient years, emphasizing the importance of early action planning. Despite the need for immediate intravenous hydrocortisone therapy and fluid resuscitation to reverse such life-threatening attacks, prevention through education of the patient remains the foundation of therapy. Despite recommendations now, it is evident that large numbers of patients do experience adrenal crises, indicating a need for further study to delineate the condition and develop effective preventive measures. Recognition and management of the multifactorial etiology of adrenal crises will be essential to reducing the resultant morbidity and mortality in such groups.

Test Your Knowledge

1. What are the key differences between Type 1 and Type 2. Diabetes Mellitus?
2. What are the main causes and symptoms of hypothyroidism, and how is it diagnosed?
3. Compare and contrast the differences between primary and secondary adrenal insufficiency.

8.3. Common Metabolic Disorders

Learning Outcome

1. Describe obesity and metabolic syndrome
2. Understand hyperlipidemia
3. Explain gout and uric acid metabolism

General metabolic disorders comprise a wide variety of conditions that are often intimately related to hormonal and energy disturbances within the body. Most prominently featured among these are AN and obesity, two diseases that illustrate the diverse pathophysiology of metabolic disease. Obesity, which is an excess of body fat, has become epidemic in current society, killing approximately 17% of U.S. children and adolescents. This multifactorial condition arises from an impairment of energy homeostasis with a plethora of comorbidities, including type 2 diabetes and CVD. The interconnection of obesity and endocrine dysfunction necessitates holistic treatment modalities that address not only weight management but also fundamental metabolic processes, highlighting the importance of multidisciplinary clinical paradigms for treating such diseases (Ciobanu et al., 2020). Contrarily, AN presents a vastly different scenario, reflecting the psychological profile of metabolic disorders. A highly self-imposed starvation and a disturbed body image are characteristics of the disorder that predominantly affects young women and manifests as extreme caloric restriction. The endocrine effect of anorexia can lead to serious complications, like functional amenorrhea as a result of the disruption of the hypothalamic-pituitary-ovarian axis. Interestingly, while such endocrine adjustments are reversible under proper intervention, long-standing nutritional deficiencies pose dire threats to reproductive health and fetal-maternal outcomes in future potential pregnancies (Ciobanu et al., 2020). This highlights the importance of learning about metabolic disorders as intricate disorders for which therapeutic interventions of a generic nature will not be adequate, requiring selective therapy that targets both physical and psychological well-being. Successful management of common metabolic disorders is further hindered by the need for a multifactorial management program that includes behavior modification, dietary intervention, and, when indicated, pharmacological management. In obesity, conventional forms of therapy are generally of limited value, particularly in the more severe cases where prevention becomes the focus rather than intervention. Just one medication, orlistat, is FDA-approved for long-term use in adolescents, highlighting the deficit in pediatric treatment (Ameer et al., 2018). The treatment of anorexia requires not only reconstitution of nutrition but also psychological counseling to counteract the destructive effects of the disease on the mind. Therefore, the resolution of generalized metabolic disorders requires a comprehensive strategy that maximizes interdisciplinary interaction among clinicians, promoting the interdependence of metabolism, endocrinology, and mental well-being.

8.3.1. Obesity and Metabolic Syndrome

The growing prevalence of obesity has been significantly linked with the onset of metabolic syndrome, and it has been identified as a key public health issue. Obesity, which is an energy dysregulation chronic illness, is widespread among many individuals, and severe obesity is more and more worrisome since it now affects nearly 6% of children in the US. Pathophysiologic mechanism of obesity extends beyond fat accumulation; it encapsulates a complex interaction of metabolic and hormonal derangements culminating in insulin resistance and other associated health risks. Type 2 diabetes and CVD are directly proportional to the extent of obesity, implying that optimal prevention and management are the pillars of individual and population health status. Thus, the fight against obesity must be directed towards comprehensive programs involving behavioral therapy, diet, and physical activity to manage this complex condition (Ameer et al., 2018). Obesity and metabolic syndrome are also complicated by conditions like polycystic ovary syndrome (PCOS), where insulin resistance tends to overlap with the clinical presentation of obesity. Studies have shown that phenotypes of PCOS exhibit varying degrees of insulin resistance, with a significant percentage of affected females showing evidence of obesity. The classic phenotype, characterized by hyperandrogenism, long-duration oligoanovulation, and polycystic ovaries, is highly vulnerable to elevated insulin resistance, observed in approximately 80.4% of the affected group. This intricate relationship implies that obesity not only escalates the risk of metabolic syndrome but also impacts its expression among different populations.

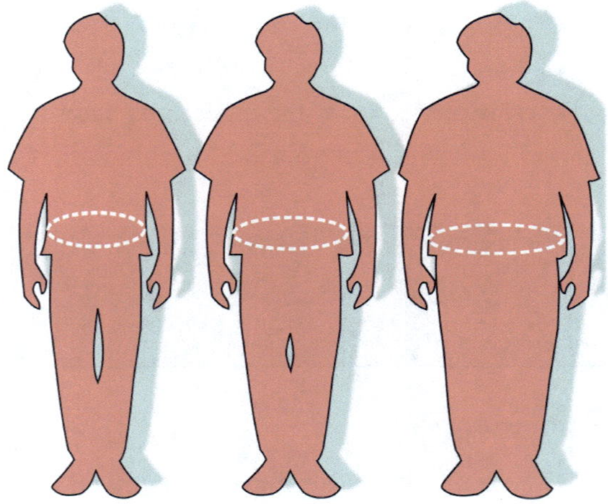

Figure 8.8. Illustration of obesity and waist circumference.

Source: https://upload.wikimedia.org/wikipedia/commons/thumb/0/08/Obesity-waist_circumference.svg/800px-Obesity-waist_circumference.svg.png.

Therefore, recognition of the distinctive phenotypic manifestations of PCOS is critical to implement specific metabolic screening and interventions, ensuring treatment directly targets high-risk populations (Bonin et al., 2013). As understanding of obesity and associated metabolic complications grows, there is an urgent need for more clinical approaches aimed at addressing these compounding problems. Sustained weight control remains a challenging problem, with conventional therapeutic measures having limited effectiveness. Existing pharmacologic treatment, in the form of agents such as orlistat, raises a growing demand for new treatment models to lead patients through the epidemic of obesity. Also, practitioners should be careful about those drugs having the potential to cause weight gain, which could further complicate the comorbidities of obesity and metabolic syndrome (Figure 8.8).

An integrative management that combines pharmacotherapy with lifestyle modification and individualized patient care will be essential in averting the dangers of obesity and its related complexities, ultimately promoting QoL and health outcomes among individuals affected (Ameer et al., 2018) (Figure 8.9).

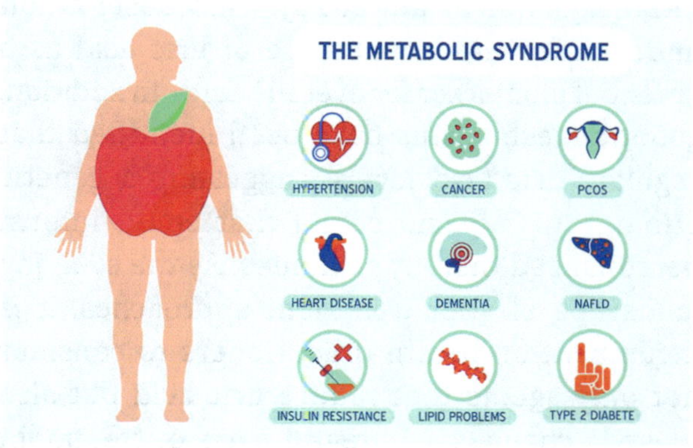

Figure 8.9. The metabolic syndrome.

Source: https://oxyjon.s3.ap-south-1.amazonaws.com/blog/wp-content/uploads/2023/07/07073041/Metabolic-Syndrome-and-Diabetes.jpg.

8.3.2. Hyperlipidemia

Hyperlipidemia, a high level of lipids in the blood, is one of the significant risk factors for most endocrine and metabolic illnesses, particularly CVD. Hyperlipidemia tends to be divided based on what type of lipid is elevated—cholesterol, triglycerides, or both. The consequences of hyperlipidemia extend beyond simple lipid disorder; they can lead to hazardous health effects like atherosclerosis, pancreatitis, and fatty liver disease. Recent studies have indicated the interconnection of hyperlipidemia with metabolic syndrome and complicating factors that present challenges in the treatment of the patient in clinic visits. With increasing realization among medical professionals about the very interconnected nature of hyperlipidemia, a unified approach of treatment consisting of lifestyle modifications, drug management, and follow-up will be necessary to overcome the associated risks. Hyperlipidemia management needs to be tailored to individual risk factors such as genetic predispositions and comorbidities. Statins are likely the most commonly prescribed medications for cholesterol lowering, but their efficacy is influenced by concurrent medical conditions such as diabetes or obesity. The relationship between hyperlipidemia and psychiatric disorders, particularly schizophrenia, has been underscored in recent publications. Schizophrenia patients have an increased rate of hyperlipidemia and related conditions, for the most part caused by the side effects of the use of antipsychotic drugs (Saari et al., 2005). Antipsychotic medication has the potential to increase cholesterol and triglyceride levels, adding to the reason why medical doctors need to monitor lipid levels regularly for this group of individuals. An understanding of these correlations can guide more effective treatments for both mental disease and metabolic disease. Furthermore, increasing the prevalence of hyperlipidemia highlights the importance of prevention and early intervention in public health strategies. Prevention and early intervention campaigns for healthy living and exercise may significantly contribute to changing lipid levels and general metabolic status among the population. Novel evidence introduces the systemic nature of hyperlipidemia, primarily its link with metabolic syndrome and cardiovascular comorbidities (Altschul et al., 2024). The bio-systemic interaction between lipid metabolism and endocrine function highlights the need for integrated healthcare management that caters to both nutritional and pharmacological interventions. By focusing on education and proactive management principles, the healthcare community can help reduce the negative consequences of hyperlipidemia and enhance overall patient outcomes when managing endocrine and metabolic diseases (Figure 8.10).

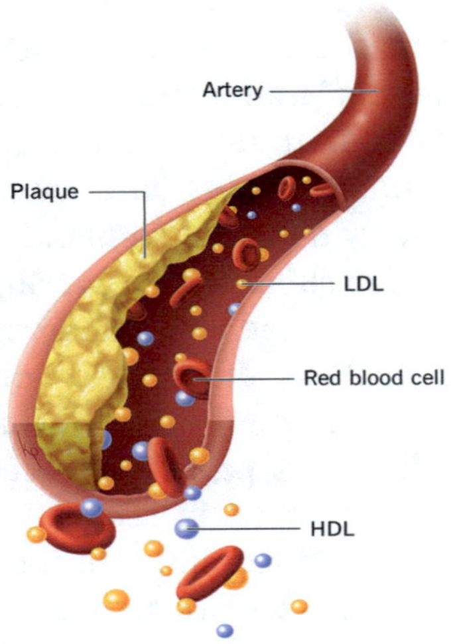

Figure 8.10. Hyperlipidemia illustration.

Source: https://my.clevelandclinic.org/-/scassets/images/org/health/articles/21656-hyperlipidemia-illustration.ashx.

8.3.3. Gout and Uric Acid Metabolism

Gout, an inflammatory form of arthritis, is characterized mainly by the presence of monosodium urate crystals within joints as a result of elevated levels of serum uric acid, or hyperuricemia. Uric acid is a purine metabolite, and its formation is tightly controlled in a normal individual. Excess production of uric acid may result from causes such as diminished renal excretion or increased dietary purine intake. Understanding the metabolic pathways that lead to the production and excretion of uric acid is important for properly diagnosing and treating gout. Long-term contact with high levels of uric acid may not only lead to the painful attacks of gout but also the risk of CKD and cardiovascular conditions, indicating timely and proper interventions and treatment modalities in the management of these interrelated conditions (Osorio-Alonso et al., 2016).

The linkage of hyperuricemia with the spectrum of metabolic disorders, such as hypertension and CVD, has been the subject of extensive research interest. Epidemiological evidence supports that hyperuricemia is implicated in the pathogenesis of various clinical disorders, with recent findings suggesting an intimate correlation between elevated serum urate and conditions such as hypertension and CKD (Agarwal et al., 2018). This observation underscores the prominence of uric acid as a potential biomarker for overall health. In addition, genetic mechanisms have been identified that regulate uric acid levels, suggesting a genetic etiology to hyperuricemia that could inform personalized therapy regimens. As the evolving landscape of gout treatment approaches, it is incumbent on health practitioners to consider not only agents that reduce uric acid but also lifestyle changes as integral parts of treatment plans. Antioxidant therapy may be a practical approach to decreasing the oxidative stress associated with hyperuricemia.

The biochemical intricacy of uric acid metabolism intersects with oxidative stress pathways, especially in CKD patients, in whom high levels of uric acid drive inflammatory processes (Osorio-Alonso et al., 2016). Recent research data have indicated that interventions, including dietary antioxidants and pharmacologic therapy to reduce uric acid levels, are feasible and can lower oxidative stress and improve renal function. As evidence accumulates for the associations of hyperuricemia with various adverse health outcomes, the inclusion of antioxidant therapies could be beneficial to gout and comorbid condition treatment. Longitudinal studies in the future would be necessary to examine the efficacy of such interventions while elucidating the complex interplay among uric acid metabolism, inflammatory responses, and oxidative stress to optimize treatment outcomes for patients with metabolic diseases (Figure 8.11).

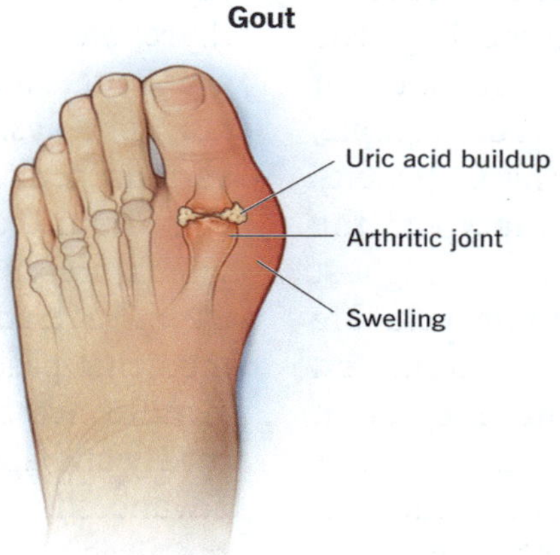

Figure 8.11. Gout.

Source: https://my.clevelandclinic.org/-/scassets/images/org/health/articles/gout.

Test Your Knowledge

1. What is metabolic syndrome, and how is it linked to obesity?
2. Describe the role of uric acid metabolism in the pathogenesis of gout and identify factors that contribute to hyperuricemia.

8.4. Diagnostic Approaches

Learning Outcome

1. Understand the role of blood tests and hormone level assessments
2. Describe imaging techniques for gland evaluation
3. Focus on genetic testing and its relevance

A sound diagnostic approach is critical in the management of endocrine and metabolic disorders, as they often present with overlapping syndromes that need a thorough evaluation. Clinicians must use an arsenal of diagnostic tools, including long patient histories, physical examinations, and advanced laboratory testing. For instance, disorders such as AN directly impact endocrine function, with complications arising as amenorrhea and alterations in reproductive potential due to dysfunctions in the hypothalamic-pituitary-ovarian axis. Early diagnosis of such presentations is vital since most of the physiologic changes are reversible if addressed in a timely way. Thus, a proper understanding of the disorder's clinical presentation enhances diagnostic accuracy and allows for the implementation of best treatment practices that can mitigate risk for long-term complications, e.g., reproductive dysfunction, in affected individuals (Ciobanu et al., 2020). In addition, the characterization of particular phenotypes in disorders like PCOS demonstrates the usefulness of personalized diagnostic approaches. Through evaluation of diagnostic criteria set by the Rotterdam consensus, clinicians can distinguish between PCOS phenotypes based on specific features such as hyperandrogenism and menstrual disturbance. Such classifications not only aid in the diagnosis of the condition but also guide the assessment of metabolic risk for each phenotype. For example, research depicts profound genetic heterogeneity of insulin resistance across phenotypes; the most common phenotype exhibits the highest rate of insulin resistance, providing valuable information for building individualized management plans. Therefore, the integration of targeted diagnostic evaluations provides the opportunity for individualized treatment and prevention, enhancing patient outcome in metabolic health (Bonin et al., 2013). Use of both biochemical and imaging tests also further enhances clinical assessments in endocrine disorder diagnosis. The application of hormonal assays can reveal dysregulations in hormone secretion levels, while imaging processes such as ultrasound or MRI can detect alterations in endocrine gland structures. For example, ovarian morphology measurement in women suspected of having PCOS is essential in diagnosing and determining the extent to which such conditions affect metabolic function. Additionally, the combination of these diagnostic modalities allows for a better appreciation of the patient's overall health, enabling earlier implementation of interventions and more optimal treatment strategies. Finally, an integrated diagnostic approach, which combines clinical evaluation with high-tech examination, must be employed to navigate the array of endocrine and metabolic diseases and to promote greater long-term health in those afflicted with them.

8.4.1. Blood Tests and Hormone Level Assessments

Blood tests and endocrine and metabolic disorder evaluations of hormone levels are essential diagnostic and management tools for endocrine and metabolic disorders. The blood tests provide useful information about the hormonal regulation necessary to ensure homeostasis. For instance, thyroid function tests, which measure thyroid-stimulating hormone (TSH) and free thyroxine (fT4), are essential in the detection of hypothyroidism or hyperthyroidism. Thyroid hormone dysregulations can potentially lead to serious health outcomes, including metabolic compromise and cardiovascular comorbidities, which necessitate accurate assessment for effective treatment. For this reason, general medicine practitioners need to understand the significance of these tests in order to institute timely and appropriate interventions. Secondly, advances in laboratory methods have enhanced the precision and reproducibility of hormone assays, which are imperative in the evaluation of heterogeneous endocrine disorders. Methods such as liquid chromatography with mass spectrometry (LC-MS) have increased the sensitivity of testing for hormone levels, allowing small traces of hormones to be detected in the blood. This is particularly beneficial for diseases that may involve subtle hormonal imbalances, i.e., adrenal insufficiency or PCOS. Moreover, as more is discovered through research, clinicians must stay abreast of changing guidelines on interpreting hormone levels to optimize patient care. Implementation of EBPs into clinical practice enhances decision-making and, by default, patient outcomes in endocrine medicine. There is substantial evidence that calls for an assessment of environmental factors in relation to hormone levels. Research has proven that exposure to certain environmental pollutants, including polybrominated diphenyl ethers (PBDEs) and polychlorinated biphenyls (PCBs), influences hormonal status and can cause conditions like hypothyroxinemia. For example, a study demonstrated that domestic dogs exposed to the pollutants exhibited alterations in thyroid hormone levels, which means that such trends would be present in humans exposed to them. Therefore, understanding the larger picture of hormone level measurements in relation to environmental factors is important for medical professionals, as it can provide better insight into the possible etiologies of endocrine diseases and guide prevention efforts. The integrated process supports the importance of complete blood checks and hormone measurement in the treatment of endocrine and metabolic disorders (Blum et al., 2018; Kass et al., 2017) (Figure 8.12).

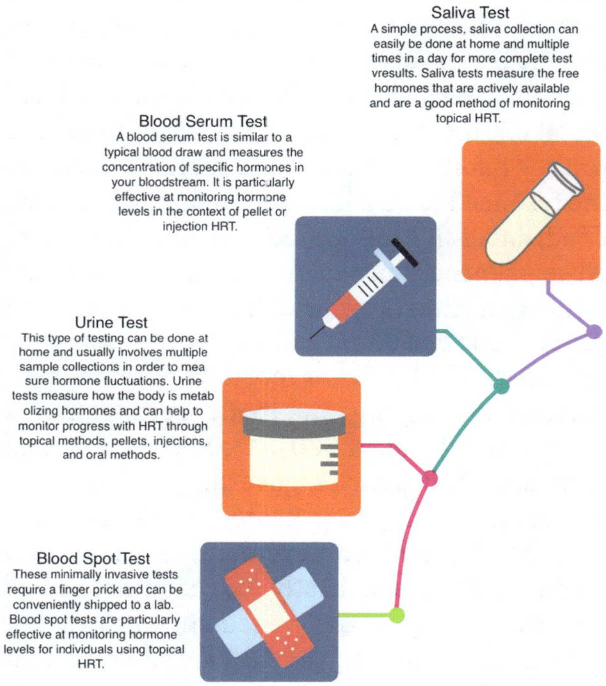

Figure 8.12. Types of hormone tests.

Source: https://www.bodylogicmd.com/wp-content/uploads/2020/04/types-of-hormone-tests.jpg.

8.4.2. Imaging Techniques for Gland Evaluation

Evaluation of glands in the context of endocrine and metabolic conditions relies significantly on advanced imaging modalities to enhance diagnostic accuracy and the outcome of treatment. Traditional modalities such as CT and ultrasound have been an integral part of standard practice for decades, offering information on the morphology of the glands. The latest advancements in imaging modalities, such as MRI and AFI, are revolutionizing gland evaluation. This is particularly relevant in assessing conditions such as thyroid diseases, where correct localization and characterization of nodules are crucial. AFI, for instance, exploits the intrinsic fluorescence of tissues to facilitate real-time feedback intraoperatively, enhancing the ability to differentiate between parathyroid and thyroid tissues, a significant factor in reducing complications in thyroid surgeries (Aigner et al., 2020). Additionally, the unique advantage of AFI as an up-and-coming tool for gland examination outside traditional applications, and especially within the realm of endocrinology, has been made increasingly apparent. While AFI has long been utilized in ophthalmology, its clinical application is being expanded to thyroid and parathyroid assessments. Studies have revealed that skin autofluorescence is an indicator that can be used to predict systemic conditions like diabetes and cardiovascular health, thus further confirming the multifunctional applications of this method in the assessment of gland function and homeostasis (Aigner et al., 2020). In addition, the increased sensitivity and resolution in imaging now allow for pathology identification at an earlier phase, thus resulting in enhanced patient management results. Specifically, the development of these technologies is a paradigm shift toward individualized medicine with imaging at the forefront of developing treatment protocols based on detailed gland evaluations. Despite the promising developments in imaging techniques, several challenges are present to standardize these techniques for clinical use across the board. The heterogeneity of imaging techniques and the lack of regulatory guidelines can make comparability across studies challenging, leading to variability in clinical outcomes. The introduction of new technologies, such as AFI, into day-to-day practice necessitates rigorous testing to implement standardized protocols that enhance the reproducibility of results in diverse clinical environments.

Moreover, although the initial results of AFI's effectiveness in discriminating glandular tissues during surgery are encouraging, further studies are warranted to fully account for its potential and improve its accuracy in different operating environments. Continued studies on these imaging modalities will be required to refine their applications in appropriately assessing the gland in the treatment of endocrine and metabolic diseases.

8.4.3. Genetic Testing and Its Relevance

The rationale of genetic testing in the context of endocrine and metabolic disorders runs deep, particularly in the early diagnosis of diseases such as Type II Diabetes Mellitus. The increasing incidence of the disorder, more so in children, makes genetic predisposition increasingly a crucial factor. Genetic testing can explain familial patterns, identify those at heightened risk, and lead to early intervention strategies. Knowledge of the genetic underpinnings of this heterogeneously expressed disorder allows clinicians to individualize treatment and prevention plans, focusing on modifiable risk factors like diet and exercise. As indicated in current studies, early detection and intervention can drastically counteract risk for severe comorbidities like cardiac disease and renal failure, inevitably resulting from extended diabetes treatment (Kapke et al., 2015). Therefore, genetic testing is a critical tool in averting the long-term consequences of metabolic disorders. Genetic testing is also a crucial tool in treating and diagnosing endocrine disorders, as it facilitates the identification of syndromic disorders resulting from genetic mutations. For instance, specific genetic abnormalities have been linked to adrenal insufficiency or thyroid disease, where identifying the underlying genetic cause influences therapeutic interventions. Patients presenting with signs consistent with these disorders may undergo genetic testing not only for diagnostic purposes but also to guide the management approach. In the clinical environment, detecting patterns of endocrine abnormalities through genetic profiles can help adopt a more individualized care approach. Such personalized approaches may comprise personalized doses of hormone replacement therapies (HRTs) or intervention on specific gene-associated pathways, optimizing patient outcomes in treating endocrine disorders. Other than its therapeutic and diagnostic advantages, genetic testing also poses key ethical issues that need to be seriously considered in endocrine and metabolic disease management. Issues of genetic privacy, informed consent, and equitable access to the test need to be addressed so that the benefits of advances in genetic medicine are available to all segments uniformly. For instance, in patients with acanthosis nigricans and suspected genetic backgrounds, caution is necessary, as demonstrated by case reports of patients with various underlying metabolic derangements (Vincentiis et al., 2020). Developing ethical standards and policies governing the practice of genetic testing can protect patients while promoting scientific developments in such a fast-evolving field. Lastly, the significance of genetic testing in daily medicine comes not only from enhancing diagnosis and treatment but also from constructing an ethical and fair system of healthcare for managing endocrine and metabolic diseases (Figure 8.13).

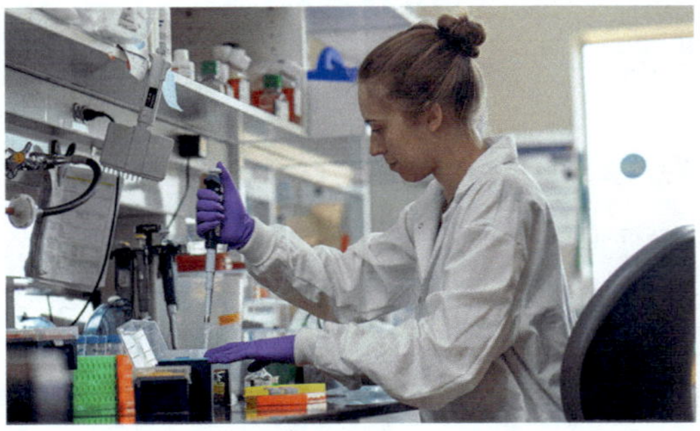

Figure 8.13. Genetic testing.

Source: https://www.ashg.org/wp-content/uploads/2025/04/Photo-Laboratory-imagery-744x444-1.png.

Test Your Knowledge

1. What are the common blood tests and hormone assays used to diagnose thyroid disorders?
2. Which imaging techniques are most effective for evaluating the structure and function of endocrine glands such as the pituitary, adrenal, and thyroid glands?

8.5. Treatment Modalities

Learning Outcome

1. Explain how pharmacological interventions play a pivotal role in managing endocrine and metabolic disorders
2. Focus on lifestyle modifications and dietary management
3. Understand surgical options for endocrine disorders

Effective treatment modalities are required for the treatment of endocrine and metabolic disorders, which range from a plethora of conditions such as diabetes, obesity, and hormone-related conditions. Hormone replacement therapy is an essential strategy, particularly in trans populations attempting to synchronize their physical characteristics with their gender identity. The Endocrine Society has established protocols that endorse hormone therapies, such as estrogens with antiandrogens for trans women and testosterone for trans men. Beyond encouraging desired physical change, these therapies also encourage great psychological benefits, including enhanced mental health and reduced anxiety and depression symptoms. Using a multidisciplinary treatment modality, healthcare providers personalize hormone therapies based on each patient's specific needs, thereby maintaining both body and mind well-being during the transition, as seen in recent literature on gender-affirming interventions (Arcelus et al., 2018). In addition to hormone therapies, lifestyle interventions remain the mainstay of metabolic disorders, particularly type 2 diabetes control. Despite guidelines emphasizing regular exercise, adherence in high-risk groups is less than satisfactory. New treatment interventions like whole body vibration training (WBVT) have recently been presented as potential alternatives for traditional exercise, specifically targeted towards those who have difficulty performing traditional workout exercises. Early research indicates that WBVT is capable of enhancing insulin sensitivity, as indicated by a considerable reduction in homeostasis model assessment of insulin resistance (HOMA-IR) after a structured training program. This kind of study emphasizes the importance of examining varied and accessible physical activities suitable for different groups of patients, as nonadherence to traditional exercise prescriptions can otherwise negate health benefits in patients at risk of endocrine metabolic disorders (Babraj et al., 2017). Moreover, pharmacological treatment becomes paramount in the treatment of endocrine disorders other than hormone therapy. Medications that correct problems such as hyperthyroidism or insulin resistance are needed to restore balance and optimize metabolic function. For instance, medicines like thionamides or radioactive iodine can be employed in thyroid disease to reduce excessive hormone production. Similarly, medications like metformin are commonly used to correct insulin resistance, effectively controlling blood glucose in type 2 diabetes. Such pharmacotherapy not only alleviates short-term symptoms but also corrects chronic complications of such disorders. Strategic use of pharmacologic drugs, combined with changes in lifestyle and hormone replacement, depicts an integrated approach to endocrine and metabolic disorders, thus improving QoL and patient outcomes.

8.5.1. Pharmacological Interventions

Pharmacological management is at the core of the management of endocrine and metabolic disorders and plays a vital role in QoL in patients. Pharmacological management is directed towards restoring hormonal imbalances and metabolic derangements, resulting in symptomatic relief and long-term prevention of complications. For instance, insulin and oral hypoglycemic therapy is at the core of managing type 2 diabetes, where glucose control is critical to prevent severe complications such as nephropathy and neuropathy. Similarly, thyroid hormone replacement is essential in the management of hypothyroidism, keeping metabolic activity at its optimum functioning. As the pharmacological environment evolves, research continuously assesses the safety and effectiveness of new drugs for treatment, continually enhancing patient outcomes.

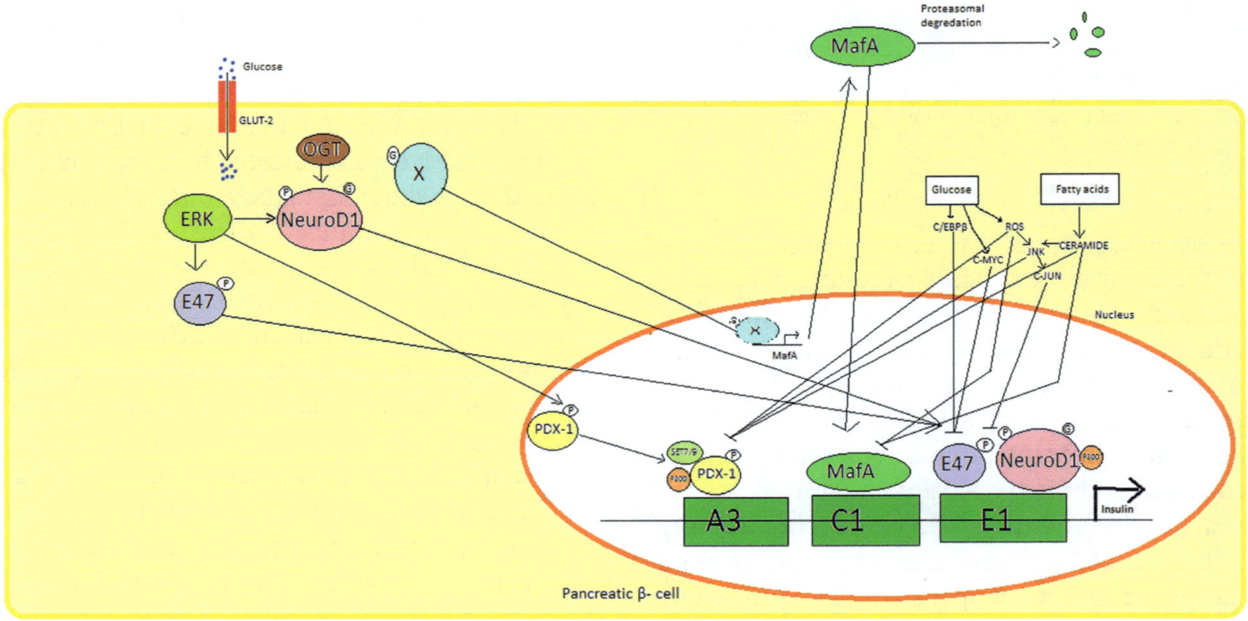

Figure 8.14. Diagram of insulin regulation upon high blood glucose.

Source: https://upload.wikimedia.org/wikipedia/commons/6/6a/Insulin_gene_activation.png.

Cushing's syndrome is just one of many examples of how pharmacologic management of endocrine disease may be complicated. It is a result of excess production of cortisol and is characterized by many disabling signs and symptoms and complications. The treatments are usually surgical, but when surgery is not feasible, drug therapy is the priority. Cortisol synthesis inhibitors such as ketoconazole and metyrapone have proven effective in reducing cortisol. The treatments address most of the metabolic complications of the syndrome, including glucose intolerance, hypertension, and obesity. The importance of early diagnosis and prompt pharmacological treatment cannot be overstated, as they play a vital role in restricting the pathogenicity of the condition and improving overall patient survival rates (Biller et al., 2016). Further, pharmacological treatment is increasingly intertwined with behavioral and psychological factors, especially about the psychological repercussions of most endocrine disorders. It is well evident that chronic disease management extends beyond the physical to include the psychological well-being of patients as well. Chronic stress and endocrine imbalances support the need for holistic treatment regimens. Therefore, healthcare professionals must integrate a holistic process by applying pharmacological modalities combined with treatments such as cognitive behavior therapy to address mental well-being. This integration is required, as Estrine et al. (2006) state that stress has a significant impact on the development of endocrine diseases. A multidimensional perspective enables practitioners to treat both the biological and psychological factors of endocrine and metabolic diseases simultaneously (Figure 8.14).

8.5.2. Lifestyle Modifications and Dietary Management

Effective treatment of PCOS demands a multi-dimensional approach, particularly in the form of lifestyle interventions and diet control. Weight loss is a significant intervention, even for women who may not necessarily present with obesity as the main symptom. Studies have established that modest weight loss is enough to enhance insulin sensitivity and regularize menstrual cycles, which enhances many of the symptoms associated with PCOS. Certain dietary modifications, such as reducing saturated fat intake and balancing unsaturated fats, could also accompany weight loss and augment metabolic function. The combination of a healthy diet and weight management not only controls the chief metabolic complications of PCOS but is also beneficial for symptoms like hirsutism and the management of acne, thus overall well-being (Ghazeeri et al., 2021). In addition, the role of diet in controlling PCOS cannot be overemphasized. Evidence indicates that high GI foods are detrimental to insulin sensitivity, which contributes to type 2 diabetes, a prevalent comorbidity in PCOS women. Thus, following a diet of low-GI foods like whole grains, green vegetables, and legumes may control blood glucose and alleviate insulin resistance. Nutritional treatment in medicine has also become an important method, with the potential of customized diet interventions that take into account the statuses of different individuals and their preferences. Utilization of dietary measures raises the efficacy of PCOS symptom control, underlining the importance of individualized dietary planning in a comprehensive treatment plan (Namoosi et al., 2024). Besides diet control, daily physical exercise is a fundamental component in the overall management of PCOS. Exercise has been proven to enhance insulin sensitivity, weight control, and general physical health. It is suggested that a minimum of 150 minutes of moderate-intensity aerobic exercise weekly can be highly beneficial. In addition, the inclusion of resistance training can also enhance metabolic effects by stimulating lean muscle mass. Behavior modification that maintains both physical activity and diet not only assists in symptom control but also prevents long-term PCOS complications. By application of a holistic management approach including these dimensions, PCOS women can benefit with significant health and quality-of-life outcomes, thus highlighting the importance of a multi-factorial approach in overall medicine for endocrine and metabolic diseases (Ghazeeri et al., 2021).

8.5.3. Surgical Options for Endocrine Disorders

Surgery has a significant role to play in the treatment of most endocrine disorders, particularly in cases where conservative management fails. Endocrine surgery is also most commonly indicated for conditions such as hyperparathyroidism, thyroid neoplasms, and adrenal neoplasms. Thyroidectomy or lobectomy may effectively relieve symptoms and avert cancer dissemination in benign thyroid nodules or malignancies. In addition, parathyroidectomy is a routine surgical intervention in cases of PHPT, particularly symptomatic HM. By removing the hyperfunctioning gland(s), these procedures not only eliminate immediate health problems but also improve long-term outcomes. These procedures underscore the importance of early surgical intervention in offering the overall QoL in patients with endocrine diseases. Another broad area of endocrine surgery is the management of pancreatic neuroendocrine tumors (PNETs). Although comparatively rare, these tumors can manifest with a range of behaviors from benign to highly malignant and hence need personalized surgical care. Whipple operations and enucleations are two of the surgical techniques employed, depending on the size, location, and general health status of the patients. Surgical resection is the most successful mode of treatment of localized PNETs, capable of producing curative outcomes. Besides, refinement of minimally invasive surgeries has become the modern vogue, offering patients shorter recovery times and fewer surgical hazards. All this is a trend towards a more scientific and patient-oriented approach to the management of complex endocrine ailments, underlining the relevance of surgical expertise in contemporary endocrinology. Surgical interventions for endocrine disorders extend beyond tumor resection and embrace operations for hormone regulation and metabolic balance. For example, bariatric surgery has been proven to be an effective treatment for the management of morbid obesity and associated metabolic disease, as obesity is well known to enhance a multitude of endocrine dysfunctions. This option is particularly pertinent for adolescents, with recent evidence recognizing obesity as a chronic illness that has a complex impact on energy homeostasis, as underscored in more recent research. Operations such as gastric bypass or sleeve gastrectomy not only induce significant weight reduction but also lead to increases in insulin sensitivity and a decrease in type 2 diabetes prevalence in patients. Furthermore, understanding the endocrine effects of such procedures emphasizes the importance of incorporating surgical treatment into a comprehensive strategy for endocrine and metabolic disorders, ultimately improving patient outcomes and long-term health prospects (Figure 8.15).

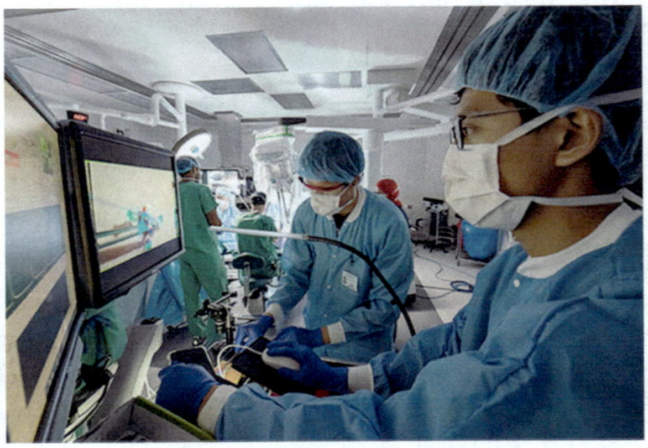

Figure 8.15. Endocrine surgery.

Source: https://health.ucdavis.edu/media-resources/contenthub/health-library/treatments/endocrine-surgery-marquee.jpg.

Test Your Knowledge

1. How do lifestyle modifications, including diet and exercise, contribute to the management and prevention of metabolic syndrome?
2. In which endocrine disorders is surgery considered a primary or adjunctive treatment, and what are the common surgical procedures involved?

8.6. Emerging Research and Future Directions

Learning Outcome

1. Understand the advances in hormone replacement therapies
2. Focus on genetic research and personalized medicine
3. Deal with innovations in metabolic disorder management

New literature in the field of endocrine and metabolic disorders indicates the extreme interaction between psychosocial status and physical health outcomes. Recent research suggests that stressors experienced throughout the lifespan, particularly among elderly individuals, are recognized to exacerbate conditions like diabetes and obesity. The link highlights the need for a multidimensional treatment approach involving medical and psychological therapy. With scientists exploring these correlations further, understanding the influence of chronic stress on metabolic pathways holds promise to unlock new avenues in treatment. Importantly, this coming together of metabolic management and behavioral health can allow for more personalized care, improving patient outcomes and general well-being, particularly in those population segments that are most vulnerable, e.g., the elderly individual who may carry a high load of stress and attendant health issues (Estrine et al., 2003). As the field of medical research continues to evolve, technology and data analysis take center stage in broadening our understanding of endocrine and metabolic disorders. The use of big data and machine learning techniques is revolutionizing the practice of diagnosis and treatment algorithms, enabling them to target patient care more specifically. New technology can facilitate easier identification of biomarkers for specific disorders, leading to earlier diagnosis and treatment. Also, wearables and health apps are propelling real-time monitoring of metabolic metrics, delivering patients and clinicians unprecedented insights into personal health patterns. The innovations also produce models of care that can integrate evidence-based care more appropriately, enabling patients to receive cutting-edge care supported by the latest research evidence (Estrine et al., 2006). In the coming days, the focus on avoiding endocrine and metabolic diseases will definitely gain momentum. Research increasingly highlights the contribution of lifestyle factors, such as sleep and physical activity, to maintaining metabolic well-being. It has been observed in aging individuals that chronic insomnia can be associated with a spectrum of health ailments, and this calls for comprehensive sleep tests to be included as a part of metabolic disorder programs (Estrine et al., 2003). The way forward will undoubtedly include population-based health promotion programs that promote education about these lifestyle factors. Moreover, interdisciplinary collaboration among endocrinologists, nutritionists, and mental health professionals could contribute to the efficacy of treatment in the provision of diverse support that appeals to the specific needs of the patients. Preventive care, education, and integrated care methods will be imperative in addressing the growing burden of endocrine and metabolic disorders.

8.6.1. Advances in Hormone Replacement Therapies (HRTs)

The evolving picture of the HRT has become a significant problem in internal medicine for the management of endocrine and metabolic disease. Advances in HRT are particularly relevant to populations with hormonal deficiency, such as postmenopausal women and breast cancer survivors. While traditional hormone treatments have been the norm, new data warn against their administration in women with a history of breast cancer because of the risk potential. It has been reported by Davis et al. (2017) that non-hormonal therapies like selective serotonin/noradrenaline reuptake inhibitors and gabapentin are now effective treatments for menopausal symptoms such as vasomotor symptoms (VMS). Transitioning to non-hormonal therapies is required not only to alleviate symptoms but also to prevent related health risks, highlighting the importance of individualized treatment approaches concerning both QoL and safety in treating patients. Furthermore, the progress of HRTs extends beyond the symptomatic treatment of postmenopause. The incorporation of new modes of treatment, particularly genetic and molecular treatments, has the potential to significantly improve patient outcomes. An example of this is evident in recent news stories on Duchenne muscular dystrophy (DMD), where multidisciplinary approaches involving endocrine management are central to enhancing patient QoL and survival. This evolution requires a better understanding of how hormone therapies should be optimized based on emergent scientific evidence and individual patient needs. Such integration is a sign of a paradigm shift towards predictive diagnostics and curative treatments designed to restore hormonal homeostasis and address indiscriminate health concerns. Finally, the discussion of enhancements in HRTs also extends to treating such disorders as vulvovaginal atrophy (VVA) and osteoporosis. Female patients who previously may have been precluded from standard HRT due to breast cancer now seek these novel treatments, including low-dose vaginal estrogen and new options like vaginal laser therapy, which, though still being studied, holds promise (Davis et al., 2017). Patient safety and treatment efficacy need to be at the forefront of minds, especially as practitioners experiment with these alternatives within the complicated field of endocrine disorder treatment. An integrated strategy for HRT not only embraces pharmacologic advances but also mandates continuous reflection of the evolving evidence base to ensure that patients are provided with the best and safest available therapeutic regimens (Figure 8.16).

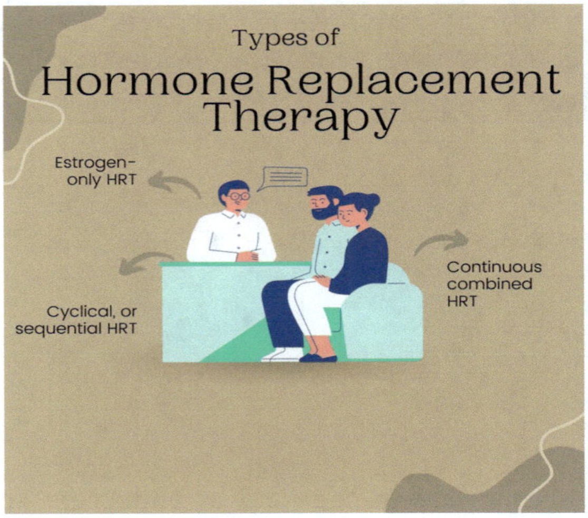

Figure 8.16. Types of hormone replacement therapy.

Source: https://renewmespa.com/wp-content/uploads/2021/11/Hormone-Replacement-Therapy-1024x1024.png.

8.6.2. Genetic Research and Personalized Medicine

The intricate relationship between genetic research and individualized medicine is particularly pertinent when endocrine and metabolic disease is involved. Personalized medicine aims to tailor treatment according to individual genetic traits, which could potentially enhance treatment effect and outcome. As an example, it has been shown that PCOS patients present heterogeneously, and genetic, environmental, and lifestyle factors influence presentation. This complexity calls for an advanced understanding of the PCOS genetic foundation in developing suitable, patient-specific management regimens. With its progression in genetic research, it is now critical to identify specific biomarkers that will guide clinicians in selecting the most appropriate interventions for any patient, thereby improving management and QoL in such women with this syndrome (Namoosi et al., 2024). The significance of incorporating genetic data into treatment protocols becomes apparent when one considers the different ways individuals react to changes in life and diet. The present evidence suggests that specific diet regimes, such as ketogenic diets, have been shown to assist with symptom relief in PCOS. However, the effectiveness of these interventions can vary substantially between individuals, requiring an individualized treatment approach. With an understanding of the genetic influences on metabolic reactions, healthcare workers can make dietary recommendations specific to the individual patient's profile. Not only will this approach alleviate the current symptoms, but it also facilitates long-term health enhancement by preventing possible complications from endocrine disorders (N/A, 2018). Further breakthroughs in genetic research, yet to be discovered, also promise to reshape the choice of therapies available for endocrine and metabolic diseases. Ongoing research into molecular and genetic mechanisms that regulate response to various treatment modalities can more effectively meet the complexities of conditions like PCOS. An awareness of this can form the basis for creating new interventions that are not just responsive but also preventive in nature. Future studies need to focus on longitudinal research to gain an in-depth understanding of the impact of individualized nutritional and lifestyle interventions on healthcare outcomes over the long term. Lastly, a genetically informed strategy for personalized medicine can lead to more sustainable and effective shields for endocrine and metabolic diseases, synthesizing therapy with the unique biological settings of the individual patient (Namoosi et al., 2024).

8.6.3. Innovations in Metabolic Disorder Management

Management of metabolic disorders has seen a paradigm shift over the years through newer approaches that focus on patient-centered care and better therapeutic modalities. These developments, particularly in the field of drug therapy and management of lifestyle, have revolutionized the way healthcare professionals treat diseases such as diabetes, obesity, and metabolic syndrome. For instance, continuous glucose monitoring has changed the way diabetes is managed by allowing real-time measurement of blood glucose. Such technology allows patients to make well-informed decisions regarding their insulin doses and food consumption, thereby optimizing glycemic control. Furthermore, the improvement in pharmacotherapy, as evidenced by the introduction of GLP-1 receptor agonists and SGLT2 inhibitors, has enhanced therapy efficacy through novel mechanisms of action, allowing for weight loss and cardiovascular effects in the presence of metabolic disease. Accordingly, such innovations have a tremendous effect in hampering disease progression and improving QoL. In addition to technological innovation, an important development in metabolic disorder care is the growing focus on multidisciplinary models of care. Through the facilitation of interaction among endocrinologists, dietitians, exercise physiologists, and mental health professionals, the models introduce a more integrated model of treatment. This model of combined care allows for comprehensive assessments and tailored interventions addressing the multi-determination of the biological, psychological, and social determinants of metabolic disease. As an example, in integrated models of care, mental healthcare is becoming more recognized as a central component, such as in programs monitoring drug use and promoting wellness strategies in comorbid psychiatric illness and metabolic disease. The development of systems that facilitate coordination of care ensures consistent messaging and support to patients, which in turn enhances adherence to treatment plans and improves health outcomes in general (Bruce et al., 2012). However, there remain impediments in the application of novel techniques in managing metabolic disorders. Among these challenges is the unpredictability of adrenal crisis (AC) in patients with adrenal insufficiency, which remains a critical concern for health professionals. A focus on more intensive attention and education on prevention has been noted in recent studies, but this alone may not sufficiently decrease the risk of AC events. This is a challenge that requires constant innovation in educational resources and patient monitoring systems. Establishing standardized definitions and methodologies for AC can harmonize research efforts to understand the efficacy of prevention strategies better and improve clinical outcomes in this group of patients (Falhammar et al., 2017). By breaking through these barriers, the specialty can continue to evolve, making effective management of metabolic disorders achievable and adaptable to the needs of diverse patient populations (Figure 8.17).

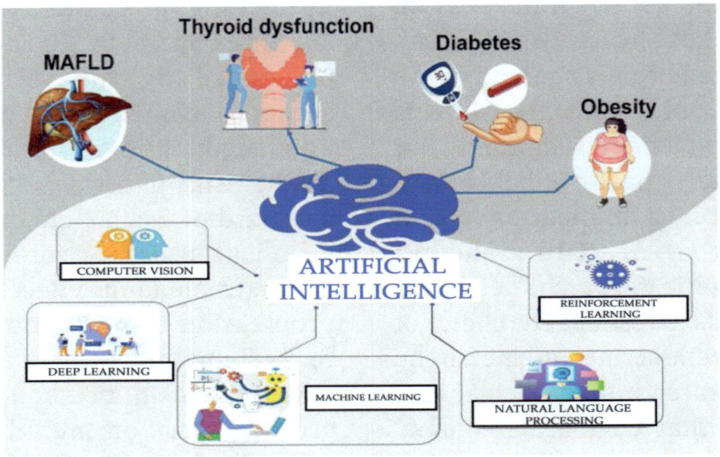

Figure 8.17. Artificial intelligence in the management of metabolic disorders.

Source: https://media.springernature.com/lw685/springer-static/image/art%3A10.1007%2Fs40618-025-02548-x/MediaObjects/40618_2025_2548_Fig1_HTML.png.

Test Your Knowledge

1. What recent advances in hormone replacement therapies have improved outcomes for patients with endocrine disorders such as diabetes or thyroid disease?
2. How is genetic research influencing the development of personalized medicine approaches in the diagnosis and treatment of metabolic disorders?

SUMMARY

There is a call to value the complexity of endocrine and metabolic disorders and their extensive contribution to patients' health outcomes. The high prevalence of hypertension in South Africa, with approximately 6 million of its population affected, is proof that incorporating lifestyle change is central in managing these conditions. The South African Hypertension Society guidelines favor increased physical activity and weight control, emphasizing anticipatory interventions as a means of delaying or even eliminating the need for pharmacotherapy. It not only addresses the inherent medical problems involved but also fosters an awareness of how lifestyle change can prevent complications in long-term illnesses (Collard et al., 2014). Lastly, it focuses on the necessity of educational interventions for both healthcare providers and patients regarding their management. Moreover, the intricate interaction of metabolic disorders with their phenotypes necessitates a more stratified approach to treatment and diagnosis. Phenotyping PCOS into metabolic and hormonal types based on characteristics highlights the urgency of therapeutic interventions tailored to individual needs. According to a single study of women with PCOS by Rotterdam criteria, discordant prevalence of insulin resistance between phenotypes argues against the likelihood that a single approach will prove adequate (Bonin et al., 2013). By considering the unique metabolic profiles suggested by these phenotypes, clinicians are more likely to identify patients at higher risk and employ matching interventions, which would significantly impact long-term health and well-being positively. In combining the data on endocrine and metabolic disorders, it becomes clear that interdisciplinary models of care are crucial for effective management. Endocrinologists, nutritionists, and behavioral health practitioners can assemble multidisciplinary teams to meet the unique needs of patients. By promoting integrated care models, the patients are likely to respond to individualized treatment plans based on their unique physiological and lifestyle conditions. Encouraging patients to participate in their own healthcare generates a sense of responsibility and ownership of lifestyle choices, ultimately leading to greater long-term health improvements. Therefore, the application of these perspectives not only maximizes patient care but also enhances integration with broader public health goals aimed at relieving the burden of chronic diseases (Bonin et al., 2013; Collard et al., 2014).

The pathogenesis of endocrine and metabolic diseases is multifactorial and necessitates an interdisciplinary approach to effectively address and treat them. Dysregulation of hormones, a characteristic of most endocrine diseases, can lead to various symptoms affecting physiological systems. Diabetic mellitus and hypothyroidism, for instance, are characterized by a sudden alteration in the metabolic process, with complications developing in the overall system. In addition, most of these disorders intersect with environmental risk factors, i.e., toxic chemical exposure, which tend to increase health effects. More specifically, research has shown that exposure to toxic chemicals can harm development, leading to long-lasting effects, from learning disorders to behavioral disorders. This highlights the need for broad health policies that consider both biological and environmental health determinants to avert risks of endocrine and metabolic dysfunction (Hitchcock et al., 2011). Stress, in addition, cannot be overlooked as a cause and factor in the development of endocrine disorders. The HPA axis of the body is activated by chronic stress, secreting glucocorticoids, hormones that may impact normal metabolic functions. This stress response can progress to diseases like Cushing's syndrome, in which excessive cortisol leads to severe health effects. CNS response and endocrine function must be recognized as intertwined by healthcare providers. Wholesome treatment strategies that provide for both mental and physical wellness need to be applied to manage the multifaceted nature of these disorders. Closing this gap between the disciplines will enhance overall treatment effectiveness of the strategies, stressing that there should be a holistic approach to treating endocrine and metabolic disorders (Estrine et al., 2006). In conclusion, treatment for endocrine and metabolic disorders must be undertaken through an integrated framework that addresses biological, environmental, and psychological factors. The interrelationship of these factors underscores a need for a comprehensive understanding of how they interact to influence health outcomes. A comprehension by healthcare providers of the multifactorial etiology of these disorders will enable more effective, individualized treatment regimens. Throughout the evolution of public health, policy overhaul will be essential in countering the effects of toxic environmental contaminants while simultaneously mitigating the psychological pressures that adversely affect endocrine well-being. An integrated approach of this nature can reduce the incidence and severity of endocrine and metabolic illnesses in the populace (Estrine et al., 2006; Hitchcock et al., 2011).

KEY TERMS FROM THIS CHAPTER

- Addison's disease
- Adrenal insufficiency
- Anorexia nervosa (AN)
- Endocrine disorders
- Endocrine homeostasis
- Histological effects
- Human endocrine system
- Hypoglycemia
- Metabolic balance disturbances
- Adrenal cortex
- Adrenocorticotropic hormone (ACTH)
- Antioxidant therapy
- Endocrine function
- High-fiber diets
- Hormone production
- Hyperthyroidism
- Luteinizing hormone (LH)
- Metabolic derangements

CRITICAL THINKING QUESTIONS

1. **Which hormone is primarily responsible for lowering blood glucose levels?**
   a. Glucagon
   b. Insulin
   c. Cortisol
   d. Growth hormone
2. **Which of the following is a common cause of hyperthyroidism?**
   a. Hashimoto's thyroiditis
   b. Graves' disease
   c. Addison's disease
   d. Cushing's syndrome
3. **A patient presents with increased thirst, frequent urination, and unexplained weight loss. Which disorder is most likely?**
   a. Type 1. Diabetes Mellitus
   b. Hypothyroidism
   c. Addison's disease
   d. Acromegaly
4. **Which gland secretes cortisol?**
   a. Pituitary gland
   b. Thyroid gland
   c. Adrenal gland
   d. Pancreas
5. **Metabolic syndrome includes all the following features EXCEPT:**
   a. Abdominal obesity
   b. Hypertension
   c. Hyperglycemia
   d. Hypotension

Short Answer Questions

1. What are the primary endocrine glands involved in metabolic regulation, and what hormones do they secrete?
2. Explain the pathophysiology and clinical features of diabetes mellitus types 1 and 2. How do their treatments differ?
3. Describe the mechanisms and consequences of thyroid hormone imbalances, including hypothyroidism and hyperthyroidism.
4. What are the diagnostic criteria and management strategies for metabolic syndrome?
5. Discuss the role of the adrenal glands in endocrine disorders such as Addison's disease and Cushing's syndrome.
6. How does obesity contribute to the development of insulin resistance and other metabolic disturbances?
7. Outline the diagnostic approach, including laboratory tests and imaging, used to evaluate patients suspected of having endocrine disorders.

Answers to Critical Thinking Questions

1. (b); 2. (b); 3. (a); 4. (c); 5. (d)

REFERENCES

1. Chow, J., Rahman, J., Achermann, J. C., Dattani, M. T., & Rahman, S. (2016). Mitochondrial disease and endocrine dysfunction. *Nature Reviews Endocrinology, 13*(2), 92–104. https://doi.org/10.1038/nrendo.2016.151Agarwal, A., Wright, A. F., Gifford, A., Spiliopoulou, A., Benjamini, Y., Cadzow, M., et al. (2018). Phenome-wide association study (PheWAS) on the genetic determinants of serum urate level and disease outcomes in UK Biobank. https://core.ac.uk/download/429731779.pdf (accessed on 27th June 2025).
2. Aigner, F., Pratschke, J., Schumann, T., Stockmann, M., et al. (2020). Recent advances and the potential for clinical use of autofluorescence detection of extra-ophthalmic tissues. https://core.ac.uk/download/323257980.pdf (accessed on 27th June 2025).
3. Altschul, D. J., Azzam, A. Y., Essibayi, M. A., Mohamed, A., et al. (2024). Epidemiological patterns, treatment response, and metabolic correlations of idiopathic intracranial hypertension: A United States-based study from 1990 to 2024. https://core.ac.uk/download/654947402.pdf (accessed on 27th June 2025).
4. Ameer, B., Weintraub, H., et al. (2018). Pediatric obesity: Influence on drug dosing and therapeutics. https://core.ac.uk/download/155271623.pdf (accessed on 27th June 2025).
5. Arcelus, J., Gooren, L., Klink, D., T'Sjoen, G., et al. (2018). Endocrinology of transgender medicine. https://core.ac.uk/download/162667742.pdf (accessed on 27th June 2025).
6. Armanini, D., Bordin, L., Camozzi, V., Donà, G., et al. (2015). Transient hypercortisolism and symptomatic hyperthyroidism associated to primary hyperparathyroidism in an elderly patient: Case report and literature review. https://core.ac.uk/download/53518371.pdf (accessed on 27th June 2025).
7. Babraj, J., & Hawkey, A. (2017). Improved insulin sensitivity following a short-term whole body vibration intervention. https://core.ac.uk/download/228177866.pdf (accessed on 27th June 2025).
8. Badiali, D., Bruno, G., Ribichini, E., Rossi, M., et al. (2019). Role of fiber in nutritional management of pancreatic diseases. https://core.ac.uk/download/231748461.pdf (accessed on 27th June 2025).
9. Ball, P., Morrissey, H., & Solanki, V. (2018). Disease-modifying effects of type 2 diabetes mellitus and bipolar disorder comorbidity. https://core.ac.uk/download/158352052.pdf (accessed on 27th June 2025).
10. Biller, B. M. K., Colao, A., De Martino, M. C., Isidori, A. M., et al. (2016). Complications of Cushing's syndrome: State of the art. https://core.ac.uk/download/54532161.pdf (accessed on 27th June 2025).
11. Blum, M. R., Dekkers, O. M., Den Elzen, W. P. J., Du Puy, R. S., et al. (2018). Study protocol: A randomized controlled trial on the clinical effects of levothyroxine treatment for subclinical hypothyroidism in people aged 80 years and over. https://core.ac.uk/download/161514514.pdf (accessed on 27th June 2025).
12. Bonin, C., Bonora, E., Dall'Alda, M., Di Sarra, D., et al. (2013). Divergences in insulin resistance between the different phenotypes of the polycystic ovary syndrome. https://core.ac.uk/download/55800175.pdf (accessed on 27th June 2025).
13. Bruscalupi, G., & Gnocchi, D. (2017). Circadian rhythms and hormonal homeostasis:

Pathophysiological implications. https://core.ac.uk/download/98342817.pdf (accessed on 27th June 2025).

14. Carnevale, I., De Santis, E., Limana, F., Perrone, A., et al. (2015). One special question to start with: Can HIF/NFkB be a target in inflammation? https://core.ac.uk/download/54248898.pdf (accessed on 27th June 2025).
15. Ciobanu, C., Fica, S., Poterasu, M., Rowland, M., et al. (2020). Anorexia nervosa and reproduction: Connecting brain to gonads. https://core.ac.uk/download/304672903.pdf (accessed on 27th June 2025).
16. Collard, J., Gafane, L., Nell, T., Rennie, D., et al. (2014). Physical activity and hypertension in South African adults. https://core.ac.uk/download/29852228.pdf (accessed on 27th June 2025).
17. Davis, S. R., Gompel, A., Lumsden, M. A., Pinkerton, J. V., et al. (2017). Managing menopausal symptoms and associated clinical issues in breast cancer survivors. https://core.ac.uk/download/96884955.pdf (accessed on 27th June 2025).
18. De Vincentiis, L., Di Paolo, M., Iacovelli, A., Mezzaroma, M., et al. (2020). A case of acanthosis nigricans in a HIV-infected patient. https://core.ac.uk/download/323192484.pdf (accessed on 27th June 2025).
19. Donaldson, P. L., Garshnek, V., Hooke, L. R., Rowe, L., et al. (2025). *USSR Space Life Sciences Digest, Issue 18.* https://core.ac.uk/download/pdf/42831902.pdf (accessed on 27th June 2025).
20. Estrine, J., & DeLisle, L. (2006). Stress: Putting the brain back into medicine. https://core.ac.uk/download/71356692.pdf (accessed on 27th June 2025).
21. Estrine, J., & O'Brien, N. (2003). Sleep, health, and aging. https://core.ac.uk/download/71356671.pdf (accessed on 27th June 2025).
22. Falhammar, H., Rushworth, R., & Torpy, D. (2017). Adrenal crises: Perspectives and research directions. https://core.ac.uk/download/80534615.pdf (accessed on 27th June 2025).
23. Gardiner, A., & Hilton, A. (2016). Managing constipation in adults with co-morbidities. https://core.ac.uk/download/151161237.pdf (accessed on 27th June 2025).
24. Ghazeeri, G., Hmedeh, C., et al. (2021). Nutritional management in polycystic ovary syndrome: Challenges and opportunities. https://core.ac.uk/download/161103740.pdf (accessed on 27th June 2025).
25. Gianfrilli, D., Graziadio, C., Hasenmajer, V., Isidori, A. M., et al. (2018). Glucometabolic alterations in secondary adrenal insufficiency: Does replacement therapy play a role? https://core.ac.uk/download/188824845.pdf (accessed on 27th June 2025).
26. Hirata, A., Marigliani, B., Aguiar-Yamaguchi, G., Miguel, G., Borborema, J. F., Azevedo, J. L., et al. (2011). Structural changes in intestinal enteroendocrine cells after ileal interposition in normal rats. https://core.ac.uk/download/pdf/290516.pdf (accessed on 27th June 2025).
27. Hitchcock, E., & Madsen, T. (2011). Growing up toxic: Chemical exposures and increases in developmental disease. https://core.ac.uk/download/71358334.pdf (accessed on 27th June 2025).
28. Kapke, D. R. (2015). Childhood type II diabetes: The risks and complications. https://core.ac.uk/download/58826199.pdf (accessed on 27th June 2025).

29. Kass, P., Lau, G., Puschner, B., Walter, W., et al. (2017). Comparison of polybrominated diphenyl ethers (PBDEs) and polychlorinated biphenyls (PCBs) in the serum of hypothyroxinemia and euthyroid dogs. https://core.ac.uk/download/323070337.pdf (accessed on 27th June 2025).
30. Michael, J. R. (2017). The relations of metabolic syndrome to anxiety and depression symptoms in children and adults. https://core.ac.uk/download/84397711.pdf (accessed on 27th June 2025).
31. Osorio-Alonso, H., Pedraza-Chaverri, J., Scholze, A., Sánchez-Lozada, L. G., et al. (2016). New pathogenic concepts and therapeutic approaches to oxidative stress in chronic kidney disease. https://core.ac.uk/download/pdf/50717190.pdf (accessed on 27th June 2025).
32. Saari, K. (2005). Hyperlipidemia and metabolic syndrome in schizophrenia: A study of the Northern Finland 1966 birth cohort. https://core.ac.uk/download/628860256.pdf (accessed on 27th June 2025).
33. Sarmidi, M. R. (2012). Food is our medicine. https://core.ac.uk/download/11801185.pdf (accessed on 27th June 2025).
34. Winchester, B. R., Brahm, N. C., et al. (2012). Development of a medication monitoring system for an integrated multidisciplinary program of assertive community treatment (IMPACT) team. https://core.ac.uk/download/pdf/26995413.pdf (accessed on 27th June 2025).

RENAL AND GENITOURINARY SYSTEM: DISORDERS, DIAGNOSTIC APPROACHES, AND TREATMENT OPTIONS

9

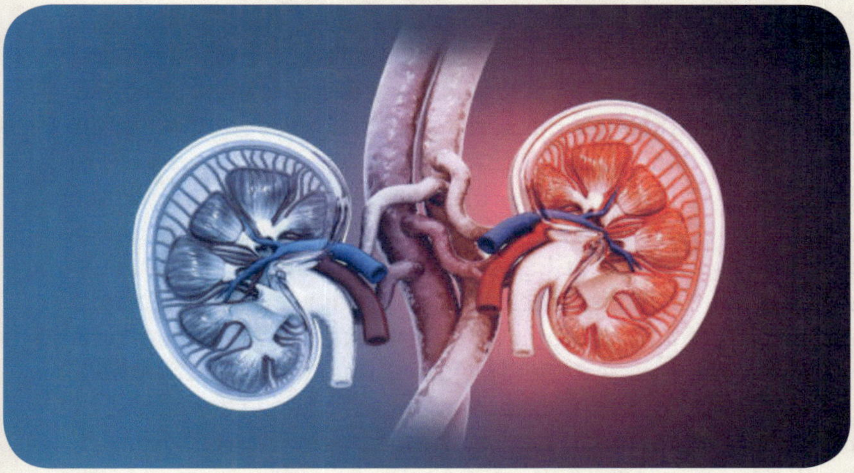

LEARNING OBJECTIVES

After studying this chapter, you will be able to:

1. Describe the anatomy of the renal system
2. Explain the physiology of the renal system
3. Understand common renal and genitourinary disorders
4. Focus on diagnostic approaches in in the realm of renal and genitourinary medicine
5. Define treatment options for renal and genitourinary medicine

Introduction

Understanding the subject of general medicine, particularly the renal and genitourinary system, is necessary for comprehending the intricate interplay of various physiological and pathological mechanisms affecting these organs. The renal system is primarily responsible for body fluid control, maintenance of electrolyte balance, and waste removal, while the genitourinary system consists of both the reproductive organs and the urinary passage. Understanding these systems is not only important for treating illnesses such as renal malignancy, UTIs, or CKD, but also for addressing more general health issues caused by these organs. By exploring the interaction between renal function and overall health, including metabolic and blood pressure regulation, physicians can recognize the need for early diagnosis and patient-centered treatment strategies. In the pursuit of renal and genitourinary system-specific disorders, one must consider the constantly evolving developments in diagnostic technologies and treatment strategies. Imaging modalities such as CT and ultrasonography have facilitated the diagnosis of renal tumors and other pathologies with better sensitivity, enabling us to better differentiate between indolent and aggressive types of tumors. For instance, a recent study unveils the development of a nomogram that can predict indolent renal cortical tumors through the integration of CT features and clinical data, with a high concordance index after external validation (Asnis-Alibozek et al., 2016). These are valuable tools in guiding clinical practice, tailoring treatment strategies, and ultimately optimizing patient care. As EBP is adopted by healthcare practice, it is therefore critical that practitioners remain current with these innovations and their implications on patient management. Additionally, the effect of shared decision-making cannot be overstated in renal and genitourinary system care. As the treatment paradigm has shifted towards personalized medicine, understanding patient preferences and values optimizes the efficacy of therapeutic interventions. For example, the use of various types of anesthetics in processes such as transcatheter aortic valve replacement (TAVR) highlights the necessity of striking a balance between clinical success and cost-effectiveness in patient care (Aksoy et al., 2017). Inclusion of such patient-centered measures enhances understanding of treatment environments, such as striking a balance between potential risks and expected outcomes. Lastly, blending clinical excellence with patient involvement will shape the future of general medicine for the genitourinary and renal system, ushering in a new epoch in integrated delivery of healthcare.

Definition of the Renal and Genitourinary System

The genitourinary system, including the kidneys, ureters, bladder, and urethra, plays a vital role in the body's homeostasis. The complex system is primarily responsible for blood filtration, electrolyte regulation, and waste product excretion through urine. The kidneys play a crucial role in filtering toxins from the blood, reabsorbing essential nutrients, and regulating blood pressure by the renin-angiotensin-aldosterone mechanism. Furthermore, the renal system is intricately integrated into numerous other body functions, influencing overall health, fluid balance, and electrolyte status. It is therefore of critical importance to understand this system in general medicine, as conditions such as CKD and UTIs can have a significant impact on patient outcomes. In practice, an adequate knowledge of the genitourinary and renal system also involves its interaction with other systems of the body. For instance, the kidneys are involved in regulating hemoglobin production through the secretion of erythropoietin and in calcium metabolism via vitamin D activation. Because the kidneys possess bidirectional functions, their impairment would initiate a series of health disorders outside the urinary system, including cardiovascular disorders and metabolic derangement. An acceptable illustration of this is the manner in which diabetes has been discovered to be connected to the renal system. According to recent research, nearly half of diabetic patients present with kidney function comorbidities, reflecting the importance of monitoring kidney status in managing chronic disease (Bolt et al., 2015). More importantly, the genitourinary aspect of this system includes reproductive health, again equating the importance of renal processes with general health. Diseases like prostate hypertrophy, bladder cancer, and venereal diseases may directly affect renal function, resulting in a complex clinical situation. A multidisciplinary approach is usually needed in the comprehensive evaluation and management of renal and genitourinary conditions due to the way these systems interplay with the whole body. A greater understanding of the genitourinary and renal system allows for expansion of overall medical treatment, allowing doctors to develop targeted interventions for patients whose medical complications are multifaceted (Burity et al., 2014). The interconnectedness of this system highlights its role in sustaining overall wellness and underscores the importance of ongoing education and research in this field.

Importance of General Medicine in Renal Health

The general medicine function in ensuring renal well-being is essential, as it involves the holistic management of many chronic illnesses that significantly affect renal function. General medicine-trained doctors are capable of identifying and managing the numerous factors that influence renal well-being, such as diabetes, hypertension, and CVD. They are not independent conditions; instead, they often coexist and complicate one another in intricate ways, with the ability to potentiate renal impairment. Understanding how these chronic conditions interact can enable GPs to introduce preventative interventions and therapeutic interventions tailored to the needs of an individual patient. This not only enhances patients' QoL but also reduces the burden on healthcare systems by avoiding progression of renal disease. In this regard, the overall medical framework serves as an infrastructure for coordinated care, ensuring careful observation and control of renal status. Additionally, detection and care of comorbid conditions are of utmost importance in preventing renal failure. Studies have indicated that multimorbidity affects a significant proportion of the population, particularly diabetes patients, with up to 26 million patients likely having to manage more than one chronic disease that affects their treatment and well-being. For instance, conditions such as CHF and obesity have been revealed to hinder patients from reaching important diabetes care goals, including controlling blood pressure and lipids. This interrelatedness highlights the importance of general medicine doctors being able to evaluate and manage multiple chronic conditions simultaneously, thereby optimizing health gain for patients at risk of kidney disease. Ultimately, a general medicine approach not only optimizes patient compliance with treatment but also refines the methods adopted in renal healthcare, aligning with prevailing trends in the management of chronic diseases within the healthcare industry (Bolt et al., 2015). Equally important is education and awareness within the general practice of renal health. GPs are in an ideal position to advise patients on the importance of kidney function and the impact of lifestyle factors on renal health. This involves prompting a healthy diet, a regimen of physical activity, and periodic health check-ups, all of which are crucial to the early detection of renal issues. In addition, general medicine integrates patient participation practices to optimize adherence to prescribed treatment protocols and lifestyle modifications. As complications related to the kidneys may develop subtly, patient education in self-care and the maintenance of kidney function can lead to improved results. Together with evidence-based guidelines and regular monitoring, the general medical practitioner can be a key driving force for renal health and serve a vital role in the patients' overall well-being, thus identifying the importance of a holistic strategy in the management of the genitourinary system (Burity et al., 2014).

Overview of Common Disorders

In the area of renal and genitourinary illness, the 22q11.2 deletion syndrome (22q11.2DS) is of interest, as it is a prevalent chromosomal microdeletion disorder with a variable clinical presentation. Described as a microdeletion of chromosome 22 leading to DiGeorge syndrome, in which affected patients presented with a triad of immunodeficiency, hypoparathyroidism, and congenital heart disease, much is known about this condition. In addition to the classical presentations, 22q11.2DS patients may exhibit a range of congenital anomalies with renal impingement. The heterogeneity of presentation makes the syndrome amenable to multidisciplinary care, involving pediatrics, surgery, genetics, and counseling, among others.

If possible, detecting the syndrome in the prenatal or neonatal period increases opportunities for improved outcomes and underscores the importance of complete screening of at-risk populations (Bassett et al., 2015). The other key issue in the domain of common renal and genitourinary disorders is the increasing health load of NCDs in developing countries. Projections indicate a rapid rise in NCD mortality rates within the next several decades and hence force proactive policy intervention. Under these circumstances, economic evaluation of renal and genitourinary disorder interventions becomes necessary. A review of the financial analysis reveals significant evidence gaps, particularly in resource allocation to effective prevention and treatment interventions. Policymakers, being confronted with limited resources, can identify cost-effectiveness across various interventions, which can allow for more informed decisions. Narrowing the existing knowledge gap can aid in enhancing population health, particularly given that NCDs impose an unequal burden on developing regions (Fox-Rushby et al., 2006). In addition, psychological and developmental complications related to renal and genitourinary disease need to be addressed, especially when assessing disorders such as 22q11.2DS. Patients tend to have more instances of behavioral phenotypes, cognitive impairments, and psychiatric disorders. Where chronic health conditions intersect with mental health, there is an important area for innovation in general medicine. Patients, especially children, are bound to face resilience deficits due to the complexity of living with physical as well as psychological consequences of their ailment. A holistic treatment model involving not just medical management of renal afflictions but also integrated psychological intervention is mandatory. This type of holistic reaction guarantees that the care extends beyond urgent health requirements to entire well-being and development, enabling people to thrive despite diagnoses (Bassett et al., 2015).

9.1. Anatomy of the Renal System

Learning Outcome

1. Explain the structure of the kidneys
2. Describe the function of the ureters and bladder
3. Define the role of the urethra

The renal system, or the urinary system, plays a role in maintaining the human body in a state of homeostasis through regulating fluid and electrolyte balance, blood pressure, and acid-base balance. Comprising the kidneys, ureters, bladder, and urethra, the system's primary function is blood filtration to produce urine, which removes waste products and excess material. Approximately 1 million functional units known as nephrons exist in each kidney, which assist in the filtration process. The glomerulus within the nephrons filters blood in a way that water, ions, and small molecules pass through but large proteins and blood cells are prevented from doing so. This intricate structure indicates the kidneys' significance not only in the elimination process but also in active secretion and reabsorption processes, which contribute to systemic physiological conditions and overall health. Ureters are ducts along which urine is transported from the kidneys to the bladder through peristaltic contractions. The bladder is a temporary reservoir of urine, containing approximately 300 to 500 milliliters in adults. It consists of elastic and contractile muscular walls that store and ultimately drain urine during micturition. The urethra, on the other hand, is the final organ of the urinary tract with the voluntary function of expelling urine from the bladder out to the external environment. In men, the urethra is longer and also carries semen, a reflection of anatomical differences that have profound health implications for gender-specific health issues, including UTIs and prostate disease. Understanding the structural and functional attributes of these elements is essential for diagnosing and treating renal and genitourinary diseases in the best possible way. Anatomical abnormalities of the renal apparatus, such as agenesis or dysplasia, can have far-reaching consequences on a person's overall health. Syndromes like 22q11.2 deletion syndrome highlight the complex relationship between genetic defects and renal pathology, with patients with this condition having congenital renal abnormalities in addition to other systemic features. These renal abnormalities need an extensive, interdisciplinary treatment strategy as they have the potential to cause long-term health complications like hypertension, UTIs, and renal failure. Proper and early diagnosis plays a critical role in optimizing prognosis, with prenatal or neonatal screening proving to be important for early intervention. The anatomy of the renal systems and corresponding pathologies highlights the importance of integrating general medicine practices to optimally treat these conditions, ultimately enhancing patient care in renal and genitourinary settings.

9.1.1. Structure of the Kidneys

Kidneys are significant bean-like organs that play crucial roles in eliminating waste from the blood and maintaining homeostasis in the body. Each kidney is made up of three significant areas: the cortex, the medulla, and the renal pelvis. The outer cortex contains nephrons, which are functional units that result in urine. These nephrons consist of a glomerulus, where blood is filtered, and tubules that change the filtrate to regulate electrolyte balance, fluid volume, and removal of wastes. The inner medulla is organized in a pyramidal form with the loop of Henle and collecting ducts that are required for the concentration of urine and the conservation of water. The renal pelvis acts as a funnel through which urine is channeled to the ureter. This anatomy is important for the recognition of various nephropathies since abnormalities can indicate dysfunction or disease in the renal system. Beyond basic anatomy, the kidney's structure establishes its significance in health and disease in the system. The nephrons' intricately organized structure allows it to react properly to metabolic stimuli and the alteration of the environment, and thus not only controls fluid equilibrium but also the acid-base equilibrium of the body. Previous studies have also linked kidney function with diseases such as CKD and metabolic disorders, and have enlightened the interaction between renal architecture and overall health. For instance, nephrons can be harmed by metabolic stress, leading to kidney stones, a disease triggered by environmental and genetic factors, as discussed in current research.

As nephrolithiasis has to do with more overall systemic issues, there is a need for a deeper understanding of kidney structure and pathology, informing initiatives toward prevention as well as therapeutic intervention that takes into consideration not just the kidneys but health in general. Moreover, medical research advancements have led to information on therapeutic modalities for managing renal pathologies caused by structural issues. Kidney stones, a common urological condition, highlight the importance of understanding renal architecture, as it is directly related to treatment outcomes. Structural nephron abnormalities not only predispose the patient to stone development but also present the disease as a systemic disease with associated complications like hypertension and type 2 diabetes. Current data suggest that the study of plant therapies may provide fewer adverse effects but work directly against stone formation and associated complications. Recognition of such interrelationships is a testament to the relevance of nephron structure in understanding renal and systemic diseases and argues for the need for holistic treatment methods, as emphasized in current medical literature (Babu et al., 2019) (Figure 9.1).

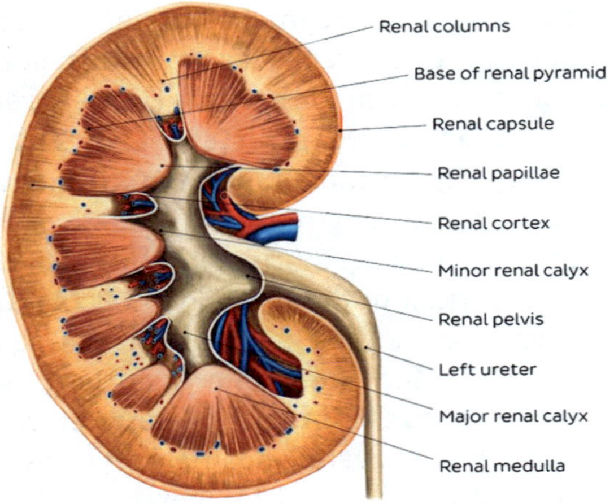

Figure 9.1. Kidney's structure.

Source: https://www.kenhub.com/thumbor/6h_vqbnkREKCXdDQX7uHtc3jI6U=/fit-in/800x1600/filters:watermark(/images/logo_url.png,-10,-10,0):background_color(FFFFFF):format(jpeg)/images/library/10923/renal-cortex_englishMA.jpg.

9.1.2. Function of the Ureters and Bladder

The ureters and bladder are crucial parts of the renal and genitourinary systems, performing vital functions in the process of urine elimination after its formation in the kidneys. Muscular tubes known as ureters, measuring approximately 25–30 centimeters in length, transport urine from the renal pelvis to the bladder via peristaltic movements. This transport is vital because it ensures urine is transported to the bladder efficiently and in a timely manner for storage, thereby preventing disruption of the homeostasis balance (Gomez-Rodriguez et al., 2010). Their smooth muscle layers enable them to achieve the rhythmic contractions necessary to expel urine, even when the body is in different positions. Furthermore, the position and length of the ureters are functionally beneficial as they facilitate urine flow under pressure from the collecting urine in the bladder and gravity, ensuring an overall efficient urinary tract. The bladder is a temporary urine reservoir that holds urine until voluntary excretion is initiated. Constructed structurally as a distensible hollow organ, the bladder can contain normally some 400–600 milliliters of urine in adults without pain. The specific muscle layer of the bladder, the detrusor muscle, is responsible for both storage and final expulsion of urine during micturition. Once the bladder has filled to a certain level of fullness, sensory nerve impulses stimulate the brain to trigger the micturition reflex by coordinating the contraction of the detrusor muscle and the relaxation of the internal sphincter (Aguirre-Avalos et al., 2018).

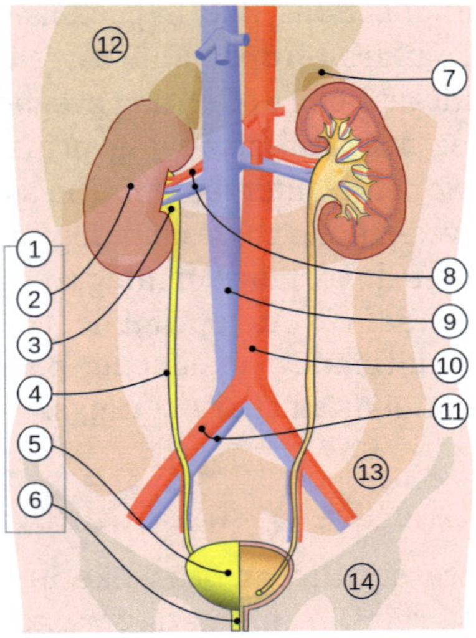

Figure 9.2. The ureters (labeled 4) are tubes that carry urine and connect the kidneys to the bladder.

Source: https://upload.wikimedia.org/wikipedia/commons/thumb/3/30/Urinary_system.svg/800px-Urinary_system.svg.png.

Such precise interaction shows the bladder's significant role within the urinary system, coordinating both the neurological and muscular components to manage the process of urination effectively. Beyond their primary roles, the bladder and ureters make a vital contribution to the general health of the urinary tract, impacting conditions that can lead to complications such as infection or injury. Obstructive uropathy from stones within the ureter, for instance, can impede urine passage and, if left untreated, can lead to extensive renal impairment. The durability of the bladders is also tested in cases such as UTIs and TB, as seen from the complications accompanying urinary tract TB and leading to severe loss of kidney function and overall health (Aguirre-Avalos et al., 2018). Understanding such related functions and hazards is important for medical professionals since it points to the need for early diagnosis and management of cases of dysfunction of the bladder or ureter, leading to contributing to patient welfare in general medicine of the renal and genitourinary system (Figure 9.2).

9.1.3. Role of the Urethra

The urethra plays a central role in the human body, particularly in the renal and genitourinary system, as the primary passage for urine elimination from the bladder. The urethra is a tubular organ that differs in length and diameter between men and women. In women, the urethra is longer and more complicated because it has the dual responsibility of urination and ejaculation. The male urethra is approximately 20 centimeters long, while the female urethra is roughly 4 centimeters long. It is essential to understand such anatomical differences in order to appreciate the consequences of urethral health and the complications of urethral dysfunction or disease. Urethral functional abnormalities may lead to serious complications like urinary incontinence or obstructive pathologies, and hence the significance of complete medical attention in urethral abnormalities. Apart from its anatomical significance, the urethra is also endowed with sophisticated mechanisms for the control of urine flow, which are governed by voluntary as well as involuntary muscles. The external urethral sphincter, for example, plays a significant role in voluntary control, while the internal sphincter functions involuntarily to prevent leakage. This two-stage process comprises distinct physiological states, i.e., activity and sleep, and signifies the function of the urethra in homeostasis and general urinary health. In addition, the urethra is susceptible to a range of pathologies, from infections to strictures, which compromise its function and contribute to systemic health issues.

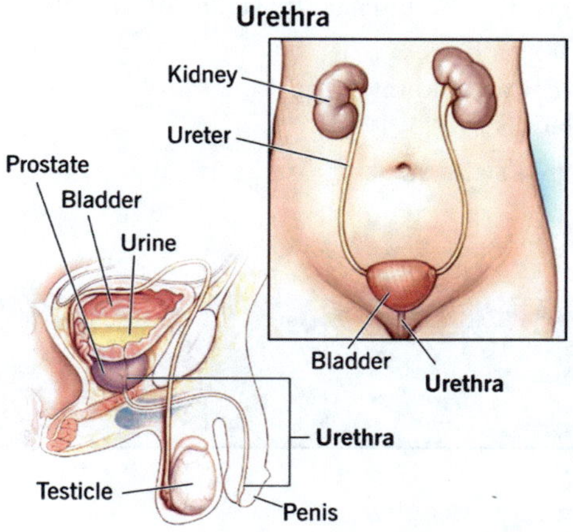

Figure 9.3. The urethra is a tubelike passage that allows urine (and semen, if applicable) to leave your body.

Source: https://my.clevelandclinic.org/-/scassets/images/org/health/articles/23002-urethra.

These issues mandate careful medical evaluation and management, underscoring the importance of urethral integrity as part of the larger picture of renal and genitourinary well-being. The role of the urethra extends beyond its functional roles in medicine; it also serves as a platform for diagnostic and therapeutic modalities. Urologic procedures, including cystoscopy, often use the urethra as a pathway to access the bladder and lower urinary tract, facilitating adequate urologic evaluation. Treatments, including catheterization, also demonstrate the significance of the urethra's role in both acute and chronic clinical conditions and its valuable aid in managing urinary retention or obstruction. With its complex functions, clinicians must possess a good understanding of its anatomy and physiology, as well as the potential complications that may arise. Awareness of these is at the heart of ensuring optimal patient results for the management of renal and genitourinary disease and requires a comprehensive understanding. It requires continued research and study in this vital area of medicine (Figure 9.3).

Test Your Knowledge

1. Describe the internal structure of the kidney, including the cortex, medulla, nephrons, and their functional significance.
2. What are the main functions of the ureters, and how do they transport urine from the kidneys to the bladder?
3. Explain the structure and function of the urinary bladder in urine storage and elimination.

9.2. Physiology of the Renal System

Learning Outcome

1. Understand the filtration process in the nephrons
2. Discuss the regulation of electrolytes and fluid balance
3. Focus on hormonal control of renal function

The renal apparatus, which primarily consists of the kidneys, ureters, bladder, and urethra, is tasked with keeping the human body in a state of homeostasis. The filtration of blood to produce urine, thereby regulating electrolytes, fluid content, and the body's pH, is the responsibility of the kidneys. There are about a million nephrons in each kidney, and these are the functional units on which the filtration of blood takes place. In the nephron, the mechanisms such as glomerular filtration, tubular reabsorption, and tubular secretion interact synergistically to control the volume and composition of body fluids. These are significant since an imbalance in renal physiology may lead to extreme physiological derangements, ultimately affecting well-being and health. This intricate system highlights the importance of renal function not just in excretion but also in participating in a variety of metabolic processes that allow for survival. Moreover, the physiological processes of the renal system are intrinsically linked to systemic blood pressure regulation. The kidneys help maintain blood pressure via the renin-angiotensin-aldosterone system (RAAS) when there is reduced blood flow to the kidneys. Renin, an enzyme released by the juxtaglomerular cells, facilitates the conversion of angiotensinogen to angiotensin I, which is then converted to angiotensin II. Angiotensin II is a potent vasoconstrictor that raises blood pressure and causes the release of aldosterone from the adrenal glands, promoting the reabsorption of sodium and water in the kidney. This relationship indicates the dual role of the kidney in excretion and homeostasis, which has repercussions on cardiovascular well-being. Therefore, knowledge of the renal system's impact on blood pressure can be used to guide therapeutic intervention of diseases such as heart disease and hypertension, and is a significant area of investigation in general medicine of the renal and genitourinary system. Furthermore, the pathophysiologic foundation of renal function may encompass an understanding of CKD and its systemic effects. Since kidney function declines with age, waste products and blood toxins create uremic syndrome, whose signs may range from fatigue to impaired mentation. CKD also includes alterations in mineral metabolism that affect bone health through renal osteodystrophy. With escalating diabetes and hypertension rates, the healthcare burden imposed by CKD is considerable, warranting emphasis on its early diagnosis and integrated management strategies. Therefore, renal physiology not only lays a foundation for the understanding of the kidneys but also highlights the importance of preventive therapy and early intervention to minimize the long-term consequences of renal disease in general medicine for the genitourinary and renal system.

9.2.1. Filtration Process in the Nephrons

The filtering process in the nephrons, the functional units of the kidney, is complex but indispensable for maintaining body homeostasis. This complex process starts in the glomerulus, where blood passes from the afferent arteriole. The glomerular capillaries, lined with fenestrated endothelial cells, allow water and small solutes to pass through but block the passage of large molecules such as proteins and blood cells. This initial sieving results in the generation of glomerular filtrate, a process susceptible to the afferent and efferent arteriole pressure difference. Interference in this pressure can generate abnormal filtration, which calls for a proper grasp of the mechanical as well as biochemical parameters regulating the nephron function. Overall, the integrity of the filtration process is most critical because it lays the foundation for subsequent tubular reabsorption and secretion processes and directly impacts renal health. After the glomerular filtration process, the nephron is subjected to a multitude of reabsorptive and secretory processes in the tubular system, which includes the proximal convoluted tubule, loop of Henle, distal convoluted tubule, and collecting duct. Every segment is specialized in the reabsorption of different solutes like sodium, chloride, glucose, and water, and the excretion of waste products. The proximal convoluted tubule, for instance, reabsorbs approximately 65% of filtered sodium and water, whereas the loop of Henle creates a concentration gradient that enables water and potassium ion reabsorption. This particular control maintains essential compounds within and eliminates toxins and metabolic wastes economically. This fine appreciation for such tubular processing is critical, especially in cases of kidney function pathology, where differential reabsorption can significantly manage fluid and electrolyte balance in the body.

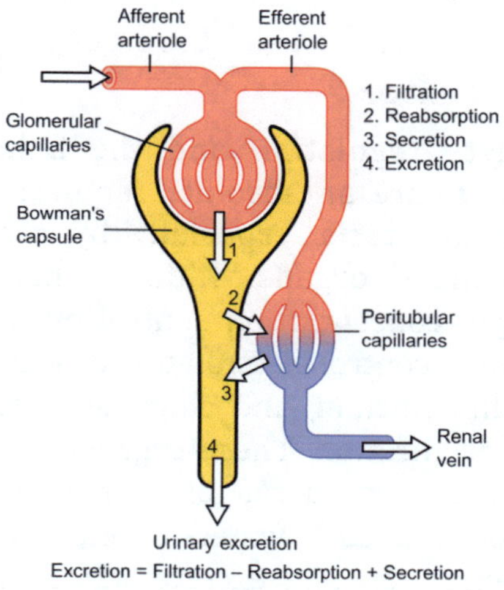

Figure 9.4. Steps involved in urine formation.

Source: https://s3-us-west-2.amazonaws.com/courses-images/wp-content/uploads/sites/1940/2017/05/31172653/physiology-of-nephron.png.

The nephron's function to filter and alter the renal filtrate is essential not only for the elimination of waste but also for the overall fluid and electrolyte balance. Research has shown that it is possible for various factors, like the expression of certain proteins in the renal tubular cells, to affect both the rate of filtration and the reabsorption functions of the nephron. For instance, TMIGD1, a receptor expressed in kidney epithelial cells, is essential for cell survival and morphology, highlighting the critical role of cellular integrity in optimal nephron function (Arafa et al., 2016). Moreover, learning about the conservation of filtration mechanisms between species through a comparative analysis of vertebrate and planarian excretory systems highlights the significance of nephron function in evolutionary systems and its potential to inform human health (Alexander et al., 2015). With such interdisciplinary study of nephron function, the benefits of conservation of these processes come into view, especially as it pertains to kidney disease and failure (Figure 9.4).

9.2.2. Regulation of Electrolytes and Fluid Balance

Electrolyte regulation and the balance of body fluids are an absolute requirement for body homeostasis, especially by renal and genitourinary organs. Kidneys mainly do electrolyte concentration control by the body. The kidneys control electrolytes such as sodium, potassium, calcium, and chloride in terms of their concentration. These organs function by complex nephron arrangements, which filter the blood, reabsorb water-soluble substances and electrolytes, and excrete waste products. Electrolyte imbalance is liable to induce severe health issues, including cardiovascular instability and neuromuscular disturbances. The dynamic control of fluid balance is underscored by the kidneys' ability to adjust electrolyte excretion in accordance with nutritional requirements and hormonal regulation. The RAAS, for example, controls sodium reabsorption and, therefore, circulating blood volume, demonstrating the intricate interplay between renal function and worldwide fluid balance in maintaining systemic health. Hormonal regulation plays a significant role in the kidneys' management of electrolytes and fluid balance. Two of these hormones are antidiuretic hormone (ADH) and aldosterone, which stimulate the retention of water and sodium, respectively. ADH, released by the posterior pituitary gland, increases the permeability of the collecting ducts of the kidneys, resulting in water reabsorption and consequently concentrating urine. Alternatively, aldosterone affects the distal tubules' reabsorption of sodium and excretion of potassium, which plays an essential role in the maintenance of cell membrane electrical potential across. The balance between the hormones is necessary for the occurrence of normal physiology and can be affected by numerous conditions like HF or dehydration. Understanding of these hormonal mechanisms is critical for health professionals when they manage fluid balance among patients with renal or cardiovascular disorders and the interconnectedness of body systems. Additionally, fluid balance management is influenced by the body's response to disease conditions. For instance, CKD can lead to abnormal electrolyte regulation and therefore leads to hyperkalemia and hyponatremia, which further exacerbate cardiovascular complications. Failure of the kidneys to excrete adequate quantities of fluid can lead to edema, hypertension, and HF. Conversely, conditions such as diabetes insipidus, which lead to excessive water loss, can result in hypernatremia and increased plasma osmolality, indicating a failure in maintaining fluid retention. Clinicians must integrate such data in determining appropriate therapeutic interventions for patients with electrolyte imbalance. By thoroughly understanding the pathological and physiological mechanisms of fluid balance, physicians can effectively address the finer points of renal and genitourinary health and the necessity for targeted interventions in these vital systems.

9.2.3. Hormonal Control of Renal Function

The endocrine control of renal function is multifaceted, involving several regulatory hormones that oversee different body physiologies. The kidneys, through their delicate network of nephrons, respond to hormonal signals to maintain body fluid, electrolyte, and acid-base homeostasis. Key hormones to this process are ADH, aldosterone, and NPs. ADH plays a critical role in water reabsorption by increasing the permeability of the renal collecting ducts, which is essential in dehydration states or when there is an increase in plasma osmolarity. Aldosterone, which is released from the adrenal cortex, controls reabsorption of sodium in the collecting duct and distal convoluted tubule, hence increasing blood pressure and volume. Both of these hormones aid in maintaining renal function to accommodate the physiological demands and environmental changes. Along with direct regulation of water and electrolyte homeostasis, hormonal actions on renal function extend to other systems, particularly in response to metabolic changes. For instance, androgens were shown to influence renal physiology, but their action is not typically attributed directly to renal function. Indications point towards androgen receptors possibly being involved in other forms of cancer, bringing into light the possibility of a correlation between hormonal modulation and kidney function. While largely associated with prostate cancer, the androgen response is manifest in various tissues that affect overall metabolism, and therefore renal health. Also, endocrine ailments, such as those involving altered androgen sensitivity, may present with renal manifestations, highlighting the interrelatedness of hormonal homeostasis and renal function (Kurzrock et al., 2014). Moreover, studies on some patient populations illustrate how alterations in hormones lead to severe renal consequences. In spinal and bulbar muscular atrophy (SBMA), however, patients, for instance, exhibit a spectrum of hormonal derangements and renal features. In such groups of patients, research mentions elevated levels of creatine kinase and deranged glucose metabolism, which point towards the impact of hormonal status on renal and genitourinary function (Angelini et al., 2016). Apart from this, lower urinary tract symptoms, prevalent among the patient group in question, emphasize the importance of understanding hormonal control in intricate clinical situations. Therefore, the identification and management of hormonal regulation of renal function enhances our ability to develop comprehensive treatment strategies in the broad context of general medicine of the renal and genitourinary tract (Figure 9.5).

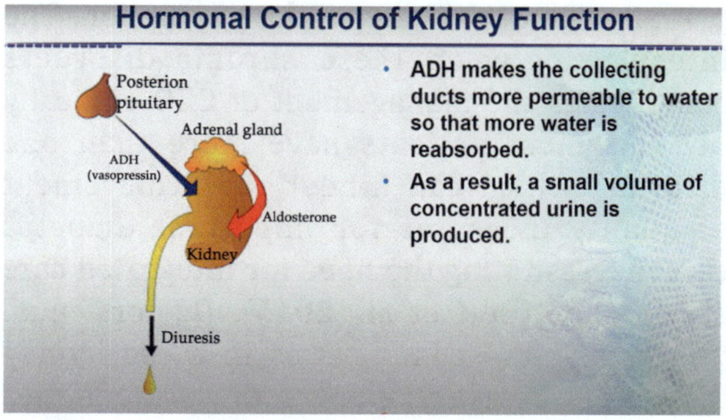

Figure 9.5. Hormonal control of kidney function.

Source: https://i.ytimg.com/vi/VDt96M0-_Wg/hq720.jpg?sqp=-oaymwEhCK4FEIIDSFryq4qpAxMIARUAAAAAGAElAADIQj0AgKJD&rs=AOn4CLA6OKoUp1dsogWKHDfc6Cd2kCEhfQ.

Test Your Knowledge

1. How do the kidneys regulate sodium, potassium, and calcium levels to maintain electrolyte balance in the body?
2. Which hormones are involved in renal function regulation, and how do they affect kidney activity?

9.3. Common Renal Disorders

Learning Outcome

1. Describe chronic kidney disease (CKD)
2. Understand acute kidney injury (AKI)
3. Define kidney stones

The kidneys play a vital role in homeostasis but are susceptible to a myriad of disorders that can dramatically compromise their function. The most prevalent renal disorders include CKD, glomerulonephritis, and kidney stones, all with their own pathophysiological sophistication and requiring personalized management strategies. CKD, a progressive loss of renal function, is generally the consequence of diabetes and hypertension, two of the most prevalent comorbidities of the population. The interplay between these chronic disorders complicates the management of CKD clinically because most patients have more than one disorder, which can hinder the achievement of quality measures for important diabetes care, necessitating the need for integrated care approaches (Bolt et al., 2015). Doctors must understand the complexities in these kidney diseases to devise proper treatment modalities and maximize outcomes. Glomerulonephritis, a common renal disease, represents inflammation of the kidney's filtering units that could be caused by infection, autoimmune mechanisms, or certain medications. The condition could be acute or chronic and could afflict patients of all ages. Acute glomerulonephritis can develop with a sudden onset, presenting symptoms and signs of hematuria, edema, and hypertension, where timely intervention should be done to prevent irreversible damage to the kidneys. Conversely, glomerulonephritis has a slow course with progressive renal insufficiency that may lead to failure of the kidneys. Treatment of glomerulonephritis involves an exhaustive diagnostic procedure of serological investigations and renal biopsy to identify the etiology and tailor therapy based on it. That is why early identification and correct referral to nephrology specialists for sophisticated treatment modalities are important. Kidney stones are a frequent but often preventable renal disease, characterized mainly by the formation of mineral aggregations within the renal system. Lifestyle dietary habits, fluid balance, and metabolic derangement contribute to the very significant development of stones. Agonizing acute attacks are a common experience for patients, who primarily require emergent care for analgesia and potential surgery in obstructing stones. While the majority of kidney stones pass spontaneously, the frequent recurrence of stones causes additional problems, which can lead to chronic damage to the renal parenchyma. Thus, patient education regarding modification of lifestyle, including increased fluid intake and dietary modification, becomes mandatory for preventing recurrence. Furthermore, understanding the determinants of kidney stones in terms of their metabolic and genetic causes can determine targeted prevention measures and restrict the possibility of recurrence, ultimately improving patient QoL (Burity et al., 2014).

9.3.1. Chronic Kidney Disease (CKD)

Chronic kidney disease (CKD) is a significant global public health problem and is characterized by a gradual loss of kidney function over time. CKD can be due to various etiologies like diabetes, hypertension, and glomerulonephritis, and is usually asymptomatic in the early stages. As CKD progresses, the kidneys lose their ability to filter out the waste products of metabolism from the blood, leading to a buildup of toxins and resulting in complications such as fluid overload, electrolyte imbalance, and metabolic acidosis. The increasing prevalence of CKD mandates greater awareness and active intervention by the healthcare community, particularly because CKD commonly coexists with other chronic illnesses. Thus, the awareness and identification of CKD symptoms are essential in the early treatment and to prevent irreversible renal failure that will ultimately necessitate renal replacement therapy by dialysis or transplant. CKD implications extend beyond a person's health and have far-reaching implications on healthcare services and society at large. With the rising prevalence of CKD, healthcare expenditures for its management, including hospitalization and outpatient services, mount substantially. A comparison of ED visits reveals that patients who are transplant recipients, particularly kidney transplant recipients, tend to experience a wide variety of and intricate symptoms, hence a high rate of hospitalization (Benedetti et al., 2009). This represents the intricate link between CKD and other systemic illnesses, which calls for the adoption of an elaborate method to care delivery by the healthcare practitioners. In addition, the social and psychological impacts of CKD on patients, such as anxiety and compromised QoL, present an additional layer of complexity to the public health issue and must be addressed through multi-faceted management strategies. Electrolyte imbalance in sodium (Na+) and potassium (K+) is prevalent among CKD patients and poses a significant risk to their overall health. The kidneys are crucial in the regulation of electrolyte balance, and whenever their function is disrupted, it can result in disturbances in serum electrolytes. Such disturbances may result in serious consequences, such as cardiac arrhythmias, neurological disturbances, and even death in extreme cases (Lombardi et al., 2022). Current studies indicate that slight alterations in electrolyte balance can influence prognosis and outcomes of patients, highlighting the imperative for meticulous monitoring and handling of such disturbances in patients with CKD. For health practitioners, awareness of these possible threats is critical as the stability of electrolytes can prevent secondary complications and improve treatment of victims with CKD (Figure 9.6).

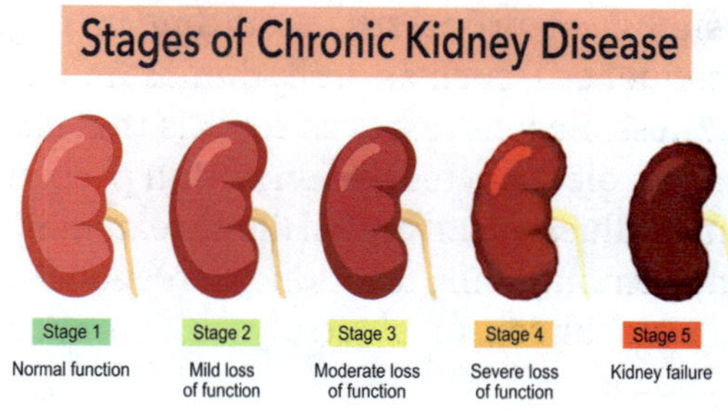

Figure 9.6. Stages of chronic kidney disease.

Source: https://www.carehospitals.com/ckfinder/userfiles/images/chronic-kidney-disease.webp.

9.3.2. Acute Kidney Injury (AKI)

Acute kidney injury (AKI) is characterized by an abrupt loss of renal function that can cause a variety of clinical manifestations, including electrolyte disturbances, fluid overload, and uremic phenomena. AKI with an acute presentation can be caused by numerous etiologies, which are traditionally classified as prerenal, intrinsic, and postrenal. Prerenal AKI usually arises from conditions that compromise renal perfusion, e.g., dehydration or CHF. In contrast, intrinsic AKI may arise by virtue of direct renal parenchymal injury, e.g., acute tubular necrosis and glomerulonephritis. Postrenal AKI usually arises from urinary tract obstruction, e.g., kidney stones or neoplasms, ultimately with consequent interference with urine flow. Early recognition and intervention are critical, with severity and duration of AKI predicting long-term renal prognosis. It is important to appreciate these mechanisms to have proper management strategies in the renal and genitourinary tract. The association between electrolyte imbalances and AKI is well illustrated, highlighting the vital role of the kidneys in maintaining homeostasis. Electrolyte derangements, with sodium and potassium being the most common, are commonly observed in AKI patients. Either high or low levels of serum electrolytes can interfere with essential physiological processes, resulting in negative consequences, such as arrhythmias and muscle weakness. Recent research reveals that changes in serum electrolytes—even within presumably normal values—can foretell life-threatening renal events, emphasizing the kidney's responsiveness to disturbances in electrolytes (Lombardi et al., 2022).

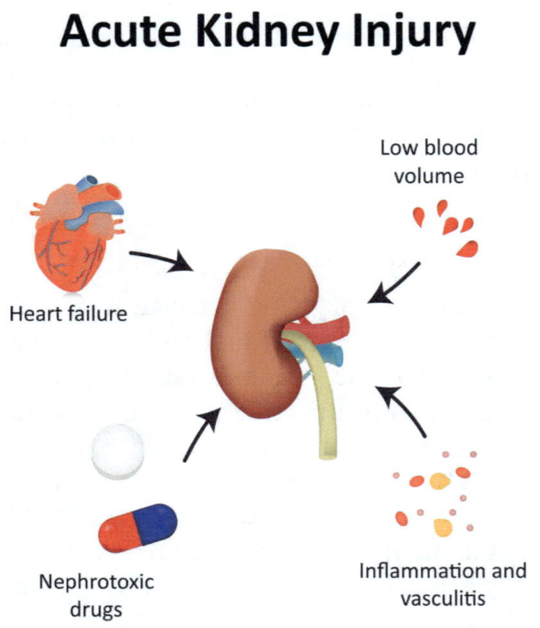

Figure 9.7. Acute kidney injury.

Source: https://wp04-media.cdn.ihealthspot.com/wp-content/uploads/sites/464/2024/08/Acute-Kidney-Injury-1.jpg.

Consequently, maintaining optimal electrolyte levels is of paramount importance in managing AKI, and clinicians must closely monitor these parameters to mitigate complications and enhance patient prognosis. Moreover, the implications of AKI extend beyond immediate renal damage, influencing the overall health trajectory of affected individuals. Notably, conditions such as BK polyomavirus nephropathy have demonstrably increased incidence in kidney transplant recipients and can complicate AKI outcomes. Although commonly detectable in transplanted kidneys, BKVN can occur in native kidneys, particularly in patients with prior histories of other organ transplants (Aggarwal et al., 2023). Grasp of the intricacies of such comorbid conditions is at the core of clinicians providing care for patients with AKI, enabling timely interventions and specially crafted therapeutic approaches. Because AKI may progress to CKD and other systemic diseases, a thorough assessment that considers underlying factors like infections and viral nephropathies is necessary in renal care management and in achieving optimal outcomes in the broader context of general medicine for the renal and genitourinary system (Figure 9.7).

9.3.3. Kidney Stones

Kidney stones or nephrolithiasis are a significant problem in the renal and genitourinary systems due to their increasing prevalence and healthcare costs. Nephrolithiasis is a calcified mineral deposits that form within the kidneys and can be of different sizes and compositions, but is typically composed of calcium oxalate, uric acid, and struvite. Risk factors encompass genetic, dietary, and environmental factors, such as dehydration, overeating foods high in oxalate, and certain metabolic conditions. The mechanism of stone production is a multifactorial process that includes supersaturation of the urine with stone material, decreased urinary inhibitor, and altered urinary pH, all leading to crystal precipitation. These mechanisms need to be understood to develop preventative interventions and therapeutic regimens, especially for susceptible populations, to decrease renal colic attacks and the development of CKD (Burity et al., 2014). Clinical manifestations of kidney stones vary widely based on their size and location within the urinary tract. Patients may present with acute pain, typically in the form of flank pain, and hematuria, nausea, and vomiting. Acute presentation of these symptoms usually brings patients in for emergency assessment, during which imaging techniques, such as ultrasound or

CT, are employed for diagnosis. Although small stones can pass spontaneously with adequate hydration, larger stones are more likely to cause complications, such as urinary obstruction, hydronephrosis, or infection. Treatment choices range from conservative strategies, including water intake enhancement and analgesia, to interventions like extracorporeal shock wave lithotripsy or ureteroscopy, depending on the type of stones and symptoms in the patient. Their presence is necessary for proper care and prevention of recurrence (Andreoli et al., 2018). Prevention of kidney stone recurrence is essential, particularly in individuals who have recurrent episodes. Total management includes educating the patient on dietary modifications, increased fluid intake, and medication treatment as required. Dietary modification should focus on decreasing sodium intake, regulating protein intake, and increasing fluid intake to produce a minimum of two liters of urine daily. For some stones, medication can be administered to correct metabolic disturbances or reduce saturation of the stone-forming substances in urine. Regular follow-up and monitoring of urinary parameters can also guide individualized prevention strategies, enabling patients to manage their condition optimally. Focusing on prevention by health professionals can significantly reduce the burden of recurrent nephrolithiasis and its complications, while also supporting overall kidney function in the population (Burity et al., 2014) (Figure 9.8).

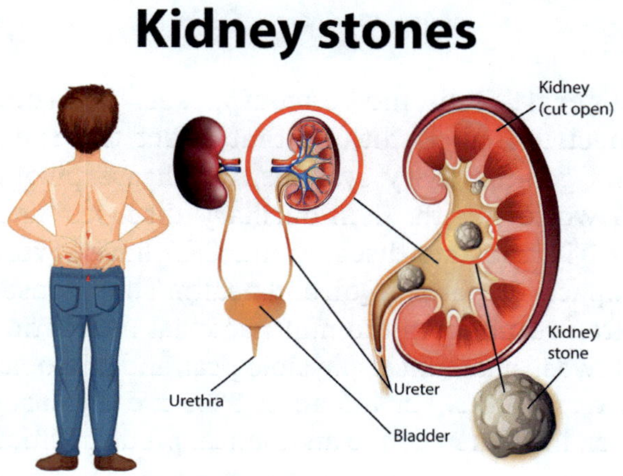

Figure 9.8. Understanding kidney stones.

Source: https://handehospital.org/wp-content/uploads/2024/04/Kidney-Stones-scaled.jpg.

Test Your Knowledge

1. What are the major causes and risk factors for the development of chronic kidney disease (CKD)?
2. How is acute kidney injury (AKI) classified, and what are the key differences between prerenal, intrarenal, and postrenal causes?

9.4. Genitourinary Disorders

Learning Outcome

1. Describe urinary tract infections (UTIs)
2. Discuss prostate disorders
3. Explain how Incontinence issues represent a significant challenge within the broader context of renal and genitourinary

General medicine encompasses a broad spectrum of conditions that affect the renal and genitourinary systems, which are pivotal to world health. Genitourinary diseases such as UTI, prostate disease, and CKD have severe impacts on patient QoL and health. The diseases often result from the multifactorial interaction between anatomical, physiological, and microbial determinants. For instance, UTIs are primarily seen in women due to anatomical predisposition and cause symptoms of dysuria and frequency. Prompt treatment is necessary; delayed treatment can lead to ascending infection with pyelonephritis or sepsis. In turn, identification of risk factors and preventive approaches is imperative to improving genitourinary health patient outcomes, and therefore, the need for successful screening and education programs in primary care settings. CKD constitutes another important group of genitourinary conditions that pose a growing health risk, particularly for the elderly. CKD's insidious progression is often asymptomatic until late presentation, making early detection paramount. Varying parameters, like proteinuria and glomerular filtration rate (GFR), are employed to quantify renal function and the extent of kidney injury. Comorbidities like hypertension and diabetes facilitate increasing renal impairment, resulting in conditions like CVD. Multifactorial treatment protocols for these comorbidities are found to enhance CKD care outcomes, according to research. For instance, diabetic patients are supported by condition-specifically designed intervention that caters to their individual health needs, as reflected in the study showing that individuals with depression have a more difficult time in achieving glycemic control (Bolt et al., 2015). This emphasizes integrated thinking in the management of genitourinary disease. Furthermore, there is no denying the intersection between genitourinary illness and mental health, as the psychological state directly influences the management of long-term conditions. Genitourinary patients endure social stigmatization and suffering in their emotional lives, which may hinder their reaction to treatment. Effective communication between healthcare professionals and patients is the solution to such barriers, but most practitioners lack the necessary skills to manage the psychosocial aspects of care. Further, evidence indicates that psychiatric disorders are associated with both treatment regimen non-compliance and the achievement of health goals in the management of chronic disease (Burity et al., 2014). Therefore, the inclusion of mental health screening and supportive counseling in the management of genitourinary conditions is necessary, enabling a general treatment regimen that considers physical and psychiatric well-being as well as improved patient outcomes.

9.4.1. Urinary Tract Infections (UTIs)

Urinary tract infections (UTIs) are a significant illness, typically of the renal and genitourinary tracts. With UTIs and bacterial proliferation in the urinary tract, the condition can have multiple symptoms, from dysuria to more generalized presentations such as fever and malaise. In certain populations, particularly the elderly, presentation is less typical and generally leads to overdiagnosis and overtreatment due to nonspecific clinical manifestations. Urinalysis remains a common diagnostic method, but its validity is undermined in older patients, where asymptomatic bacteriuria may not be treated. Thus, clinicians must exercise careful clinical acumen in distinguishing genuine infection from innocent bacteriuria, particularly by using local guidelines that address resistance patterns and recommend narrow-spectrum antimicrobial therapy, thereby minimizing exposure to inappropriate antibiotics (Beveridge et al., 2011). UTI management needs to be an EBP, underpinned by shifting clinical guidelines to bridge gaps in methodology and empirical treatment regimens. Current consensus statements, founded on systematic reviews and collaborative consultation among global experts, show the lack of high-quality data surrounding UTI management. Less than one in four questions regarding prevention, diagnosis, and treatment led to unambiguous guidance. The disparity here emphasizes the need for ongoing research and clinical trials on UTI interventions that can provide solid, evidence-based recommendations. In addition, the emphasis on clinical review and not firm recommendations for much of UTI care captures the complexity and the nuance involved in this ubiquitous but multifaceted illness (Abdul-Azim et al., 2024).

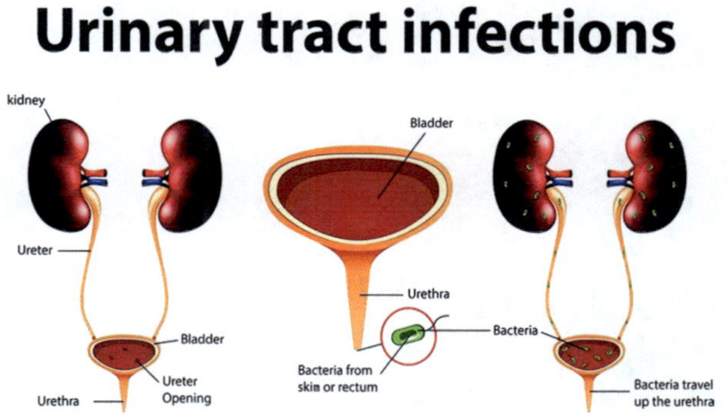

Figure 9.9. Urinary tract infections (UTIs).

Source: https://www.apexhospitals.com/_next/image?url=https%3A%2F%2Fbed.apexhospitals.com% 2Fuploads%2FUTI_3d1a698556.png&w= 1920&q=75.

In addition to encouraging general awareness of UTIs, there is a need to review prevention strategies that can inhibit infection risk, especially in at-risk individuals. These include observing good hygiene habits, maintaining adequate fluid intake, and properly controlling indwelling catheters, which are most commonly associated with catheter-associated UTIs. Recent findings show that reducing catheter use and opting for alternative options can significantly decrease infection prevalence. Therefore, prevention must be integrated into clinical practice, as it can benefit not only individual patients but also alleviate the burden of UTIs on healthcare systems. As the field continues to evolve, increased emphasis on antimicrobial stewardship and narrow-spectrum agents will also be important in successfully and responsibly treating UTIs (Beveridge et al., 2011) (Figure 9.9).

9.4.2. Prostate Disorders

Diseases of the prostate are a crucial aspect of men's health, and conditions such as benign prostatic hyperplasia (BPH), prostatitis, and cancer of the prostate are of special concern. BPH is the enlargement of the prostate gland, which is most commonly identified in older men and which may result in urinary symptoms, including a delay in initiating urination, frequency, and nighttime urination. Statistics indicate that at age 60 years, approximately 50% of men will experience symptoms of BPH, hence making it a significant field of study in general medicine. Understanding the pathophysiology of BPH, which is believed to be due to hormonal and growth factor changes, is essential for effective management and treatment using drugs and surgery based on the intensity of the symptoms. Prostatitis, or inflammation of the prostate, can occur at any age and is classified as acute and chronic. Acute bacterial prostatitis is a condition that requires emergency treatment due to its potential to cause systemic complications. Chronic prostatitis (CP) presents a complex issue, which is often associated with pelvic pain and has significant impairment of QoL. There is some evidence to suggest that CP may be non-infectious in origin and, therefore, challenging to treat. The interconnection between psychological morbidity and patient symptom perception in the case of CP also suggests a multidisciplinary approach to care, with a focus on combining urology, psychology, and physical therapy services in order to treat it effectively. Another serious condition within the prostate disorder category is erectile dysfunction. It is the most frequent cancer diagnosis in men, particularly men above 50 years of age. Though actual causation remains unclear, genetic predisposition, diet, and exposure to some environmental agents are associated with increased risk. Early detection and improved survival occur with repetitive screening through prostate-specific antigen (PSA) testing and digital rectal exam. However, the complexity of treatment options like active surveillance, surgery, and radiation therapy requires detailed counseling between healthcare professionals and patients regarding intended benefit versus risk. With increasing knowledge about prostate cancer through investigations, identification of the molecular and genetic characteristics of prostate cancer can unveil new therapeutic advances that can redirect management for this prevalent disorder from the perspective of general medicine of the renal and genitourinary tract (Figure 9.10).

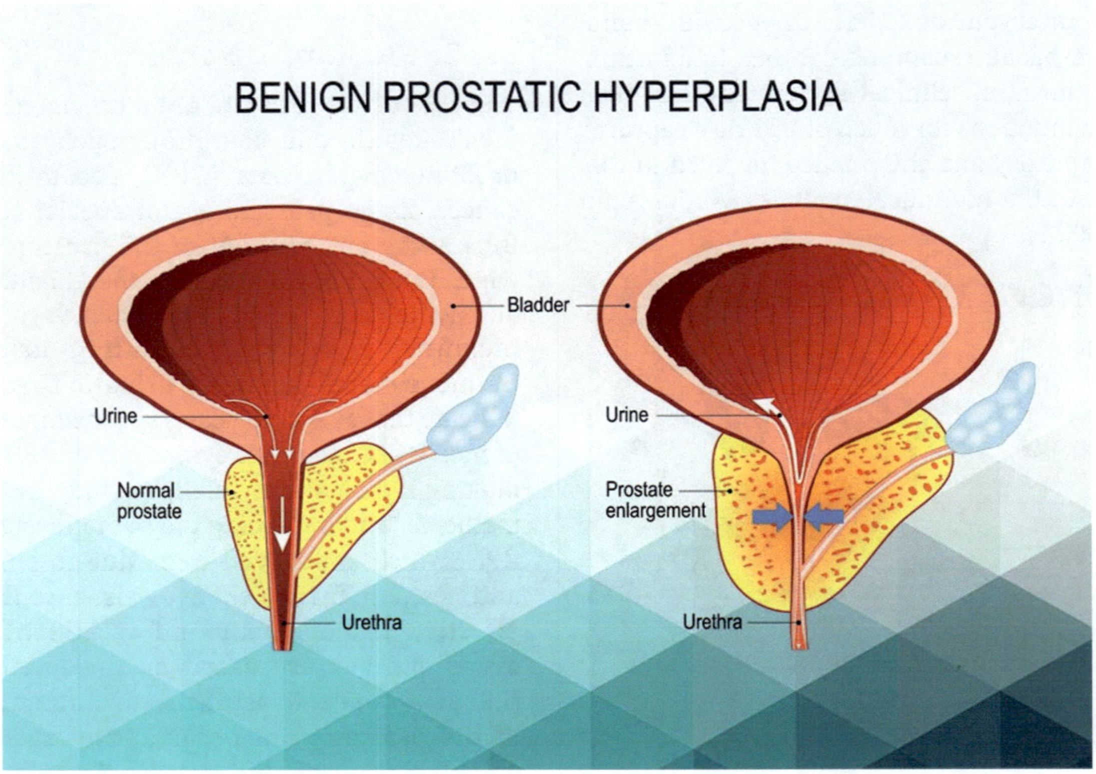

Figure 9.10. Benign prostatic hyperplasia.

Source: https://advuro.com/wp-content/uploads/2021/01/benign-prostatic-hyperplasia-graphic.jpg.

9.4.3. Incontinence Issues

Incontinence issues are a significant issue in the overall picture of renal and genitourinary well-being, crossing all age demographics. Incontinence issues can arise due to many reasons, including age, sex, and overall medical issues. Although urinary incontinence is often perceived as an independent issue, it typically coexists with other medical issues, including metabolic syndrome and pelvic floor dysfunction. For instance, in females, the complications of surgical interventions of conditions like uterine fibroids might aggravate incontinence symptoms, hence complicating the clinical presentation. This serves to highlight the importance of clinicians adopting a holistic approach to incontinence management, whereby all intersecting medical conditions are treated and controlled appropriately, since incontinence, if left untreated, can lead to compromised QoL and increased healthcare use. Aside from that, the complexities of incontinence are not only bodily but also psychosocial. Incontinence traditionally results in embarrassment and social withdrawal on the part of patients, making them resistant to treatment. Recent studies have indicated that most people with urinary incontinence do not report their incontinence to health professionals, primarily due to misinterpretation of the controllability of the condition. This pattern is most evident among younger groups, where the stigma of incontinence is perhaps more pronounced. Practitioners need to recognize these dynamics, as these emphasize patient education and open communication about incontinence interventions. With improved communication and care support, health professionals can empower patients to tackle these challenges without fear of judgment, resulting in better health outcomes. In addressing the clinical treatment of incontinence, recent advances in treatment strategies hold promising avenues for successful intervention. It is suggested by study results that rehabilitation programs tailored to individuals, along with appropriate surgical interventions, can effectively reduce incontinence symptom severity and associated dysfunctions. For instance, individualized rehabilitation following hysterectomy surgery has proved the regression of symptoms like stress urinary incontinence and pelvic floor failure, employing hormone treatments and specific pelvic floor exercise. These multifaceted interventions not only address the physical symptoms but also enhance overall QoL in patients with these illnesses. Despite current solutions, the ongoing challenges in detecting and diagnosing incontinence necessitate further research and the evolution of streamlined processes, particularly within transitional care settings. Clearer guidelines will be important to ensuring patients receive comprehensive and continuous care throughout their lifetime, ensuring proper control over incontinence conditions in accordance with their holistic health needs, as noted by Bavendam et al. (2017) and Proshchenko et al. (2022) (Figure 9.11).

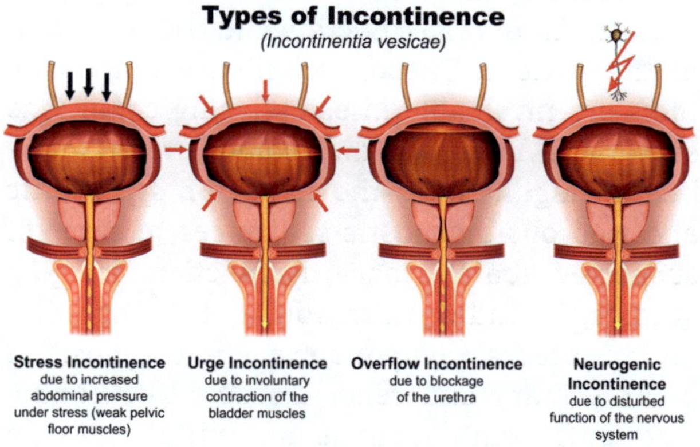

Figure 9.11. Types of incontinence.

Source: https://cdn2.webdamdb.com/1280_UzC6dpmQiMI48o7E.jpg?1673548883.

Test Your Knowledge

1. What are the common causative organisms of urinary tract infections (UTIs), and what factors predispose individuals to recurrent UTIs?
2. Describe the different types of prostate disorders.

9.5. Diagnostic Approaches

Learning Outcome

1. Understand urinalysis and blood tests
2. Describe imaging techniques for renal and genitourinary systems
3. Define biopsy procedures

Diagnostic approaches in renal and genitourinary medicine are crucial to successful patient management and response to treatment. Diagnostic approaches involve various methodologies that include urine and blood tests, imaging modalities, and, in some instances, invasive procedures like biopsies. Accurate patient history and physical exam frequently offer the first step toward diagnosis, allowing clinicians to identify signs and symptoms that may lead to specific renal disease or urologic illnesses. Subsequently, non-invasive tests such as urinalysis and serum creatinine assay permit assessment of renal function and overall health of the patient. These preliminary diagnostic tools are invaluable in establishing conditions such as CKD or UTI that could affect kidney health, highlighting the need for systematic and rigorous diagnostic sequences in cases of suspected genitourinary dysfunction. Imaging studies, including ultrasound, CT, and MRI, are an integral component of the diagnosis of genitourinary and renal disease. Ultrasound, frequently employed as an initial imaging modality, provides valuable information regarding kidney size and structure, while CT scans can yield more advanced visual displays of renal tumors or obstructions. The use of MRI, where exposure to ionizing radiation is a limiting factor, also improves the diagnostic process by allowing the evaluation of abnormalities in soft tissues as well as vascular structures. Each modality has its own strengths and weaknesses, and therefore, clinicians must identify the most suitable technique for use depending on the specific patient case. Moreover, integration of imaging findings with clinical data enhances diagnostic sensitivity, which enables appropriate and timely interventions in the management of renal and genitourinary disease. Besides traditional diagnostics, advances in genetic diagnosis and molecular diagnosis have offered a critical element of renal disease knowledge. For instance, the detection of diseases such as 22q11.2 deletion syndrome illustrates the overall significance of genetic disorders in renal and genitourinary health. Studies have indicated that the syndrome goes hand in hand with a variety of congenital anomalies, including malformations in the kidneys, hence the need for comprehensive screening and genetic counseling among the affected (Bassett et al., 2015). The progress further demonstrates the importance of using a multidisciplinary approach in treating the condition, integrating specialties such as pediatrics, surgery, and genetics to provide cohesive care. By recognizing the complexity introduced by genetic factors and the connection to renal function, physicians can better tailor diagnosis and treatment protocols that address the immediate threat while also incorporating long-term patient management and outcome optimization.

9.5.1. Urinalysis and Blood Tests

Urinalysis is a valuable diagnostic tool in the evaluation of renal and genitourinary function, enabling clinicians to screen for many conditions, including UTIs, renal dysfunction, and metabolic disease. Through analysis of urine samples, which can be obtained with methods such as midstream clean catch or catheterization, the physician can determine aspects like specific gravity, pH, protein, glucose, and the presence of pathologies such as bacteria and leukocytes. Of note, urine culture remains the gold standard for diagnosing UTI, and research has indicated that a well-designed symptom cluster will often eliminate culture in certain situations, as demonstrated by recent data indicating high sensitivity and specificity with symptom-based diagnosis (Lamond et al., 2006). Thus, urinalysis, in addition to enabling early detection and intervention, is a cost-effective method of delivering healthcare in managing urinary conditions. Blood work is also a key component of the diagnosis of kidney and urinary health, yielding information about renal function and systemic disease. Markers such as serum creatinine, BUN, and electrolytes are repeatedly monitored to measure kidney function and detect renal impairment. They serve as markers of GFR and are essential for determining the effectiveness of the kidneys at filtering waste from the blood. Besides, urinalysis increases the diagnostic significance of blood analysis for nephritis, AKI, and CKD. More sophisticated testing procedures, such as those probing the interaction of analyses of the results from blood and urine samples, can enhance diagnostic processes significantly, as suggested by studies with enhanced predictive values derived from extensive screening tests (Kabilan et al., 2017). Thus, mixing blood analysis with urinalysis yields a balanced approach to renal and genitourinary health maintenance. For pediatric health in particular, blood testing and urinalysis necessitate special consideration due to the diagnostic challenges inherent with younger populations. In children with UTI symptoms, studies have shown that more frequent urinalysis with complete investigations, such as urine white blood cell count and Gram stain, is more sensitive compared to routine investigations (Kabilan et al., 2017). This is particularly important, as early treatment and diagnosis prevent potential complications of untreated urinary infection. Moreover, blood testing in this population, though less common, is instrumental in the detection of systemic infection or complications of renal disease. By using a judicious combination of advanced urinalysis techniques and selective blood sampling, healthcare practitioners can establish a sounder and more effective model for diagnosis and treatment of urinary disease in children, such that interventions are timely and appropriate for this high-risk patient group (Figure 9.12).

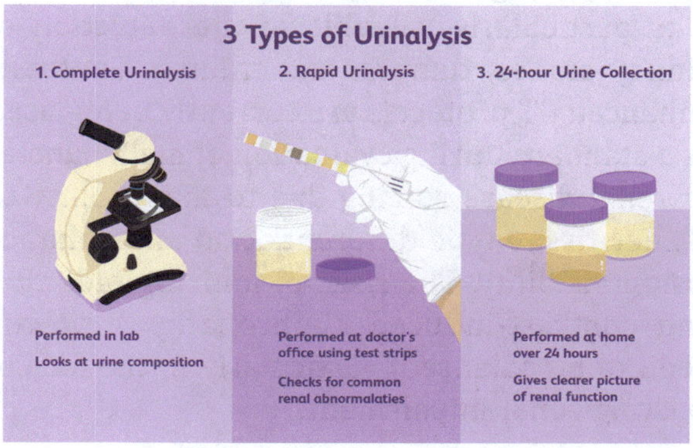

Figure 9.12. Types of urinalysis.

Source: https://www.verywellhealth.com/thmb/1CSy-NkV6JJb8uiD6w03FdENyzs=/1500x0/filters:no_upscale():max_bytes(150000):strip_icc()/3156950_color-5ba560b4c9e77c008233667f.png.

9.5.2. Imaging Techniques (Ultrasound, CT, MRI)

Imaging modalities play a crucial role in the management and assessment of renal and genitourinary disease. Of all the modalities used, ultrasound is most frequently utilized due to its non-invasive nature and ability to be employed for real-time imaging. The modality is excellent in assessing renal anatomy, presence of renal masses, and conditions such as hydronephrosis or renal cysts. Its non-ionizing nature and low cost are benefits of ultrasound; therefore, it is a first-line tool, especially in pediatrics and obstetrics. Also, recent advances in ultrasound technology, e.g., Doppler imaging, further enhance its use in evaluating blood flow and vascular impairment within the kidney and adjacent structures to provide a more comprehensible picture of the renal condition. While ultrasound is an excellent initial imaging modality, CT significantly increases diagnostic value, especially in difficult situations. CT scans provide detailed high-resolution images and allow for viewing the renal and urinary tract anatomy in greater detail than ultrasound. It is particularly valuable in the detection of kidney stones, tumors, and trauma. Contrast-enhanced CT protocols are currently being used as a standard during evaluation of malignancies or renal disease staging due to their ability to render tissue type differentiation and enhance lesion visibility. The risks of ionizing radiation and contrast-induced nephropathy, however, need to be balanced, particularly in the face of existing renal impairment.

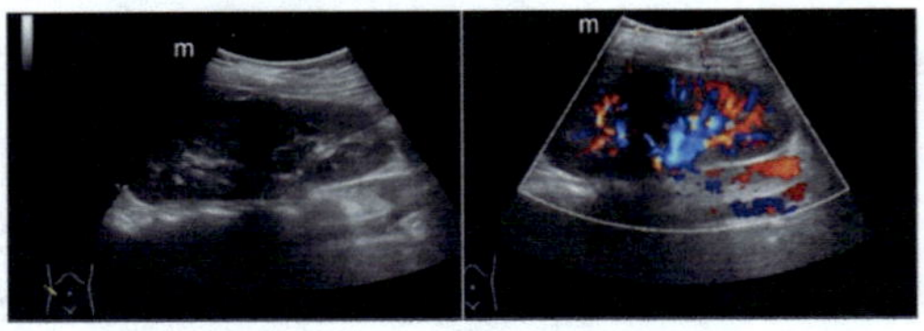

Figure 9.13. Ultrasound of the patient's urinary system showed the right kidney was visible.

Source: https://www.researchgate.net/publication/355739770/figure/fig2/AS:1084311923105792@1635531516342/The-ultrasound-of-the-patients-urinary-system-showed-that-the-right-kidney-was-visible.jpg.

Therefore, appropriate risk-benefit analyses are needed in the selection of CT scanning in the context of renal and genitourinary examinations. MRI provides another powerful addition to the diagnostic armamentarium for renal and genitourinary disease, particularly when contrast involving soft tissue is most important. MRI is especially valuable in staging renal tumors, detecting lesions, and diagnosing pelvic floor disorders due to its improved resolution of soft tissues and the lack of ionizing radiation. MRI is particularly advantageous in patients with contraindications to CT contrast material as it employs gadolinium-based contrast agents, which tend to be safer for this group of patients. Moreover, fMRI techniques, such as diffusion-weighted imaging (DWI), yield data on tumor characterization and response to therapy, enhancing individualized treatment plans. Thus, the addition of MRI in imaging allows for a more robust approach to understanding complex renal and genitourinary pathologies, as illustrated by recent evidence of its applicability in clinical practice (N/A, 1987; Burity et al., 2014) (Figure 9.13).

9.5.3. Biopsy Procedures

Biopsy procedures are a critical part of renal and genitourinary disease diagnostic investigation, and they are required to provide histological evidence for appropriate management. Two primary types of biopsies used in such situations are needle biopsy and surgical biopsy. Biopsies using a needle are performed by percutaneously inserting a needle to sample tissues from the kidney or covering tissues, offering an option with minimal invasiveness and reduced recovery times. Generally performed as ultrasound or CT-guided procedures, needle biopsies allow for the diagnosis of conditions such as glomerulonephritis or kidney cancers. In-depth access to the targeted region for obtaining tissue samples will enable pathologists to provide positive diagnoses that are essential in therapeutic considerations and prognostic estimates important for patient care. Not only are biopsy methods used in diagnosis, but they are also used in the management of renal and genitourinary illnesses. For instance, the evaluation of abnormal renal masses identified by imaging studies at times involves a biopsy to distinguish between malignant and benign lesions. Accurate histological assessment via biopsy has the capability of changing treatment protocols significantly; for example, a diagnosis of non-secretory multiple myeloma diagnosed through a colonic biopsy illustrated just how crucial biopsies are not just in diagnosing conditions but also in detecting complications, such as the one leading to renal failure (Delicata et al., 2013). Moreover, with the management of chronic illness, such as end-stage renal disease and chronic viral hepatitis, biopsies can shed light on underlying pathologies that eventually shape management plans and improve patient care (Breaban et al., 2018). Altogether, biopsy procedures are prevalent within the practice of general medicine concerning renal and genitourinary systems, enabling a greater understanding of various diseases. The success of such protocols relies on their ability to provide meaningful information about tissue pathology and cellular features, which inform clinical decisions. With advancements in imaging technology and biopsy techniques, the precision of biopsies only continues to rise, with the potential for enhanced patient outcomes through early and targeted interventions. The integration of biopsy with clinical data enhances risk stratification and therapeutic care in patients, representing a critical convergence of imaging, pathology, and treatment approaches in modern medicine.

Test Your Knowledge

1. What key components of urinalysis help in diagnosing renal and genitourinary disorders, and how do abnormal findings guide further investigation?
2. Which blood tests are most commonly used to assess kidney function and detect genitourinary diseases, and what do their results indicate?

9.6. Treatment Options

Learning Outcome

1. Discuss pharmacological interventions in the management of conditions about the renal and genitourinary systems
2. Understand the surgical landscape in the renal and genitourinary system
3. Explain the concept of lifestyle modifications

In renal and genitourinary medicine, treatment is multi-faceted due to the complexity of conditions in this body system. Treatment can differ with the diagnosis, etiology, and overall health of the patient. To illustrate, patients with CKD may be managed by behavioral changes such as diet and exercise, in addition to pharmacological therapy to control hypertension and diabetes, the most frequent comorbidities. In addition, ACE inhibitor administration has been found to slow CKD progression and thus become a foundation for CKD management. This patient-specific therapeutic approach emphasizes that healthcare professionals should conduct diligent evaluations to guide sound treatment modalities and address specific patient needs and preferences. Surgical interventions are also a necessary component in the platform of treatment for renal and genitourinary disease. Renal tumors or intensive obstruction due to calculi may necessitate procedures ranging from minimal laparoscopic intervention to more robust open surgery. Additionally, robot-assisted surgeries have boosted accuracy in procedures, reducing recovery times and enabling better patient outcomes. For end-stage renal disease, renal transplantation continues to be the preferred option, giving patients hope to have a normal life without needing dialysis. However, the success of such procedures relies upon an entirely clear comprehension of the patient's condition and associated risks, increasing the part played by multidisciplinary teams in creating worldwide regimens of treatment. In consideration of the non-surgical treatments, therapeutic pharmacology has extensively widened the scope of accessible therapies for numerous renal and genitourinary diseases. For instance, novel advances in immunosuppressive therapy have improved patient results in kidney transplants, overcoming such drawbacks as rejection. New drugs for the treatment of urinary incontinence and BPH have also emerged, resulting in improved QoL for affected individuals. With increasingly more treatment modalities being uncovered through continuous research, particularly of NCDs as observed in more recent studies, medical practitioners should be vigilant to determine the cost-effectiveness of these treatments. This is so that not only are new therapies beneficial from their clinical relevance but also sustainable within the constraints of limited healthcare resources (Fox-Rushby et al., 2006). Ultimately, evolution in treatment depends on an active and reactive health community that is prepared to change based on emerging evidence and patient need.

9.6.1. Pharmacological Interventions

Pharmacotherapeutic treatment is a significant element in treating renal and genitourinary system-related conditions. The systems are so complex that multiple components are necessary to treat them, and both the chronic and acute forms of drug treatment are usually involved. Such drugs as ACE inhibitors and diuretics are commonly utilized for the management of hypertension and fluid overload, which are frequent among patients with renal disease. Moreover, treatments of CKD may also involve erythropoiesis-stimulating agents (ESAs) to counteract anemia, a frequent complication that arises as a consequence of reduced erythropoietin production by the kidneys. The accurate choice and management of these drug agents require a thorough understanding of their pharmacodynamics and PK, particularly regarding renal function, as improper dosing may result in drastic side effects or exacerbation of the disease. Surgical operations within the genitourinary system usually require the use of antibiotic prophylaxis to prevent postoperative infection complications. The rationale for using antibiotics before and during surgeries is highlighted by the risk of infection, which plays a significant role in determining the patient's outcome. For instance, when conducting surgery on the kidneys or bladder, empirical antibiotic prophylaxis is essential. Individualizing the selection of antibiotics to patient-specific profiles and comorbidities, such as renal insufficiency, is paramount. In addition to preventing infection, it also addresses the growing problem of antibiotic resistance. Prophylactic antibiotic use is also informed by economic affordability and clinical efficacy considerations, which optimizes the result of therapy while reducing the likelihood of complications due to multidrug-resistant (MDR) pathogens (Farkhodovich et al., 2023). Moreover, congenital condition treatment, like in the 22q11.2 deletion syndrome, requires an interprofessional team that provides a combination of pharmacological approaches with surgery and psychological therapy. Patients with the syndrome are mainly prone to several complications, including renal abnormalities, which require prompt diagnosis and an individualized therapeutic scheme. The clinical variability highlights the necessity of personalized pharmacotherapy, particularly in treating cognitive, behavioral, and renal abnormalities (Bassett et al., 2015). Effective management relies on a prompt diagnosis that facilitates timely intervention with pharmacological treatment, addressing the physiological and psychological features of the syndrome. Therefore, it is important to combine pharmacological treatments with surgical and general management strategies in order to improve overall patient outcomes in general medicine for the renal and genitourinary tract (Figure 9.14).

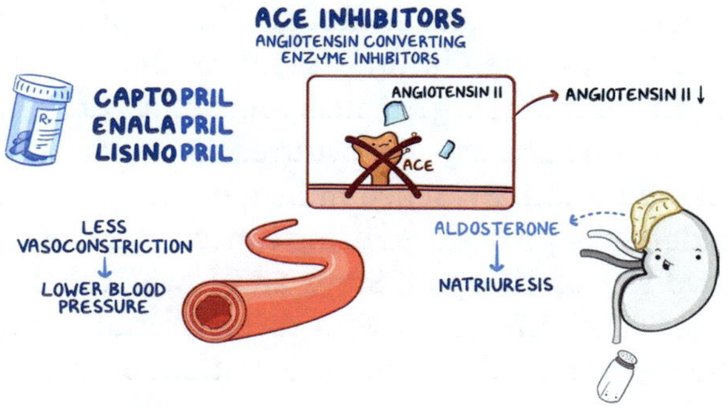

Figure 9.14. ACE inhibitors.

Source: https://d16qt3wv6xm098.cloudfront.net/B3ZRfzxyRDCK3r-Ed-egwQ7JQmyqCXT0/_.jpg.

9.6.2. Surgical Procedures

The field of surgery in the renal and genitourinary tract includes a wide range of procedures necessary for correcting various conditions. Urologists perform operations that address disorders such as kidney stones, prostate cancer, and urinary incontinence, whereas nephrologists specialize in kidney-specific procedures. Some of the common surgeries are nephrectomies, cystectomies, and prostatectomies. All of these procedures can be performed with the traditional open technique or minimal invasive techniques such as laparoscopy or robotic-assisted surgery, which not only reduce tissue damage but also reduce recuperation time, making it possible for patients to return to normal function earlier. Consequently, more patients are increasingly opting to have surgery rather than conservative treatment plans, so it is necessary to become well-versed in the operative method, indications, and selection criteria for patients involved. One of the changes in surgical practice is the move towards the use of more conscious sedation for procedures, as in the case with TAVR for cardiac treatment, indicating an overall trend in surgical specialties. Conscious sedation is a state of induced sedation with control that allows patients to remain awake, thus enhancing faster recovery and fewer complications compared to general anesthesia. Although the application of conscious sedation is more defined in cardiovascular surgery, its applicability to renal and genitourinary procedures is an area of consideration. Evidence indicates that patients undergoing procedures using conscious sedation have shorter hospital stays and lower costs of care. This shift aligns with recent initiatives in the medical field of enhancing patient outcomes while being cost-effective in the utilization of healthcare resources, an integrating approach critical to the evolving nature of surgery in the renal and genitourinary domain (Aksoy et al., 2017). The administrative aspect of surgery in the renal and genitourinary apparatus also warrants consideration, particularly in relation to healthcare expenditure and patient outcomes. With the narrowing of resources, information regarding cost-effectiveness in different surgical methods is essential. A critical analysis of outcomes associated with different procedures, including hospitalization and follow-up, is required for optimizing surgical procedures. There is a necessity to incorporate EBP that not only ensures patient safety and satisfaction but also incorporates costs. Lastly, the marriage of innovative surgical techniques with cost-effective protocols lends to greater aggregate effectiveness throughout the health system, which provides the impetus for continued improvement in surgical technique aimed specifically at the renal and genitourinary specialties. By optimizing both the twin goal of quality care and economic sustainability, the field can optimize the QoL for patients alongside learning the nuances of modern medicine (Burity et al., 2014).

9.6.3. Lifestyle Modifications

In general medicine, and more specifically in the renal and genitourinary systems, adopting lifestyle modifications is crucial for disease prevention and treatment. Multiple lifestyle problems—be it diet and exercise, stress reduction, and so on—play a vital part in the upkeep of healthy kidneys and prevention of such complications as hypertension. Research indicates that dietary modifications can bring a dramatic impact to blood pressure levels; for example, an oral Nigella sativa seed extract trial demonstrated a significant reduction of systolic and diastolic blood pressure of patients, highlighting the therapeutic potential of nutrition in the management of renal-associated hypertension (Kamkhah et al., 2008). However, these findings highlight the need to place dietary interventions as part of regular kidney care regimens. Physical activity is also an essential component of lifestyle modification that can profoundly promote renal function and general health. Apart from maintaining weight, physical activity also promotes heart health, which in turn is deeply linked with kidney disease. At least 150 minutes of moderate-intensity aerobic physical activities such as walking, cycling, or swimming per week is normally recommended to maintain optimal kidney function.

This exercise regimen has been shown to minimize disorders like obesity and diabetes, which are key risk factors in renal decline. Additionally, stress-reduction interventions like mindfulness and yoga can enhance an individual's mental health status, leading to improved lifestyle practices and renal health outcomes. All of these integrative approaches emphasize the multifaceted nature of lifestyle interventions in improving renal as well as genitourinary system health. In addition, the social environment of lifestyle determinants also must be considered, particularly in communities where urbanization and lifestyle changes are happening at an accelerated rate. In China, for instance, increased CVD among women reflects underlying lifestyle determinants associated with industrialization, such as poor diets and lower physical activity levels (Cao et al., 2008). Recognizing these trends, public health interventions should emphasize education on modifiable risk factors and incorporate culturally sensitive methods for behavior change. Evidence-based interventions for community participatory approaches to intervention can increase awareness, which can be translated into active management of renal and CVD risk factors. By addressing both individual behavior and more general social determinants of health, overall lifestyle change programs have the potential to make a significant difference in population health indicators for the genitourinary and renal system.

Test Your Knowledge

1. What are the common pharmacological treatments used for managing chronic kidney disease and acute kidney injury?
2. Describe the surgical options available for kidney stones and prostate disorders, including indications and expected outcomes.

SUMMARY

It is important to understand the nuances of the genitourinary and renal tract systems to be able to manage effectively in the clinical practice. The subject encompasses a range of disorders, from congenital issues to prevalent diseases like UTIs and nephrolithiasis. With continuous advancement by medical professionals in the diagnostic and treatment procedures, it is important to maintain a wide, multidisciplinary approach to the care of patients. Smooth specialty overlap, e.g., pediatrics and adult urology, may attain improved patient outcomes in situations where patients are transitioning from childhood to adulthood, especially with complex cases like in the case study where pediatric urologists consented strongly to ongoing specialized treatment of such patients (Cain et al., 2015). Furthermore, one-on-one care cannot be overemphasized because patients have different clinical profiles that need individualized treatment strategies. In menopausal medicine, for instance, hormone therapy is of significant value, particularly among symptomatic postmenopausal women younger than specific age thresholds (Davis et al., 2015). However, in line with guidelines today, clinicians must weigh the harms and benefits of these treatments against the values of the patients in an effort to optimize outcomes. It is this patient-focused style that not only encourages adherence to clinical guidelines but also leads to a deeper understanding of the specific requirements of each individual presenting with renal and genitourinary conditions. There is an imperative for future research and teaching in renal and genitourinary medicine. Continued research in new therapies and technology will be critical to advance modalities of therapy, especially with population demographics shifts that highlight the rising prevalence of urologic disease. Enhanced education for urologists and medical caregivers with a focus on transitional care is critical in bridging the gap between pediatric and adult care (Cain et al., 2015). By fostering a culture of learning that emphasizes EBP and collaborative practice, the medical community can improve patient care in this vital health area to the highest degree. Ultimately, the goal is still simple: to elevate the quality of care for individuals with renal and genitourinary conditions.

The genitourinary and renal systems play crucial roles in controlling most body functions and maintaining homeostasis. Understanding the anatomy and physiology of the systems is critical in grasping their significance to health in general. The kidneys, which filter out blood and eliminate waste products, play a significant role in maintaining electrolyte and fluid balance. In addition, the urinary system, including the ureters, bladder, and urethra, facilitates the discharge of wastes while ensuring effective urinary function. The dual functionality of these systems reflects their significance in upholding not only physical health but also affecting other body systems through feedback mechanisms. The frequency of prevalent renal and genitourinary system diseases, such as CKD, UTI, and nephrolithiasis, indicates these systems' vulnerability and complexity. CKD develops due to diabetes and hypertension, shows the systemic importance of kidney failure, and can lead to deadly complications if uncontrolled. At the same time, recurrent UTIs and stone development block normal functioning and create pain and even the need for surgery. Healthcare providers must know about these conditions to implement appropriate management strategies and improve patient outcomes, highlighting the interdependent relationship between renal health and overall health. Therapeutic interventions for disease in the renal and genitourinary systems are multifaceted and encompass an evolved understanding of both medical and surgical treatments. Pharmacological treatment, including the application of diuretics and antibiotics, is a component of the treatment for acute and chronic illness, tailored to the needs of the patient. Moreover, advances in surgical techniques, including minimally invasive techniques to remove stones, are significant advances toward the care of patients. As this type of therapy continues to evolve, it is increasingly vital that medical professionals stay informed about new advances and research techniques. Knowing about the different forms of treatment in depth allows practitioners to offer patients with issues in the renal and genitourinary tracts the best type of effective and all-encompassing care, thereby improving their lives (N/A, 1990, 1991).

KEY TERMS FROM THIS CHAPTER

- Acid-base balance
- Acute kidney injury (AKI)
- Antidiuretic hormone (ADH)
- Chromosomal microdeletion disorder
- Chronic prostatitis (CP)
- CKD symptoms
- Clinical data
- Crystal precipitation
- Doppler imaging
- Electrolyte balance
- Electrolyte imbalance
- General urinary health
- Genitourinary disease
- Genitourinary system
- Glomerulonephritis
- Hypoparathyroidism
- Indolent renal cortical tumors
- Kidney stones

CRITICAL THINKING QUESTIONS

1. **Which of the following is the most common cause of acute kidney injury (AKI) in hospitalized patients?**
   a. Glomerulonephritis
   b. Polycystic kidney disease
   c. Acute tubular necrosis
   d. Renal artery stenosis
2. **Which diagnostic test is considered the gold standard for evaluating kidney function?**
   a. Urinalysis
   b. Serum creatinine and estimated glomerular filtration rate (eGFR)
   c. Ultrasound of kidneys
   d. Kidney biopsy
3. **Which condition is characterized by the presence of proteinuria, hematuria, and red blood cell casts on urine microscopy?**
   a. Glomerulonephritis
   b. Nephrotic syndrome
   c. Acute pyelonephritis
   d. Interstitial nephritis
4. **Which of the following is the most common cause of chronic kidney disease (CKD)?**
   a. Polycystic kidney disease
   b. Diabetes mellitus
   c. Urinary tract infection
   d. Nephrolithiasis
5. **What is the hallmark symptom of nephrotic syndrome?**
   a. Hematuria
   b. Polyuria
   c. Dysuria
   d. Proteinuria

Short Answer Questions

1. What are the common causes and clinical features of chronic kidney disease (CKD) and acute kidney injury (AKI)?
2. Describe the pathophysiology, symptoms, and management of urinary tract infections (UTIs).
3. What diagnostic tests, including urinalysis and blood tests, are essential for evaluating renal function and genitourinary disorders?
4. Compare and contrast imaging techniques such as ultrasound, CT scan, and MRI in diagnosing renal and genitourinary diseases.
5. Explain the indications, procedures, and risks associated with renal and prostate biopsies.
6. What pharmacological treatments are commonly used for managing kidney stones, UTIs, and prostate disorders?
7. How do lifestyle changes and dietary modifications help in preventing and managing renal and genitourinary conditions?

Answers to Critical Thinking Questions

1. (c); 2. (b); 3. (a); 4. (b); 5. (d)

REFERENCES

1. Nelson, Z., Aslan, A. T., Beahm, N. P., Blyth, M., Cappiello, M., Casaus, D., Dominguez, F., Egbert, S., Hanretty, A. Khadem, T., Olney, K., Abdul-Azim, A., Aggrey, G., Anderson, D. T., Barosa, M., Bosco, M., Chahine, E. B., Chowdhury, S., Christensen, A., . . . Lora, A. J. M. (2024). Guidelines for the prevention, diagnosis, and management of urinary tract infections in pediatrics and adults. *JAMA Network Open*, *7*(11), e2444495. https://doi.org/10.1001/jamanetworkopen.2024.44495Aggarwal, N., Ajene, G., Fedson, S., Kulkarni, A., et al. (2023). Native BK polyomavirus nephropathy in an orthotopic heart transplant patient. https://core.ac.uk/download/643778648.pdf (accessed on 27th June 2025).
2. Aguirre-Avalos, G., & Amaya-Tapia, G. (2018). Urinary tract tuberculosis. https://core.ac.uk/download/322436565.pdf (accessed on 27th June 2025).
3. Aksoy, O., Benharash, P., Fernandez, J., Johansen, H., et al. (2017). Improved costs and outcomes with conscious sedation vs general anesthesia in TAVR patients: Time to wake up? https://core.ac.uk/download/323076994.pdf (accessed on 27th June 2025).
4. Alexander, R., Alvarado, A., Lakshmanaperumal, N., McClain, S., et al. (2015). Stem cells and fluid flow drive cyst formation in an invertebrate excretory organ.
5. Andreoli, G., Bonci, E., Celani, C., Marrucci, L., et al. (2018). Long-term renal function and hypertension in adult survivors of childhood sarcoma. https://core.ac.uk/download/159268194.pdf (accessed on 27th June 2025).
6. Angelini, L., Bello, L., Bertolin, C., Briani, C., et al. (2016). Non-neural phenotype of spinal and bulbar muscular atrophy: Results from a large cohort of Italian patients. https://core.ac.uk/download/53525604.pdf (accessed on 27th June 2025).
7. Arafa, E. (2016). Determining cellular and biochemical function of a novel adhesion molecule in kidneys. https://open.bu.edu/bitstream/2144/16062/1/Arafa_bu_0017N_11077.pdf (accessed on 27th June 2025).
8. Asnis-Alibozek, H., Cardone, M., Hindman, K., Karlo, K., et al. (2016). Renal cell carcinoma: A nomogram for the CT imaging-inclusive prediction of indolent, non-clear cell renal cortical tumors. https://core.ac.uk/download/188829181.pdf (accessed on 27th June 2025).
9. Babu, P. V. V., Balaji, B., & Subrahmanyam, C. V. S. (2019). Nephrolithiasis–most debilitating renal disorder. https://core.ac.uk/download/230499548.pdf (accessed on 27th June 2025).
10. Bassett, A. S., Emanuel, B. S., Marino, B., McDonald-McGinn, D. M., et al. (2015). *22q11.2 Deletion Syndrome*. https://core.ac.uk/download/188828218.pdf (accessed on 27th June 2025).
11. Bavendam, T., Dicianno, B. E., Dosa, N. P., Gomez-Lobo, V., et al. (2017). Research needs for effective transition in lifelong care of congenital genitourinary conditions: A workshop sponsored by the National Institute of Diabetes and Digestive and Kidney Diseases. https://core.ac.uk/download/161627514.pdf (accessed on 27th June 2025).
12. Benedetti, E., Edison, M., Gehm, L., Orsay, E., et al. (2009). A descriptive analysis of 1251 solid organ transplant visits to the emergency department. https://core.ac.uk/download/pdf/8280523.pdf (accessed on 27th June 2025).
13. Beveridge, L. A., Davey, P. G., McMurdo, M. E. T., Phillips, J., et al. (2011). Optimal management of urinary tract infections in older people. https://core.ac.uk/download/20450519.pdf (accessed on 27th June 2025).

14. Bolt, D. M., Fink, J., Greenlee, R. T., Magnan, S., et al. (2015). The relationship of individual comorbid chronic conditions to diabetes care quality. https://core.ac.uk/download/323070914.pdf (accessed on 27th June 2025).

15. Breaban, I., Ciulei, G., Cozma, A., Negrean, L., et al. (2018). Thrombocytopenia in end-stage renal disease and chronic viral hepatitis B or C. https://core.ac.uk/download/216809666.pdf (accessed on 27th June 2025).

16. Burity, J., Fonte, I. B. da, & Melo, P. B. de. (2014). Radiological Society of North America (RSNA) 3D printing Special Interest Group (SIG): Guidelines for medical 3D printing and appropriateness for clinical scenarios. https://core.ac.uk/download/212867900.pdf (accessed on 27th June 2025).

17. Cain, M. P., Large, T., Misseri, R., Szymanski, K. M., et al. (2015). Current opinions regarding care of the mature pediatric urology patient. https://core.ac.uk/download/129148791.pdf (accessed on 27th June 2025).

18. Cao, Y., Davidson, P., Digiacomo, M., Du, H., et al. (2008). Cardiovascular disease in Chinese women: An emerging high-risk population and implications for nursing practice. https://opus.lib.uts.edu.au/bitstream/10453/17158/1/2010003421.pdf (accessed on 27th June 2025).

19. Davis, S. R., Gompel, A., Lumsden, M. A., Murad, M. H., et al. (2015). Treatment of symptoms of the menopause: An Endocrine Society clinical practice guideline. https://core.ac.uk/download/42367511.pdf (accessed on 27th June 2025).

20. Delicata, J., & Farrugia, D. (2013). An unusual case of multiple myeloma. https://core.ac.uk/download/46603947.pdf (accessed on 27th June 2025).

21. Farkhodovich, R. F., & Shavkatovich, B. B. (2023). Experimental prophylaxis of antibiotics in urological patients. https://core.ac.uk/download/612988412.pdf (accessed on 27th June 2025).

22. Fox-Rushby, J., Mulligan, J., & Walker, D. (2006). *Economic Evaluations of Non-Communicable Disease Interventions*. https://core.ac.uk/download/334300.pdf (accessed on 27th June 2025).

23. Gomez-Rodriguez, J. C., Marttos, A. C., McKenney, M. G., Ogilvie, M. P., et al. (2010). A review of ureteral injuries after external trauma. https://core.ac.uk/download/pdf/8384046.pdf (accessed on 27th June 2025).

24. Kabilan, S. (2017). *Enhanced Urinalysis as A Screening Test for Urinary Tract Infection in Children Aged One Month to Twelve Years*. https://core.ac.uk/download/288215588.pdf (accessed on 27th June 2025).

25. Kamkhah, A. F., & Roghani Dehkordi, F. (2008). Antihypertensive effect of *Nigella sativa* seed extract in patients with mild hypertension. https://core.ac.uk/download/143841955.pdf (accessed on 27th June 2025).

26. Kurzrock, R., Munoz, J., & Wheler, J. J. (2014). Androgen receptors beyond prostate cancer: An old marker as a new target. https://core.ac.uk/download/323066033.pdf (accessed on 27th June 2025).

27. Lamond, E. (2006). *Toward New Criteria for The Laboratory, Clinical, And Presumptive Diagnosis of UTI*. https://core.ac.uk/download/159565075.pdf (accessed on 27th June 2025).

28. Lombardi, G. (2022). *Electrolytes Variability and Clinical Outcomes, In-Hospital Mortality and Acute Kidney Injury*. https://core.ac.uk/download/543577182.pdf (accessed on 27th June 2025).

HEMATOLOGY AND ONCOLOGY

10

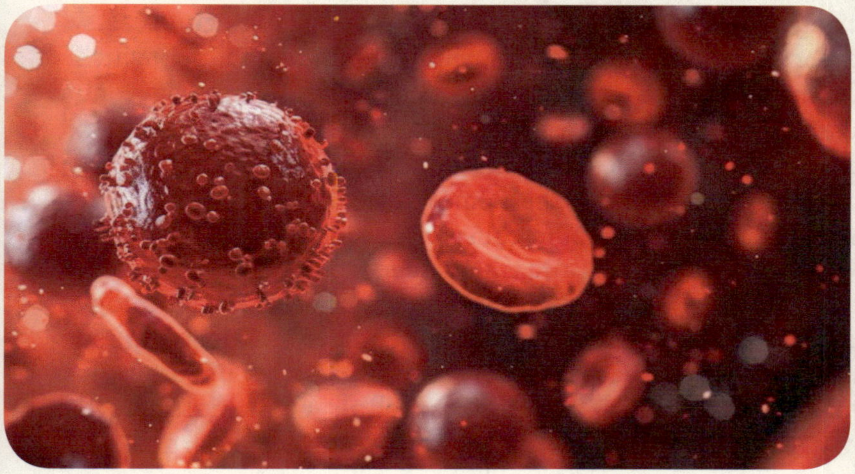

LEARNING OBJECTIVES

After studying this chapter, you will be able to:

1. Explain the role of hematology and oncology in patient car
2. Describe common hematological disorders
3. Understand common cancers in oncology
4. Discuss advances in hematology and oncology
5. Focus on challenges in hematology and oncology

Introduction

The related specialty fields of hematology and oncology are crucial to the understanding and therapy of blood disorders and cancer, respectively. Hematology is the specialty involved explicitly with blood, blood-organ-producing organs, and their associated illnesses, including anemia, coagulation disorders, and the leukemias. Oncology, however, involves multiple forms of cancer that may arise from various origins within the body. The intersection of these sciences is particularly evident in hematologic cancer therapy, both lymphomas and multiple myelomas. With advancements in diagnostic technology and therapeutic devices, the prognosis for patients has greatly improved, and customized medicine plays an increasingly significant role in tailoring treatments. Such innovations aim to enhance therapeutic success with fewer side effects, highlighting the dynamic and crucial role of hematology and oncology in current medical treatment. When pediatric oncology is utilized, there is a clear-cut differential set of problems and variables. Pediatric cancers, although less common than in adults, exhibit unique biological behavior and treatment results. The arena of pediatric malignancies encompasses a range of disorders such as leukemias and cerebral tumors, each necessitating focused clinical management strategies (Deb et al., 2025). Coordination of new therapeutic modalities such as chemotherapy, radiation, and newer agents is critical to maximize patient outcomes. Moreover, the psychosocial factors influencing care are increasingly recognized, necessitating support to patients as well as their families during and post-treatment. This holistic approach brings out the importance of ongoing research and the sensitization of healthcare professionals to the evolving trends in pediatric hematology and oncology. Hematological disorders typically result in fatal complications, which must be managed immediately with accurate management. A significant complication is febrile neutropenia, a common and dangerous condition among patients with underlying hematologic malignancies, most significantly during chemotherapy therapy (Al-Shawy et al., 2025). Identification and prompt treatment of the etiologic agents are essential to decrease risk and improve survival among such high-risk groups. Incorporation of new technology, such as advanced diagnostic systems, such as blood culture systems and antimicrobial susceptibility testing, enhances the ability of the clinician to react appropriately. Knowledge of the microbial spectrum in the patient is also important to develop effective therapy and supportive care guidelines. As it develops further, the focus on antimicrobial stewardship in hematology and oncology reflects the dual goals of controlling infections while preserving the efficacy of existing antibiotics, thus providing the patient with the best possible care for tackling such difficult concerns.

Definition of Hematology

Hematology, the clinical science that deals with the study of blood, involves the diagnosis, therapy, and prevention of blood disorders, integrating laboratory and clinical sciences. Hematology is vital for understanding various pathologies like anemia, bleeding and clotting diseases, and cancers like leukemia. With the significant role blood plays in general health, hematologists research to understand the underlying pathophysiologic mechanisms of hematological disorders in a bid to improve therapy and improve patient outcomes. The complexity of hematologic disease requires comprehensive knowledge of hemostasis, hematopoiesis, and immune function, which are essential for integrating hematology and oncology. Understanding the overlap between these disciplines is crucial, particularly since many of the hematological disorders have the potential to cause or occur in conjunction with cancer and thus need integrated treatment and investigative techniques. Hematology is particularly important for certain blood diseases; it forms the basis of oncology in general. The interaction of hematopoietic systems with neoplasms, and more particularly in the case of blood neoplasms such as leukemia and lymphoma, illustrates this synergy. As one can observe from recent research, such as that on acute lymphoblastic leukemia (ALL), treatment protocols must incorporate not only effective chemotherapy but also a system for understanding the toxic side effects of such treatments, ensuring that patient care is holistic and complete (Attarbaschi et al., 2016). Hematologists collaborate actively with oncologists in developing all-encompassing treatment protocols aimed at mitigating risk while improving patient response. This collaborative method promotes innovation in customized medicine where treatments are tailored to the patient's profile, ensuring maximum success and minimum side effects. In addition to their function in the clinic, hematologists promote innovation in diagnostics and treatment of oncology through scientific research. Advances in the discovery of biomarkers, such as studies in protein tyrosine phosphatase receptor gamma (PTPRG), illustrate the potential of targeted therapy in hematologic malignancies (Sayab et al., 2017). With further advances in research, the way is being paved for improved diagnostic methods and more innovative treatment approaches, underlining the fundamental interdependence between hematology and oncology. Continuous research into the molecular basis of such diseases not only informs science but also improves clinical use, promoting more efficient patient management strategies. Finally, the discipline of hematology constantly evolves to address the dynamic complexities and challenges of blood disorders, making it an essential part of the oncology field (Figure 10.1).

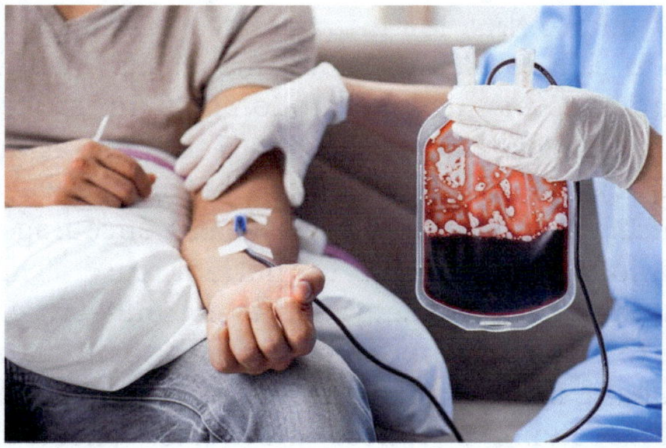

Figure 10.1. Illustration of hematology.

Source: https://www.news-medical.net/image-handler/ts/20220905093840/ri/750/src/images/Article_Images/ImageForArticle_745_16624283204238538.jpg.

Definition of Oncology

The term oncology refers to the medical specialty concerned with the diagnosis, treatment, and research of cancer. Oncology is a multidisciplinary field that unites various specialties in medicine, including surgery, radiology, and medical therapy, to treat cancer patients successfully. Oncology is not only interested in the direct therapy of tumors but also in palliative care to offer a holistic approach to patient health. The expansion of the field has been consistent with advances in science, with increasing therapeutic options available, such as targeted therapies and immunotherapy, developed to achieve maximal treatment with minimal toxicity. The intense profundity of cancer necessitates continuous education and adaptation of oncologists as newer understanding in cancer biology and treatment strategies emerges. A key aspect of oncology is understanding the patient's experience throughout the cancer continuum, the psychological, physical, and social issues that accompany cancer diagnosis. Research has shown that cancer fatigue (CRF) heavily impacts the QoL for patients and survivors and has varying prevalence at varying stages of treatment. In a study of patients with early-stage breast cancer who were undergoing chemotherapy, researchers found fatigue peaked during therapy.

They persisted afterwards, with a significant correlation between CRF and psychological morbidity such as depression and anxiety. Awareness of these aspects is critical in oncology because holistic treatments that take into account physical as well as emotional well-being play an essential role in enhancing patient outcome and QoL (Cognetti et al., 2017). The next scope extension includes a focus on healthcare workforce dynamics, particularly the dynamics of oncology nurses, who are pivotal in delivering care to patients. The job strain that oncology nurses encounter has been identified as a key problem in research, exemplifying how the work environment shapes care quality and performance. For instance, a cross-sectional study comparing public and private Saudi cancer hospitals revealed that nurses in publicly owned hospitals reported higher job strain and poor job performance, highlighting the importance of effective coping strategies in high-stress environments. This connection between patient care outcome and job strain indicates the necessity for systemic change in oncology care models to enhance the working conditions of nurses, which indirectly benefits healthcare workers and the patients they serve (Wazqar et al., 2015) (Figure 10.2).

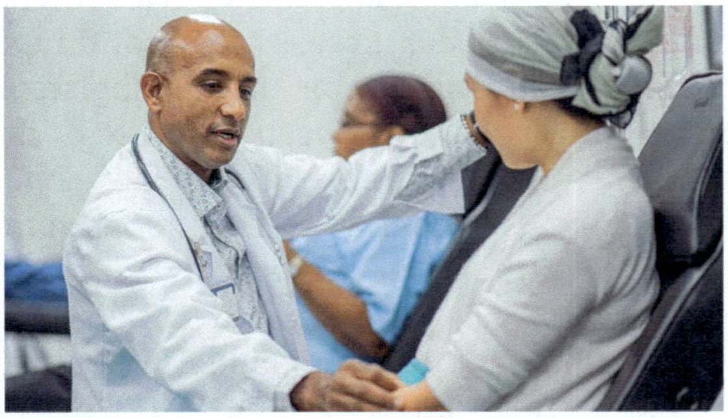

Figure 10.2. Oncologists discussing with cancer patient.

Source: https://i0.wp.com/post.medicalnewstoday.com/wp-content/uploads/sites/3/2020/02/iStock-1181263174edit-1024x575.jpg?w=1155&h=1528.

Importance of the Fields in Medicine

Hematology and oncology are at the core of today's medicine and have a significant impact on treatment and outcomes for patients. Hematology encompasses the diagnosis and treatment of blood disease, a wide range of illnesses, including anemia, coagulation disorders, and leukemia. As the understanding of the pathophysiology of blood evolves, so does the capability to accurately diagnose and effectively treat such disorders, resulting in an improved patient prognosis. Also, integration of EBP in hematology is necessary; it enables patients to receive care according to the most current scientific advancements. With medical training evolving, integration of hematology in training programs becomes increasingly necessary, particularly for students who may not be exposed to these essential specialties in their usual rotations. The establishment of a mandatory hematology rotation would further solidify fundamental knowledge in blood diseases and thus prepare future physicians to handle cases with educated assurance (Mahmood et al., 2016). Oncology, specifically cancer pathology, is one of the most challenging specialties of medicine due to the intricacy and diversity of these diseases. The rapid evolution of treatment modalities from chemotherapy and radiation to immunotherapy requires a deep understanding of tumor biology and malignancy processes. Hematology and oncology are, of course, inextricably linked here, especially when treating blood cancer like lymphoma and leukemia. Research in oncology is necessary as it informs the creation of personalized medicine strategies, individualizing the treatment through patient-specific profiles for enhanced therapeutic efficacy. The importance of understanding the regulation of gene expression by microRNAs, for instance, lies in their role in B cell development and malignancy, which underscores new methodologies in cancer management and treatment (Fernando et al., 2012). Interdisciplinary collaboration between oncologists and hematologists also encourages a holistic approach to patient care. This interspecialty collaboration is not only critical in the formulation of effective treatment plans but also in addressing the psychosocial demands of receiving a cancer diagnosis. Oncology and hematology need to be coordinated to collaborate with patients through complex treatment regimens, with attention to QoL. For instance, as patients navigate through the implications of blood cancers, the combination of psychological support service intervention and palliative care can significantly improve their care experience. Moreover, continuous breakthroughs in genetic studies and molecular biology further reinforce the value of such fields, as they pave the way for revolutionary treatments against the distinctive aspects of blood cancers. The growth of hematology and oncology as spheres in healthcare markets reflects their critical contribution to enhancing medical treatment for patients.

10.1. The Role of Hematology in Patient Care

Learning Outcome

1. Understand the diagnosis of blood disorders
2. Describe treatment options for hematological conditions
3. Explain the impact of hematology on overall health

In hematology, patient care involves an integrated approach, addressing not only the biomedical factors that cause hematologic diseases but also the social factors of health that directly influence patient outcomes. The crossroads of socioeconomic status and health disparities in hematologic conditions are stark, such as the undertreatment of pain in sickle cell disease patients due to implicit bias and structural racism in healthcare systems. This is a key challenge to hematologists and allied healthcare professionals to seek continuous education and self-reflection to minimize biases. Initiatives, such as the Health Equity Rounds at the University of California, San Francisco, aim to shed light on these disparities by creating discussion out of real cases and applying EBP to ensure balanced care for populations disproportionately affected by hematologic disorders (Jain, 2024). The importance of attending to the psychosocial requirements of hematologic patient care is no less critical. Hematology is often marked by complex, emotionally laden cases, for instance, the therapy of blood cancers and chronic blood illnesses, which can produce immense psychosocial suffering for the families and patients involved. This distress not only foretells higher morbidity and mortality but also affects the quality of care provided by clinicians, most of whom have their own rates of burnout. Curricula that focus on intensive psychosocial training, like the Artful Oncology program, highlight the necessity for hematology and oncology fellows to learn communication skills that address these complexities. By equipping healthcare professionals with the necessary tools to manage these challenges, patient care quality is enhanced, leading to improved general patient satisfaction and outcomes (Al-Mondhiry et al., 2024). Furthermore, integration of hematology into overall cancer care planning demonstrates the need for interprofessional collaboration in today's medicine. Since hematologic conditions frequently emerge in the practice of oncology, hematologists' tasks extend beyond treatment and diagnosis to critical functions of integrating care. By collaborating with oncologists, social workers, and other members of the clinical team, hematologists can influence personalized treatment plans based on the intricate needs of a patient. Through collaboration, an integrative approach is enabled in capturing patient care by addressing both the biological and psychosocial features of disease. With the evolving medical field, it is clear that hematology is an integral component of a well-balanced, patient-centered approach to care in oncology, warranting the necessity of ongoing learning and interdisciplinary interaction in the field (Jain, 2024).

10.1.1. Diagnosis of Blood Disorders

Diagnosis of blood disorders is the most crucial aspect of hematology and oncology, involving a blend of clinical assessment and laboratory study. Identification of the pathogenesis of hematopoiesis and the pathology of blood malignancies is essential to provide the correct diagnosis. For instance, chronic myeloid leukemia (CML) could be diagnosed based on specific genetic mutations and aberrant expression of various biomarkers. As indicated in the latest studies, PTPRG, a receptor gene of protein tyrosine phosphatase, appears to be a future marker of CML. The intricate cooperation between PTPRG expression and the presence of Philadelphia chromosome-positive cells determines the need for implementing sophisticated methodologies in the diagnostic process. Thus, the development of proper antibodies, such as TPγ B9-2, can enhance diagnostic accuracy and monitoring in patients with blood disorders, allowing for the implementation of timely and effective treatment modalities (Sayab et al., 2017). Moreover, the cross-link between autoimmune disorders and hematological malignancies also makes the diagnosis of blood disorders more complex. Clinical presentation tends to overlap, thereby rendering it challenging to diagnose and treat conditions like autoimmune hemolytic anemia (AHA) in chronic lymphocytic leukemia (CLL) and non-Hodgkin lymphomas (NHL) patients. Evidence indicates that AHA is a frequent event associated with lymphoproliferative disorders, where the neoplastic clone can promote antibody production. Therapeutic use with rituximab, an anti-CD20 monoclonal antibody, has been promising, though its efficacy in NHL-associated AHA has to be investigated further. By combining an appreciation of autoimmune phenomena with traditional hematology diagnostics, doctors can adopt a more integrated approach to managing this complex interplay, thereby enhancing patient outcomes (Fozza et al., 2011). Finally, the development of molecular diagnostics has transformed the horizon of diagnosing blood disorders from traditional hematology into a more specific one. More advanced techniques such as flow cytometry, NGS, and immunohistochemistry are increasingly being utilized to determine the exact genetic and molecular etiology of most blood diseases. For CML, understanding how PTPRG is downregulated at diagnosis can dictate highly specific individualized treatments, with the potential to monitor treatment response through biomarker levels. This shift towards individualized diagnostics not only provides for the convenience of early identification but also gives health experts the ability to craft therapeutic interventions that have a significant influence on patient prognosis and QoL. As research continues to evolve, the integration of these advanced methods will undoubtedly enhance the diagnostic process in the field of hematology and oncology (Sayab et al., 2017) (Figure 10.3).

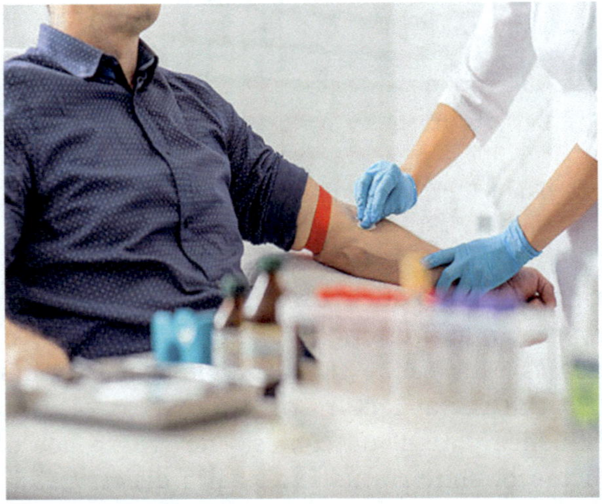

Figure 10.3. Collecting a blood sample for the diagnosis of blood disorders.

Source: https://www.ayushmandiagnostics.com/departments/image/hematology.jpg.

10.1.2. Treatment Options for Hematological Conditions

The management of hematologic disorders is an extensive array of treatment options; each suited for the specific disorder type and patient. One of the primary approaches is the use of targeted agents, particularly for conditions like CML, where the BCR-ABL fusion protein is the primary etiology of the disease. Imatinib, a tyrosine kinase inhibitor, revolutionized the treatment regimen of CML, but resistance tends to develop due to mutations within the BCR-ABL kinase domain. Recent evidence shows that pre-existing mutations may be identified within $CD34^+$ stem cells and correlate robustly with imatinib resistance (Aleem et al., 2011). This recognizes the pressing need for screening for mutations at diagnosis to guide treatment and optimize patient-specific outcomes, allowing for progression to more tailored practice in hematology. Another significant treatment option for hematologic disorders is the use of supportive treatments, particularly in myelodysplastic syndromes (MDS). MDS is a heterogeneous disease condition in which patients might struggle with anemia management, requiring chronic transfusions for QOL. Transfusion medicine is a key part of the overall approach as it alleviates symptoms caused by low hemoglobin. Iron overload and other complications due to transfusion dependency can add to the cost of MDS treatment (Berger et al., 2008). Management of such issues entails a process of structured risk stratification, allowing clinicians to effectively modify treatment plans by balancing supportive care with the application of potential disease-modifying treatments.

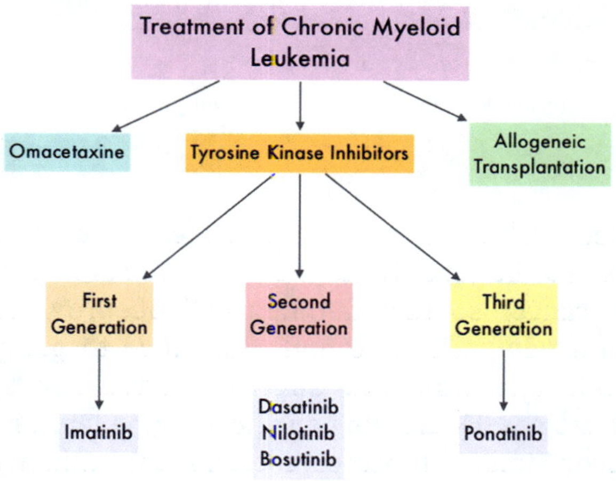

Figure 10.4. Treatment of chronic myeloid leukemia (CML).

Source: https://www.oncoprescribe.com/app/uploads/_1437626007.jpg.

Additionally, new therapies such as hypomethylating drugs and newer immunotherapies continue to reshape the therapeutic landscape of hematology and oncology. Hypomethylating drugs such as azacitidine and decitabine have demonstrated their efficacy in certain MDS subtypes, with the option to improve bone marrow function and hematopoiesis. In addition, the advent of immunotherapy has opened up new doors for the treatment of hematological malignancies, particularly acute myeloid leukemia (AML) and lymphomas. The newer strategies highlight the interactive nature of treatment methods and the importance of patient-specific therapies, considering not only disease pathophysiology but also the unique status of each patient. With constant research and clinical trials, the prospect for better results increases every year in hematology and oncology (Figure 10.4).

0.1.3. Impact of Hematology on Overall Health

Hematology, which is the study of blood, blood organs, and blood diseases such as anemia and leukemia, is a critical area of education in comprehending overall health. Hematological disease can have a significant impact on both the QoL and survival of a patient. For instance, hematologic malignancy patients like acute leukemia have heterogeneous outcomes based on the modality of treatment, where recent studies have shown mixed survival rates between bone marrow and umbilical cord blood transplant. The susceptibility to developing graft-versus-host disease (GVHD) complications underscores the importance of hematology in determining effective therapeutic practices and informing clinical choices in donor selection based on disease severity and patient considerations (Abdel-Azim et al., 2019). Therefore, integrating hematological well-being in routine assessments is crucial for prevention and enhanced patient care. Further, the development of new diagnostic technologies such as circulating tumor DNA (ctDNA) analysis illustrates the revolutionary potential in hematology. By identifying genetic mutations in hematological malignancies, clinicians can infer tumor behavior and therapeutic targeting. For instance, understanding mutations like TP53 and KRAS through the analysis of ctDNA is now essential in tailoring treatment strategies for diseases like pancreatic ductal adenocarcinoma (PDAC), a very aggressive disease that tends to present in advanced phases (Fanta et al., 2019). Since ctDNA analysis is indicative of clinical outcomes, it underlines hematology's synergistic potential to oncological practice, emphasizing how markers within the blood may be employed as available but informative indicators of disease advancement and response to treatment. The synergy eventually enhances the precision of oncological treatment. Lastly, hematology's impact on overall health transcends the treatment outcomes in question, representing an intricate specialism that is intertwined with the general pattern of preventive medicine. Ongoing monitoring of blood health can detect underlying conditions, such as chronic inflammation or nutritional deficiencies, which pose risk factors for future complications, including malignancies. Furthermore, patients with hematological disorders also require interdisciplinary management with nutritionists and psychiatrists to address the well-being of the whole. Through early detection and treatment of hematological disorders, health systems can prevent the aggravation of health conditions, leading to improved patient outcomes and reduced healthcare costs in the long term. The increased importance of hematology, thus, helps to accentuate its vital relevance not only to oncology but to the management of health in general, validating its intrinsic role in medicine.

Test Your Knowledge

1. What are the key diagnostic tests used in hematology to identify common blood disorders?
2. How do hematological disorders impact overall health and what are the potential systemic complications if left untreated?

10.2. The Role of Oncology in Patient Care

Learning Outcome

1. Understand the process of diagnosing cancer
2. Discuss treatment modalities in oncology
3. Focus on palliative care and supportive services

The role of oncology in patient management is central when considering the complexity of managing cancer. Oncology not only encompasses overt medical care but also a critical emphasis on educating the patient and the family as a unit. Because the diagnosis of cancer is intimidating, particularly in children, clear communication is essential. An interprofessional model, as recommended by the Children's Oncology Group Nursing Discipline, expects that education concerning diagnosis and treatment is to be family-oriented and patient-focused. This stresses that healthcare providers need to be sensitive to the psychosocial impact of cancer so that families will be provided with adequate time and assistance to grasp their situation and apply effective coping strategies. By creating an encouraging learning environment, healthcare teams can enhance patient results through effective education (Ahern et al., 2016). In addition to educational interventions, sharing information about prognosis is crucial to oncology patient care. Pediatric oncology nurses are usually integral to the communication process as facilitators, but their role has not been universally recognized. As identified in research, effective prognosis-related communication (PRC) needs to be achieved through interdisciplinary collaboration, yet nurses are usually excluded from essential discussions. This not only undermines their potential for contribution but also affects the overall experiences of patients and families. A paradigm change is needed that allows oncology nurses to be more proactive in PRC so that they are better poised to support families through challenging conversations about the cancer diagnosis and treatment as well as prognosis. Increased collaboration and education of physicians and nurses can significantly improve communication outcomes in oncology settings (Haglund et al., 2019). Furthermore, the emotional and psychological dimensions of cancer care cannot be overstated. The inclusion of psychosocial support in cancer treatment is vital to building resilience for patients and their families. As the treatment progresses, addressing patients' emotional needs becomes increasingly vital as they go through the challenges of living with cancer. Psychosocial coping and mental health interventions need to be integrated into treatment. The value of an integrated model of care with medical treatment combined with mental and emotional support cannot be overstressed, as this integrated model, in the end, is what adds to QoL and compliance with treatment. Through providing an environment centered on psychosocial health, oncology can significantly improve patient care and establish better health results for cancer patients (Ahern et al., 2016).

10.2.1. Diagnosis of Cancer

The cancer diagnostic process is complex and involves using a spectrum of diagnostic modalities necessary to accurately define the disease. Primary investigations typically begin with a thorough clinical assessment, where physicians take a complete medical history and conduct a physical examination. After this, imaging studies such as X-rays, CT scans, MRIs, and PET scans are employed, providing invaluable visual data on potential malignancies. Every imaging modality has its own strengths in revealing the presence and nature of tumors, serving as the foundation for subsequent treatments. Besides imaging, tissue biopsies offer a sure diagnosis through histopathological examination, which is critical in differentiating benign from malignant masses. The synergy of these diagnostic procedures serves as a platform for targeted treatment strategies, highlighting the importance of timely and precise cancer detection. Biomarkers increasingly play a pivotal role in the diagnosis and monitoring of cancer treatment, as they reflect markers of biological activity driving cancer. For instance, in hepatocellular carcinoma, advanced imaging techniques such as DWI and perfusion imaging (MRP) can assess early changes of therapy as well as estimate progression-free survival (PFS). It has been demonstrated recently that DWI and MRP parameter alterations are sensitive biomarkers that are better than conventional measures in quantifying treatment response. Notably, in one study, a marked change in K_{trans}, a measure of vascular permeability, after two weeks of treatment, was correlated with favorable clinical results. This illustrates how the addition of sophisticated imaging biomarkers to the clinic can improve diagnosis and direct therapy, ushering in personalized medicine for oncology (Ancukiewicz et al., 2013). With the constantly evolving landscape of cancer diagnosis, improving technology and new therapies shape the future of patient care. The advent of immune-based therapies like checkpoint inhibitors and CAR T-cell therapy has changed treatment trends, accompanied by the increased need for monitoring and diagnosing associated complications. Immune-related adverse events (irAEs) need careful identification and management since they can manifest multifocal symptoms that cut across organ systems. Management of the complications is premised on early diagnosis, interventions, and interdisciplinary collaboration among the health team. Besides, the evolution of imaging modalities, along with standard diagnostic techniques, provides a more accurate understanding of disease progression and reaction to treatment in relevant hematological neoplasms. This diagnostic melting pot of innovation and treatment will undoubtedly be an essential factor in enhancing cancer care for future generations (Brém et al., 2020) (Figure 10.5).

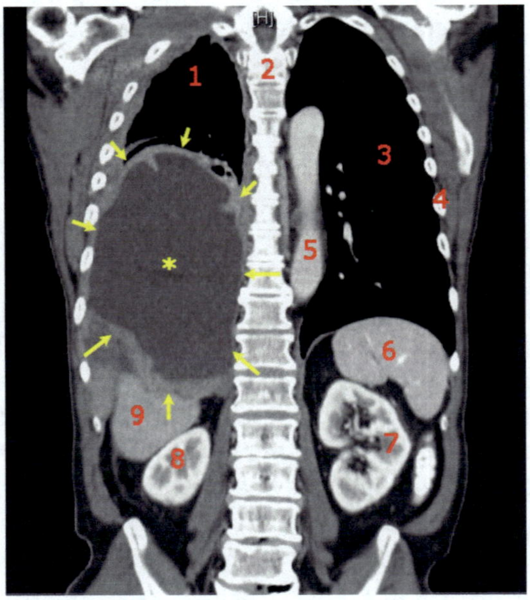

Figure 10.5. A coronal CT scan showing malignant mesothelioma, indicated by the asterisk and the arrows.

Source: https://upload.wikimedia.org/wikipedia/commons/5/56/Tumor_Mesothelioma2_legend.jpg.

10.2.2. Treatment Modalities in Oncology

The treatment environment has evolved immensely, with numerous modalities to treat the unique biological characteristics of cancer. The most common treatment methods are chemotherapy, radiotherapy, surgery, targeted therapy, and immunotherapy. Chemotherapy, employing cytotoxic agents to destroy fast-growing cells, remains the cornerstone for most malignancies. Notably, the latest development in personalized medicine has refocused attention on the targeted therapies designed against specific molecular targets of cancer. This is intended to enhance efficacy without increasing toxicity, thereby maximizing patient outcomes. For instance, the use of aromatase inhibitors in postmenopausal women with estrogen receptor-positive breast cancer has proved promising as an initial treatment modality, indicative of a growing trend towards a highly individualized approach in oncology (Agarwal et al., 2014). In pediatric oncology, the management of malignant germ cell tumors (GCT) exemplifies the use of combined therapeutic regimens. The development of cisplatinum chemotherapy has dramatically improved survival, but it also highlights the need for therapeutic decision-making to consider individual patient factors such as age and tumor type. In particular, within gonadal tumors, the possibility of primary complete resection provides the promise of cure, while more extensive nongonadal tumors generally necessitate neoadjuvant chemotherapy treatment before surgery. By employing adaptive treatment methods utilizing imaging and marker assessments, oncologists can maximize management results, illustrating how tailored regimens of treatment can influence the prognosis in children with GCT (Calaminus et al., 2002).

As advancements in genomics and treatment modalities continue to develop, integrating these variables into treatment regimens will remain essential. Current clinical guidelines involve risk stratification of tumor biology, histology, and first-line treatment response, which aids in tailoring treatment based on the individual needs of the patient. The future also sees a growth in interest in biomarkers to predict treatment outcomes, for example, in the study investigating p53 expression in elderly breast cancer patients (Agarwal et al., 2014). By developing an improved understanding of the biology of cancer, oncologists can shift away from universal trends toward precision medicine models. Not only does this shift have the potential to improve survival rates in heterogeneous populations, but it also reduces unnecessary interventions, making cancer therapy more similar to the individual patient's disease profile (Figure 10.6).

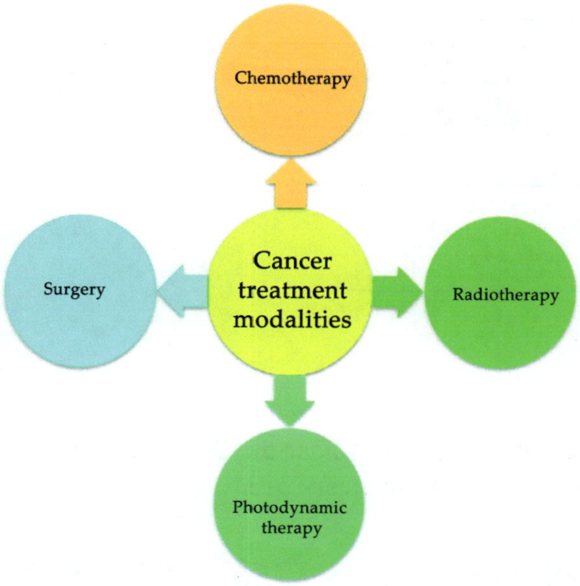

Figure 10.6. Fundamental and significant cancer treatment modalities.

Source: https://www.researchgate.net/publication/328395083/figure/fig1/AS:683627914473472@1540001004706/Fundamental-and-significant-cancer-treatment-modalities.png.

10.2.3. Palliative Care and Supportive Services

In hematology and oncology, palliative and supportive care services are precious to patient QoL improvement. These services cater to the complexities of patient needs, particularly when working with life-threatening blood cancers and associated diseases. Through the incorporation of an interdisciplinary model, palliative care teams are able to de-alienate physical distresses like pain and fatigue that patients undergoing intense treatments like chemotherapy often experience. In addition to managing the symptoms, this integrated model is focused on the psychological and emotional care needed by patients and their families throughout this ordeal. The inclusion of palliative care early in treatment planning significantly increases overall patient satisfaction, directly addressing the concerns and well-being of patients with life-changing diagnoses. The need for effective support services is significantly increased in the event of anemia caused by chemotherapy, a common occurrence among oncology patients. As shown by recent recommendations, the use of ESA is one effective method of managing anemia, particularly when hemoglobin levels fall sharply. Interventions of this kind can enhance the patient's QoL through reducing the likelihood of red blood cell transfusion, thus allowing them to maintain their course of treatment effectively. But it is equally important to assess other such needs, such as iron supplementation, that can further tailor the response to treatment and improve the overall well-being of patients. Such an individualized approach to supportive care is essential in managing anemia and its complications, ultimately influencing treatment outcomes in patients with hematology and oncology (Bohlius et al., 2019).

Palliative care is more than symptom relief; it also deals with the psychological, social, and spiritual components of care, which are typically overlooked in standard treatment protocols. Patients with life-threatening illnesses tend to experience intense physical and emotional distress, a circumstance that underscores the importance of delivering well-rounded support. Studies have indicated that palliative care interventions reduce suffering and enable improved communication among healthcare providers and patients, thus improving overall care. These services are linked with lower hospitalization rates and increased family satisfaction, revealing the potential cost savings of integrating palliative care in treatment modalities. As health systems strive to provide high-quality, patient-oriented care, it is crucial to highlight the roles of palliative care and supportive services in hematology and oncology, ensuring that patients receive integrative care to meet their complex needs (Elk et al., 2017) (Figure 10.7).

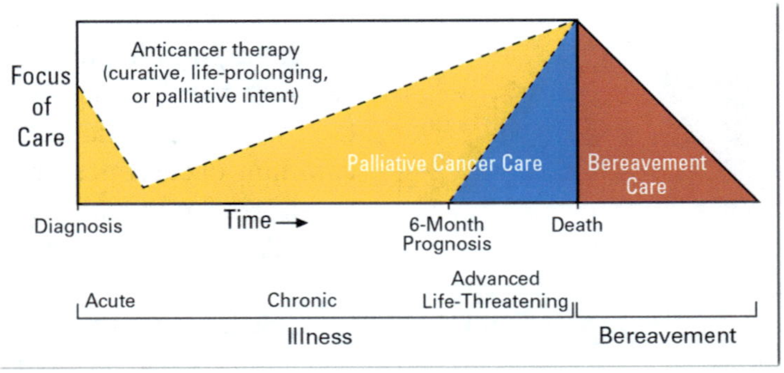

Figure 10.7. Model of palliative cancer care.

Source: https://www.researchgate.net/profile/Florian-Strasser-4/publication/24436253/figure/fig2/AS:339836276887564@1458034690752/Model-of-palliative-cancer-care.png.

Test Your Knowledge

1. What are the primary diagnostic tools and methods used in oncology to detect and stage different types of cancer?
2. Describe the main treatment modalities in oncology, including surgery, chemotherapy, radiation therapy, and targeted therapies.
3. How does palliative care complement oncological treatment?

10.3. Common Hematological Disorders

Learning Outcome

1. Describe anemia
2. Understand hemophilia, an inherited bleeding disorder
3. Explain leukemia, a malignant hematological disorder

The specialty of hematology extensively investigates ordinary hematologic diseases, which exert an enormous impact on patient health and well-being. Among these illnesses, anemia, a reduction in red blood cells (RBCs) or hemoglobin, is one of the most frequent. Anemia is caused by a variety of reasons, from nutrient deficiency syndromes of iron, vitamin B12, and folate to chronic conditions and bone marrow disorders. Clinical presentation is usually non-specific and can include fatigue, pallor, and dizziness, making it challenging to diagnose. Diagnosis includes determining the etiology of anemia for which effective control is essential; neglecting to treat the cause can lead to disabling manifestations and healthcare costs. Diagnosis approaches to anemia involve comprehensive blood examinations, such as CBCs and reticulocyte counts, which help establish the precise cause and type of anemia, guiding treatment measures from supplementation to more aggressive interventions like transfusions. Thrombocytopenia, a common hematological disorder, is defined by a reduced platelet count below the norm due to various reasons, such as bone marrow disease, heightened destruction, or sequestration of the platelets in the spleen. This condition is significant because it has grave hemorrhagic complications or spontaneous bleeding, particularly in cases where platelet counts drop to critical levels. Thrombocytopenia diagnosis would typically continue with a detailed history review, physical checkup, and certain laboratory tests that help define the etiology, e.g., idiopathic thrombocytopenic purpura (ITP) or MDS. Management often involves addressing the cause and may include platelet transfusions in acute cases. Knowledge of the nuances of thrombocytopenia is essential to doctors as they customize the treatment options while balancing potential damage from interventions and ensuring that patient safety is always ensured. Leukemia, a disease of the blood cells, is another dangerous hematological disorder with wide-ranging implications for those who suffer from it. This category includes acute and chronic forms of the disease, typically marked by an overproduction of irregular white cells that can disrupt regular hemopoiesis. Symptoms may be variable but most commonly include inappropriate tiredness, frequent infections, and spontaneous bruising or bleeding. Leukemia investigation is typically obtained by means of blood examinations, bone marrow biopsies, and cytogenetic analysis, all of which collectively determine disease subtype and stage. Treatments differ by the type and phase of leukemia and may involve chemotherapy, radiation, and stem cell transplant. Of specific interest is the continuous research into the development of targeted therapies with hopes of improved results. Leukemia needs a multidisciplinary team; hematologists, oncologists, and supportive care clinicians collaborate to render total care individualized to each patient while maximizing the QoL during therapy (Abenhardt et al., 2010; Campioni et al., 2013).

10.3.1. Anemia

The absence of red blood cells or hemoglobin, known as anemia, is a challenging situation in hematology and oncology. Numerous factors like nutritional deficiency, chronic illness, and bone marrow disorders usually bring about anemia. Anemia among cancer patients usually results as a consequence of chemotherapy, where it induces myelosuppression, hence hampering the body's ability to produce enough red blood cells. The developing weakness and fatigue can profoundly impact a patient's QoL, and hence, early and effective treatment is essential. Furthermore, detecting the etiology of anemia is necessary for tailored treatment planning and optimizing outcomes, making hematologic assessment an essential component of cancer treatment. Anemia management in oncology has been revolutionized with the introduction of ESAs. These medications work to stimulate bone marrow to increase red blood cell output, serving as a critical second option for anemic patients with chemotherapy. Current recommendations from respective professional organizations, such as the American Society of Clinical Oncology and American Society of Hematology, suggest ESA use in patients with hemoglobin levels below 10 g/dL during the treatment of non-curative cancers. Interestingly, research indicates that iron supplementation in conjunction with ESA therapy can enhance hematopoietic response and decrease red blood cell transfusion needs, optimizing total treatment efficacy (Bohlius et al., 2019). This combined approach to anemia treatment aligns with the growing recognition of the value of supportive care in oncology to reduce risk and optimize patient benefit. Furthermore, the psychological and physical effects of anemia should not be overlooked since they may significantly influence the QoL of patients. Anemia has been known to cause chronic fatigue, decreased activity level, and psychological distress, which contribute to the suffering of cancer patients. The development of PRO instruments is necessary to quantify these effects on life, especially for diseases like pyruvate kinase deficiency, which share aspects with anemia (Ionova et al., 2018). By using proper assessment tools, clinicians will better comprehend the multitude of effects of anemia and be able to make suitable therapeutic modifications. Engaging patients in their care plans and understanding the subjective nature of anemia are critical initial steps toward enhancing the overall care being provided within hematology and oncology settings (Figure 10.8).

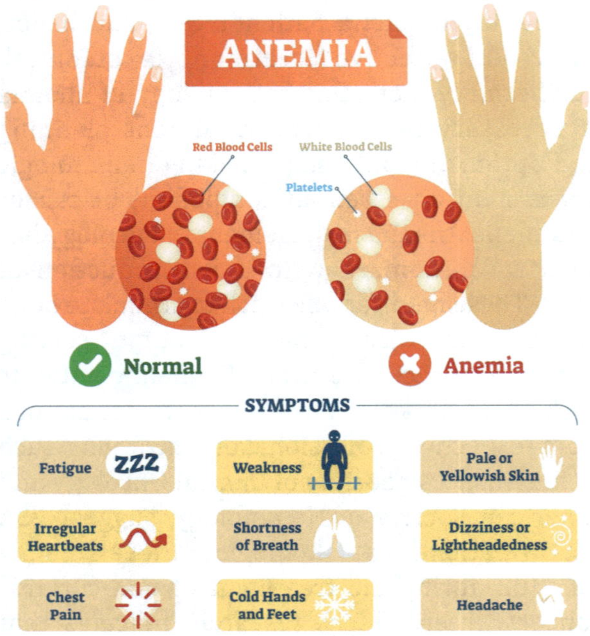

Figure 10.8. Anemia and its symptoms.

Source: https://productimages.withfloats.com/actual/61934c2a7c59fa00010f3cb8.jpg.

10.3.2. Hemophilia

Hemophilia is a genetic bleeding disorder resulting from a deficiency of specific coagulation factors in the blood that are absolutely crucial for obtaining normal blood clotting. Hemophilia occurs in two leading forms: Hemophilia A (factor VIII deficiency) and Hemophilia B (factor IX deficiency), both with mutations in the genes regulating blood coagulation. Patients with such conditions have prolonged bleeding episodes, which can cause extensive complications such as damage to joints and bleeding to the point of life-threatening levels. In addition to the physical challenges, hemophilia also presents extensive psychological challenges to patients and their relatives. The nature of the disease usually requires frequent medical attention, impacting daily life and mood. Continuous understanding of hemophilia is essential in the fields of hematology and oncology, as these fields are extensively interrelated, particularly in terms of best management and therapeutic approach. Advances in the management of hemophilia have significant promise for improving patients' QoL. Traditional therapies were primarily based on factor replacement, where the missing clotting factor was administered to patients to prevent or treat bleeding. However, these methods are time-consuming and costly, and researchers are seeking to create new approaches such as gene therapy. Gene therapy has the potential to cure the inherent genetic defects responsible for hemophilia. Through the use of viral vectors or other advanced delivery systems, normal copies of the defective genes can be delivered into the patient's cells. This groundbreaking approach not only has the potential to reduce both the incidence and severity of bleeding attacks but also to lead to the long-term cure of the disease. The potential importance of such discoveries underlines the growing necessity for the integration of genetic research into hematology and oncology clinical practice (Figure 10.9).

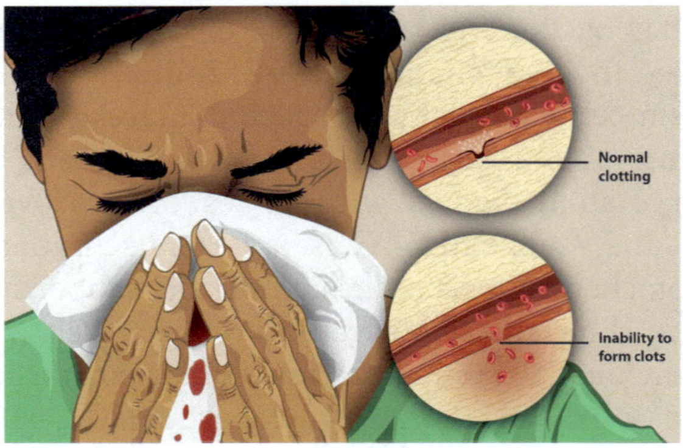

Figure 10.9. An illustration of a woman with hemophilia.

Source: https://upload.wikimedia.org/wikipedia/commons/thumb/8/89/A_woman_suffering_from_Hemophilia.png/330px-A_woman_suffering_from_Hemophilia.png.

The future of hemophilia treatment could be further transformed by research in cell therapy.

It is a process that aims to transplant healthy cells that secrete the necessary coagulation factors, thereby restoring normal hemostasis. Techniques with induced pluripotent stem cells are showing vast potential in this regard. These cells possess the unique ability to differentiate into various types of cells, including those that possess the ability to secrete the necessary clotting factors. Moreover, cell therapy is also synergistically used with gene therapy to provide a multi-modal treatment for hemophilia. With further studies validating the efficacy of such new treatments, it is clearer that hemophilia is particularly under the wing of hematology and oncology. With ongoing research on new treatments, the future for hemophilia patients is bright, bringing hope to the individuals afflicted with this genetic disorder (Astermark et al., 2012; Gaban et al., 2012) (Figure 10.10).

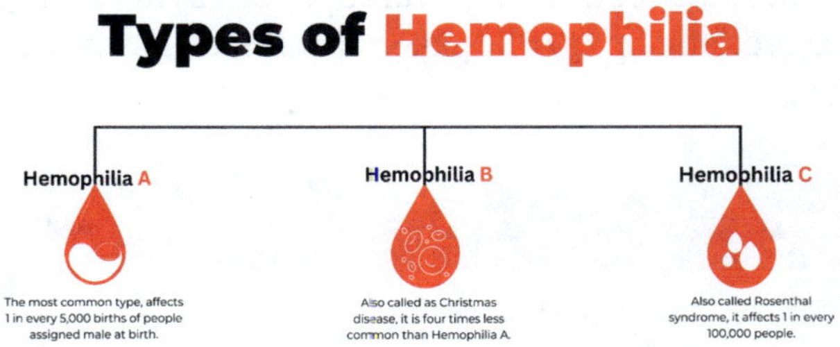

Figure 10.10. Types of hemophilia.

Source: https://www.google.com/url?sa=i&url=https%3A%2F%2Fwww.lalpathlabs.com%2Fblog%2Fhaemophilia%2F&psig=AOvVaw2FEcSi0g0KQqnwm7F-IoBC&ust=1749731981136000&source=images&cd=vfe&opi=89978449&ved=0CBcQjhxqFwoTCLCY4OGx6Y0DFQAAAAAdAAAAABAE.

10.3.3. Leukemia

Leukemia, a malignant disease of the blood, is characterized by uncontrolled proliferation of abnormal white blood cells. This cancer is normally classified into acute and chronic leukemias, which are further subclassified into lymphocytic or myeloid leukemias. Acute leukemia is rapid in onset and must be treated right away, while chronic leukemia progresses slowly and may be noted prior to needing treatment. The pathogenesis of leukemia involves genetic mutations disrupting regular hematopoiesis, most often leading to an accumulation of defective or immature cells. The identification of unique genetic markers and chromosomal alterations has shed more light on the nature of the leukemia subtypes, several of which, like CML, are associated with the BCR-ABL fusion gene, which is very promising for targeted therapy (Accurso et al., 2019). Modern therapy for leukemia is multidisciplinary and involves chemotherapy, targeted therapy, and hematopoietic stem cell transplantation. For instance, individuals with CML have experienced improved outcomes with the administration of tyrosine kinase inhibitors (TKIs), such as imatinib. Research indicates that the reduction of BCR-ABL1/ABL1IS transcript levels below 10% within three months or 1% within six months of treatment is correlated with significantly better prognosis, and the necessity of observing these molecular responses should not be exaggerated (Accurso et al., 2019). In advanced phases, where initial therapies fail, other strategies, including stem cell transplantation, may offer a promise of a cure. This therapeutic adaptability not only presents a chance for remission but also highlights the pivotal position of individually tailored treatment regimens based on individual genetic profiles and therapeutic responsiveness. Additionally, the complex management of leukemia mandates ongoing monitoring for minimal residual disease (MRD) to predict relapse and guide therapy. In patients undergoing hematopoietic stem cell transplantation, for example, those with AML and MLL translocations, MRD assessments conducted by advanced PCR technologies can provide valuable information concerning the quality and longevity of remission (Figure 10.11).

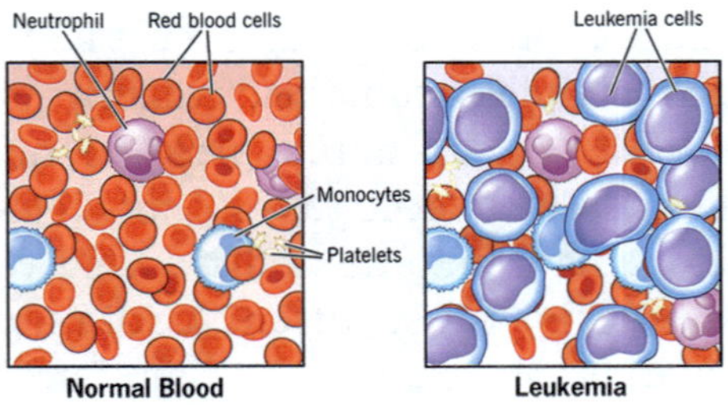

Figure 10.11. Illustration of normal blood and leukemia.

Source: https://my.clevelandclinic.org/-/scassets/images/org/health/articles/4365-leukemia.

The capacity to detect residual leukemic cells following transplant is central to tailoring follow-up therapy, which can be intensified immunotherapy for the avoidance of relapse. Through the integration of MRD monitoring into patient care, practitioners can leverage the challenge presented by high-risk leukemias, offering an improved proactive and personalized approach to treatment and survivorship. This strategic focus highlights the impressive advances in hematology and oncology, accelerating improved patient outcomes within the constantly evolving landscape of leukemia therapy (Figure 10.12).

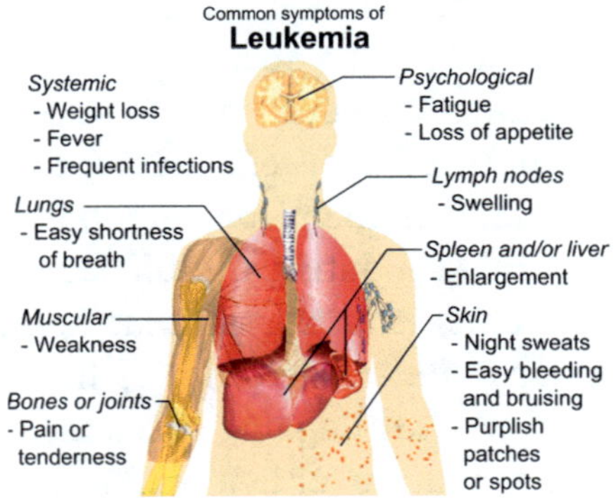

Figure 10.12. Symptoms of leukemia.

Source: https://upload.wikimedia.org/wikipedia/commons/thumb/3/3a/Symptoms_of_leukemia.png/500px-Symptoms_of_leukemia.png.

Test Your Knowledge

1. What are the different types of anemia, and how do their causes and clinical presentations differ?
2. Explain the pathophysiology of hemophilia and its impact on the blood clotting process.
3. How do acute and chronic leukemias differ in terms of progression, treatment, and prognosis?

10.4. Common Cancers in Oncology

Learning Outcome

1. Discuss breast cancer
2. Understand lung cancer
3. Describe colorectal cancer

Among the most prevalent cancers diagnosed in the field of oncology, PDAC and leukemia stand out since they possess characteristic biological characteristics and treatment challenges. PDAC, in its initial stage, usually does not express symptoms, progresses normally at an advanced stage, thus being among the leading causes of death due to cancer globally. Recent advances in NGS platforms have begun to illuminate the genomic underpinnings of PDAC, particularly the prevalent alterations in genes such as TP53 and KRAS detected by ctDNA analysis. This has revealed significant correlations between elevated ctDNA alteration levels and poor prognostic outcomes, highlighting the necessity for early diagnosis and directed therapeutic interventions. Its high incidence underscores the need for quick research in the field of personalized oncology treatment programs and the development of new therapeutic strategies (Fanta et al., 2019). In contrast, leukemia is a great challenge in hematology due to its complex pathology and heterogeneous subtypes, i.e., ALL and CLL. Early detection and appropriate treatment of leukemia have been tough, especially in environments where specialty care access is variable. Evidence has demonstrated that system factors, including the unequal distribution of health resources and delayed diagnosis, actually impact patient outcomes. Significantly, patients actually face psychological stressors and financial burden that complicate their treatment. These matters are dealt with by comprehensive health policy changes to ensure better access to well-equipped medical centers and provision of emotional support to the patients, which ensures a better environment for the effective management of leukemia (Alizadeh et al., 2015). Moreover, the convergence of hematology and oncology generates better insights into both frequent and rare malignancies, enabling the unification of effective treatment modalities. Multidisciplinary treatment of cancer includes early diagnosis, targeted therapy, and coordinated treatment strategies based on both oncologic and hematologic experience. For instance, the management of cancers like lymphoma can combine chemotherapy, radiotherapy, and immunotherapy, tailored for the individual patient and disease features. The multidisciplinary principle not only maximizes therapeutic benefit but also optimizes survival across various malignancies. As oncology science continues to progress with the latest technology and treatment modalities, unrelenting emphasis on research and education remains the bedrock for improving patient outcomes in hematology and oncology, particularly for prevalent malignancies like PDAC and leukemia.

10.4.1. Breast Cancer

The biology of breast cancer is not the only complexity, as it intersects with socio-economic as well as psychological dimensions. It is a multifactorial disease that not only requires precision in treatment but also understanding of patient inequalities, particularly in low- and middle-income contexts. Early diagnosis has been shown by research to enhance prognoses significantly, but obstacles like the unavailability of healthcare facilities and unawareness tend to act as roadblocks. In regions where healthcare centers are disproportionately segmented, as in the case of studies on leukemia patients in Iran, disparities can similarly be anticipated in breast cancer patients. Absence of psychological care and suboptimal funding for treatment contributes to the issue. Mitigation of these challenges with targeted health policies is essential for enhancing the quality of care and survival of breast cancer patients across all socioeconomic backgrounds (Alizadeh et al., 2015). Early detection and screening are most essential in the fight against breast cancer, as research indicates that routine mammography can significantly contribute to reducing death among high-risk groups. The majority of healthcare organizations suggest annual screening for women over 40 years, with a priority placed on early detection. These guidelines are easily forgotten under the influence of factors like misinformation and lack of resources. Learning these factors is vital as they lead to late diagnosis and poorer health. The process of patients battling leukemia, highlighted by Alizadeh et al. (2015), represents a significant trend in oncology where timely medical intervention is central. Sensitizing the community and providing tangible educational literature on the issue of breast cancer can, thus, prove to be a device for empowering women to seek preventive care, leading in turn to early detection and increased survivorship in the population. Over the last few years, advances in personalized medicine and molecular oncology have seen a new era in the management of breast cancer. Targeted drugs based on genetic profiling have revolutionized treatment regimens, enabling more subtle management according to the specific needs of each patient. Immune checkpoint inhibitors and hormone therapies are among the advances that have broadened the scope of treatment beyond conventional chemotherapy, bringing encouragement to patients with aggressive or advanced disease states. However, access to these cutting-edge treatments is still unequal, particularly for under-resourced regions. As evident from hematology and oncology practice studies, there is a resource deployment lag that is detrimental to patient care. It is essential to bridge the gap, which requires collaborative action by policymakers, healthcare professionals, and civil society stakeholders to enable equitable access to novel treatment options among breast cancer patients (Alizadeh et al., 2015) (Figure 10.13).

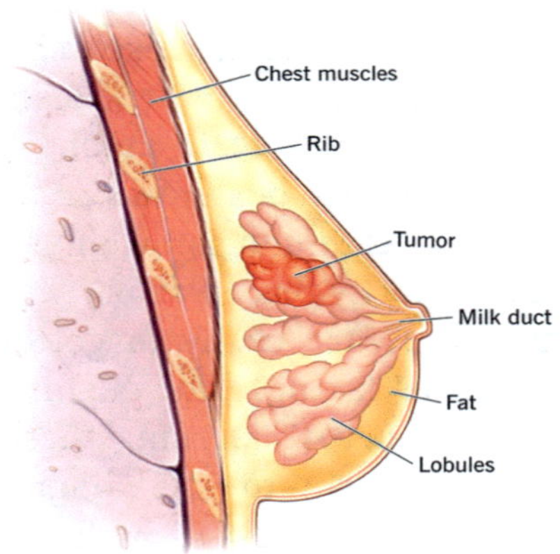

Figure 10.13. An illustration of breast cancer.

Source: https://my.clevelandclinic.org/-/scassets/images/org/health/articles/3986-breast-cancer.

10.4.2. Lung Cancer

The epidemiology of lung cancer outlines a multifactorial interaction of risk factors that highly influences its prevalence and prognosis. Cigarette smoking is the primary causal factor, accounting for 85% of all lung cancers. This is attributed to the carcinogenic chemicals in tobacco smoke that can produce genetic mutations and tumorigenesis of lung tissue. Along with smoking, secondhand smoke exposure, radon, asbestos, and other toxins in the environment increase lung cancer risk. Hereditary predispositions and family histories that increase lung cancer susceptibility have been recognized in recent studies, necessitating an extensive understanding of environmental and hereditary factors. This multi-faceted strategy is crucial for designing targeted prevention programs, particularly in high-risk groups, and thereby hopefully reducing the occurrence of lung cancer and improving prognosis in those affected. Detection of lung cancer typically involves advanced imaging modalities and histopathological examination for accurate identification and staging of the cancer. CT scanning is imperative, as it allows precise visualization of pulmonary nodules and adjacent structures, while biopsies are indicated for malignancy establishment and tumor histology. Histologic separation between non-small cell lung cancer (NSCLC) and small cell lung cancer (SCLC) is essential as a function of treatment, given that each has a differential biologic behavior and prognosis with therapy. In addition, the novel frontier of circulating tumor cells (CTCs) in lung cancer diagnosis is a promising but daunting one. CTCs are non-invasive biomarkers and provide real-time assessment of tumor development over a period of time. Recent reports indicate that methods like the High Throughput Vortex Chip have dramatically transformed the capture and analysis of CTCs, rendering them progressively valuable for clinical decision-making and personalized treatment (Che et al., 2016). With the progress in the therapy of lung cancer, the paradigm shift towards personalized medicine emphasizes the importance of molecular profiling and targeted therapy. Genomic sequencing technology has identified actionable mutations that guide the use of specific drugs, making the therapy more effective for patients. Mutagen-targeted drugs, on the other hand, have changed the ground for patients with identified mutations of the EGFR gene and have led to dramatic gains in response and survival. Exploring new pharmacologic drugs, including immunotherapy that utilizes the body's own immune system, further extends therapeutic modalities in the treatment of lung cancer. Recent research has also posited the potential of targeting co-occurring mutations to enhance response rates and limit resistance development, enabling personalized combination treatments driven by unique tumor signatures and reinforcing greater patient benefit (Anderson et al., 2014) (Figure 10.14).

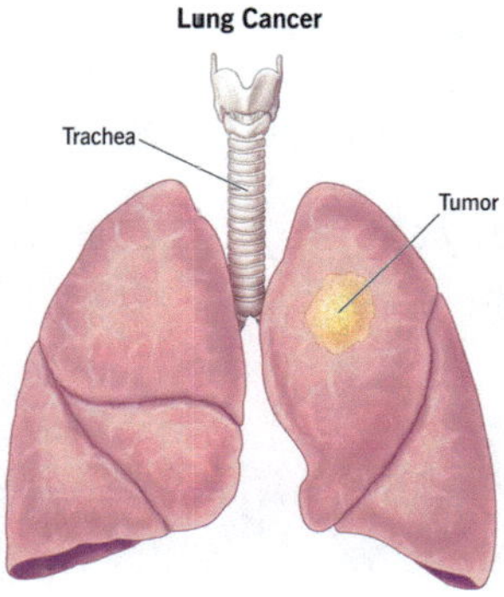

Figure 10.14. Lung cancer.

Source: https://my.clevelandclinic.org/-/scassets/images/org/health/articles/4375-lung-cancer.

10.4.3. Colorectal Cancer

Understanding colorectal cancer requires an in-depth analysis of its epidemiology, risk factors, and presentation. Colorectal cancer, occurring in the colon or rectum, is a leading cause of cancer morbidity and mortality worldwide. In terms of epidemiology, colorectal cancer is the third most common cancer and the second leading cause of cancer-related death in the United States. It is caused by a combination of several factors, including age, genetic factors, and lifestyle factors such as diet and inactivity. Interestingly, inflammatory conditions such as ulcerative colitis and Crohn's disease are linked with increased risk of developing colorectal cancer. Early detection and risk factor awareness are significant since early colorectal cancer is symptom-free and is associated with a considerable delay in treatment and diagnosis, which compromises patient outcomes and survival. Refinements in treatment modalities of colorectal cancer have been encouraging, particularly in cases of resistance to conventional treatments. New research points to the possible function of immunotherapy, that is, with checkpoint inhibitors in microsatellite instability-high (MSI-H) tumors, a subgroup of colorectal cancer with special genetic markers. Historically regarded as palliative, surgery in cancer can also have a dual function. For example, patients with malignant bowel obstruction and fistula development are most likely to be treated with surgical procedures that not only give symptomatic relief but also act as a bridge to immunotherapy, enhancing the overall prognosis and patient experience. The convergence of palliative approaches with new treatment modalities is a true reflection of the evolving landscape of colorectal cancer treatment. It underscores the importance of individualized treatment modalities based on tumor genetic makeup, as evidenced by recent findings in treatment paradigms that demand a review of the conventional approach (Bold et al., 2020). Furthermore, liquid biopsy platforms, such as interrogation of ctDNA, are transforming the practice of colorectal cancer diagnosis and monitoring. The kinetic character of ctDNA interrogation offers real-time monitoring of tumor evolution and response to treatment, offering valuable insights into the disease's biological underpinnings. At a more advanced disease stage, higher concentrations of quantifiable ctDNA have been linked with worse survival outcomes, and this is now recognized as a key prognostic factor for patient policy management. The capacity of ctDNA to reveal individual genetic mutations can direct targeted therapies and assist in building a more tailored treatment regimen, making research in this area even more necessary (Fanta et al., 2019). As increasingly is discovered about these molecular events, it is increasingly clear that the future of controlling colorectal cancer will be to integrate genomics with traditional oncology interventions to optimize patient outcomes and survival (Figure 10.15).

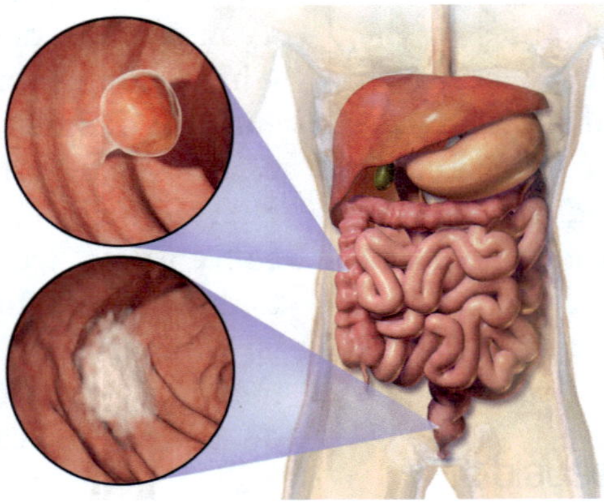

Figure 10.15. Location and appearance of two example colorectal tumors.

Source: https://upload.wikimedia.org/wikipedia/commons/thumb/1/12/Blausen_0246_ColorectalCancer.png/800px-Blausen_0246_ColorectalCancer.png.

Test Your Knowledge

1. What are the common risk factors associated with breast cancer?
2. What are the main histological types of lung cancer, and how do they differ in prognosis and treatment?
3. What are the major genetic and environmental risk factors contributing to colorectal cancer?

10.5. Advances in Hematology and Oncology

Learning Outcome

1. Focus on research and clinical trials in hematology and oncology
2. Discuss innovations in treatment approaches
3. Understand the role of technology in diagnosis and treatment

The field of hematology and oncology has witnessed significant development in recent years, particularly in the treatment of patients with hematological malignancies for viral infections. Respiratory viral infections in the community-acquired pattern (CARV) are of utmost danger to such vulnerable groups, with high morbidity and mortality rates. The findings from the EPICOVIDEHA-EPIFLUEHA registry are that among 1312 patients with hematological malignancies diagnosed with CARV in winter 2023–2024, 59.5% were hospitalized, with the unusually high ICU admission rate of 13.5%. These findings highlight the need for effective prevention and treatment measures to prevent the overwhelming incidence of CARV among these patients. Consequently, additional research into early diagnosis and tailored therapies is essential to maximize patient outcomes and create efficient protocols for future respiratory virus seasons (Monika et al., 2025). In oncology, establishing therapeutic methods for malignancies like follicular lymphoma (FL) reflects an increasing understanding of disease biology and the personalization of care. Despite FL having been characterized as an indolent neoplasm, it is problematic due to its variability and potential for early disease progression. An improved grasp of the treatment landscape for relapsed and refractory FL identifies several recent innovative therapies being investigated. The shift towards personalized medicine provides clinicians with more options when designing treatment protocols, enhancing the potential for successful results. Nevertheless, it is important that the health professionals weigh the potential advantages and limitations of these new treatments and make them harmonious with the specific patient's condition and aspirations (Muñoz et al., 2024). As progress in hematology and oncology grows each day, a detailed plan that includes improvements in treatment and supportive care will be the norm of the day. Sustained research efforts are required to address unmet patient needs, particularly those with their individual disease presentations such as lymphoproliferative disorders and hematological malignancies. The new therapies' impact on the management of matters complication-related as infections and treatment-related toxicities depends on understanding patient care dynamics. Future investigations must not only improve survival rates but improve the QoL for patients with these diseases. As the future of hematology and oncology opens up, cooperation between researchers, clinicians, and patients is essential to optimize treatment streams and design flexible healthcare systems that can accommodate the burden of these diseases.

10.5.1. Research and Clinical Trials

The clinical trial and research environment in hematology and oncology is continually evolving with new opportunities for effective treatment modalities. These trials are necessary for setting up new therapies and understanding the safety and effectiveness of new drugs. Current advances, particularly in the area of immunotherapy, have revolutionized treatment protocols, exemplified by novel modalities like immune checkpoint blockade. For instance, in the treatment of melanoma, combination immunotherapy with cytotoxic T-lymphocyte-associated protein 4 (CTLA-4) and programmed death 1 (PD-1) blockade is a good example of how clinical trials have significantly improved outcomes for patients. Despite this, the developments indicate that there remains an ongoing need for further research to improve and enhance access to treatments for all patients with hematologic malignancies and solid tumors (Daud et al., 2015). In addition, pediatric oncology has distinct challenges and opportunities in research and clinical trial designs. Cancer patients in childhood have been included predominantly in high-income countries historically in clinical trials, and many have had limited access to potentially curative treatments. However, cooperative efforts in pediatric oncology, like the development of national and international collaborative groups, have become increasingly critical in bridging the gap. The Indian Pediatric Oncology Group (InPOG) is a forward-thinking movement toward strengthening research infrastructure and outcomes in Indian children with cancer. The development of disease-specific subcommittees and the initiation of multi-center studies on disorders such as Hodgkin lymphoma and ALL show the strength that follows collaboration in establishing treatment protocols and ensuring equitable access to cutting-edge therapies (Arora et al., 2016). In hematology and oncology, research findings need to be translated into practice to enhance patient management continuously. Clinical trials not only guide treatment algorithms but also play a pivotal role in disease biology comprehension, patient stratification, and optimization of outcomes. The cycle of research, clinical research, and application continues to allow clinicians to provide more personalized and efficient interventions. Furthermore, with the progress in the area towards customized medicine, data-driven decision-making within clinical trials would be inevitable. Translational research studies coupled with emerging technologies could potentially make new therapeutic modalities available and ultimately improve the survival rates of patients afflicted with various hematologic diseases and cancers. In this regard, the significance of carefully planned research and clinical trials cannot be overestimated in developing new treatment modalities (Figure 10.16).

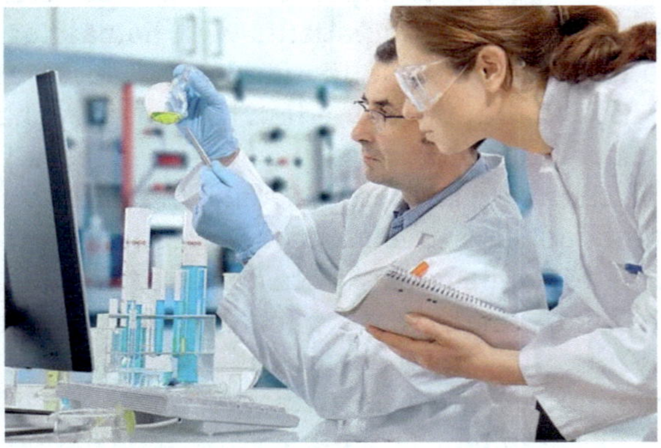

Figure 10.16. Clinical trials in oncology.

Source: https://ohcare.com/wp-content/uploads/2017/05/clinical-trial.jpg.

10.5.2. Innovations in Treatment Approaches

The field of hematology and oncology has seen formidable leaps in the areas of treatment methodologies, particularly with the entry of immunotherapy. One of the strongest advancements has been the use of monoclonal antibodies against specific cancer biomarkers, thereby fortifying the body's immune system against the malignant cells. Recent studies indicate that pembrolizumab, an anti-PD-1 antibody, significantly improves overall survival in advanced NSCLC compared to standard chemotherapeutic agents like docetaxel. In the KEYNOTE-010 trial, pembrolizumab-treated patients had better QoL scores and a reduced rate of treatment deterioration compared to standard chemotherapy-treated patients. This demonstrates the potential of immunotherapy not only to prolong survival but also to enhance patients' overall QoL (Ahn et al., 2019). Such a new approach is an indication of how personalized therapy can transform patient outcomes in hematology and oncology and divert attention from the one-size-fits-all treatment modality. In addition to immunotherapy, there has also been a remarkable turnaround in the therapeutic strategy for most malignancies with advances in the area of targeted therapies. Targeted agents are explicitly designed to recognize cancer cells based on their genetic and molecular characteristics with less toxicity to normal tissues. For instance, in the area of pancreatic cancer, researchers have explored the activity of the heat shock protein 27 (Hsp27)-targeting antisense oligonucleotide apatorsen in combination with established chemotherapy regimens. Although the incorporation of apatorsen was not linked with significant improvement in overall survival in unselected patient populations, it did yield a valuable assessment of the prognostic value of serum Hsp27 levels (Al-Hazzouri et al., 2017). This finding suggests that further research on biomarker-targeted approaches may yield personalized treatments that optimize efficacy in specific subpopulations of patients, paving the way for more successful interventions against advanced cancers. Moreover, the application of new treatment approaches such as gene therapy is beginning to revolutionize the treatment of hematology and oncology. Gene therapy aims to correct or remove genetic flaws responsible for disease onset, promising cures for certain hematologic disorders and cancers. Better trials are showing promise in using gene-editing tools such as CRISPR-Cas9 to silence oncogenes in leukemia patients. This approach not only aims to completely eliminate cancer cells but also to establish long-term resistance against future recurrences. The importance of such revolutionary techniques is massive, as they mark a shift towards curative instead of palliative therapy. As technologies continue to improve, they can initiate a new era of targeted therapy in hematology and oncology, significantly impacting patient care and survival (Figure 10.17).

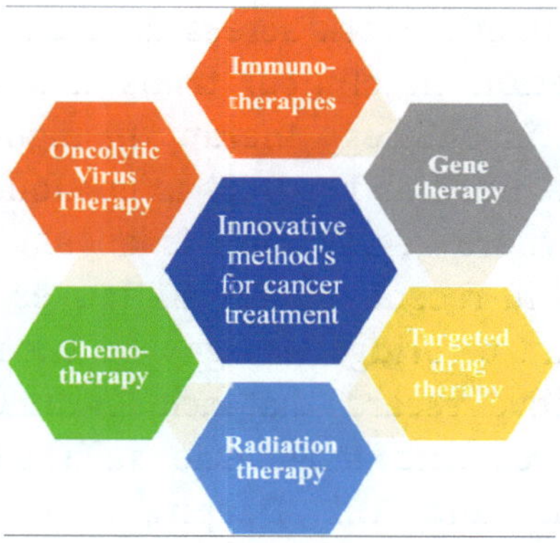

Figure 10.17. Innovative methods for treating cancer.

Source: https://www.researchgate.net/profile/Ankit-Verma-70/publication/380006529/figure/fig1/AS:11431281238192819@1713871185314/nnovative-methods-for-treating-cancer.png.

10.5.3. Role of Technology in Diagnosis and Treatment

The implementation of technology in diagnosis and treatment regimens is fundamentally transforming the hematology and oncology discipline. Technologies such as novel imaging modalities, MRI, and PET scanning enhance the ability to detect malignancies at an earlier stage and to implement interventions at the right time. Furthermore, digital pathology with high-resolution imaging and AI simplifies analysis, allowing for quicker and more accurate diagnosis of blood diseases and malignancies. By enabling pathologists to read slides more precisely, such technologies significantly reduce the likelihood of human error, ultimately optimizing patient outcomes. Furthermore, the availability of diagnostic technology in suburban and rural healthcare settings is paramount for equitable cancer treatment, as inequities often involve access to timely treatment across different regions (Alizadeh et al., 2015). Besides diagnostic advancements, technology has also revolutionized treatment modalities in hematology and oncology. Personalized treatments, facilitated by genomic sequencing, enable the use of medicine approaches tailored to target specific mutations in a person's tumor. An instance is the application of ctDNA analysis, as illustrated in recent studies, as a novel method for monitoring therapeutic response and detection of MRD. This "liquid biopsy" not only provides insights into tumor dynamics but also counteracts the shortcomings of traditional tissue biopsies, including invasiveness and the risk of complications. The identification of actionable genetic alterations by clinicians enables them to select appropriate targeted therapies, thereby maximizing treatment efficacy and preventing unnecessary side effects in patients (Fanta et al., 2019). With the increase in the scope of technology in hematology and oncology, changes to the medical system are necessary to implement these innovations to their full potential. It is a coordinated effort in sensitizing medical practitioners about the utility and application of these advanced diagnostic tests and forms of treatment. Equally significant is addressing the infrastructural needs to host such technologies, particularly in resource-limited settings. Prolonged diagnosis due to the unequal division of medical centers is a significant challenge that must be addressed to make a meaningful impact on patient care. Improved policies regarding training, resource distribution, and psychologic support for patients can allow for a more integrated approach towards cancer treatment such that gains from technology are indeed transferred to every patient with hematologic malignancies (Alizadeh et al., 2015).

Test Your Knowledge

1. How have recent clinical trials impacted the development of targeted therapies in hematologic malignancies?
2. What is role of technology in diagnosis and treatment?

10.6. Challenges in Hematology and Oncology

Learning Outcome

1. Discuss access to care challenges
2. Understand patient compliance and education
3. Explain ethical considerations in treatment

The field of hematology and oncology is faced with numerous challenges that are complicating both patient care and treatment outcomes. Among the foremost issues is the fast development in precision medicine, which, although offering promising therapy, offers principal challenges regarding execution. The transition from traditional cytotoxic therapies to targeted therapies necessitates extensive tumor profiling as well as interpreting complicated genomic data.

This process frequently draws on the services of interprofessional groups, e.g., molecular tumor boards (MTBs) that analyze tumor genomes to inform treatment decisions. The heterogeneity in the organization and deployment of MTBs across institutions can potentially generate unequal access to precision oncology gains, which, in turn, influences patient care differently depending on the healthcare setting. This conflict points to the need for universal methods that can ensure equal access to new therapy among all patients regardless of geographical or institutional variation (Grove et al., 2020). A second pressing problem is the inclusion of diverse patient populations in clinical trials, which is necessary to demonstrate that treatments work across different groups. Participation in clinical trials has become standard in oncology therapy in high-income countries. But this progress is not followed in LMICs, where registration is abysmally low. As noted in recent reports, initiatives like the InPOG aim to bridge this gap by encouraging collaborative research that includes multi-center trials for pediatric malignancies such as Hodgkin lymphoma and ALL. Despite these efforts, success will depend on clearing infrastructural hurdles, including a lack of funding, access to appropriate healthcare resources, and educational disparities among the healthcare professionals. Eradicating these challenges is essential in order to achieve maximum cure rates for pediatric cancer globally and illustrates the significance of fair clinical research (Arora et al., 2016).

Moreover, evolving patterns of treatment modalities and increasing complexities of the treatment of hematological malignancies call for continuous education and adjustment in healthcare providers. With the advent of new therapies like immunotherapies and gene therapies, clinicians must keep up with shifting patterns of practice and guidelines. Furthermore, new drug launches often trigger the need for pharmacists to take on leadership roles in genomic sequence interpretation, treatment choice, and off-label medication procurement. Integration of oncologists with pharmacists is not common and is another area of issues faced within the field. Having well-trained pharmacists involved in patient care is necessary to maximize the effectiveness of these advanced treatments.

The need for flexibility and responsiveness in hematology and oncology also addresses the imperative requirement for interdisciplinary collaboration in dealing with highly complex problems (Grove et al., 2020) (Figure 10.18).

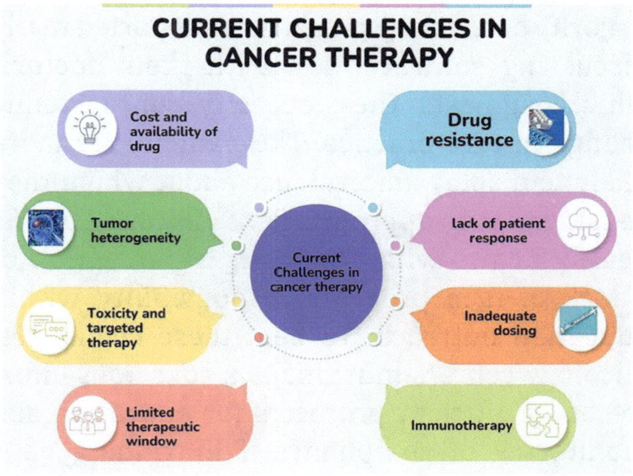

Figure 10.18. Current challenges in cancer therapy.

Source: https://ars.els-cdn.com/content/image/1-s2.0-S2667022424002810-gr2.jpg.

10.6.1. Access to Care

Treatment access is a central component in the hematology and oncology environment, as it directly affects patient outcomes and the success of treatment regimens. Inequalities in healthcare access have the potential to create wide variations in disease rates, disease development, and survival among different population groups. Patients with barriers to timely and appropriate care are susceptible to delayed diagnosis and treatment, hence worsening their health status, particularly in illnesses such as cancer, where early intervention is imperative. Such disparities are subject to socioeconomic status, geographic location, and insurance status, which makes it imperative that multi-faceted approaches address these multi-layered issues. To support equal access to hematology and oncology treatment, healthcare policies must reduce barriers and emphasize early detection and timely treatment as fundamental means of improving patient prognosis. The use of novel educational strategies is a principal aspect of improving access to care within hematology and oncology settings. Training courses designed to enhance training, such as distance learning courses, not only enhance the level of skills of medical professionals but also extend their coverage in underserved areas. For instance, implementation of new methods of curricula, such as in most ACGME-accredited emergency medical services training programs, demonstrates that properly customized learning material can actually help meet specific community needs. Through increased deployment of trained hematologists and oncologists, these programs will be able to reduce disparities in access to care that surround rural or economically disadvantaged regions. Building a solid infrastructure of health professionals capable of delivering specialized treatment is the necessary step for achieving the promise of equal access, ultimately leading to improved health outcomes and an educated patient population (Colella et al., 2020). Furthermore, institutional process difficulty, such as obtaining Institutional Review Board (IRB) approval, can inadvertently suppress early participation in clinical trials and treatment in hematology and oncology. Research has shown that delayed IRB approval times often stem from a heavy workload, complex rules, and ancillary reviews, leading to unacceptable delays in the opening of clinical trials. As a result, patients who seek more advanced treatments may wait longer than necessary, missing valuable opportunities at intervention. Decreasing these approval times through a quality improvement initiative might enable patients to access experimental therapy faster and receive the most up-to-date care possible. Efforts to reduce bureaucratic barriers by maintaining ethical standards are crucial for improving access to hematology and oncology care, creating a more responsive healthcare system capable of effectively responding to patient needs (Allen et al., 2017).

10.6.2. Patient Compliance and Education

Effective patient compliance and education are critical determinants in the care of patients undergoing treatment in hematology and oncology. Both of these determinants play a significant role in health outcomes, the success of treatment, and the overall health of the patients. Patients should be adequately informed about their disease, treatment, and the adverse effects of therapies to allow them to comply with proper treatment protocols appropriately. But divergent practices among oncology clinicians in discussing critical aspects of care can hinder effective education. As a case in point, conversations on contraception screening in adolescent girls with cancer show that many clinicians focus more on diagnosing pregnancy than on preventive practices such as appropriate contraceptive counseling. These communication gaps can lead to unplanned pregnancy, which can complicate the treatment of cancer and cause tragic repercussions for the patients at a pivotal point in their lives (Lindsay et al., 2018). The effects of inadequate patient education do not just extend to contraceptive needs; they extend as well to broader aspects of cancer care, including awareness of treatment regimens, side effect management, and indicators of disease progression. Compliance is usually determined by how well a patient understands their treatment plan and what is expected in terms of outcomes. Extensive educational interventions aimed at patients can maximize participation and collaboration in the treatment process. By using organized education programs that take into account the voice and needs of patients, healthcare professionals can successfully manage barriers to compliance. Involving interprofessional team members such as oncologists, but also social workers and nurses, is central to guaranteeing collaborative discussion, raising patient compliance and thus knowledge. Therefore, improving these education systems takes priority to enhance patient outcomes in hematology and oncology practice (N/A, 1986). Barriers to effective cancer care communication have significant potential to influence patient compliance and consequently overall treatment success. For example, the study made it clear that the majority of oncology patients had reported rarely discussing contraception with their doctors, which suggests the necessity for systemic change in care practice. The patients are more likely to display ambivalence about whom they consider most appropriate to discuss specific health factors with, reflecting a perception of a lack of firm provider responsibility within education outreach. To beat these challenges, oncology centers must make a conscious effort to set up efficient protocols for education and monitoring of compliance. Filling these gaps not only empowers patients but also creates a more cohesive healthcare setting, where patients feel nurtured and educated during their care process. Ultimately, improved patient compliance through education provides avenues for better therapeutic outcomes and QoL in patients combating the complexities of hematology and oncology (Lindsay et al., 2018).

10.6.3. Ethical Considerations in Treatment

Management of ethical concerns in hematology and oncology is crucial, particularly in relation to the distribution of resources. Increasing expenditure on new cancer treatment raises significant ethical considerations, as health systems attempt to meet rationing requirements for scarce resources. Principles of justice call for fair distribution and access to beneficial health gains. The methods of dealing with limited resources—rationalization, rationing, and prioritization—ensure that critical considerations like fairness and urgency shape the extent of treatment. For instance, rationing may involve withholding treatments due to financial constraints, an issue that seriously questions the ethics of providing care based on financial considerations. The existing controversy surrounding these ethical issues necessitates open policies and extensive engagement with society to build trust and equity in oncology treatment (Winkler et al., 2011). Our ethical issue of treating an aging population complicates the hematology and oncology situation even further. With the population aging, it is important to consider the effects of age on treatment options. The ageist ideology, which uses age as the determining criterion for the quality of care or access to care, threatens ethical medical practice. In these cases, incorporation of multidisciplinary geriatric evaluation before providing treatment is not only reasonable but also ethically required. These evaluations, which evaluate frailty and support, can assist clinicians in tailoring treatments for older adults based on their needs. However, the misapplication of these assessments manifests the dilemma of balancing ethical intention and experiential limitation within the healthcare setting (Lampugnane et al., 2017). Healthcare practitioners must solve these dilemmas to uphold the ethical aspect of providing equal and efficient care to oncogeriatric patients. Furthermore, ethical principles are observed in informed consent and patient autonomy in hematology and oncology practice. Life-changing diagnoses in patients require them to deal with complex treatment options and natural risks, which necessitate open and complete communication from providers. Informed consent is not just signing on the dotted line; it is a respectful conversation taking into account patients' values, preferences, and understanding of their health condition. Ethical practice requires oncologists to prioritize patients' subjective experiences, encouraging autonomy in decision-making, especially in cases of intensive treatment regimens. Ensuring that the patients are adequately informed allows them to make decisions based on their personal values and goals, thus making the entire therapeutic relationship more effective. This ethical requirement also highlights the importance of collaborative models of care, which facilitate mutual decision-making as a foundation of good oncology care (Winkler et al., 2011).

Test Your Knowledge

1. What are the main barriers to accessing hematology and oncology care in underserved populations?
2. How does patient compliance impact treatment outcomes in cancer therapy, and what strategies can improve adherence?
3. Discuss the ethical challenges involved in informed consent for experimental cancer treatments and clinical trials.

SUMMARY

Cooperation of experts in the provision of care is essential in the treatment of blood cancers. Children's dentistry practice, as evident in their management of leukemia patients, identifies the importance of collaboration among fields. Evidence indicates that pediatric dentists can have significant contributions to children's oral and overall health, and this pertains particularly to complications arising from cancer' therapies. Inclusion of prevention education by such professionals not only enhances patient care but also alleviates oral sequelae commonly inherent in treatment protocols. As highlighted in the study, including dental treatment in the treatment protocol for pediatric oncology patients is a step ahead in providing holistic healthcare to the vulnerable population (Rustin et al., 2018). Furthermore, long-term survivor research, such as examining renal impairment in survivors of pediatric sarcoma, offers an understanding of the chronic complications after treatment. The findings underscore that whereas one group of survivors showed CKD, others were resistant to nephrotoxicity when not receiving other chemotherapeutic agents. Such heterogeneity necessitates continued monitoring and long-term follow-up research to understand such late consequences of cancer treatments better. A comprehension of the health outcomes following therapy can help tailor follow-up care that is most applicable to individual patients' needs, thus improving their QoL in the coming years (Andreoli et al., 2018). Lastly, the findings of dental and long-term health studies underline the greatest need for multidimensional care in hematology and oncology. Addressing the multifaceted needs of patients—from managing oral complications during treatment to reducing the long-term impact of health consequences—requires an integrated team of specialists. Evidence of medical practitioners' attitudes towards the deliverability of holistic care indicates an increasing trend towards global care management strategies. Through interdisciplinary collaboration, the healthcare practitioner can enhance patient outcomes, not only for short-term care but also for long-term health and wellness of survivors of hematological malignancies (Andreoli et al., 2018; Rustin et al., 2018).

In oncology and hematology, understanding the molecular dynamics of diseases such as CML is crucial for effective treatment management. A point of concern in this aspect is the monitoring of BCR-ABL1 mRNA levels as response biomarkers to TKIs. Studies have shown that doubling times (DTs) of BCR-ABL1 transcripts can distinguish between unimportant increases in oncogene expression and real resistance to treatment. In a study involving 305 patients with chronic-phase CML, it was confirmed that the longer the DT, the lower the chances of resistance to imatinib mesylate among patients with shorter DT. This separation is crucial for early interventions, emphasizing the role of molecular monitoring in optimizing patient outcomes in the management of CML, thereby aligning the therapy strategy with the patient's requirements (Antolino et al., 2019). ALL is another area of hematologic malignancies where outcomes assessment also needs to take into consideration the toxic effects of the treatment. Although children with ALL as a group have excellent survival, they endure high acute toxicities of treatment regimens. In the Delphi research by a number of international childhood ALL trial groups, 14 major toxic effects, such as asparaginase hypersensitivity and high-dose methotrexate-related nephrotoxicity, are nevertheless not adequately controlled in present protocols. The findings indicated the heterogeneity of definitions of such toxicities across treatment guidelines, which necessitates uniform definitions and similar outcomes. Expert opinion consensus definitions will allow for better assessment of treatment toxicities, therefore enhancing quality care for pediatric ALL patients (Attarbashi et al., 2016). Collectively, these CML and ALL revelations indicate the delicate balance to be achieved between maximizing therapeutic efficacy and minimizing treatment-related toxicity in hematology and oncology. Molecular monitoring of CML serves both to distinguish among treatment effects and as a predictive indicator for modification of patient-specific therapy. Conversely, the acute toxicities agreement in ALL is focused on patient QoL and safety as important factors in complete treatment modalities. By reviewing these key points, healthcare workers will be able to create more effective management strategies that save lives and enhance patient welfare for hematological malignancies. These twin foci of the field are such that there is a developing oncology that emphasizes integrative and individualized patient care (Antolino et al., 2019; Attarbaschi et al., 2016).

KEY TERMS FROM THIS CHAPTER

- Acute myeloid leukemia (AML)
- Anemia
- Biomarker levels
- Blood disorders
- Blood-organ-producing organs
- Breast cancer
- CD20 monoclonal antibody
- Clinical sciences
- Clinical team
- Clinical trial
- Coagulation disorders
- Customized medicine
- Cytotoxic T-lymphocyte-associated protein 4 (CTLA-4)
- Flow cytometry
- General health
- Genetic mutations
- Germ cell tumors (GCT)
- Graft-versus-host disease (GVHD)

CRITICAL THINKING QUESTIONS

1. **What is the primary role of hematology in patient care?**
   a. Diagnosing and treating infections
   b. Diagnosing and managing blood disorders
   c. Performing surgery
   d. Managing psychiatric illnesses
2. **Which of the following is a common hematological disorder?**
   a. Asthma
   b. Diabetes mellitus
   c. Leukemia
   d. Osteoporosis
3. **Which cancer is most commonly diagnosed worldwide?**
   a. Lung cancer
   b. Prostate cancer
   c. Colorectal cancer
   d. Breast cancer
4. **What is the primary challenge in managing hematological malignancies?**
   a. Lack of diagnostic tools
   b. High rate of infections and complications due to immunosuppression
   c. Ineffective chemotherapy agents
   d. Excessive patient compliance
5. **Which blood test is commonly used to diagnose anemia?**
   a. Complete blood count (CBC)
   b. Blood glucose test
   c. Liver function test
   d. Kidney function test

Short Answer Questions

1. What is the role of hematology and oncology specialists in the multidisciplinary care of cancer patients?
2. Identify and describe three common hematological disorders and their clinical significance.
3. How do hematological malignancies differ from solid tumors in terms of diagnosis and treatment approaches?
4. What are the most common types of cancers encountered in oncology practice, and how are they generally classified?
5. Discuss the importance of early detection and screening in improving outcomes for common cancers such as breast, lung, and colorectal cancer.
6. What are some key challenges faced by healthcare providers in delivering effective hematology and oncology care?
7. How do patient-related factors such as compliance and education impact treatment success in hematology and oncology?
8. Explain how advances in technology and research have helped address some of the current challenges in hematology and oncology.

Answers to Critical Thinking Questions

1. (b); 2. (c); 3. (d); 4. (b); 5. (a)

REFERENCES

1. Mehta, R. S., Holtan, S. G., Wang, T., Hemmer, M. T., Spellman, S. R., Arora, M., Couriel, D. R., Alousi, A. M., Pidala, J., Abdel-Azim, H., Ahmed, I., Aljurf, M., Askar, M., Auletta, J. J., Bhatt, V., Bredeson, C., Chhabra, S., Gadalla, S., Gajewski, J., . . . Weisdorf, D. J. (2019). GRFS and CRFS in alternative donor hematopoietic cell transplantation for pediatric patients with acute leukemia. *Blood Advances, 3*(9), 1441–1449. https://doi.org/10.1182/bloodadvances.2018 030171Abenhardt, W., Artmann, A., de Rivera, I. G., Harbeck, N., et al. (2010). Prospective multicenter randomized phase III study of weekly versus standard docetaxel (D2) for first-line treatment of metastatic breast cancer. https://core.ac.uk/download/16432400.pdf (accessed on 27th June 2025).
2. Accurso, V., Antolino, A., Di Raimondo, F., Forte, S., Impera, S., Malato, A., Mannina, D., et al. (2019). Clinical implications of discordant early molecular responses in CML patients treated with imatinib. https://core.ac.uk/download/287859267.pdf (accessed on 27th June 2025).
3. Agarwal, V., Cawkwell, L., Drew, P. J., Fox, J., et al. (2014). Clinical response to primary letrozole therapy in elderly patients with early breast cancer: Possible role for p53 as a biomarker. https://core.ac.uk/download/151156899.pdf (accessed on 27th June 2025).
4. Ahern, J., Barakat, L. P., Bhatia, S., Bingen, E., et al. (2016). Patient/family education for newly diagnosed pediatric oncology patients. https://core.ac.uk/download/213078812.pdf (accessed on 27th June 2025).
5. Ahn, M. J., Barlesi, F., de Castro, G., et al. (2019). Health-related quality of life in KEYNOTE-010: A phase II/III study of pembrolizumab versus docetaxel in patients with previously treated advanced, programmed death ligand 1-expressing NSCLC.
6. Al Sayab, A., Al-Dewik, N., Fiorini, Z., Holyoake, T., et al. (2017). A new monoclonal antibody detects downregulation of protein tyrosine phosphatase receptor type γ in chronic myeloid leukemia patients. https://core.ac.uk/download/84148497.pdf (accessed on 27th June 2025).
7. Aleem, A., Qayyum, A., Jamil, A., Taj, A., Khalid, A., Tahir, A., Shah, I., et al. (2011). Detection of BCR-ABL kinase domain mutations in CD34+ cells from newly diagnosed chronic phase CML patients and their association with imatinib resistance. https://core.ac.uk/download/pdf/290490.pdf (accessed on 27th June 2025).
8. Al-Hazzouri, A., Bendell, J. C., DeBusk, L. M., Earwood, C., et al. (2017). A randomized, double-blinded, phase II trial of gemcitabine and nab-paclitaxel plus apertures or placebo in patients with metastatic pancreatic cancer: The RAINIER trial. https://core.ac.uk/download/323073315.pdf (accessed on 27th June 2025).
9. Alizadeh, S., Azad, M., Biniaz, R. B., Fard, A. D., et al. (2015). Short view of leukemia diagnosis and treatment in Iran. https://core.ac.uk/download/52205810.pdf (accessed on 27th June 2025).
10. Allen, K., Buscher, N., Caligiuri, M., Denney, R., et al. (2017). A multisite study of performance drivers among institutional review boards. https://core.ac.uk/download/323066081.pdf (accessed on 27th June 2025).
11. Al-Mondhiry, J., Walker, K. L., Bires, J., Caulkins, L. A., Hughes, C., Mohess, D., & Wadlow, R. (2024). Artful oncology: A comprehensive psychosocial oncology curriculum for hematology/oncology fellows. *Journal of Clinical Oncology*. https://www.semanticscholar.org/paper/5cf0

59209e77ad998430e9e29aad3eb5e2b184db (accessed on 27th June 2025).

12. Al-Shawy, H. A., & Jumaa, A. K. (2025). Neutropenic fever in patients with hematologic malignancies: Microorganisms and antimicrobial susceptibility. https://core.ac.uk/download/640062993.pdf (accessed on 27th June 2025).
13. Ancukiewicz, M., Catalano, O. A., Duda, D. G., Hayano, K., et al. (2013). Magnetic resonance imaging biomarkers in hepatocellular carcinoma: Association with response and circulating biomarkers after sunitinib therapy. https://core.ac.uk/download/28946070.pdf (accessed on 27th June 2025).
14. Anderson, P., Benjamin, R. S., Brown, R. E., Janku, F., et al. (2014). Novel secondary somatic mutations in Ewing's sarcoma and desmoplastic small round cell tumors. https://core.ac.uk/download/323065923.pdf (accessed on 27th June 2025).
15. Andreoli, G., Bonci, E., Celani, C., Marrucci, E., et al. (2018). Long-term renal function and hypertension in adult survivors of childhood sarcoma. https://core.ac.uk/download/159268194.pdf (accessed on 27th June 2025).
16. Antolino, A., Di Gregorio, S., Di Raimondo, F., Impera, S., Mannina, D., Manzella, L., Martino, B., et al. (2019). BCR-ABL1 doubling-times and halving-times may predict CML response to tyrosine kinase inhibitors. https://core.ac.uk/download/287859290.pdf (accessed on 27th June 2025).
17. Arora, R. S., & Bakhshi, S. (2016). Indian Pediatric Oncology Group (InPOG)–Collaborative research in India comes of age. https://core.ac.uk/download/pdf/82622201.pdf (accessed on 27th June 2025).
18. Astermark, J., Berntorp, E., Gitlin, S., Hastings, C., Hill, E., Kaushansky, K., Safa, O., et al. (2012). Outcomes of mentored, grant-funded fellowship training in hemostasis/thrombosis: Findings from a nested case–control survey study. https://deepblue.lib.umich.edu/bitstream/2027.42/91228/1/j.1365-2516.2011.02626.x.pdf (accessed on 27th June 2025).
19. Attarbaschi, A., Barzilai, S., Escherich, G., Frandsen, T. L., et al. (2016). Consensus definitions of 14 severe acute toxic effects for childhood lymphoblastic leukemia treatment: A Delphi consensus. https://core.ac.uk/download/42370388.pdf (accessed on 27th June 2025).
20. Berger, K., Gattermann, N., Hofmann, W. K., Meeßen, B., et al. (2008). Myelodysplastic syndromes: Aspects of current medical care and economic considerations in Germany. https://core.ac.uk/download/16432340.pdf (accessed on 27th June 2025).
21. Beyer, J., Blau, I. W., Burmeister, T., Friedrichs, B., et al. (2012). Molecular monitoring of minimal residual disease in two patients with MLL-rearranged acute myeloid leukemia and haploidentical transplantation after relapse. https://core.ac.uk/download/14523669.pdf (accessed on 27th June 2025).
22. Biernat, M. M., Bilgin, Y. M., Criscuolo, M., Del Principe, M. I., Falces-Romero, I., Fracchiolla, N. S., et al. (2025). Respiratory viruses in patients with hematological malignancy in boreal autumn/winter 2023–2024: EPICOVIDEHA-EPIFLUEHA report. https://core.ac.uk/download/649883056.pdf (accessed on 27th June 2025).
23. Bohlius, J., Bohlke, K., Castelli, R., Djulbegovic, B., et al. (2019). Management of cancer-associated anemia with erythropoiesis-stimulating agents: ASCO/ASH clinical practice guideline update. https://core.ac.uk/download/225130659.pdf (accessed on 27th June 2025).

24. Bold, R. J., Canter, R. J., Cho, M., Fakih, M., et al. (2020). The role of palliative surgery for malignant bowel obstruction and perforation in advanced microsatellite instability-high colorectal carcinoma in the era of immunotherapy: Case report. https://core.ac.uk/download/323311015.pdf (accessed on 27th June 2025).

25. Brém, E., Koyfman, A., & Long, B. J. (2020). Oncologic emergencies: Immune-based cancer therapies and complications. https://core.ac.uk/download/305124082.pdf (accessed on 27th June 2025).

26. Calaminus, G., Göbel, U., Haas, R. J., Schmidt, B., et al. (2002). Management of germ cell tumors in children: Approaches to cure. https://core.ac.uk/download/16432376.pdf (accessed on 27th June 2025).

27. Campioni, D. C., Cuneo, A., Farge, D., Fiamenghi, L., et al. (2013). Individual quality assessment of autografting by probability estimation for clinical endpoints: A prospective validation study from the European Group for Blood and Marrow Transplantation. https://core.ac.uk/download/54707944.pdf (accessed on 27th June 2025).

28. Che, J., Dhar, M., Di Carlo, D., Garon, E., et al. (2016). Classification of large circulating tumor cells isolated with ultra-high throughput microfluidic Vortex technology. https://core.ac.uk/download/323080454.pdf (accessed on 27th June 2025).

29. Cognetti, F., Fabi, A., Falcicchio, C., Giannarelli, D., et al. (2017). The course of cancer related fatigue up to ten years in early breast cancer patients: What impact in clinical practice? https://core.ac.uk/download/231747323.pdf (accessed on 27th June 2025).

30. Colella, M. R., Gaither, J., Schulz, K., Smith, M., et al. (2020). Innovative approaches to emergency medical services fellowship challenges. https://core.ac.uk/download/287621995.pdf (accessed on 27th June 2025).

31. Daud, A. I., & Tsai, K. K. (2015). Nivolumab plus ipilimumab in the treatment of advanced melanoma. https://core.ac.uk/download/323074185.pdf (accessed on 27th June 2025).

32. Deb, T. R., & Jahan, A. (2025). A comprehensive study on various cancer occurred in pediatric unit. https://core.ac.uk/download/656178867.pdf (accessed on 27th June 2025).

33. Elk, R. (2017). The need for culturally-based palliative care programs for African American patients at end-of-life. https://core.ac.uk/download/132289944.pdf (accessed on 27th June 2025).

34. Fanta, P., Kato, S., Kurzrock, R., Lanman, R. B., et al. (2019). Clinical correlates of blood-derived circulating tumor DNA in pancreatic cancer. https://core.ac.uk/download/323065613.pdf (accessed on 27th June 2025).

35. Fernando, T. R., Rao, D. S., & Rodriguez-Malave, N. I. (2012). MicroRNAs in B cell development and malignancy. https://core.ac.uk/download/4894914.pdf (accessed on 27th June 2025).

36. Fozza, C., & Longinotti, M. R. (2011). Use of rituximab in autoimmune hemolytic anemia associated with non-Hodgkin lymphomas. https://core.ac.uk/download/11691963.pdf (accessed on 27th June 2025).

37. Gaban, A. S., Liras, A., & Segovia, C. (2012). Advanced therapies for the treatment of hemophilia: Future perspectives. https://core.ac.uk/download/33104213.pdf (accessed on 27th June 2025).

38. Grove, M., Kiel, P. J., Kim, P., Raheem, A., et al. (2020). Precision genomic practice in oncology: Pharmacist role and experience in an ambulatory care clinic. https://core.ac.uk/download/333956949.pdf (accessed on 27th June 2025).
39. Haglund, K., Newman, A. R., & Rodgers, C. C. (2019). Pediatric oncology nurses' perceptions of prognosis-related communication. https://core.ac.uk/download/228028413.pdf (accessed on 27th June 2025).
40. Ionova, T., Johns, J., Oliva, E. N., Salek, S., et al. (2018). Appraisal of patient-reported outcome measures in analogous diseases and recommendations for use in phase II and III clinical trials of pyruvate kinase deficiency. https://core.ac.uk/download/287581341.pdf (accessed on 27th June 2025).
41. Jain, R. (2024). Health Equity Conference Series: An educational approach to combat implicit bias and structural racism in pediatric hematology/oncology. *Blood*. https://www.semanticscholar.org/paper/e231caa87d0f63a4e4e0553c6724d207e39897a7 (accessed on 27th June 2025).
42. Lampugnale, C. A. (2017). Surgical assessment of the geriatric oncology patient. https://open.bu.edu/bitstream/2144/26707/5/Lampugnale_bu_0017N_13146.pdf (accessed on 27th June 2025).
43. Lindsay, S. (2018). Understanding facilitators and barriers to contraception screening and referral in young women with cancer. https://open.bu.edu/bitstream/2144/32681/7/Lindsay_bu_0017N_14014.pdf (accessed on 27th June 2025).
44. Mahmood, A., Mandan, J., & Singh Sidhu, H. (2016). Should a clinical rotation in hematology be mandatory for undergraduate medical students? https://core.ac.uk/download/77016166.pdf (accessed on 27th June 2025).
45. Muñoz, J., Trotman, J., & Zinzani, P. L. (2024). Current and future therapies for follicular lymphoma. https://core.ac.uk/download/654520326.pdf (accessed on 27th June 2025).
46. N/A. (1985). 216 Jewish Hospital of St. Louis. https://core.ac.uk/download/70380865.pdf (accessed on 27th June 2025).
47. Rustin, H. (2018). Assessing feasibility and effectiveness of pediatric dental provider's role in oral health and prevention education in the care of children with leukemia. https://core.ac.uk/download/215483185.pdf (accessed on 27th June 2025).
48. Wazqar, D. Y. (2015). Job strain, coping strategies, and work performance among oncology nurses working in Saudi oncology care settings. https://core.ac.uk/download/61662508.pdf (accessed on 27th June 2025).
49. Winkler, E. (2011). *Rationalisierung, Rationierung, Priorisierung: Terminologie und Ethische Begründungsansätze Zur Allokation Bei Begrenzten Ressourcen In der Hämatologie/Onkologie*. https://core.ac.uk/download/16432321.pdf (accessed on 27th June 2025).

RHEUMATOLOGY AND MUSCULOSKELETAL DISORDERS

11

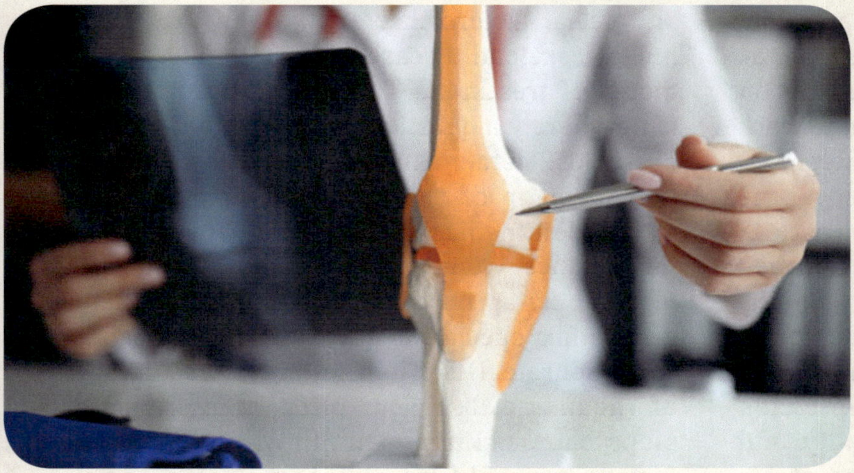

LEARNING OBJECTIVES

After studying this chapter, you will be able to:

1. Understand the anatomy and physiology of the musculoskeletal system;
2. Describe common rheumatological disorders;
3. Discuss about diagnostic approaches in rheumatology;
4. Define treatment modalities;
5. Explain the role of physical therapy in management;
6. Focus on challenges in rheumatology.

Introduction

Rheumatology is a specialist branch of medicine that is concerned with a broad spectrum of musculoskeletal system and connective tissue disorders. It encompasses common disorders like arthritis and systemic illnesses like lupus and scleroderma, which significantly impact the patients' QoL. The pathophysiology, clinical presentation, and management of rheumatological diseases are so complex that an in-depth knowledge of these aspects is needed. Rheumatologists, who have specialist knowledge in diagnosing and treating such ailments, form the core of providing individualized care to improve functional outcomes in patients. As the number of musculoskeletal conditions is increasing among geriatric patients, rheumatology is likely to play an even more significant role within the overall framework of general medicine, necessitating ongoing education and awareness among both healthcare providers and patients. In the management of rheumatological conditions, a biopsychosocial model has been significant, emphasizing the interplay among biological, psychological, and social factors. The multicomponent perspective is particularly significant in considering work-related upper limb disorders (ULDs), one of the grand challenges in the field of rheumatology. Effective management is more than just biomedical treatment; multimodal interventions aim to address both the physical and psychosocial dimensions of disease. Evidence indicates that engaging employers and patients in care plans leads to enhanced working outcomes, highlighting the importance of partnership interventions (Burton et al., 2008). In addition, intervention in psychosocial problems such as stress and mood can have a profound impact on recovery and allow individuals to return to work earlier, highlighting the need for an integrated treatment model in rheumatology. Moreover, the presentation of common conditions such as neck pain illustrates the complex interplay between physical and emotional health factors, and thus requires holistic management methods. It has been found that patients with neck pain typically present high comorbidities, such as depression and anxiety, which aggravate disability and make recovery more difficult (Souza et al., 2004). Identifying these links allows healthcare workers to develop more effective plans for management, such as psychological counseling and patient education materials. This not only reduces symptoms but also yields greater overall patient satisfaction with care. The integration of psychosocial considerations into the clinical model of rheumatology, therefore, is an important step in the practice of managing musculoskeletal disease, aligning with the broader objectives of general medicine.

Definition and Scope of Rheumatology

Rheumatology is a medical subspecialty that focuses mainly on the diagnosis and care of musculoskeletal disorders (MSDs) and autoimmune diseases. Rheumatology encompasses a wide array of conditions like arthritis, lupus, scleroderma, and other inflammatory joint diseases. What lies at the core of rheumatology is the awareness that such diseases can significantly impair a person's QoL through chronic pain, disability, and loss of mobility. Hence, rheumatologists employ a multidisciplinary approach, balancing biomedical knowledge with psychosocial factors to manage these complex diseases effectively. The evolving definition of rheumatology is a reflection of the necessity not just to cure the bodily expressions but also the psychological and social factors that manifest in long-term musculoskeletal disease, toward an integrated model of treatment. The art of rheumatology is not merely a question of managing joint and musculoskeletal pain, but rather the overall management of the patient and extending into other medical specialties. Treating RA, for instance, would require coordination with physical therapists, occupational therapists, and even other specialists such as dermatologists and nephrologists. The multifactorial etiology of rheumatic disorders often necessitates a biopsychosocial treatment, in which biological factors, psychological functioning, and social environment are relevant to successful management. Current literature shows that isolated biomedical treatments or isolated stand-alone ergonomic treatments are not sufficient to achieve the best outcomes. A multimodal approach, emphasizing interprofessional collaboration, lies at the heart of enhancing patient outcomes, particularly regarding return-to-work interventions and overall reintegration into society (Burton et al., 2008). Progress in the rheumatology discipline over the past few years has centered on maximizing treatment strategies for spondyloarthritis (SpA) and psoriatic arthritis (PsA). Recognizing that treatment targets are still under development, expert opinion has led to recommendations to initially establish remission or low disease activity as the primary goals in treating these diseases. Utilizing previously outlined treat-to-target approaches not only promotes disease control but also facilitates easier shared decision-making by patients regarding their regimen. Although there may be insufficient evidence for specific management strategies in SpA and PsA, the need for ongoing assessment of disease activity and associated comorbidities highlights the role of rheumatology in supporting enhanced patient treatment (Baraliakos et al., 2013). Overall, rheumatology remains an advancing and growing specialty, underscoring the need for comprehensive, multidisciplinary treatment regimens to manage the intricacies of musculoskeletal disease.

Importance of Musculoskeletal Health

The significance of musculoskeletal health cannot be overemphasized, particularly in the context of general medicine and rheumatology. MSDs are prevalent and can manifest as severe aspects of multimorbidity, defined as the coexistence of two or more chronic conditions. Because so many individuals live with these comorbid health conditions, the impact of MSDs goes far beyond painful and irritating symptoms; it also consists of decreases in overall QoL, increased healthcare utilization, and adverse effects on productivity in society. Understanding the role of musculoskeletal wellness in this expanded overall health continuum is essential for healthcare providers who wish to offer holistic care and treatment options that address the complexity of multimorbidity. By prioritizing musculoskeletal health, clinicians can contribute to improved patient outcomes and reduce the economic cost of managing chronic disease (Agoritsas et al., 2017). Moreover, musculoskeletal conditions such as RA, OA, and osteoporosis are leading causes of physical disability globally. These conditions are both recognized as national priorities for health in most nations due to their widespread incidence and their chronic impact, directly influencing public health policy and planning for resources. Musculoskeletal conditions tend to facilitate the loss of dexterity and mobility, long-term pain, and restrictions on physical functioning, affecting not only individual patients but also their families and communities in general. This widespread impact underscores the imperative to integrate musculoskeletal health into primary care, in a way that practitioners can address them best in complicated healthcare systems (Brown et al., 2014). By adopting evidence-based targeted intervention and preventive methods, the health system can minimize the extensive personal and economic burdens of the conditions. The integration of a multidisciplinary musculoskeletal strategy is crucial for optimizing patient care and developing long-term health. Rheumatologists, physical therapists, and other clinicians integrate their efforts through this approach to address the multiple aspects of musculoskeletal illnesses comprehensively. Pain-free treatment regimens, customized to incorporate physical rehabilitation and lifestyle modifications, aim not only to relieve symptoms but also to enable patients to become active participants in managing their own care. Furthermore, public education on musculoskeletal health will promote preventive practices, such as exercise and nutrition, necessary for musculoskeletal integrity. Through the awareness of the interconnectedness of musculoskeletal health and overall health outcomes, policymakers and healthcare providers alike can better serve individuals who struggle with these prevalent disorders, ultimately enhancing affected populations' QoL (Agoritsas et al., 2017).

Overview of Common Rheumatological Conditions

Rheumatologic diseases are a wide range of disorders that are primarily localized to the muscle, joint, and connective tissue. OA or degenerative joint changes with inflammation limiting motion is one of the most prevalent. The patient may present with stiffness, swelling, and pain over an area and this significantly impacts daily function and QoL. Management also includes non-steroidal anti-inflammatory drugs (NSAIDs) such as diclofenac, which has been shown to significantly alleviate symptoms associated with OA. Notably, topical formulations of diclofenac provide a less risky alternative with less systemic side effects and relief from pain without the GI and renal risks of oral administration. Thus, understanding development in the treatment of OA and similar conditions, in particular the transition to topical treatments, for optimal care (Banning et al., 2008) is crucial. Another rheumatological condition that is commonly encountered is RA, an autoimmune disorder with chronic inflammation of the joints. Unlike OA, RA is typified by systemic disease and potentially affects patients of all ages with symmetric pain in the joints and fatigue. The pathogenesis of RA remains multifactorial, involving genetic susceptibility and environmental influences. The clinical course has the potential to result in severe joint deformity and significant loss of function. Multidisciplinary treatment strategies for RA generally include disease-modifying antirheumatic drugs (DMARDs) and biologic agents with the hope of halting disease progression. Continuous monitoring and therapeutic regimen adjustments are necessary to optimize results and reduce drug-related side effects. Clearly, there is a need to understand the intricacies of RA to cater to the needs of such patients effectively. Chronic back pain (CBP) is also a major challenge in rheumatology, a condition that is as complex as it is seemingly uncomplicated musculoskeletal discomfort. CBP is heterogeneous in its underlying causes from degenerative disc disease to psychosomatic in origin, hence resulting in varying patient outcomes and experience. Research has indicated that existing therapeutic interventions are nonspecific, reinforcing the development of more specific interventions to address the heterogeneity of the condition. Population research incorporating clinical assessment has prioritized physical symptoms, mental status, and overall patient functioning. This wider realization of the unique population of people with CBP calls for subgroup-specific treatment and diagnostic indicators, resulting in eventual innovation in coping with CBP (Gerhardt et al., 2013). With evidence-based, methodologically sound research, clinicians are better placed to treat the associated complexities of CBP and improve patients' outcomes.

11.1. Anatomy and Physiology of the Musculoskeletal System

Learning Outcome

1. Explain the structure of bones and joints
2. Understand the function of muscles and connective tissues
3. Deal with the interaction between the musculoskeletal system and the immune response

The musculoskeletal system consists of bones, muscles, cartilage, tendons, and ligaments, which function in cooperative interdependence to provide structure, support, and movement to the human body. Bones serve as a permanent framework, offering protection to vital organs and permitting mobility by articulating against one another at joints. The bone consists of a dense outer layer of cortical bone and a spongy internal framework, referred to as trabecular bone, which contains marrow for hematopoiesis. The most essential is the organization of bone tissue, as it contains minerals like calcium and phosphorus that contribute to bone development and bone density (Hoppmann et al., 2022). Furthermore, the study of musculoskeletal anatomy is not only for the skeletal system but also for the relationship between bones and muscles, which is crucial for effective movement and exercise to ensure overall health (Hoppmann et al., 2022). Muscle tissue, classified as three kinds—skeletal, smooth, and cardiac—is an essential agent of movement and support. Skeletal muscles, being under voluntary control, attach to bones by direct connection via tendons and possess the ability to move the body. The muscles contract to produce movement, maintain the body in a position, and generate heat, which is essential for thermoregulation. Physiological processes of muscle contraction involve complex biochemical pathways, in which neuromuscular junctions facilitate the transmission of nervous impulses to the muscle fibers. Understanding how these muscles act upon skeletal systems plays a significant role in diagnosing mobility-affecting disorders, such as muscular dystrophy or inflammatory myopathies, which extensively deteriorate muscle function and general health (Meryl et al., 2022). Besides, the roles played by tendons and ligaments within the musculoskeletal system are crucial, as they are connective tissues used to stabilize joints and transmit muscle forces to bones. Ligaments connect bone to bone while also assisting in resisting abnormal movement, which is required to prevent injuries. Tendons join muscles to bones and play a central role in translating muscle forces into movements. Both of these structures are essential to musculoskeletal integrity and are often the site of pathologies—sprains, strains, and degenerative changes—that lead to dysfunction and pain. There must be a vast knowledge of these components for efficient management of MSDs because it dictates treatment modalities that will restore function and enhance mobility for the affected population (Hoppmann et al., 2022).

11.1.1. Structure of Bones and Joints

The human skeleton is a complex system of joints and bones that serves a vital role to provide movement, protection, and support. Bones, the chief constituents, are constantly dynamic tissues that are remodeled throughout life through the influence of mechanical stress and biological forces. Such remodeling helps a lot in maintaining bone density, and dysregulation leads to conditions like osteoporosis, which significantly increases the risk of fractures, especially among older adults. Clinical evidence highlights that increasing bone loss increases fragility, and therefore it is critical for healthcare professionals to implement frequent screening and management protocols to minimize the risk of fractures for high-risk groups, particularly those over 50 years of age (Meryl et al., 2022). Understanding of this anatomic arrangement and the implications for musculoskeletal health is paramount in the effective management of rheumatological disease (Figure 11.1).

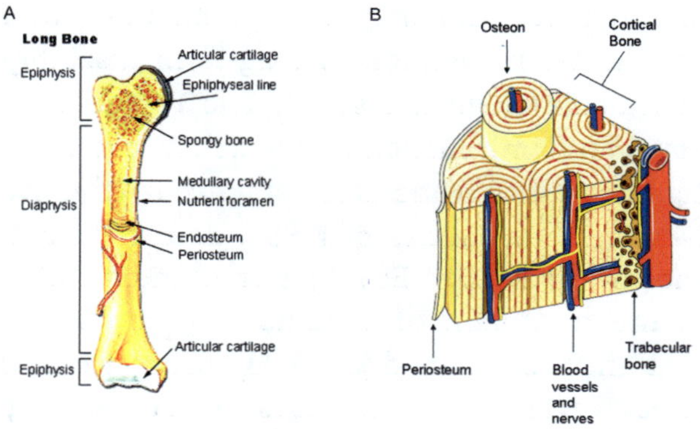

Figure 11.1. Structure and components of a long bone. (A) Long bones are longer than they are wide, consisting of a long shaft (the diaphysis) plus two articular (joint) surfaces called epiphyses. (B) A 3D representation of the structure and organization of trabecular and compact bone.

Source: https://www.researchgate.net/profile/Helen-Owen-Roberts/publication/33053455/figure/fig1/AS:669510117892106@1536635059285/Structure-and-components-of-long-bone-A-Long-bones-are-longer-than-they-are-wide.ppm.

Joints are the articulations of bones that provide movement as well as stability. They are divided into several types, i.e., synovial, cartilaginous, and fibrous joints, each with different structures and functions. Synovial joints, for instance, are the most mobile type, comprising a fluid-filled synovial capsule that lubricates articular surfaces to allow free movements. The integrity of these joints' structure is essential to overall musculoskeletal function; however, they are often compromised in OA and RA, resulting in stiffness, pain, and limited mobility. The management and treatment of the disease conditions of the joint might involve both pharmacologic and nonpharmacologic therapeutic approaches targeting the symptoms as well as structural alterations at the underlying level (Adam et al., 2022). Patient education about joint maintenance and health plays an important role in the prevention of long-term disability in rheumatological disease. The relationship between joint function and bone structure has significant implications for practice in effective treatment modalities of MSDs. Extracorporeal shockwave therapy (ESWT) is a new intervention in the treatment of a number of conditions that affect bones and joints. By using acoustic shockwaves, ESWT induces tissue healing, relieves pain, and can augment bone remodeling, especially in conditions like calcific tendinopathy and plantar fasciitis.

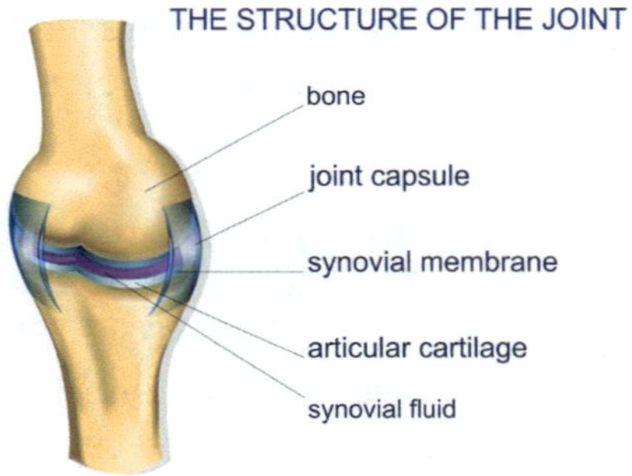

Figure 11.2. Structure of joint.

Source: https://3dmusclelab.com/wp-content/uploads/2019/11/synovial-joint.jpg.

Through the processes by which shockwave therapy works, these consist of stimulating angiogenesis and collagen production, which are instrumental to the repair and regeneration of both bony and soft tissue structures. With advancing understanding of musculoskeletal conditions, the incorporation of novel therapies like ESWT into clinical practice may help to better manage patients with chronic pain and loss of function, ultimately towards the goal of enhanced QoL and mobility (Adam et al., 2022) (Figure 11.2).

11.1.2. Function of Muscles and Connective Tissues

Muscles and connective tissues form the fundamental structures of the musculoskeletal system, facilitating movement, stabilizing, and protecting internal organs. The muscles are classified into three types: skeletal, cardiac, and smooth. They play a primary role in voluntary and involuntary movement, with the skeletal muscles of top concern regarding locomotion and everyday activity. These fibers contract and relax due to neural stimulation, enabling both fine and gross motor activities. Along with muscles are the connective tissues of tendons, ligaments, cartilage, and fascia, which provide the flexibility and support required for the musculoskeletal system to function. How muscle and connective tissue work together is necessary for posture control and balance and for coordinated movement performance. Understanding this dynamic relationship is crucial to the management of many rheumatological disorders affecting muscle and joint function. Muscle and connective tissue integrity are commonly disrupted by conditions such as RA and OA, and may cause profound functional impairment (Figure 11.3).

Rheumatic diseases usually manifest as inflammation around and within joints, leading to pain, stiffness, and reduced mobility. RA, for instance, manifests with inflammation of the synovium that not only affects joint tissue but may also result in muscle atrophy and weakness secondary to disuse. Connective tissues also lose strength with age and repetitive stress, leading to conditions like tendinitis or bursitis that impair the function of affected muscles. Such issues are generally treated by a multidisciplinary team that combines physical therapy and potentially novel treatment approaches like endogenous tissue engineering, which aims to induce the body's natural repairing mechanisms (Adam et al., 2012).

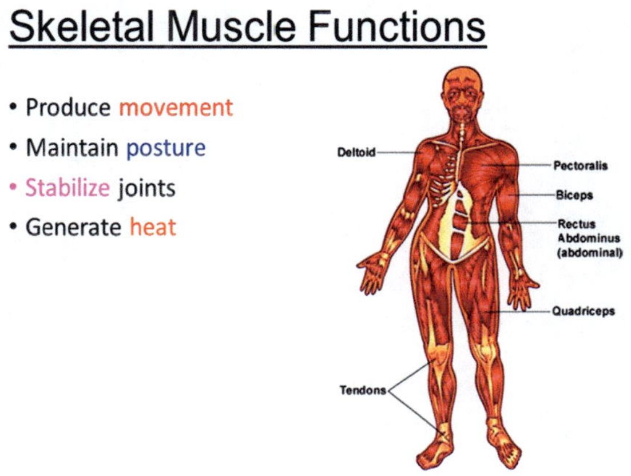

Figure 11.3. Skeletal muscle function.

Source: https://slideplayer.com/9286029/28/images/slide_1.jpg.

Thus, enhancing our understanding of muscle function and connective tissue health is core to the management of MSDs. In practice settings, the interplay between muscle and connective tissues extends beyond movement to encompass an integrated understanding of patient health, particularly in rheumatology. Interdisciplinary cooperation among providers of medical care, including rheumatologists and physiatrists, highlights rehabilitation programs tailored to each patient's requirements. Modalities of treatment, such as individualized exercises, forms of physical therapy, and adjunctive techniques like therapeutic ultrasound and laser therapy, were utilized to enhance tissue recovery and function. Education programs that allow active patient participation can improve treatment outcomes remarkably, particularly with temporomandibular joint and other overused joint conditions (Krapac et al., 2010). Patient participation not only makes it easier to follow through with therapeutic measures but also educates patients and allows them to take active responsibility in the preservation of musculoskeletal well-being, leading eventually to better QoL (Figure 11.4).

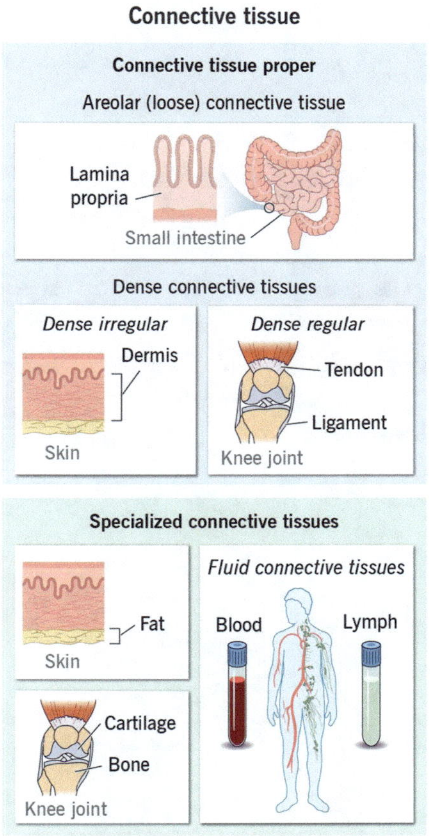

Figure 11.4. Connective tissue.

Source: https://my.clevelandclinic.org/-/scassets/images/org/health/articles/connective-tissue.

11.1.3. Interaction Between the Musculoskeletal System and Immune Response

The musculoskeletal-immune system interaction is a particularly significant area of study within rheumatology, and particularly in the context of autoimmune diseases like RA and inflammatory myopathies. The immune system plays a role in maintaining the body's health in musculoskeletal terms, defending against infection, and contributing to the breakdown of musculoskeletal tissues when it becomes dysregulated. While invading synovial tissues, immune cells can potentially promote the inflammatory milieu that is responsible for conditions like RA. Dysregulation of immune activation in this case could lead to the production of pro-inflammatory cytokines, perpetuating a vicious cycle of inflammation, pain, and joint destruction. This pathological interaction finally culminates in significant morbidity, which is a rationale for unmasking immune mechanisms responsible for musculoskeletal disease in therapeutic strategies.

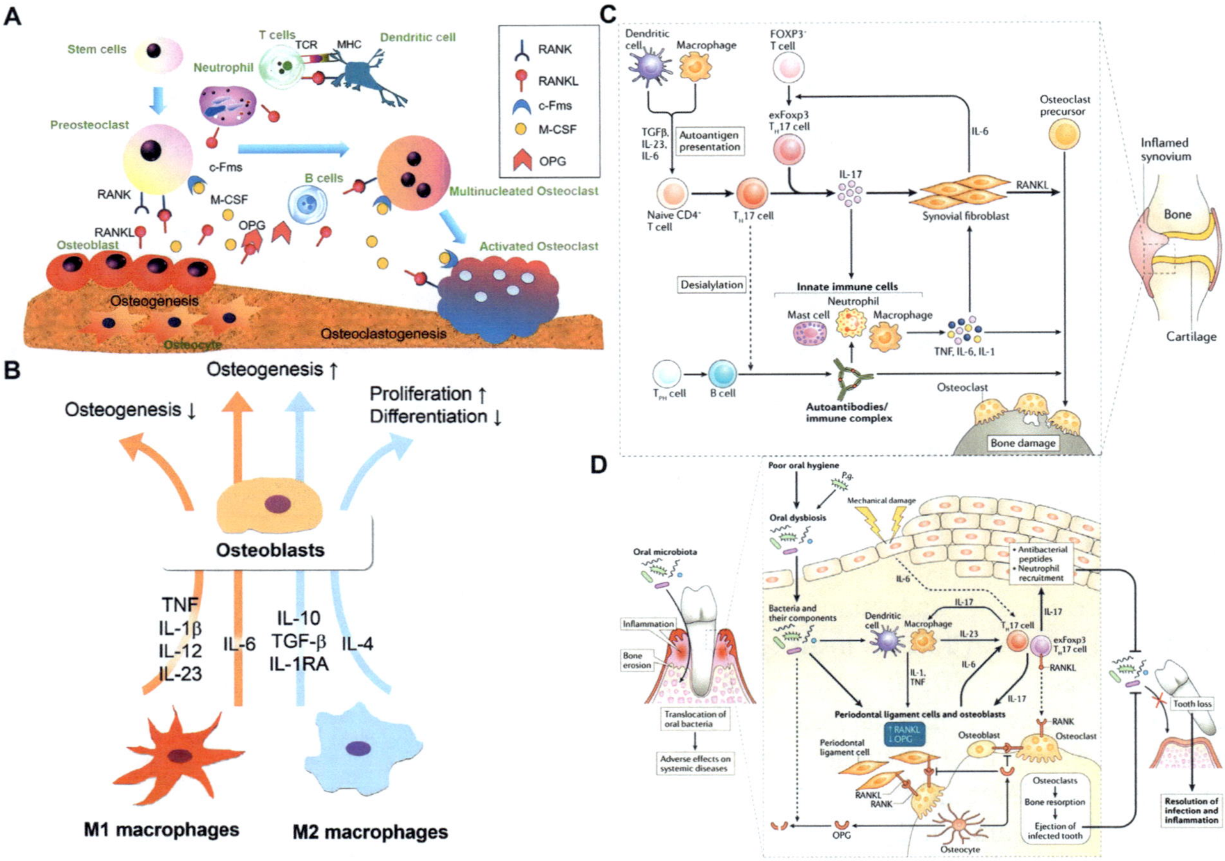

Figure 11.5. The interaction of the skeletal system and the immune system. (A) Interaction between skeletal and immune cells by secreting related factors. (B) M1 and M2 interact with osteoblasts through cytokines such as IL-6, IL-23, IL-10, and TGF-β. (C) The role of T cells, macrophages, and neutrophils in RA-induced bone erosion. (D) The role of T cells, macrophages, and DCs in bacterial periodontitis-induced bone erosion.

Source:

Besides, the advent of immunotherapies, namely immune checkpoint inhibitors, has revealed novel dimensions of the interplay between the immune system and MSDs. These treatments, designed to enhance the body's anti-cancer immune response, can unintentionally trigger autoimmune side effects, particularly in the presence of existing immune system abnormalities. An examination of the current literature indicates that neurological side effects and other autoimmune diseases can arise following such treatments, suggesting an effect by which enhanced immune function proves to be uncontrolled and targets not only the tumor but the patient's own tissues as well. The clinical significance of such findings underscores the need for careful surveillance and control of side effects that may arise in patients receiving immunotherapy for cancers, especially as immunotherapies are increasingly used in the treatment of cancer (Dalakas et al., 2018). Moreover, emerging evidence indicates that micronutrients such as vitamin D may influence the immune system and affect musculoskeletal health. Vitamin D has come into prominence in recent years for its immunomodulatory role and potential to prevent autoimmune phenomena. Deficiency of vitamin D has been reported in a number of rheumatic diseases, and it therefore appears that peak levels may be beneficial not only to bone but also to immune homeostasis. While a "more-is-better" approach to supplementation is tempting, vitamin D and immune function are complex and deserve a conservative evaluation of both therapeutic risk and benefit. Future research will be needed to determine the relevance of vitamin D status in children with rheumatic disease, emphasizing integrated approaches that consider both immune and musculoskeletal factors (Burnham et al., 2011) (Figure 11.5).

Test Your Knowledge

1. Describe the primary structural components of a long bone and explain the function of each part.
2. Compare and contrast the three major types of joints in the human body, including examples and their range of motion.
3. Explain the roles of different muscle types (skeletal, cardiac, and smooth) in the musculoskeletal system.

11.2. Common Rheumatological Disorders

Learning Outcome

1. Describe rheumatoid arthritis
2. Explain osteoarthritis
3. Understand lupus and other autoimmune disorders

Rheumatological conditions are a broad spectrum of conditions that primarily involve the joints, muscles, and connective tissue and cause significant morbidity. Among these, OA is the most prevalent and is defined by cartilage loss and bone remodeling. OA manifests as chronic pain and stiffness in the weight-bearing joints, such as the knee and hip. Traditional management involves pharmacologic and non-pharmacologic treatments, including physical therapy and lifestyle changes, along with pharmacologic treatments such as NSAIDs. Of special note, diclofenac topical formulations have become well-liked due to their effectiveness at pain relief while reducing the systemic side effects of oral NSAIDs. Research emphasizes that local diclofenac can be very effective in alleviating pain and stiffness in OA patients while not eliciting the colossus GI or renal damage that its oral counterparts cause, making it a promising therapeutic agent in symptom relief in this disease (Banning et al., 2008). Another of the most common rheumatological ailments is RA, an autoimmune disease caused by persistent inflammation of the synovial joints. This disease is often associated with systemic manifestations, including malaise and fatigue, which complicate its treatment. The inflammatory process of RA can lead to joint damage and disability if left untreated and needs to be treated early. DMARDs are standard pharmacologic treatments aimed at suppressing the autoimmune process and preventing progressive joint destruction. The introduction of biologic therapies has dramatically altered RA treatment, targeting distinct immune response pathways to offer maximum control over the disease. However, the response to treatment can be heterogeneous, underscoring the importance of personalized therapy in treating RA in a productive way, which is significant in enhancing patient outcomes in this complex disease (Gerhardt et al., 2013). CBP is also a significant problem among rheumatological and MSDs, with consequences extending beyond physical anguish to broader socio-economic aspects. Its heterogeneity typically defines CBP because the patients come with varied symptomatology that complicates treatment approaches. The limitations of current treatment strategies lie in the lack of targeted therapies aimed at specific patient groups because typical treatments do not affect heterogeneous groups. Recent research activity has focused on breaking such a limitation by exploring the multi-factorial aspects of CBP, including psychosocial determinants, co-morbid conditions, and varying mechanisms of pain. Such comprehensive research highlights the requirement of treatment modalities for subgroups that would enhance the potency of intervention and inform future clinical practice. Such ongoing identification of such complex relationships in the treatment of back pain is essential in informing refinement of therapeutic strategies in rheumatology (Gerhardt et al., 2013).

11.2.1. Rheumatoid Arthritis (RA)

Rheumatoid arthritis (RA) is a chronic inflammatory autoimmune disease that primarily affects the joints, producing pain, swelling, and ultimately joint damage if not adequately treated. The pathophysiology of RA involves an autoimmune response where the defense system of the body mistakenly attacks the synovial tissue, resulting in inflammation and destruction. This disease not only affects physical well-being but also significantly affects mental well-being as the patients acquire comorbidities such as depression and anxiety. Additionally, the chronic nature of RA poses challenges in the activities of daily living and QoL, thus calling for multisided management comprising drugs, physiotherapy, and patient education. As RA progresses, understanding its widespread implications is central to medical practitioners to enable them to design patient-centered interventions addressing not just the physical, but also the emotional and psychosocial needs of individuals with this disabling illness. One of the outstanding aspects of RA is its widespread impact on various body systems, predominantly on foot health. Foot disease is prevalent in RA patients and contributes significantly to global disability. It has been demonstrated through studies that despite foot disease being extremely common in RA patients, it is usually neglected in the treatment strategy. Incompetence among clinicians in dealing with complications occurring in the foot makes the neglect worse. Therefore, there is growing agreement on the need to integrate expert podiatric care into rheumatology services on an urgent basis. This integration would increase access to appropriate foot care interventions and ultimately provide better QoL for patients. Promoting greater collaboration among podiatrists and rheumatologists would encourage better management strategies that address the foot diseases, and therefore decrease chronic pain and enhance mobility so that patients remain active members of their community. Furthermore, fatigue is often an overlooked and important component of RA, similar to comments in other rheumatological conditions such as ankylosing spondylitis.

Fatigue can occur in several areas, affecting physical vigor, mood, and mental well-being. The patients grow fatigued physically, irritated emotionally, and low psychologically, generating a multivalued interaction of the complexities in treatment. Current management of RA-related fatigue is generally unsatisfactory, and much is done by patients without guidance or framework. Evidence supports rising interest in the use of psychological interventions for this refractory fatigue. It shows up the possibility of the need for individually adapted methods of working with it, with mind-based treatments one likely option. Implementing evidence-based interventions that work on both the emotional and physical causes of fatigue can empower patients, eventually leading to improved overall health results in treating RA (Figure 11.6).

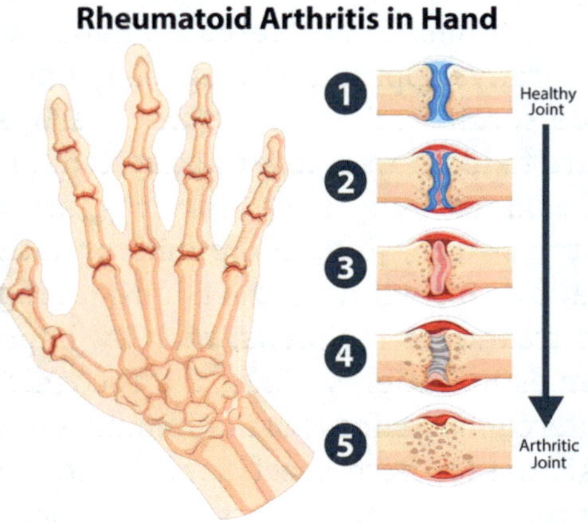

Figure 11.6. Rheumatoid arthritis in hand.

Source: https://anova-irm.com/images/jch-optimize/rs/768/images_Rheuma_Rheuma__Hand__Skizze.webp.

11.2.2. Osteoarthritis (OA)

Osteoarthritis (OA) is a top area of interest in rheumatology and musculoskeletal diseases research, involving the destruction of cartilage and bone. The condition often occurs in the form of pain, stiffness, and functional impairment, which is usually experienced by weight-bearing joints such as knees, hips, and the spine. OA often starts with aging, obesity, and repetitive joint stress, which may lead to increasing medical and social costs. Early diagnosis and treatment are crucial, as they can diminish symptoms and improve the quality of patients' lives. Research highlights the multifactorial etiopathogenesis of OA, including genetic, environmental, and mechanical features. An understanding of these factors is significant for designing effective therapies with an emphasis on limiting the disease burden and ensuring optimal patient care in rheumatology (Paoloni et al., 2017). OA treatment options involve an assortment of pharmacologic and non-pharmacologic interventions, depending on the extent and localization of the illness. The NSAIDs are typically administered to treat pain and inflammation; however, they pose threats, particularly in the geriatric population. Physical rehabilitation, such as exercise regimens and weight management projects, is crucial in re-establishing functional status to the joint as well as alleviating pain. Innovating modalities, including intra-articular injection of hyaluronic acid or corticosteroids, offer an alternative pain pathway for patients who are not responding sufficiently to conventional management. Of note, recent studies point out spa therapy, which combines physical rehabilitation with natural mineral treatment, as a comprehensive treatment of musculoskeletal pathologies like OA (Paoloni et al., 2017). This extensive treatment strategy emphasizes the necessity of individualized patient care in rheumatology. Increased research on OA is essential to improve treatment protocols further and enhance understanding of pathophysiology. With ongoing biomedical research unearthing new therapeutic targets and interventions, the fight against OA becomes increasingly sophisticated. New epidemiological findings suggest rising prevalence rates of OA on a global scale, most frequently reported in conjunction with lifestyle determinants of sedentary life and obesity, raising awareness for prevention. Further, the dynamic between OA and comorbidities, such as fibromyalgia, highlights the complex process of managing comorbid patients with identical symptoms. The synthesis of holistic treatment modalities addressing both physical and psychosocial domains is essential to enhance patient outcomes. With the progress in the field, the development of expert consensus statements, for example, as in rheumatotherapy, will continue to support EBP that aims to optimize care for those suffering from this prevalent disorder (Paoloni et al., 2017) (Figure 11.7).

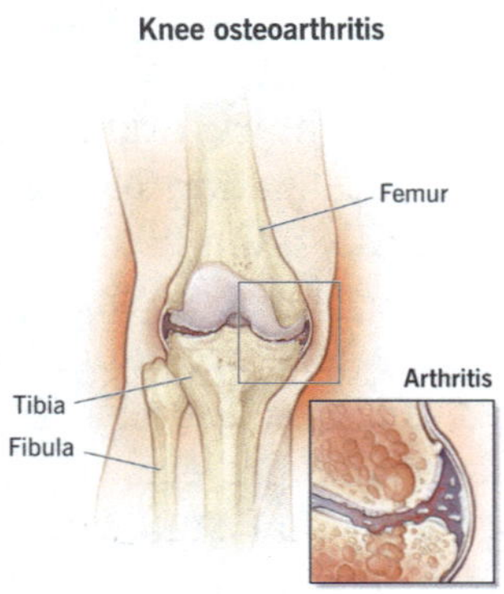

Figure 11.7. Knee osteoarthritis.

Source: https://my.clevelandclinic.org/-/scassets/images/org/health/articles/knee-osteoarthritis.

11.2.3. Lupus and Other Autoimmune Disorders

Autoimmune illnesses, like lupus, are a complex and heterogeneous group of conditions characterized by the immune system's faulty identification of the body's own tissues as foreign. This abnormal immune response can cause widespread inflammation and damage to numerous organ systems, including: the skin, the joints, the kidneys, and the CNS. Systemic lupus erythematosus (SLE) is the most common form of lupus and is classically observed with heterogeneous presentation, ranging from minimal manifestations to widespread organ involvement. The clinical presentation of SLE is variable, and it is challenging to diagnose and manage, necessitating a keen understanding of the disease to implement successful rheumatological treatment modalities. With the multisystem nature of lupus, clinicians must remain vigilant for signs of multisystem involvement, since in failing to recognize these subtleties, patients can suffer significant morbidity and diminished QoL. Recognition of the relationship between lupus and other autoimmune illnesses is significant for gaining insight into their pathophysiology and management strategies. Many autoimmune illnesses share standard mechanisms, such as genetic predisposition, environmental influences, and dysregulation of the immune system. For instance, systemic conditions like Sjögrens syndrome and RA are often associated with lupus, complicating patient presentation and therapeutic decision-making. The coexistence of these syndromes underscores the importance of an integrative approach to diagnosis, which may include serological and imaging investigations that are tailored to assess multisystem disease. Furthermore, vigilance for co-presenting symptoms—e.g., joint symptoms or fatigue—can allow for clinical decision-making and adapt treatment regimens, thereby improving outcomes in patients. Thus, the recognition of the interconnectedness of autoimmune illnesses is essential for both practitioners and patients to appreciate the multiplicity of such conditions. A significant but oftentimes neglected aspect of autoimmune illnesses like lupus is their potential impact on auditory and vestibular function, thereby underscoring the necessity for a multidisciplinary management. Research has determined that sensorineural hearing loss and vestibular dysfunction are possible in systemic autoimmune disorders due to the autoimmune process directed towards the inner ear. The auditory symptoms may present variably, and clinicians must differentiate primary inner ear conditions from secondary conditions such as lupus. Prompt treatment and diagnosis, such as with the administration of corticosteroids, can bring about significant improvement in symptoms, emphasizing the need for increased awareness among clinicians. Even though current case study literature is limited, identification of the need for the evaluation of auditory and vestibular function in lupus patients can encourage more effective, coordinated care approaches to mitigate the diverse consequences of autoimmune disease (Adelchi et al., 2018; Mok et al., 2014) (Figure 11.8).

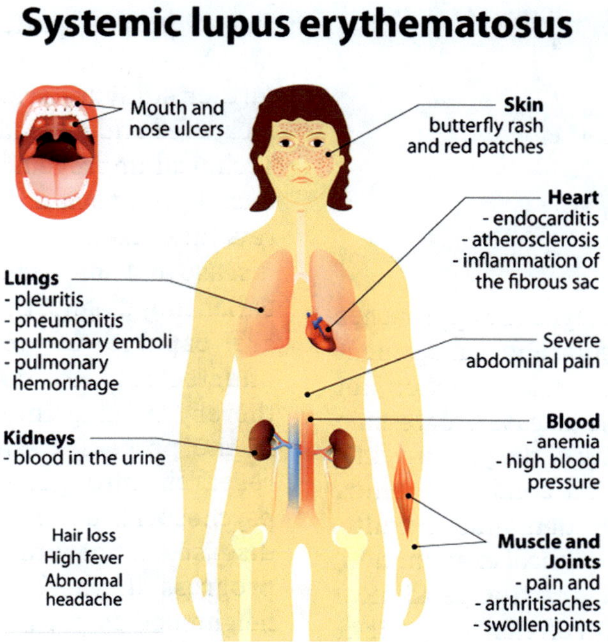

Figure 11.8. Systemic lupus erythematosus (SLE).

Source: https://medlineplus.gov/images/PX0000PC_PRESENTATION.jpeg.

Test Your Knowledge

1. What are the key pathological differences between rheumatoid arthritis and osteoarthritis?
2. How does the autoimmune process contribute to joint damage in rheumatoid arthritis?
3. What are the common risk factors and primary symptoms of osteoarthritis?

11.3. Diagnostic Approaches in Rheumatology

Learning Outcome

1. Discuss clinical evaluation and patient history in diagnosing and managing rheumatology and musculoskeletal disorders
2. Explain laboratory tests and imaging techniques for rheumatology and musculoskeletal disorders
3. Focus on the differential diagnosis of musculoskeletal disorders

In rheumatology, effective diagnostic approaches are central to the early detection and management of musculoskeletal disease. Early detection not only avoids the chance of the disease progressing but also enhances the quality of the patient's life. The type of rheumatological conditions tends to be complex, and hence demands a multi-modal technique including clinical examination, laboratory studies, and imaging studies. Clinical assessments, with comprehensive patient history and physical examination, can provide initial data regarding the pathogenesis of musculoskeletal pain. However, integration of serologic analysis of biomarkers, e.g., rheumatoid factor (RF) and anti-CCP antibodies, is crucial to establishing definitive diagnoses such as RA. Hence, the integration of these strategies is mandated in order to traverse the clinical landscape smoothly, patients receiving optimal and targeted interventions in the end. Moreover, rheumatological diagnostic strategies must have a biopsychosocial orientation, particularly for conditions that may be of either biological or psychosocial etiology. This is particularly applicable in the diagnosis and management of fibromyalgia, among other complicated syndromes. Through this broad outlook, clinicians can better understand the interplay between physiological symptomatology and psychological parameters, necessary for chronic pain and fatigue diseases. Whereas the pathophysiology of fibromyalgia is still not very well known, research shows that abnormal pain processing forms an integral component of the condition's diagnosis and treatment (CDC, 2017). As such, the utilization of psychosocial testing in conjunction with traditional diagnostic practice can lead to more effective treatment and improved patient outcomes. Moreover, the evolving nature of rheumatology calls for further study in terms of enhancing diagnostic measures and expanding treatment modalities. Technical improvements in diagnostic imaging techniques, such as MRI and ultrasound, have revolutionized visualization of inflammatory disease and soft tissue pathology within joints, enhancing diagnostic accuracy. The techniques are capable of detecting minor changes undetectable by conventional radiography, thereby making intervention possible earlier in the process. Besides these imaging tools, research into genetic, environmental, and psychosocial determinants of rheumatological diseases is of utmost urgency. Along with progress in the sector, there is sure to be heightened emphasis on designing personalized medicine approaches that tailor diagnostics and treatment strategies in line with individual patient profiles, as highlighted by ingenious interventions addressing both the biology and psychosocial elements of diseases (Burton et al., 2008; Glennon et al., 2019). This systemic diagnostic model aims not only to improve clinical results but also to optimize overall QoL in individuals afflicted with rheumatological diseases.

11.3.1. Clinical Evaluation and Patient History

Proper clinical evaluation and patient history constitute the foundation for the diagnosis and management of rheumatology and MSDs. Proper patient history is important in identifying how the symptoms started, how long they last, and what they are like, such as pain, stiffness, or impairment. Physician-patient communication is an essential factor since, through this, patients can open up and provide relevant information, and also build confidence in the physician-patient relationship. Factors like the patient's occupation, lifestyle, and previous medical history also play a significant role in the identification of the potential underlying conditions of their musculoskeletal condition. Their evaluation can be utilized to differentiate between some conditions, such as inflammatory arthritis or tendinopathy, and non-specific musculoskeletal complaints, thereby affecting the subsequent diagnostic process and treatment plan. The integration of a biopsychosocial evaluation in patient evaluation further aids in the management of MSDs. This model encompasses not only the biological aspects, such as pathology and physical symptoms, but also the psychosocial aspects, which are capable of having a strong influence on a patient's outcome. For instance, psychological status, social support, and job issues are all able to influence the severity of pain as well as the patient's ability to return to work. Evidence shows that an awareness of these psychosocial factors can result in more efficient treatment strategies since they are directly associated with musculoskeletal disorder outcomes (Burton et al., 2008). Health practitioners are therefore required to remain actively engaged in the biological and psychosocial domains during evaluations for the purposes of creating comprehensive and patient-tailored treatment regimens. EBTs play an essential part in embracing clinical practice to treat musculoskeletal pathologies. A current consensus study by experts has identified varied treatment modalities that may actually supplement traditional approaches, such as Spa therapy, to enhance patients with MSDs (Paoloni et al., 2017). A clear relationship between clinical evaluation and subsequent interventions is critical in ensuring that treatment modalities are in line with each patient's unique needs and circumstances. Following proper patient evaluation, starting multimodal treatment programs with physical therapy, psychological counseling, and occupational integration is essential in optimizing recovery and improving long-term outcomes. By the strict application of an interdisciplinary approach to clinical evaluation, health professionals can significantly improve the quality of care rendered to patients with rheumatologic and MSDs (Figure 11.9).

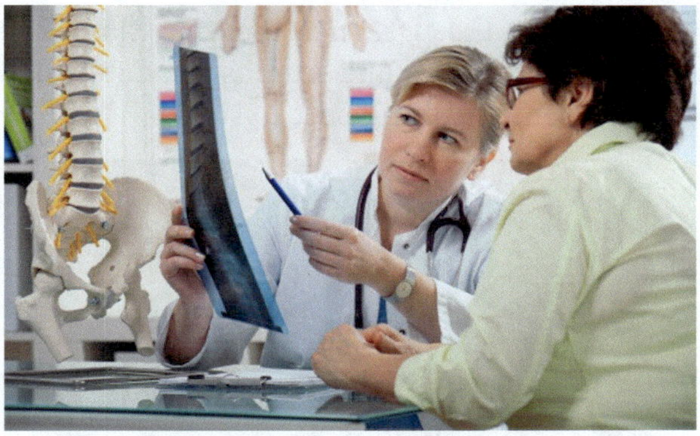

Figure 11.9. Rheumatologist evaluating patient history.

Source: https://healthtravelabroad.com/images/treatments/orthopedics.jpg.

11.3.2. Laboratory Tests and Imaging Techniques

In rheumatology and musculoskeletal diseases, laboratory tests and imaging modalities play a significant role in diagnosis and management. Such techniques not only allow clinicians to diagnose the underlying inflammatory condition but also evaluate the functional status of the musculoskeletal system. Routine laboratory tests, such as CBCs, erythrocyte sedimentation rates (ESRs), and serological tests like RF and anti-citrullinated protein antibodies (ACPA), provide very valuable information about the presence and severity of autoimmune conditions like RA. Besides, new biomarkers—such as anti-carbamylated protein antibodies (anti-CarP)—are currently being investigated for associations with cardiovascular involvement in RA patients, also demonstrating the shifting landscape of laboratory tests in this field (Alessandri et al., 2017). Imaging modalities complement laboratory testing by visualization of structural changes in joint and periarticular soft tissues. More sophisticated modalities, such as MRI and ultrasound, have enhanced the detection of missed early inflammatory arthritis on routine X-rays. MRI is particularly valuable for quantifying the integrity of articular cartilage and the presence of synovitis, while simultaneous ultrasound studies can determine the involvement of the soft tissues.

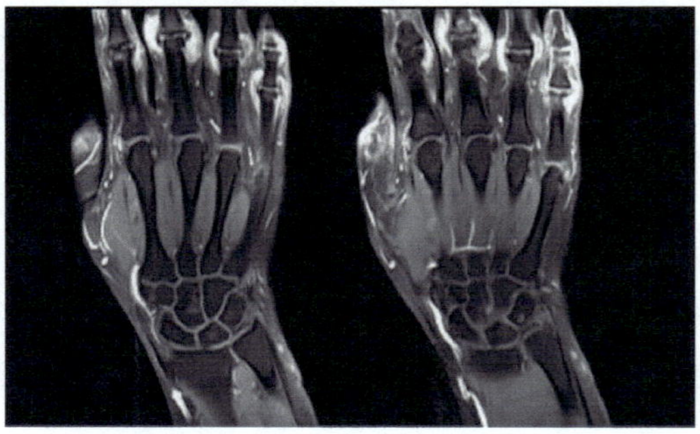

Figure 11.10. Magnetic resonance imaging-enhanced scanning: T1-weighted image contrast enhanced, showing thickened, fusiform, and not uniformly enhanced lesions, mimicking a "rheumatoid arthritis" appearance. Synovial hyperplasia or inflammation in small joints was also observed.

Source: https://www.researchgate.net/publication/321999892/figure/fig4/AS:669172514160654@1536554568503/Magnetic-resonance-imaging-enhanced-scanning-T1-weighted-image-contrast-enhanced-showing.png.

The application of these imaging modalities facilitates a more detailed evaluation of patients, allowing for early intervention that can prevent permanent joint damage. They also the monitoring of disease activity and response to treatment, with changes being made in management plans based on real-time data. Integration of imaging modalities and laboratory tests into clinical practice in rheumatology underscores the need for a multidisciplinary approach to the provision of care to patients. Notably, education programs, including online learning materials, have a pivotal role in imparting essential knowledge on such methods to medical professionals. Such sites provide an environment conducive to unstructured learning while upholding education standards offered by institutions such as EULAR, enabling practitioners to keep up with the current best practices in diagnosis and management (Armstrong et al., 2005). By bridging knowledge gaps and enhancing diagnostic competence, these programs ultimately translate into improved patient outcomes for rheumatology and MSDs (Figure 11.10).

11.3.3. Differential Diagnosis of Musculoskeletal Disorders

In rheumatology, differential diagnosis of musculoskeletal diseases is a critical component of the clinical service because it enables clinicians to identify the etiology of patients' symptoms. Because of the multifactorial nature of musculoskeletal diseases, it could be a task requiring a systematic approach, such as the coordination of clinical presentations, patients' history, and investigations. Adopting an infrastructure of effective treatment, this approach requires clinicians to differentiate between inflammatory, degenerative, metabolic, and infectious etiologies. For example, RA and OA are both diseases with many similarities in joint pain, but very different pathologies and management approaches beneath them. Making appropriate diagnoses is important because misclassification can lead to inappropriate management and negatively affect patient outcomes. The strength of such a differential diagnostic model is that it is used beyond reductionist symptom checklists, and it forces clinicians to gain an intimate knowledge of the disorders involved. Diagnostic decision support software (DDSS) is an exciting new development in enhanced diagnostic accuracy. It consists of large databases of clinical information used to aid in formulating differential diagnoses from presented patients. For instance, in a study employing SimulConsult®, significant reduction of diagnostic errors among clinicians was shown when they employed decision support within their examination process, improving the accuracy in diagnosing MSDs from 28% errors only to 15% with assistance (Athreya et al., 2016). The improvement underscores the capacity of technology to complement generalists, especially in fields such as pediatric rheumatology, where specialist availability is scarce. By enhancing clinical reasoning and providing pertinent clinical findings, DDSS can relieve specialists of part of their workload and improve patient care by enabling more precise diagnoses. Furthermore, accurate diagnosis of MSDs is particularly critical for the cases of chronic pain with connective tissue diseases (CTDs) such as SLE and SSc. Such patients are likely to experience musculoskeletal pain of varying kinds, including arthralgia and myalgia, which makes it difficult during diagnosis. Identifying the pain source in such cases is crucial to avoid over-treatment, especially when chronic widespread pain, like fibromyalgia, may be superimposed (Atzeni et al., 2015). Chronic pain not only physically disables a patient but can also have a detrimental effect on mental health and overall QoL. Accordingly, a subtle differential diagnosis taking into account the complex nature of pain in CTDs is required, not only because it affects treatment objectives but also because it impacts the overall management of these complicated patients within rheumatology (Figure 11.11).

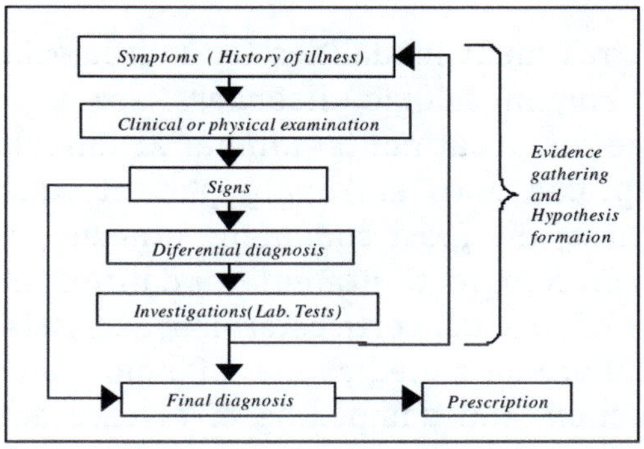

Figure 11.11. Summary of the differential diagnosis.

Source: https://www.researchgate.net/profile/Rainer-Unland/publication/221248709/figure/fig3/AS:340421285826568@1458174167211/Summary-of-the-differential-diagnosis.png.

Test Your Knowledge

1. Which laboratory tests are most commonly used to diagnose rheumatoid arthritis and how do their results guide clinical decisions?
2. What imaging modalities are preferred for detecting early joint damage in rheumatoid arthritis versus osteoarthritis?

11.4. Treatment Modalities

Learning Outcome

1. Understand pharmacological treatments in the management of rheumatological and musculoskeletal disorders
2. Discuss non-pharmacological interventions
3. Focus on emerging therapies and clinical trials

The treatment modalities for musculoskeletal and rheumatologic disorders are a broad range of treatments aimed at alleviating symptoms and improving patient function. Of these, the most commonly utilized are the pharmacologic treatment modalities in the form of NSAIDs, corticosteroids, and DMARDs, which are all aimed at the inflammation, pain reduction, and dampening of disease activity. Because the disorders are multifactorial in origin, medication may not be sufficient, however. Complementary therapy in the form of physical therapy, occupational therapy, and lifestyle modification plays significant roles in successful management strategies, stimulating greater mobility and a generally improved QoL. As medical understanding progresses, the demand for bespoke strategies that use individualized treatment plans aligned with patient profiles becomes increasingly evident, highlighting the value of the multidisciplinary approach to management. Non-pharmacological interventions are increasingly favored in the field of treatment modalities, particularly for conditions like fibromyalgia, a condition that occurs in approximately 2% of adults in the United States and consists predominantly of middle-aged women. The etiology of fibromyalgia, being multifactorial and including genetic predisposition and trauma, necessitates that treatment be addressed individually. As is borne out by recent studies, including those by the CDC, effective management can often include, in addition to drugs, psychological therapy, exercise intervention, and stress management alongside addressing the disorder itself. The negative impact of fibromyalgia on daily functioning makes it especially desirable to have comprehensive treatment approaches beyond symptom relief alone to improve the QoL overall (Glennon et al., 2019). This hybrid approach ensures that people's personal needs are being addressed, resulting in better results. One of the new therapy modalities is spa therapy, and it has been proven to help manage musculoskeletal pathologies. The agreement among medical experts indicates that spa therapy can be utilized as an effective adjunct to treatment, particularly with chronic diseases. Research conducted via a Delphi procedure involving clinicians from various clinical backgrounds has highlighted spa therapy's effectiveness in augmenting treatment efficacy for MSDs. Expert panel recommendations highlight the need to individualize the choice of treatment according to patient condition and preference (Paoloni et al., 2017). By integrating spa treatment into the regimen, medical professionals can provide patients with a therapeutic route toward symptom relief and rehabilitation, ultimately improving the overall efficacy of treatment protocols for rheumatologic disorders.

11.4.1. Pharmacological Treatments

Pharmacotherapy plays a crucial role in controlling musculoskeletal and rheumatological disorders, with pain relief and increased patient function. NSAIDs are typically the initial treatment of choice for conditions such as OA and RA, with pain reduction and reduction of inflammation. In combination with NSAIDs, DMARDs take a key position in the treatment of rheumatic inflammatory diseases as they help in suppressing the disease mechanisms, literally altering the disease course. An effective strategy can include employing a combination of drugs based on the patient's condition, considering comorbidities, previous response to treatment, and overall health status. Hence, precise pharmacologic management remains most important in QoL enhancement and the alleviation of the burden of chronic MSDs. In patients with fibromyalgia, nevertheless, drug treatment is very heterogeneous due to the complex nature of the disease. Medications such as selective serotonin reuptake inhibitors (SSRIs) and serotonin-norepinephrine reuptake inhibitors (SNRIs) have emerged as favorites for being efficacious treatments in the alleviation of widespread pain and sleep disturbance experienced with fibromyalgia. Furthermore, low doses of tricyclic antidepressants and anticonvulsants, such as gabapentin and pregabalin, are typically incorporated into treatment regimens to reverse neuropathic pain. Because fibromyalgia symptoms like fatigue and cognitive dysfunction are so complicated, interdisciplinary treatment with the addition of pharmacotherapy alongside lifestyle modification, physical therapy, and psychological counseling is traditionally recommended. This comprehensive treatment strategy acknowledges the need for more control over both the physical and psychological domains of the disorder, ultimately leading to better functional outcomes for patients. More recent developments in the pharmacological treatment of MSDs emphasize the need for individualized therapy, particularly concerning upcoming studies and advancements. Following specialist consensus, as outlined in studies investigating spa treatment, some pharmacological treatments must closely follow clinical advice, so that choice is both in relation to effectiveness and to the preference of the patient (Paoloni et al., 2017). This becomes particularly pertinent with the treatment of multifactorial conditions that require personalized interventions, such as where comorbidities involving rheumatologic disorders alongside fibromyalgia (Glennon et al., 2019) are involved. With novel therapeutic medicines becoming more accessible, ongoing clinical studies are important to establishing the safety and efficacy of such drugs. An adaptive pharmacological model, therefore, directed by newer evidence will be of greater utility to the evolving context of rheumatology and musculoskeletal disorder treatment, ultimately enhancing patient outcomes (Figure 11.12).

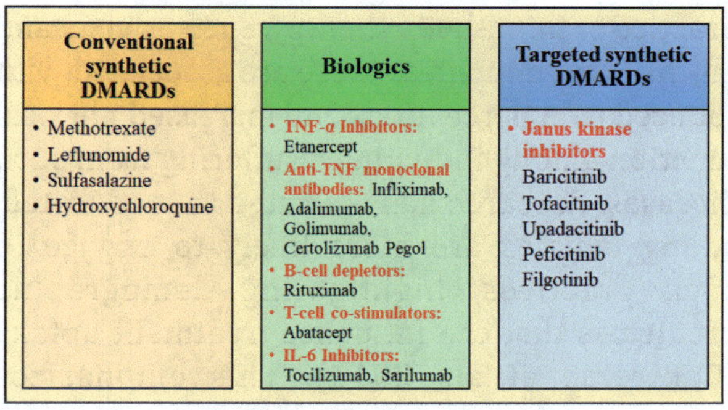

Figure 11.12. Classification of DMARDs used for the management of rheumatoid arthritis.

Source: https://www.mdpi.com/pharmaceuticals/pharmaceuticals-17-00248/article_deploy/html/images/pharmaceuticals-17-00248-g001.png.

11.4.2. Non-Pharmacological Interventions

Non-pharmacological treatments are of the highest significance in the management of rheumatological and MSDs to provide better QoL to patients without excessive drug dependence. These strategies comprise a multitude of therapeutic interventions, including physical therapy, exercise training, and integrative therapies like mindfulness and meditation. Of note, the combination of these treatments is highly effective in reducing symptoms, improving physical functioning, and improving mental health among patients with chronic pain disorders. Moreover, non-pharmacological interventions provide a holistic treatment intervention that is aligned with patients' values and lifestyle, which promotes greater involvement in their care plans. Recent evidence has also demonstrated the effectiveness of non-pharmacological treatment in the management of some conditions, like fibromyalgia, which is typified by chronic pain and fatigue. All together, these treatments—ranging from dietary management to mind-body approaches—reduce symptoms and promote general health. Notably, the increase in the practice of mind-body therapy, such as yoga and tai chi, is prominent, as these are associated with reduced pain perceptions and increased physical function among individuals suffering from such diseases. Research has indicated that educated, young females are more likely to engage in such practices, highlighting demographic predictors that can influence treatment uptake (Contreras et al., 2019). This emphasizes the need for tailoring interventions to meet diverse patient needs. Furthermore, emerging agreement among professionals regarding the appropriateness and effectiveness of alternative non-pharmacological treatments strengthens their place in clinical practice. Consensus built by a professional committee on the application of Spa therapy proves a healthy support base for such therapies, substantiating their use as treatment modalities for MSDs (Paoloni et al., 2017). This proves a general awareness among medical practitioners that non-medication avenues need to be incorporated in routine care paradigms, thereby enhancing the treatment outcomes among chronic musculoskeletal condition patients. Such an agreement not only reassures clinicians of their practice but also empowers patients with the skill to actively seek out and be involved in inclusive, multiform treatment methods.

11.4.3. Emerging Therapies and Clinical Trials

With continued progress in rheumatology, emerging treatments and results from clinical trials are starting to influence treatment patterns for MSDs. With an emphasis on SpA as an example, emerging evidence from studies indicates the importance of establishing treatment targets to maximize patient outcomes. Systematic review of the literature set down primary treatment goals, such as remission or low disease activity, which were achievable through shared decision-making between the patient and clinician. Due to insufficient evidence supporting these findings, recommendations were drafted by an expert panel in light of frequent monitoring of disease activity. These were designed to create an ordered approach towards the management of SpA, considering the complexity and heterogeneity of the disease, leading eventually to care best pathways for those suffering from such conditions (Baraliakos et al., 2013).

In addition to the development of treatment targets, the advent of biologic therapies towards the beginning of the 21st century is a pivotal turning point in RA and associated disease care. Biologics has revolutionized treatment options, yet they need to be accompanied by rigorous data collection so that their long-term efficacy and safety can be better appreciated. The establishment of national and international registries for biologics effectively achieves this purpose, as they pool information from diverse populations and treatment settings. Over 15 years ago, these registries have provided useful insights into the real-world efficacy of biologic therapies, bridging the gap between clinical trials and real clinical practice. All such detailed information would not only enhance the knowledge of biologics but also guide future treatment for MSDs (Finckh et al., 2017).

Registry data, coupled with new therapies, are required to provide appropriate treatment for complex rheumatologic diseases. All these advancements pave the way for continued research trials that explore novel therapeutic modalities, including new biologics and individualized targeted therapies for the patient at hand. As research develops, knowing the mechanisms underlying disease and the pharmacogenomics of these therapies will further define treatment protocols. The future results of these studies highlight the role of patient-directed strategies in rheumatology. By prioritizing patient involvement in treatment interventions and integrating evidence from emerging therapies, healthcare workers can optimize individuals with MSDs' well-being, resulting in better clinical response and overall well-being (Baraliakos et al., 2013; Finckh et al., 2017).

Test Your Knowledge

1. What are the main classes of pharmacological agents used in the management of rheumatoid arthritis, and how do they differ in mechanism of action?
2. How are biologic agents targeting specific immune pathways changing the treatment landscape for autoimmune rheumatic diseases?
3. What role do clinical trials play in advancing treatment options for rheumatologic disorders?

11.5. Role of Physical Therapy in Management

Learning Outcome

1. Understand the importance of rehabilitation
2. Describe techniques used in physical therapy
3. Discuss patient education and self-management strategies

The incorporation of physical therapy as part of the treatment of rheumatology and musculoskeletal conditions is an essential aspect of patient care. Physical therapists play a key role during the rehabilitation process by constructing personalized exercise programs that compensate for the limitations caused by diseases such as arthritis and chronic low back pain. These interventions aim to restore functioning, enhance mobility and pain reduction, and enhance the QoL of the patients ultimately. Personalized treatment is central to current approaches, which encourage early intervention with an emphasis on avoiding disability in the long run. As described in the literature, excellent physical therapy is of most significant benefit if initiated early after the onset of symptoms, and this assists in a patient's self-management skills considerably and reduces reliance on pharmacological management of pain (Souza et al., 2001). Physical therapy is also important in educating patients about their conditions and providing insight into the mechanics of their musculoskeletal issues. This educational component empowers patients by providing them with knowledge of pain control strategies and the importance of maintaining activity in the presence of pain. As attested to by the ongoing debate in the literature, engaging patients in their rehabilitation not only motivates adherence to exercise programs but also enhances their ability to adjust to chronic pain (Antal et al., 2008). The holistic approach taken by physical therapists, which incorporates both physical and psychosocial elements, demonstrates the importance placed on treating the complexity inherent in conditions like low back pain. Consistent with this, the role of physical therapy extends beyond physical rehabilitation to include a holistic model intended to optimize patient outcomes. Furthermore, the effectiveness of physical therapy in managing MSDs is established by the need for multidisciplinary interventions. Collaborative models of practice, involving physical therapists, rheumatologists, and other healthcare providers, offer an integrated treatment plan that addresses the physical and emotional aspects of pain. It is this interdisciplinary practice that is most crucial, particularly in the treatment of low back pain, which is often marked by psychosocial components that exacerbate the patient's condition. When clinicians recognize the limitations of monomodal therapy, they can better appreciate the need to integrate physical therapy into the overall management regimen. Consequently, future studies and clinical trials regarding the efficacy of diverse models of therapy have a lifelong endeavor in continuously refining the comprehension of how to optimize physical therapy, which consequently facilitates the reimagining of treatment paradigms (Souza et al., 2001). In sum, the active role of physical therapy enhances the care of rheumatology and musculoskeletal diseases, leading to patient-focused care and better health outcomes (Figure 11.13).

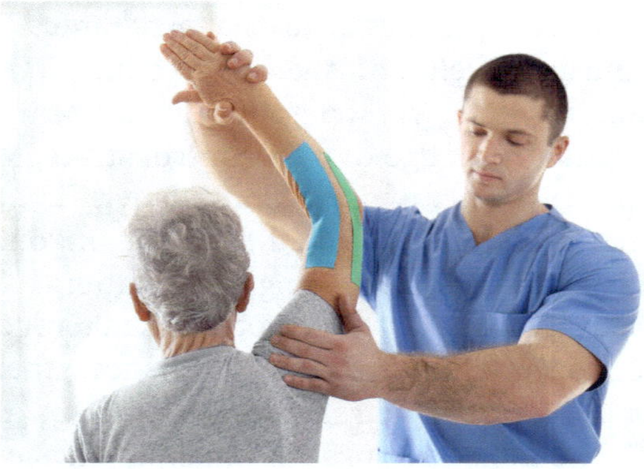

Figure 11.13. Physical therapy for rheumatoid arthritis.

Source: https://storage.googleapis.com/treatspace-prod-media/pracimg/u-2202/shutterstock_579092716.jpeg.

11.5.1. Importance of Rehabilitation

Rehabilitation is a key component in the management of patients with musculoskeletal and rheumatologic conditions, a structured process towards restoration of function and improved QoL. Despite the advancements in medical treatments, patients suffering from diseases like arthritis and ULDs will often end up with functional impairment that imposes a significant barrier to their usual activity. There is an overall rehabilitation process that includes several strategies, such as physical therapy, occupational therapy, and psychosocial support, which facilitate multi-dimensional recovery. The biopsychosocial model, especially, which incorporates biological, psychological, and social factors, focuses on addressing not just the physical but also the emotional and situational aspects present in the life of the patients. Engaging patients in rehabilitation not only enhances their physical functioning but also empowers them by fostering resilience and active participation in health management. Additionally, the efficiency of rehabilitation is further enhanced by the individualized modalities that consider the unique needs and status of each patient. Evidence-based management strategies demonstrate that multimodal interventions, where multiple treatment modalities are applied, have considerable occupational advantages. In a ULDs research study, it was found that neither biomedical treatment nor ergonomic methods are sufficient, but more so positive recovery hinges on a combined approach that can facilitate early return to work and active reintegration into the workforce. This emphasizes the importance of multidisciplinary collaboration among healthcare professionals, employers, and patients in ensuring rehabilitation occurs in an enabling work environment. By aligning treatment with the patient's professional and personal goals, rehabilitation is a central element to the process of improved health and functioning. Furthermore, rehabilitation measures such as Spa therapy have also proven to be beneficial adjuncts in the management of MSDs, as supported by clinical consensus statements. The addition of Spa therapy is not only beneficial physically but also ensures psychological health through holistic treatment. This is particularly the case in maintaining the effectiveness of rehabilitation since it can reverse pain and restore mobility, with psychosocial problems also addressed that can hinder rehabilitation. Therefore, tailored rehabilitation programs through various therapeutic modalities, like alternative therapies, are likely to produce the optimum outcome for patients who are resistant to rehabilitation from chronic diseases. Ultimately, successful rehabilitation strategies are vital not only to be symptom-free but to promote long-term health and functional autonomy of patients with musculoskeletal and rheumatologic diseases to enable them to enjoy their QoL (Figure 11.14).

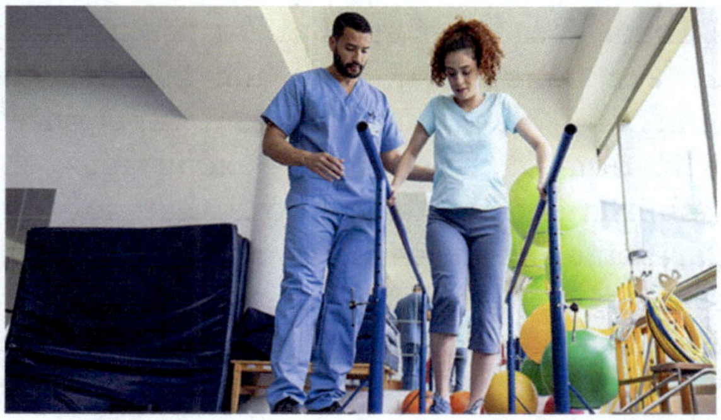

Figure 11.14. Musculoskeletal rehabilitation.

Source: https://www.hopkinsmedicine.org/-/media/images/health/2_-treatment/rehabilitative-therapy/msk-rehab-teaser.jpg.

11.5.2. Techniques Used in Physical Therapy

Several physical therapy techniques employed are of critical significance in the management and recovery of patients with rheumatologic and musculoskeletal disorders. One of these critical techniques is manual therapy, with hands-on methods designed to increase tissue mobility and reduce pain. Manual therapy also entails joint mobilization and manipulation, which can improve joint function and reduce inflammation. For patients with chronic diseases like fibromyalgia, which is widespread in approximately 2% of U.S. adults, manual therapy can offer considerable symptomatic relief through improved range of motion and reduced muscle tension. As such, these methods play a pivotal role in addressing the complex nature of chronic pain disorders and ensuring maximum overall function during daily activities, thereby enhancing the well-being of patients seeking relief from debilitating musculoskeletal pain (Glennon et al., 2019). Another key method applied in physical therapy to guarantee maximum management of rheumatological disorders is exercise therapy. Routine exercise plans can also alleviate stiffness, improve joint stability, and enhance cardiovascular health. Physical therapists prefer to customize exercise regimens to an individual patient's needs by incorporating strength training, flexibility exercises, and aerobic conditioning to create a balanced recovery program. This individually based exercise approach helps with physical as well as psychological aspects of chronic pain management. For example, incorporating aerobic exercises could promote acceptance of pain and better mental health, rendering patients stronger in terms of tolerating their conditions. Such beneficial effects highlight the significance of regular exercise, as it can increase physical functions and global health in patients suffering from long-term conditions such as RA (Acharya et al., 2014). In addition, recent physical therapy strategies have increasingly leveraged technology to maximize patient outcomes in musculoskeletal rehabilitation. Modalities such as ultrasound, electrical stimulation, and laser therapy are utilized along with standard physical therapy methods to promote healing and reduce inflammation. For example, electrical stimulation may be used to control pain by interrupting pain transmissions, allowing the patients to participate more actively in their own rehabilitation. Technology-assisted methods not only facilitate effective pain control but also support patient adherence to behavioral changes. By educating patients to use these modalities responsibly, along with an integrated pain management approach, therapists can significantly improve patients' self-management of their conditions. This synergy of new and old methods enables patients to enjoy holistic care tailored to their rheumatological concerns, overall leading to better health outcomes (Acharya et al., 2014; Glennon et al., 2019) (Figure 11.15).

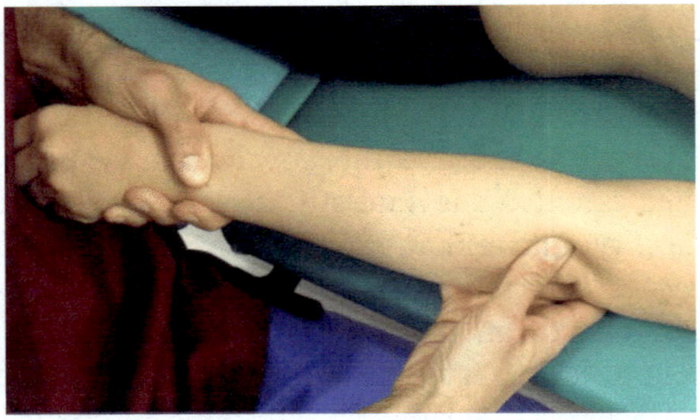

Figure 11.15. Elbow joint mobilization/manipulation.

Source: https://www.researchgate.net/publication/312411894/figure/fig4/AS:451446790463494@1484644710555/Elbow-joint-mobilization-manipulation.png.

11.5.3. Patient Education and Self-Management Strategies

An interdisciplinary patient education and self-management strategy is essential in the treatment of musculoskeletal and rheumatology disorders. Patient education, apart from enhancing patients' knowledge regarding the disease, enables patient empowerment to take an active role in their healthcare. Successful education involves communicating information about the nature of the disease, compliance with treatment, and the benefits of lifestyle modification. By delivering needs-based information, healthcare professionals can counteract feelings of uncertainty and anxiety among patients. In addition, an organized education program can promote a conducive environment where patients feel at ease inquiring and questioning. Consequently, better-informed patients are more likely to engage in self-management activities, leading to enhanced health outcomes, as seen in many examples in the context of rheumatology and musculoskeletal settings. In addition to basic education, self-management interventions must be a top priority to allow patients to manage their long-term conditions more effectively. Multimodal interventions are of value in furthering favorable occupational outcomes and reducing work loss attributable to ULDs, as seen in recent studies (Burton et al., 2008). Such interventions ought to incorporate components such as pain management strategies, physical conditioning, and ergonomic adjustments at the workplace. Furthermore, the application of the biopsychosocial model is essential because it emphasizes the harmony between biological factors and psychosocial elements in determining patient experiences. Utilization of this model encourages the establishment of interventions that not only address the physical character of pain but also the psychological barriers that may impede effective self-management. Enhancing self-management ability through skill-building sessions and peer support groups can further enable them to manage the complexity of their conditions on a day-to-day basis. Lastly, addressing behavioral and psychological factors is crucial when gearing up effective pain self-management interventions for individuals with chronic conditions, including those experiencing hemophilia-related joint pain. Research indicates that increased acceptance of pain can lead to improved QoL, and there is a need for interventions that promote such an attitude (Acharya et al., 2014). Pain management programs should help patients better understand their pain, differentiate between chronic and acute pain, and promote adherence to medications. By focusing on cognitive and affective aspects of pain, e.g., reducing negative thinking and increasing intrinsic motivation, patients can be instructed to manage pain more effectively. Not only does this integrated approach improve physical QoL, but it also enhances mental hardness, ultimately leading to a more unified and effective self-management regimen that benefits individuals with rheumatological and musculoskeletal diseases.

Test Your Knowledge

1. Why is physical therapy considered a critical component in the rehabilitation of patients with rheumatologic and musculoskeletal disorders?
2. What are some common physical therapy techniques used to improve joint function and reduce pain in patients with arthritis?
3. What role does patient education play in enhancing self-management and long-term outcomes in musculoskeletal disorders?

11.6. Challenges in Rheumatology

Learning Outcome

1. Focus on access to care challenges in rheumatology and musculoskeletal disorders
2. Discuss the management of chronic pain
3. Understand the psychological impact of rheumatological disorders

Rheumatology, as a specialist medical branch, is faced with numerous challenges emanating from the complex nature of MSDs. The first great challenge is making diagnoses that often present with overlapping symptoms and differential presentations. This is made even more complicated by the need for detailed patient evaluations beyond mere physical examinations. A good diagnosis must take into consideration one's clinical history, family history, and psychosocial concerns. There is evidence to suggest that intervention for these multifactorial factors, for instance, a biopsychosocial model, can provide improved management for patients with a spectrum of rheumatic diseases, such as those affecting the upper limbs. Unraveling the complexities behind diagnosis is essential to ensuring that treatment plans are in place and started early and effectively, reducing the burden of disease on healthcare systems and patients (Burton et al., 2008). Apart from diagnostic difficulties, the care for chronic diseases in rheumatology is highly complicated, particularly in terms of patient participation and therapeutic adherence. Many patients with conditions such as ankylosing spondylitis experience fatigue, which can have adverse effects on their QoL and complicate self-management. Participants have recognized that subjective feelings of physical exhaustion and emotional upset directly influenced their participation in therapies (Calin et al., 2013). Emotional and psychological factors are likely to lead to non-adherence or resistance to treatment when treatments include drug-based methods with side effects. This highlights the importance of standardized management regimens that focus on patient education and incorporate non-pharmacological strategies, such as psychological treatments and lifestyle modifications, to improve compliance and overall patient outcomes within rheumatology. Furthermore, the systemic problems in rheumatology include the collaboration and communication among healthcare professionals and patients. Effective management of MSDs requires a multidisciplinary approach, with interagency coordination among rheumatologists, physical therapists, and mental health experts. Communication failures and the lack of coordinated interventions can, however, hinder the creation of effective treatment plans. For instance, evidence indicates that multimodal interventions, including behavioral and ergonomic solutions, can have a profound impact on the occupational outcome of upper limb disorder patients (Burton et al., 2008). Subsequently, developing interdependent environments where all stakeholders—patients, providers, and employers—are involved is crucial in overcoming the inherent obstacles of rheumatology. Utilizing strategies aimed at improving the care team members' communication and coordination can help in better managing chronic illness, as well as in improving the quality of patient care.

11.6.1. Access to Care and Healthcare Disparities

Access to care in rheumatology and musculoskeletal disease is heavily influenced by several factors that create health disparities. Economic status, geographic location, and race all play significant roles in determining a person's ability to obtain adequate and timely care. Patients in urban areas will likely have more convenient access to specialist healthcare, whereas patients in rural areas generally face challenges such as fewer rheumatologists and limited transportation access. These disparities can lead to delayed treatment and diagnosis, exacerbating the progression of MSDs and decreasing the QoL for sufferers of such diseases. Financial constraints might also bar the necessary access to resources, like medicine or rehabilitation, thus putting additional strain on already ailing persons. This systemic disparity in healthcare access underscores the strong rationale for special initiatives aimed at reducing barriers and promoting equity in this rheumatology specialty. Furthermore, healthcare disparity in rheumatology is not solely the result of the logistical obstacles but also reflecting broader systemic determinants such as policy and insurance coverage. Variation in health insurance plans has a significant influence on the availability of rheumatological services, with the majority of patients depending on private coverage that routinely excludes certain therapies or requires them to pay substantial out-of-pocket costs. Medicaid or no insurance patients might have even more restrictive restrictions, with limited access to appropriate services and specialist referrals. Consequently, such imbalances can lead to poorer health, with the patients opting for delayed appointments or, in some cases, forgoing the treatments altogether due to expenses. To remediate these systemic inequities, a comprehensive effort has to be made that constitutes healthcare policy reform, increased financing of musculoskeletal disorder research, and enhanced education of physicians on the needs of special underprivileged populations, as described by evidence of the extent of research and investment required to eradicate these issues (Desjardins et al., 2009; Callahan et al., 2014). In addition to addressing systemic obstacles, raising awareness and providing education among healthcare providers are also critical in reducing healthcare disparities in rheumatology. Educating clinicians regarding the diverse requirements of patient populations can enhance their identification of signs of disparities and their response appropriately in the process of providing care. For instance, training programs for physicians to understand cultural competence and social determinants of health can bridge the knowledge gap and improve patient interaction. Moreover, outreach programs to underrepresented populations can foster early diagnosis and treatment, providing patients with knowledge of the condition and resources. By assisting healthcare providers to deliver more equitable care, disparities can be minimized and general health outcomes in rheumatology and MSDs can be enhanced. In the long term, what is required is cooperation between providers, policymakers, and communities to reorganize access to care and develop a more inclusive healthcare system that meets the needs of all patients.

11.6.2. Management of Chronic Pain

The treatment of chronic pain, particularly in musculoskeletal conditions and rheumatology, is a complex process that needs multiple facets. The traditional biomedical models prioritize physical pathology at the expense of the broader psychosocial determinants of pain perception and experience. The new evidence refers to multimodal intervention programs that are not only pharmacological in character but also incorporate psychological support and physical rehabilitation. Through the biopsychosocial approach, clinicians can more appropriately deal with the array of factors leading to chronic pain, with overall standards of care. Their application supports the need for integration among healthcare providers, patients, and employers, to create an integrated management plan that is aware of patients' individual situations and needs (Burton et al., 2008). In CTDs such as SLE and SSc, chronic pain is frequently an intense and incapacitating symptom. The frequency of varied pain syndromes, including arthralgia, myalgia, and fibromyalgia, underlines the importance of thorough assessment of pain etiology to direct appropriate treatment modalities. CTD pain not only handicaps the physical function of the patient but also influences mental health and social functioning similarly. Therefore, knowledge of the multifactorial pain is most important to avoid the over-treatment trap caused by concentrating on a single factor of the pain experience. Optimal management of pain according to patient profiles takes on considerable significance in improving health outcomes and QoL (Atzeni et al., 2015). To optimize the management of chronic pain within musculoskeletal and rheumatological contexts, an excellent acquaintance with best practices is essential. Healthcare providers need to educate themselves about recent research in the area of the efficacy of multidimensional intervention methods that can include physical therapy, cognitive-behavioral therapy, and medication, such as analgesics and anti-inflammatory medications. Furthermore, transitional work schedules may also facilitate a patient's return to work, hence restoring normalcy and functional independence. As more research emerges to find the answers to pain management, an engaged and informed approach will assist healthcare providers in designing integrative plans of care that treat both physical and emotional well-being (Burton et al., 2008) (Figure 11.16).

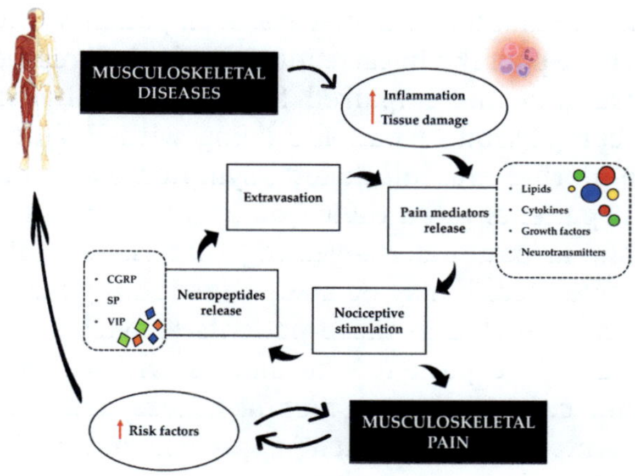

Figure 11.16. Musculoskeletal pain cycle.

Source: https://www.researchgate.net/publication/360436769/figure/fig3/AS:11431281210649773@1702064826275/Musculoskeletal-pain-cycle-Some-musculoskeletal-disorders-are-characterised-by-an.tif.

11.6.3. Psychological Impact of Rheumatological Disorders

The psychological impacts of rheumatological illness are beyond the concrete symptoms the patients manifest, significantly affecting mental health and global QoL. RA and fibromyalgia, for example, are usually accompanied by chronic pain and fatigue, which can lead to elevated rates of depression and anxiety. Because the patients undergo continuous discomfort, they can be restricted from fulfilling daily activities and social interaction. Literature finds that psychological distress in sufferers of MSDs is widespread, suggesting an interactive dynamic between mental and physical well-being. Furthermore, the impact of the disorders on QoL is wide-ranging, in the sense that patients will typically feel helpless and isolated and, as a consequence, experience more emotional distress (Davies et al., 2019). Also, evidence is presented that suggests mental health as a disease determinant in highlighting the relationship between psychological well-being and rheumatological disease. Such patients tend to have poorer clinical features, such as increased disability and impaired functional ability. In a comparison of patients living with HIV and co-morbid musculoskeletal symptomology, the UK patients rated their QoL as lower than the Zambia patients, suggesting that issues with mental health may be a key contributing factor to overall QoL in these patients (Davies et al., 2019). The patient who suffers with chronic pain combined with mental illness demands an integrative treatment approach that caters to the physical as well as the psychological requirements for optimal patient outcome. Integrated care is even more warranted in the management of Ehlers-Danlos Syndrome (HEDS), where the psychological implications are intertwined with rheumatological problems. Long-term evaluations have shown that HEDS patients have a higher prevalence of rheumatological comorbidities, and these can lead to further complications if they are not treated. This connection between excessive medical workups and identification of major rheumatological diseases emphasizes the necessity for extensive evaluation. Untreated rheumatological diseases often lead to increased symptoms and decline in physical function, which can later evolve into chronic pain and disability. Thus, healthcare providers must prioritize mental health screening and supportive interventions in rheumatological care to foster a holistic approach to patient health.

Test Your Knowledge

1. What are the main barriers to accessing rheumatologic care, and how do healthcare disparities affect patient outcomes?
2. Why is chronic pain management particularly challenging in patients with rheumatologic disorders?
3. How can integrating mental health support improve the overall management and quality of life for patients with chronic rheumatologic conditions?

SUMMARY

Rheumatology and musculoskeletal disease management, specifically for OA and RA, detects significant gaps in current practice among GPs. Even though the majority of GPs acknowledge the merit of OA monitoring, the execution of organized review processes is astonishingly low. This gap suggests that poor care is not attributed to a lack of information but is more the consequence of systemic barriers that must be addressed holistically. A majority of the practitioners choose to monitor physical function and pain, aligning their practices with the existing guidelines. Failing a unified effort to provide standardized monitoring, second-class patient care will inevitably persist, necessitating reforms in the way GPs manage OA (Bishop et al., 2013). Similarly, international management of RA suggests an overwhelming necessity for standard practices when managing the comorbidities of the disease. Studies reveal high prevalence of comorbidities in RA patients with significant variations in treatment across nations. High prevalences of comorbidities such as depression, CVD, and hyperlipidemia are reported, which means that RA patients may require more intensive healthcare than they receive. Compliance inconsistency with guidelines not only affects patient outcome but also reflects ignorance regarding the interrelated nature of such diseases. Having a systematic treatment and assessment of comorbidities can enhance patient care and slow down the progression of both RA and accompanying health conditions (Abdelwahab et al., 2013). Based on these findings, it is clear that a paradigm shift to optimize care for rheumatology and musculoskeletal disease patients is needed. The implications are not only on individual clinicians but on healthcare systems overall, requiring an integrated and proactive system of patient monitoring and education. By placing greater focus on systematic evaluations and enhancing treatment plan adherence, healthcare professionals can mitigate the adverse effects of undiagnosed comorbidities. With the evolving healthcare landscape, it is imperative that healthcare systems invest in continuous education and set guidelines of best practice, ultimately aiming at improved quality of care and improved patient outcomes for patients who are afflicted by these chronic diseases (Abdelwahab et al., 2013; Bishop et al., 2013).

Rheumatology and MSDs are treated with an all-encompassing understanding of varying factors, including biological, psychological, and social factors. Current literature emphasizes the importance of employing a biopsychosocial approach in treating ULDs. From this point of view, it is understood that even as biological interventions are essential, psychosocial factors play an important role in occupational performance and overall well-being. Evidence shows that neither solely biomedical remedies nor ergonomic interventions in isolation are sufficient; instead, multimodal formats involving multiple treatment channels must be used to achieve optimal results. For successful management to be maintained, employers and workers alike must be engaged, fostering collaboration that can maximize recovery as well as facilitate functional capacity in the work environment (Burton et al., 2008). Fibromyalgia is yet another significant field under rheumatology and MSDs, characterized by diffuse pain and co-morbid issues such as fatigue and cognitive issues. It occurs in approximately 2% of American adults, most being middle-aged women, and thus understanding the complex nature of this disease is essential in a bid to treat it efficiently. The etiology of fibromyalgia has been linked to genetic factors, infections, and trauma, although its exact cause remains elusive. Treatments vary significantly, ranging from pharmacological to stress management and exercise therapy. With ongoing studies, there is a growing development of more effective diagnostic procedures to better identify and target treatments for patients with fibromyalgia. Its impact on daily functioning underlines the need for integrative treatment strategies (Glennon et al., 2019). Multimodal interventions and differential diagnosis knowledge are crucial in the proper management of rheumatological and MSDs. Early return to work or maintenance at work is a valuable outcome that multidisciplinary teams of health professionals, employers, and employees can make feasible through the evidence. Emphasizing workplace accommodation, psychosocial support, and active rehabilitation can lead to improved patient outcomes during ULDs. Moreover, encouraging a culture shift in the perception of complaints of the upper limb and its relation to work allows for the dissemination of EBP. By putting forward a positive climate and incorporating evidence from current studies, health professionals can make interventions not only to treat symptoms but also to impact overall QoL and workplace productivity (Burton et al., 2008).

KEY TERMS FROM THIS CHAPTER

- Angiogenesis
- Biopsychosocial treatment
- Co-morbid conditions
- Disease progression
- Genetic predisposition
- Human skeleton
- Immune system
- Inflammatory myopathies
- Interdisciplinary patient education
- Autoimmune diseases
- Chronic back pain (CBP)
- Diagnostic decision support software (DDSS)
- Fibromyalgia
- Healthcare workers
- Immune checkpoint inhibitors
- Infectious etiologies
- Inflammatory process
- Internal organs

CRITICAL THINKING QUESTIONS

1. **Which of the following is the most common inflammatory arthritis affecting small joints of the hands?**
   a. Osteoarthritis
   b. Rheumatoid arthritis
   c. Gout
   d. Ankylosing spondylitis
2. **Which laboratory test is most specific for diagnosing rheumatoid arthritis?**
   a. Rheumatoid factor (RF)
   b. Erythrocyte sedimentation rate (ESR)
   c. Anti-cyclic citrullinated peptide (Anti-CCP) antibody
   d. C-reactive protein (CRP)
3. **What is the first-line treatment for acute gout attacks?**
   a. Methotrexate
   b. Nonsteroidal anti-inflammatory drugs (NSAIDs)
   c. Corticosteroids
   d. Colchicine
4. **Physical therapy in rheumatoid arthritis primarily aims to:**
   a. Cure the disease
   b. Replace medication therapy
   c. Increase inflammation for healing
   d. Improve joint function and reduce pain
5. **In osteoarthritis management, physical therapy interventions mainly focus on:**
   a. Increasing joint inflammation
   b. Immobilizing the joint permanently
   c. Surgical replacement of joints
   d. Strengthening muscles around affected joints

Short Answer Questions

1. What are the clinical features that distinguish inflammatory rheumatologic disorders, such as rheumatoid arthritis, from degenerative conditions like osteoarthritis?
2. Outline the stepwise diagnostic approach used in rheumatology, including clinical evaluation, laboratory tests, and imaging techniques.
3. Compare and contrast the pharmacological and non-pharmacological treatment modalities commonly used in managing rheumatoid arthritis.
4. How does physical therapy contribute to improving function and reducing disability in patients with musculoskeletal disorders?
5. Identify three common challenges faced by healthcare providers in managing patients with chronic rheumatologic diseases.
6. Explain the importance of patient history and clinical examination in differentiating between various musculoskeletal disorders.
7. Discuss emerging therapies in rheumatology and the role of clinical trials in advancing treatment options.

Answers to Critical Thinking Questions

1. (b); 2. (c); 3. (b); 4. (d); 5. (d)

REFERENCES

1. Dougados, M., Soubrier, M., Antunez, A., Balint, P., Balsa, A., Buch, M. H., Casado, G., Detert, J., El-Zorkany, B., Emery, P., Hajjaj-Hassouni, N., Harigai, M., Luo, S., Kurucz, R., Maciel, G., Mola, E. M., Montecucco, C. M., McInnes, I., Radner, H., . . . Kay, J. (2013). Prevalence of comorbidities in rheumatoid arthritis and evaluation of their monitoring: results of an international, cross-sectional study (COMORA). *Annals of the Rheumatic Diseases*, *73*(1), 62–68. https://doi.org/10.1136/annrheumdis-2013-204223Acharya, A., Barlow, J., Barry, M., Buhrman, B., Buzzard, M., Cour, K., Eckman, E., et al. (2014). A review of evidence about behavioral and psychological aspects of chronic joint pain among people with hemophilia. https://core.ac.uk/download/46171148.pdf (accessed on 27th June 2025).
2. Adam, C. (2012). Endogenous musculoskeletal tissue engineering–a focused perspective. https://core.ac.uk/download/10908942.pdf (accessed on 27th June 2025).
3. Agoritsas, T., Ahmadi, S., Arthritis Research UK, et al. (2017). The contribution of musculoskeletal disorders in multimorbidity: Implications for practice and policy. https://core.ac.uk/download/157858595.pdf (accessed on 27th June 2025).
4. Alessandri, C., Ciciarello, F. L., Colasanti, T., Conti, F., et al. (2017). Association between antibodies to carbamylated proteins and subclinical atherosclerosis in rheumatoid arthritis patients. https://core.ac.uk/download/98347599.pdf (accessed on 27th June 2025).
5. Antal, A., Antal, A., Delitto, A., Keller, A., Moore, A., Pascual-Leone, A., Radebold, A., et al. (2008). Chronic non-specific low back pain–sub-groups or a single mechanism? https://core.ac.uk/download/335445.pdf (accessed on 27th June 2025).
6. Armstrong, R., Hall, W., Maier, P., Ng, M., et al. (2005). Joint Zone: Users' view of an adaptive online learning resource for rheumatology.
7. Athreya, B., Newgard, C. D., Correll, C. K., Deal, C. L., Zurakowski, D., Vittinghoff, E., Ang, E. Y. N., et al. (2016). Evidence-based decision support for pediatric rheumatology reduces diagnostic errors. https://core.ac.uk/download/83049477.pdf (accessed on 27th June 2025).
8. Atzeni, F., Bazzichi, L., Casale, R., Di Franco, M., et al. (2015). Pain in systemic connective tissue diseases. https://core.ac.uk/download/54524187.pdf (accessed on 27th June 2025).
9. Banning, M. (2008). Topical diclofenac: Clinical effectiveness and current uses in osteoarthritis of the knee and soft tissue injuries. https://core.ac.uk/download/335727.pdf (accessed on 27th June 2025).
10. Baraliakos, X., Betteridge, N., Braun, J., Burgos-Vargas, R., et al. (2013). Treating spondylarthritis, including ankylosing spondylitis and psoriatic arthritis, to target: Recommendations of an international task force. https://core.ac.uk/download/55764870.pdf (accessed on 27th June 2025).
11. Bishop, A., Clarson, L. E., Daniel, R., Edwards, J. J., et al. (2013). Monitoring osteoarthritis: A cross-sectional survey in general practice. https://core.ac.uk/download/16460378.pdf (accessed on 27th June 2025).
12. Brown, L., Bywood, P. T., & Raven, M. (2014). Allied health integration: Collaborative care for arthritis and other musculoskeletal conditions. https://core.ac.uk/download/43335674.pdf (accessed on 27th June 2025).

13. Burnham, J. M., & von Scheven, E. (2011). Vitamin D supplementation in the pediatric rheumatology clinic. https://core.ac.uk/download/323072035.pdf (accessed on 27th June 2025).

14. Burton, A. K., Abasolo, L., Alizadehkhaiyat, O., Pearce, B. G., Baldwin, M., Beaton, D., Bonde, J. P., et al. (2008). Management of work-relevant upper limb disorders: A review. https://core.ac.uk/download/1649687.pdf (accessed on 27th June 2025).

15. Calin, A., van Tubergen, A., Belza, B., Cote-Arsenault, D., Dernis-Labous, E., Irvine, E., Dagfinrud, H., et al. (2013). Patient perspectives of managing fatigue in ankylosing spondylitis, and views on potential interventions: A qualitative study. https://core.ac.uk/download/16460591.pdf (accessed on 27th June 2025).

16. Callahan, L. F., Martin, K. R., Mingo, C. A., Schoster, B., et al. (2014). Individual and community socioeconomic status: Impact on mental health in individuals with arthritis. https://core.ac.uk/download/29150971.pdf (accessed on 27th June 2025).

17. Chapman, J., Dalbeth, N., Gow, P., Rome, K., et al. (2010). Podiatry services for patients with arthritis: An unmet need. https://core.ac.uk/download/1662153.pdf (accessed on 27th June 2025).

18. Chou, R. C., Dinulos, M. B. P., Gui, J., Rodgers, R., et al. (2017). Ehlers-Danlos syndrome hypermobility type is associated with rheumatic diseases. https://core.ac.uk/download/231133896.pdf (accessed on 27th June 2025).

19. Contreras, J. (2019). Utilization of mind-body practices for adults with fibromyalgia: 2017 National Health Interview Survey. https://core.ac.uk/download/231832574.pdf (accessed on 27th June 2025).

20. Croce, A., D'Aguanno, V., De Vincentiis, M., De Virgilio, A., et al. (2018). Audio-vestibular symptoms in systemic autoimmune diseases. https://core.ac.uk/download/188823057.pdf (accessed on 27th June 2025).

21. Dalakas, M. (2018). Neurological complications of immune checkpoint inhibitors: What happens when you 'take the brakes off' the immune system. https://core.ac.uk/download/213444184.pdf (accessed on 27th June 2025).

22. Davies, K. A., Martin, K., Ngalamika, O., Van de Ven, C., et al. (2019). Impact of musculoskeletal symptoms on physical functioning and quality of life among treated people with HIV in high and low resource settings: A case study of the UK and Zambia. https://core.ac.uk/download/201001131.pdf (accessed on 27th June 2025).

23. De Souza, L. H., & Frank, A. O. (2001). Conservative management of low back pain. https://core.ac.uk/download/333411.pdf (accessed on 27th June 2025).

24. De Souza, L. H., Frank, A. O., & Frank, C. A. (2004). Neck pain and disability: A cross-sectional survey of the demographic and clinical characteristics of neck pain seen in a rheumatology clinic. https://core.ac.uk/download/333427.pdf (accessed on 27th June 2025).

25. Desjardins, C., Ehrenberg, R. G., & St. Clair, E. W. (2009). The scope and scale of clinical research accomplished by rheumatologists early in their careers. https://core.ac.uk/download/5131729.pdf (accessed on 27th June 2025).

26. Finckh, A., Strangfeld, A., Zink, A., Gabay, C., et al. (2017). Biologics registers in RA: Methodological aspects, current role and future applications. https://core.ac.uk/download/83942043.pdf (accessed on 27th June 2025).

27. Gerhardt, A. (2013). Non-specific chronic musculoskeletal pain: Prevalence, spatial extent of pain, mental comorbidities, and psychophysiological patterns. https://core.ac.uk/download/32584109.pdf (accessed on 27th June 2025).

28. Glennon, M. K. (2019). Today's fibromyalgia. https://core.ac.uk/download/286697650.pdf (accessed on 27th June 2025).

29. Hoppmann, R., Mladenovic, J., Melniker, L. A., Badea, R., Blaivas, M., Montórfano, M., Abuhamad, A., et al. (2022). International consensus conference recommendations on ultrasound education for undergraduate medical students. *The Ultrasound Journal, 14*. https://doi.org/10.1186/s13089-022-00279-1 (accessed on 27th June 2025).

30. Krapac, L., & Badel, T. (2010). Paramecia temporomandibular globe–reumatološki I fizijatrijski Printup. https://core.ac.uk/download/14422628.pdf (accessed on 27th June 2025).

31. LeBoff, M. S., Greenspan, S. L., Insogna, K., Lewiecki, E. M., Saag, K. G., Singer, A., & Siris, E. S. (2022). The clinician's guide to prevention and treatment of osteoporosis. *Osteoporosis International, 33*, 2049–2102. https://doi.org/10.1007/s00198-021-05900-y (accessed on 27th June 2025).

32. Mok, T. M. Y. (2014). Immunosuppressants in systemic lupus erythematosus–treatment options and potential toxicity. https://core.ac.uk/download/38055590.pdf (accessed on 27th June 2025).

33. Paoloni, M., Bernetti, A., Brignoli, O., Coclite, A., et al. (2017). Appropriateness and efficacy of spa therapy for musculoskeletal disorders: A Delphi method consensus initiative among experts in Italy. https://core.ac.uk/download/84928671.pdf (accessed on 27th June 2025).

34. Tenforde, A. S., Borgstrom, H., DeLuca, S., McCormack, M., Singh, M., Soo Hoo, J., & Yun, P. H. (2022). Best practices for extracorporeal shockwave therapy in musculoskeletal medicine: Clinical application and training consideration. *PM&R, 14*, 611–619. https://doi.org/10.1002/pmrj.12790 (accessed on 27th June 2025).

NEUROLOGY: COMMON NEUROLOGICAL DISORDERS, DIAGNOSTIC TECHNIQUES, AND TREATMENT APPROACHES

12

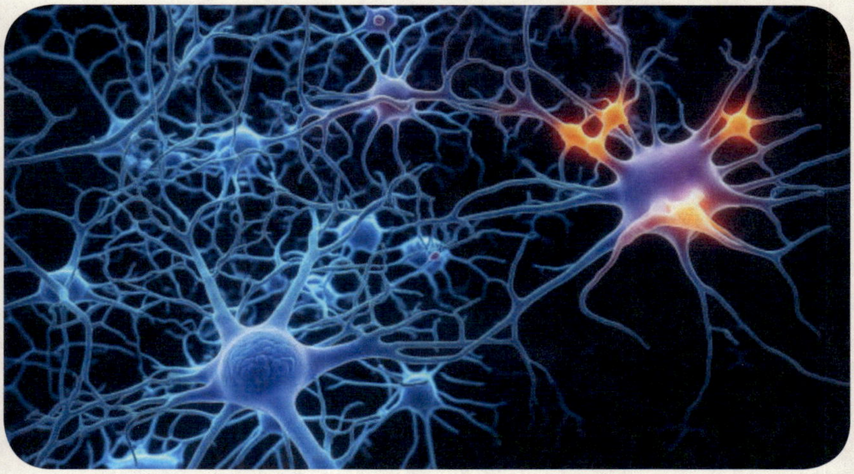

LEARNING OBJECTIVES

After studying this chapter, you will be able to:

1. Explain the structure of the nervous system
2. Describe common neurological disorders
3. Discuss diagnostic techniques in neurology
4. Understand treatment approaches in neurology
5. Define the role of neurology in mental health
6. Focus on advances in neurological research

Introduction

Neurology is the study and treatment of nervous system diseases, a complex system of the brain, spinal cord, and peripheral nerves. Not only does this branch study the structure and function of these systems, but it also studies various neurological diseases, such as epilepsy, Alzheimer's disease, and MS. Neurological knowledge is significant to the understanding of the impact of these conditions on daily function, patient QoL, and overall health outcomes. The concept of QoL, for instance, can be particularly challenging in patients with traumatic brain injury (TBI), as highlighted by research that depicts the need for specific testing tools like the QOLIBRI. These tools are necessary for measuring the effectiveness of treatment and interventions administered to patients with neurological impairment, thereby giving insight into their subjective well-being and recovery accomplishment components (Sae-Sia et al., 2013). Neurology not only includes diagnosing and treating neurological disorders but also conducting essential research focused on building knowledge in the field. A good example is Guillain-Barré syndrome (GBS), an acute condition where there is a rapid onset of paralysis and weakness. The ongoing International GBS Outcome Study (IGOS) is a landmark study to identify the clinical and biological determinants that affect the variability in GBS presentations. This multicenter study collects vast amounts of data from a diverse population of participants with a view to gaining insights into effective treatment protocols and ultimately improving patient outcomes. This kind of research highlights the importance of integrated care in neurology, where evidence-based data are key to developing new treatment protocols and comprehensive management programs aimed at focusing on individualized care for diverse populations with neurological conditions (Bateman et al., 2017). In addition, convergence of advancements in molecular biology and neuroimaging technologies continues to revolutionize neurology. Technologies such as fMRI and advanced electrophysiological methods enable unprecedented examination of brain function and disease. Such technologies, in addition to assisting with the diagnosis of several neurological disorders, also would allow researchers to follow disease progression and treatment response more accurately. With ever-evolving neurology, the connection between clinical practice and scientific research increasingly comes to light, and the need for neurologists to keep abreast of new technologies and findings rises to the top. Ultimately, the future of neurology relies on adapting to new findings so that providers can provide EBP to enhance the QoL in patients with neurological disorders.

Definition and Scope of Neurology

Neurology is a specialty branch of medicine dealing with the diagnosis and treatment of nervous system disease, including the brain, spinal cord, and peripheral nerves. It brings together anatomy, physiology, and pathology information to discuss the various neurological diseases, such as stroke, epilepsy, and neurodegenerative diseases like Alzheimer's and Parkinson's. The field is distinctive not merely in the focus on complex neural mechanisms but also in its interdisciplinarity, generally intersecting with other medical fields, as well as psychiatry, neurosurgery, and rehabilitation medicine. Because neurological illnesses frequently manifest in diverse symptoms and underlying etiology, the field of neurology involves detailed diagnosis, treatment, and management of disease in consideration of both biological and psychosocial factors. The way of evaluating and treating neurological diseases has had a significant transformation, which advancements in the fields of neuroimaging and molecular biology have driven. Modern neurologists make use of a variety of investigative technologies, such as MRI and CT scans, to monitor brain anatomy and identify pathologies. Also, the inclusion of novel treatments, including drug therapy and neuromodulation, has broadened the therapeutic range. For instance, the modified Rankin scale (mRS) is also widely employed in stroke trials to ascertain patient outcomes. However, evidence confirms the existence of considerable interobserver variability in the scoring that indicates the complexity of neurological assessment, as documented in studies of mRS scoring across observer groups (Dawson et al., 2008). Neurology is therefore not only encompassing of the pathophysiology of disease but also demands strict methodologies in arriving at sound patient assessment. The practice of neurology is not restricted to the clinical field; it also encompasses important contributions to education and research. Research efforts are continually ongoing in investigating the genetic, molecular, and environmental determinants affecting neurological disorders, insights from which could potentially give rise to new modes of therapy. The discipline further puts its weight behind the education of medical practitioners on the complexities of neurological disorders, thus raising their ability to detect and treat such conditions successfully. A historical perspective has also been created, where the examination of figures such as Socrates illustrates the crossroads of philosophy and neurology and suggests that certain neurological conditions affect conduct and systems of belief (Muramoto et al., 2018). Thus, the domain of neurology encompasses not only scientific understanding of the nervous system but also its profound implications at individual and societal levels (Figure 12.1).

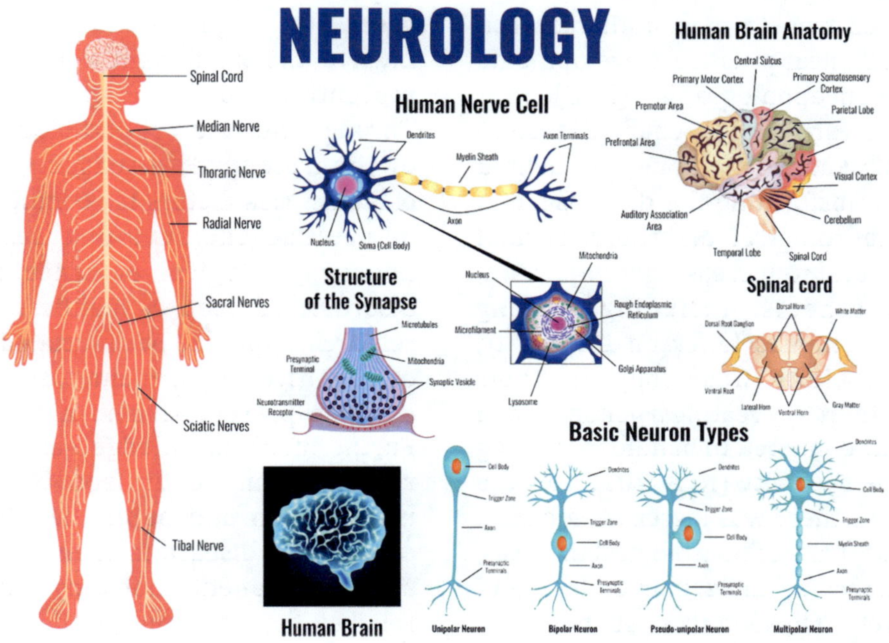

Figure 12.1. Neurology illustration.

Source: https://www.fcneurology.net/wp-content/uploads/2023/12/neurology-image.jpg.

Historical Development of the Field

The history of neurology can be traced back to ancient history when initial physicians began to hypothesize the link between the brain and behavior. Early anatomists in ancient Egypt, for example, viewed the structure of the brain as they further mummified it. These ideas were further developed by Greek thinkers like Hippocrates and Galen, who contended that mental functions were rooted in the brain, rather than in the heart, which had been supposed previously. This shift paved the way for later neurological exploration, which substantiated that the brain is the superior regulator of various physiological and psychological processes. As the centuries went on, advances in neuroanatomical understanding and disease arose together with anatomical investigations and dissections, demonstrating a progressive but meaningful change in how humans understood the nervous system's functioning. The 19th century saw a revolutionary era in the history of neurology, which was one of significant advances in clinical observation as well as experimental physiology. Pathbreakers such as Charles Brown-Séquard conducted groundbreaking work that illuminated the connections between neurological ailments and the accompanying physiological changes. Brown-Séquard's work on diabetes and its neuropathies brought the interaction between the nervous system and other functions to the forefront. His work at the Imperial Museum of Natural History highlights the collaborative aspect of scientific discovery during this period, as he engaged with influential figures like Dom Pedro II. These collaborations enabled the interchange of ideas that would not only advance clinical neurophysiology but also bring integrity and credibility to neurology as a new branch of medicine (Gomes et al., 2023). With neurology entering the 20th century, new technologies transformed both research techniques and clinical practice. Developments such as electroencephalography (EEG), first developed in the early 1920s, enabled doctors to explore cerebral activity with unprecedented sophistication, transforming the diagnosis and treatment of neurological disorders. Formal education also became increasingly important, with medical schools, including leading institutions like Thomas Jefferson University, beginning to include neurology in their curriculum and thereby creating a generation of neurologists well-equipped to handle increasing challenges in the specialty (N/A, 2017). As the discipline evolved, there was increased focus on the biological substrate of neurological diseases, in step with improving molecular biology and genetic research. These advances not only increased clinical understanding but also set in motion new therapy, reaffirming neurology as a basic branch of medicine.

Importance of Neurology in Medicine

The field of neurology has a core function in current medicine, primarily because it targets the investigation of diseases that significantly affect the quality of human life. Nervous system diseases, such as Alzheimer's disease, Parkinson's disease, and MS, are ideal examples of diseases that not only destroy intellectual and motor functions but also create emotional as well as social issues for patients and their relatives. Understanding the natural neurobiological processes allows neurologists to develop targeted therapies that can mitigate symptoms as well as improve general patient outcomes. In addition, neurology overlaps with other fields of study, expanding the medical fraternity as it promotes inter-professional practice for complex diseases requiring broad-spectrum treatments. Hence, neurologists play an integral role in enhancing healthcare provision by offering specialization that contributes to overall care suited to individual patient needs. Applications of neurology extend beyond the process of diagnosis and treatment; they also involve the significant role of neurology in preventive medicine practice and public health. Through the study of pathological foundations of neurological diseases, scientists can establish risk factors for conditions like stroke or neurodegenerative diseases. To illustrate, neurophysiological evidence indicates that disorders of sleep, as manifested in tauopathy research, appear to be associated with the onset of cognitive impairment, suggesting the role of sleep preservation in neurological health. Furthermore, knowledge gained from disease research can be utilized to guide lifestyle modification and public health policy aimed at reducing disease incidence. This preventive approach benefits not only patients but also relieves the economic burden of neurological illnesses on the health system. Therapeutically, neurology integrates more than one treatment modality, including pharmacotherapy, physical therapy, and cognitive rehab. Recent advances in dance therapy, especially for PD and postural instability, underscore the pivotal position of combined therapeutic approaches in neurological treatment. This approach has also been discovered to enhance QoL and gait function in patients with motor impairment. By treating both cognitive and somatic aspects of neurological conditions, neurologists can significantly increase patient rehabilitation outcomes. The interdisciplinarity of neurology emphasizes its value as part of the medical discipline; not only does it strive to meet the challenges of the human brain and nervous system, but it also mirrors the advanced nature of therapeutic techniques that strive to enhance patients' lives overall.

12.1. The Structure of the Nervous System

Learning Outcome

1. Understand the central nervous system (CNS)
2. Describe the peripheral nervous system (PNS)
3. Discuss neurons and glial cells

The structure of the nervous system is the foundation of learning neurology, as it allows the different functions vital for survival and interaction with the environment. Composed of the peripheral nervous system (PNS) and the CNS, the intricate system governs sensation, motor functions, and intellectual processes. The CNS, which includes the spinal cord and the brain, serves as the primary center of control and interprets messages while providing instructions. In contrast, the PNS comprises all the neural tissues beyond the CNS, i.e., spinal and cranial nerves, which transfer information between the body and brain. Structural segregation such as this delineates not only the complex organization of the nervous system but also the interdependence of its structures since the PNS acquires sensory information that directs CNS responses and thus is a holistic and dynamic system essential for efficient functioning (Anderson et al., 2015). Segregation of the nervous system into more specialized structures allows for enhanced function and flexibility. Within the CNS, the brain is subdivided into various regions that are specialized for different functions. For instance, the cerebrum coordinates higher-order cognitive functions like reasoning, memory, and emotion, while the cerebellum regulates voluntary movement and balance. The brainstem, on the other hand, regulates basic autonomic functions like heart rate and breathing. This arrangement is an advanced evolutionary adaptation to many environmental pressures, with its purpose being to maximize processing and response to information efficiency. Moreover, the interconnection between these brain regions, facilitated by extensive neural networks, demonstrates the principles governing information integration, crucial for behavior adaptation and survival, as captured in the argument regarding the hierarchical structure of brains (Gaiseanu et al., 2020). On the PNS level, organization is defined by its somatic and autonomic structures, both performing crucial but distinct roles in the body. Voluntary movement and the transmission of sensory feedback from external stimuli are the realms of the somatic nervous system, with the eventual impact on behavior and action in the immediate world. The autonomic nervous system is that which modulates involuntary body function, producing homeostasis via its sympathetic and parasympathetic divisions. This duality is required to cope with the many physiological requirements, from stress response to digestion. Furthermore, the organization of these systems is evidence that the nervous structure reflects the complexity of human experience, varying from simple reflex circuits to intricate emotional responses. The understanding of these structures and how they interact provides a full view of the nervous system and its central role in neurologic illness and health (Anderson et al., 2015).

12.1.1. Central Nervous System (CNS)

The central nervous system (CNS) is the body's regulating center for voluntary and involuntary movements, integrating sensory information to enable integration of sensory inputs. The CNS consists of the brain and spinal cord and plays a central role in homeostasis and behavioral regulation. The brain, an intricate network of glial cells and neurons, facilitates higher-order thinking, emotional responses, and motor activity. Meanwhile, the spinal cord is an avenue through which neuronal impulses are transmitted from the brain to the PNS. Understanding the complexities of CNS function provides valuable insight into neurological disease because disruption of any kind can produce enormous impairments in normal functioning. The recent scientific studies have shed light on the role of inflammation in CNS illness, which is in agreement with recent models of neurodegenerative diseases. Chronic inflammation in the CNS is a strong contributor to diseases like MS and Alzheimer's disease. Importantly, microglial activation—resident immune cells of the CNS—is an overarching factor in neuroinflammatory processes that characterize these diseases. It has been found that the occurrence of inflammatory markers is associated with neurodegeneration, further exacerbating the pathology of these diseases. The link between immune responses and neurotransmitters has emerged as a significant field of research, in line with the intricate interactions within the CNS (Giubilei et al., 2016).

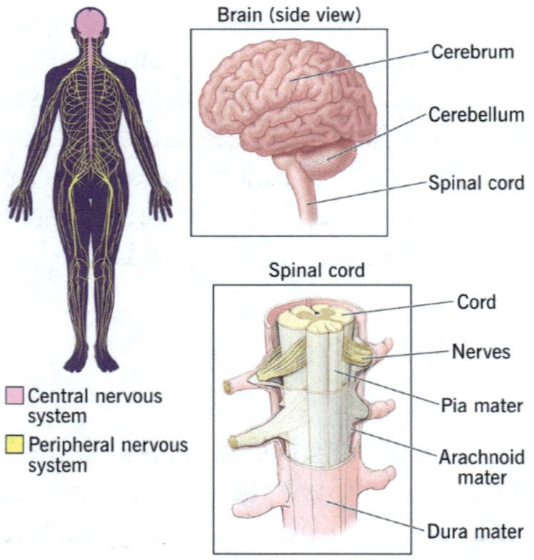

Figure 12.2. Schematic diagram showing the central nervous system and the peripheral nervous system (PNS).

Source: https://my.clevelandclinic.org/-/scassets/images/org/health/articles/central-nervous-system.

Moreover, treatment modalities with anti-inflammatory elements have emerged as a major focus in treating neurological diseases. Studies point towards the efficacy of anticoagulants and anti-inflammatory agents in the prevention of the detrimental effects of inflammation within the CNS, notably in diseases such as MS. The pro-inflammatory potential of thrombin and fibrinogen has amplified the role of the coagulation pathway in CNS pathology (Adams et al., 2018). Through research into such therapeutic possibilities, scientists aim to develop complementary therapies that not only lower inflammation but also modulate disease progression. The developing paradigm of CNS function and disease establishes the primal imperative for new methods of neurology to unleash the potential for improved patient benefits and outcomes of neurodegenerative diseases (Figure 12.2).

12.1.2. Peripheral Nervous System (PNS)

The peripheral nervous system (PNS) has a vital role of relaying sensory and motor information between the body and the CNS. It includes all neural structures outside the brain and spinal cord. The PNS comprises cranial nerves, spinal nerves, and peripheral nerves that innervate muscles and organs. The extensive system allows for voluntary and involuntary responses such that a coordinated response to external stimuli can be evoked. Further, the PNS can be divided into somatic and autonomic systems, such that the somatic nervous system deals with voluntary movement and the autonomic nervous system with involuntary body functions. Acknowledging the PNS's intricate organization is essential to comprehending how neurologic disorders can disrupt communication pathways to cause different clinical presentations requiring specific interventions. Neuropathies that arise from pathologies in the PNS tend to produce considerable morbidity in the patient, hence highlighting the need to appreciate their clinical presentation. Conditions like polyneuropathy may be caused by a diverse set of etiologies, for example, genetic factors, autoimmune illness, and toxins. For instance, polyneuropathy with monoclonal gammopathy of immunoglobulin M (IgM) is a common paraproteinemic neuropathy, involving myelin sheath damage. It is responsible for producing manifestations ranging from mild paresthesias to disabling sensory ataxia. With IgM immunoglobulins binding to glycolipids in the peripheral nerves, they initiate neuroinflammatory responses, which can lead to progressive nerve damage. These complexities highlight the value of rigorously diagnosing PNS disorders and the need for multimodal treatment regimens that treat the underlying pathophysiology, ultimately benefiting patient outcomes (Dalakas et al., 2018). The therapeutic context for PNS disorders has further evolved, driven by advances in immunological appreciation and pharmacologic treatment. Despite challenges in the case of disorders like IgM-associated neuropathy, newer treatment approaches like rituximab promise new horizons. This monoclonal antibody has promise in altering the immune response by downregulating IgM production and thereby alleviating some of the neurotoxic effects of myelin disruption. The effectiveness of these treatments remains uncertain, however, while clinical benefit is noted in some patients, others experience only transient improvement. The heterogeneity of responses to immunotherapies necessitates ongoing clinical studies to optimize treatment regimens and identify predictive biomarkers of favorable outcomes. In so doing, neurobiological understanding of PNS disorders will still drive individually tailored therapy approaches, maximizing care delivery for the so-affected individuals (Brust et al., 2014).

12.1.3. Neurons and Glial Cells

Neurons and glial cells are the fundamental structural elements of the CNS that carry out specialized yet integrated functions required for normal brain function. Neurons are specialized nerve cells responsible for conveying electrical impulses in the brain and spinal cord. They also involve complex communication processes that enable the processing of information vital to cognition, sensation, and motor control. On the other hand, there are more numerous glial cells that are responsible for providing key support, protection, and maintenance of the neuronal environment. There are different types of supportive cells, including astrocytes, oligodendrocytes, and microglia, each contributing unique functions to support neuronal viability and functioning. Having these primary cell types is essential in understanding how their interactions can be broken, the causation of neurological disorders and impairments, and how this is indicative of a balance that is part of overall CNS health. New studies have indicated complex interactions between the glial and neuron cells, with reciprocal effects on brain disease and health. For instance, astrocytes play a key role in the process of healing following TBI. There is evidence that astrocytes are actively involved in mechanisms of repair and synaptic remodeling and are not mere bystanders (Figure 12.3).

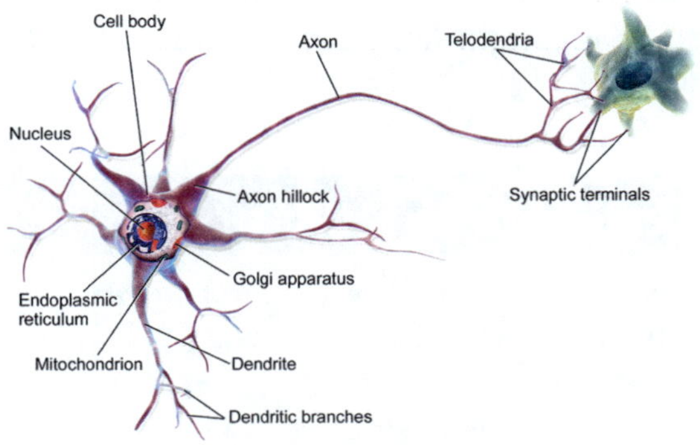

Figure 12.3. Multipolar neuron.

Source: https://upload.wikimedia.org/wikipedia/commons/thumb/1/10/Blausen_0657_MultipolarNeuron.png/1024px-Blausen_0657_MultipolarNeuron.png.

The upregulation of ephrin-B1 and other markers within astrocytes after TBI has been found to contribute to the regulation of synaptic contact and neural plasticity. This indicates an active role of glial function in modulating neuronal health, where a change in astrocytic function can greatly influence that of the neuron and recovery in case of trauma. Through examination of such interactions, researchers are increasingly conscious of the need to account for both glial cells and neurons in efforts towards effective therapeutic strategies to numerous neurological disorders (Ethell et al., 2016). In addition to providing support cells, glial cells are also involved in the modulation of inflammatory responses in the CNS. For instance, the therapy using functionalized carbon nanotubes (f-CNTs) has been shown to respond with neurons and glia by eliciting inflammatory cytokine responses. The divergent uptake of f-CNTs by astrocytes and microglia highlights the mediating function of glial cells in response to exogenous agents that can affect nerve integrity. Apart from this, the convergence of glial cell activation and neuronal survival highlights the intricate nature of the CNS milieu and the need to maintain homeostasis. Understanding these interactions is of utmost significance, as it opens up the possibility of designing specific therapies that take advantage of glial responses to mitigate harm and facilitate recovery (Bianco et al., 2013). Therefore, examination of neurons and glial cells together not only deepens our knowledge of CNS function but also holds the promise of new approaches to therapy for neurological disease (Figure 12.4).

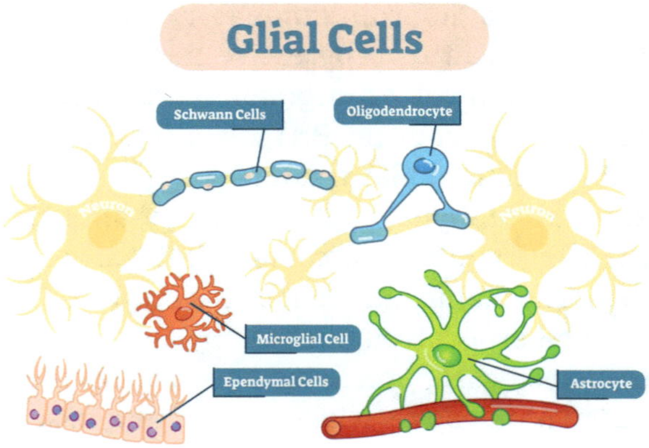

Figure 12.4. Glial cells.

Source: https://www.verywellhealth.com/thmb/KTilfCxnabrUhsp536BLMgZ_8Zk=/1500x0/filters:no_upscale():max_bytes(150000):strip_icc()/glialcellsillustration-5a94d585642dca00362568c4.jpg.

Test Your Knowledge

1. What are the main components of the central nervous system (CNS), and what are their primary functions?
2. How does the peripheral nervous system (PNS) differ structurally and functionally from the central nervous system?
3. Describe the basic structure of a neuron and explain the roles of its main parts.

12.2. Common Neurological Disorders

Learning Outcome

1. Describe Alzheimer's disease
2. Understand Parkinson's disease
3. Define multiple sclerosis

In neurology, neurologic disorders are a common phenomenon and bear a significant quality-of-life impact on the patients and a heavy burden for health systems. One of the most prevalent diseases is PD, which shows a range of motor and non-motor symptoms like postural instability and cognitive impairment. The linkage of these symptoms gives rise to stringent disabilities, thereby making therapeutic approaches for rehabilitation extremely crucial. Recent developments in therapy, including dance therapy, have been indicated as a valuable option for improving PD patients' walking and overall motor performance. Dance therapy not only deals with physical impairment but also cognitive impairment, which reinforces motor dysfunction, suggesting an integrated treatment for this disabling neurologic disorder (Agnetti et al., 2012). Another essential condition within this category is chorea, a hyperkinetic movement disorder characterized by disorganized, spontaneous movements that can disrupt normal activities. Typically associated with Huntington's disease, chorea can also occur based on many acquired or genetic causes, including autoimmune diseases, metabolic disorders, and certain medications. Chorea's complexity demands a very comprehensive clinical assessment to determine its etiology, possibly including genetic testing and diligent review of symptoms. It is also important in creating an effective treatment program to discover potential underlying causes, since treatment can vary a lot depending on the etiology of the disorder. Thus, expanding our understanding of chorea not only enriches clinical practice but also sheds light on the broader context of genetic and environmental factors affecting neurological health (Tabrizi et al., 2007). Apart from PD and chorea, other common neurological illnesses, such as MS and epilepsy, illustrate the broad spectrum of neurological disorders. MS, an autoimmune disease affecting the CNS, may be responsible for a variety of neurological signs and symptoms, such as fatigue, motor weakness, and cognitive decline. The unpredictable nature of MS relapses can significantly affect patients' daily activities and require ongoing medical attention. Similarly, epilepsy, defined by recurrent seizures, besides presenting short-term health risks, also results in long-term mental health consequences as well as social functioning. Both these illnesses stress the importance of early diagnosis, treatment methods, and a multidisciplinary care system to provide comprehensive care to individuals suffering from neurological illnesses. As we further develop our understanding of these diseases, we improve the potential for better management and QoL in patients and their families.

12.2.1. Alzheimer's Disease

Alzheimer's is a severe neurological disease, with gradual deterioration in intellectual functions, involving reasoning, memory, and speech. It is primarily seen in the geriatric population, with symptom onset after age 65. Mild forgetfulness can be the presenting feature in early-stage Alzheimer's. Still, with the advancement of the disease, the patient may become disoriented with respect to place or time, find it difficult to do everyday tasks, and exhibit mood swings and personality changes. These impairments are complex, involving not only biological etiologies like amyloid plaque deposition and tau tangles in the brain, but also psychosocial factors that manifest in the patients' lives. The complexity of Alzheimer's disease requires an interdisciplinary treatment strategy with the confluence of science from neurology, psychology, and social science to provide better patient outcomes and caregiver care. The behavioral and psychological symptoms of dementia (BPSD) in Alzheimer's aggravate the patients' as well as the caregivers' problems. The symptoms include anxiety, depression, agitation, and even psychotic manifestations, and these can present despite the cognitive impairments. Understanding the etiology of BPSD is necessary while formulating effective treatment approaches; it is one that involves a global understanding and includes individual biological, psychological, and environmental factors. The treatment models of today emphasize the importance of individualized care plans, often beginning with non-pharmacologic interventions before pharmacotherapy, exceptionally where traditional drugs may not be practical or appropriate (Figure 12.5).

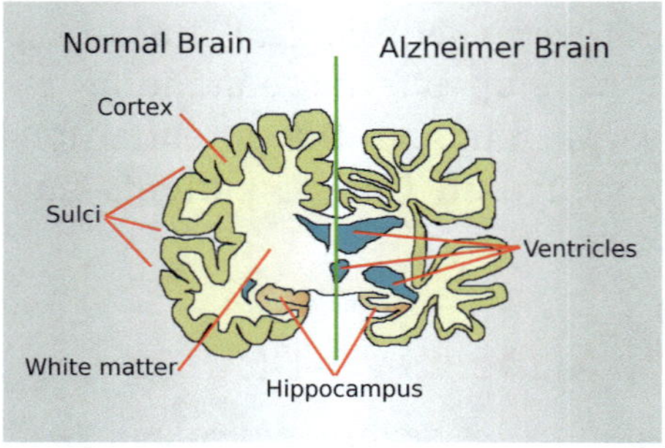

Figure 12.5. Drawing comparing how a brain of an Alzheimer's disease patient is affected to a normal brain.

Source: https://upload.wikimedia.org/wikipedia/commons/thumb/5/5f/Brain-ALZH.png/1024px-Brain-ALZH.png.

Regular management strategy reviews are required to evaluate patient response and modify accordingly. This complexity reflects the need for ongoing research and clinical debate surrounding BPSD to optimize care in the Alzheimer's population (Riese et al., 2017). Further, awareness regarding the genetic mechanisms and pathophysiology of Alzheimer's disease is also essential for future developments in diagnosis, treatment, and prevention. Current scientific research has clarified some of the genetic risk contributions to developing Alzheimer's, along with increasing evidence on biomarkers that potentially would enable earlier detection. An interesting point is that certain studies highlight the need for more specific clinical criteria and diagnostic tools that could potentially enhance the detection of atypical neurodegenerative disorder presentations (Hoeglinger et al., 2013). With the growing insight into the genetics and biochemistry of Alzheimer's disease, the development of specific treatments is increasingly feasible. Nevertheless, there are still challenges, such as the lack of effective biomarkers for diagnosis and monitoring treatment response. For this reason, further multidisciplinary cooperation and development of new research concepts are required to overcome the difficulties of Alzheimer's disease and advance patient care in neurology (Figure 12.6).

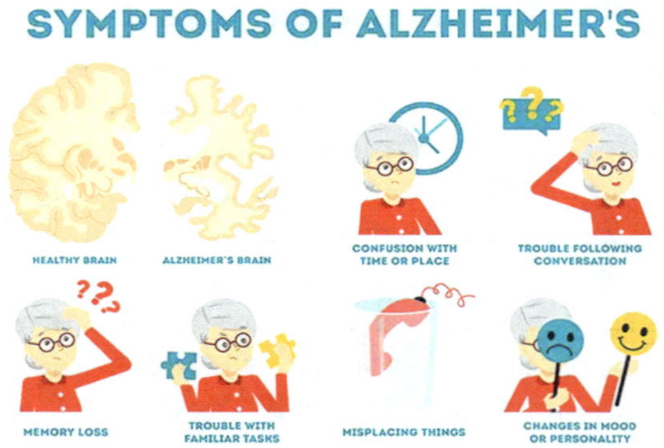

Figure 12.6. Symptoms of Alzheimer's disease.

Source: https://www.apexhospitals.com/_next/image?url=https%3A%2F%2Fbed.apexhospitals.com%2Fuploads%2Falzheimers_1_742d43a731.png&w=1920&q=75.

12.2.2. Parkinson's Disease (PD)

Parkinson's disease (PD) is a neurodegenerative disorder with both motor and nonmotor symptoms. The traditional picture of PD is the combination of bradykinesia, rigidity, and rest tremor; however, the disease encompasses more than just these motor impairments. Nonmotor symptoms such as depression, cognitive dysfunction, and sleep disturbances have become more significant for their debilitating impact on patients' QoL. These nonmotor symptoms often appear early in the disease course and may be equally debilitating, prompting an imperative for interventions effective against the worldwide needs of patients. As researchers explore various treatment modalities, understanding the relationship between motor and nonmotor symptoms is useful in the development of integrated management strategies for PD. Exercise interventions represent a new adjunct to traditional therapeutic therapy for both the motor and nonmotor symptoms of Parkinson's disease. According to research, engagement in aerobic exercise and strength training is associated with significant improvements in mood, cognition, and sleep among both healthy older adults and clinical groups. Specifically, exercise has been known to enhance mood and cognition, which is essential in light of the resultant cognitive dysfunction often associated with PD. In addition, the literature highlights the importance of integrating exercise interventions into clinical management, particularly since they represent a safe and effective treatment option aimed at diminishing a range of nonmotor symptoms. This multi-modal approach not only promotes physical exercise but also offers a considerable therapeutic benefit to PD patients, eventually improving their QoL (Cronin-Golomb et al., 2015). Cognitive rehabilitation has also been found to be feasible and potentially beneficial in the remediation of cognitive deficits associated with PD. Recent studies highlight the beneficial effects of goal-oriented cognitive rehabilitation on mood, QoL, and overall cognitive functioning over standard treatment approaches. Through systematic goal setting and tailored cognitive training, patients demonstrate significant improvements in self-rating goal attainment and satisfaction, further implying the usefulness of tailored cognitive interventions. Therefore, cognitive rehabilitation provides a new means of enhancing the cognitive functioning of PD patients and maximizing the QoL of their caregivers, who also benefit substantially. The results of such research underscore the necessity of incorporating cognitive rehabilitation into the treatment options for PD since it addresses both the needs of caregivers and patients and is an integral aspect of managing the said condition (Brand et al., 2018) (Figure 12.7).

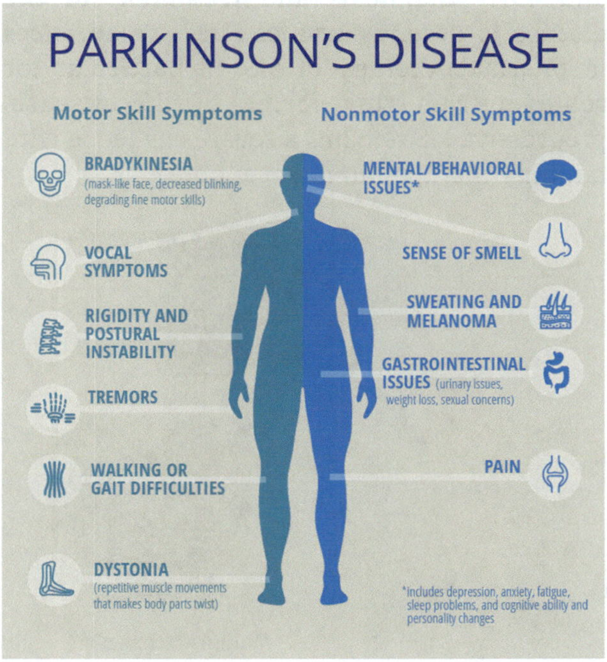

Figure 12.7. Parkinson's disease (PD).

Source: https://singaporebrain.org/wp-content/uploads/2015/08/ParkinsonsDisease.png.

12.2.3. Multiple Sclerosis (MS)

Multiple sclerosis (MS) is one of the most complex CNS illnesses, characterized by demyelination of the neurons and consequent compromise of neural transmission. It primarily occurs among young adults between 20 and 40 years of age and is characterized by a variety of neurological syndromes, such as motor and sensory deficits. This autoimmune disease occurs when the immune system of one's own body mistakenly targets the myelin sheath covering nerve fibers, leading to both inflammatory and neurodegenerative responses. The multifaceted aspect of MS demands an in-depth comprehension of its mechanisms, which continue to be explored through ongoing research. With disease progression, patients present with a range of incapacitating signs and symptoms significantly impacting their QoL, and therefore, an effective therapeutic intervention and early diagnosis and treatment of the disease is urgently needed. Despite advances in pharmacotherapy of MS, in particular for relapsing-remitting forms of the disease, progressive MS remains a severe challenge with minimal therapeutic intervention.

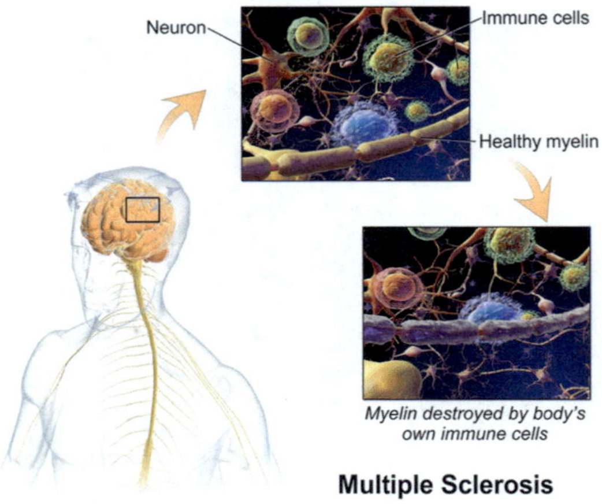

Figure 12.8. Multiple sclerosis.

Source: https://upload.wikimedia.org/wikipedia/commons/thumb/2/2a/Multiple_Sclerosis.png/800px-Multiple_Sclerosis.png.

Most of the disease-modifying therapies available today focus primarily on the inflammatory processes characteristic of relapsing MS, with a gap remaining in treatments for patients who develop the progressive forms. Research indicates that the majority of individuals with MS face great barriers as they progress through the symptomatic relief and control of the disease. There is an urgent need to research holistic management approaches to cater to the complex dynamic of symptoms that affect progressive MS patients. Through various MS societies, cooperative efforts are proposed to identify important research areas focusing on innovative therapeutic interventions, thereby maximizing the potential for meaningful improvements in treatment outcomes in the population (Baker et al., 2012) (Figure 12.8).

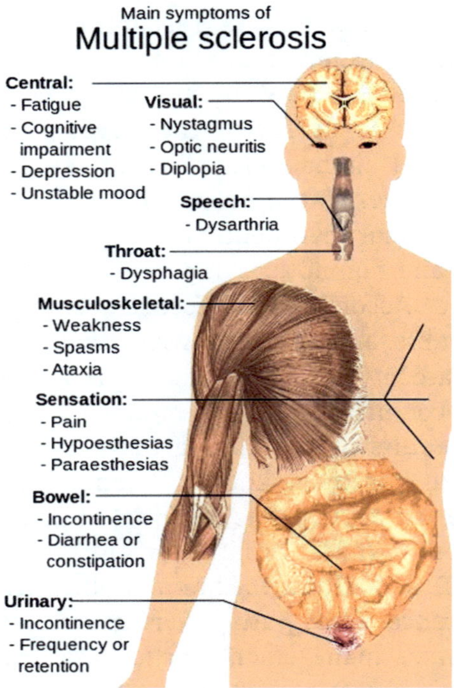

Figure 12.9. Symptoms of multiple sclerosis.

Source: https://neurosciencenews.com/files/2013/09/public-symptoms-ms.jpg.

Recent discoveries reveal the most critical areas of research to help design improved treatment strategies for every form of MS. The examination of experimental models and confirmation of targets are critical for developing forthcoming treatments that will meet the specific needs of progressive MS patients. Concurrently, proof-of-concept clinical trials must be formulated to offer insight into the efficacy of new treatment modalities without compromising volunteers' safety and well-being.

Furthermore, clinical outcomes measures that closely approximate patients' experience ought to receive a high level of priority to evaluate the performance of interventions. With the medical and scientific field remaining on an interdisciplinary path, tremendous strides can be achieved in translating research findings into applicable therapies in individuals suffering from MS. Through enhanced synergy and innovation, the prospects are up-and-coming for improving the lives of individuals suffering from this complex neurological disorder (Kay et al., 2015) (Figure 12.9).

Test Your Knowledge

1. What are the key clinical features that help differentiate Alzheimer's disease from other types of dementia?
2. Describe the primary motor symptoms of Parkinson's disease and the underlying pathophysiology.
3. What is the typical clinical presentation of multiple sclerosis, and how does its pathogenesis affect the nervous system?

12.3. Diagnostic Techniques in Neurology

Learning Outcome

1. Understand neuroimaging methods (MRI, CT scans)
2. Explain electrophysiological tests (EEG, EMG)
3. Focus on neuropsychological assessments

The field of neurology has advanced significantly with the implementation of many diagnostic tests that make it easier to understand and treat neurological ailments. Of these tests, neuroimaging has proven to be a highly significant tool, enabling physicians to look inside the brain and its structure and function. MRI and CT scans are being used more frequently to diagnose structural disease, including tumors, lesions, and malformations of blood vessels. Technological development has increased the sensitivity of these imaging techniques, allowing diseases such as MS and stroke to be diagnosed at an early stage. Functional neuroimaging, using fMRI and positron emission tomography (PET), has permitted the investigation of cerebral activity patterns, aiding in the understanding of disorders such as epilepsy and neurodegenerative diseases. Together, these imaging techniques allow for timely and accurate diagnosis, which is essential for effective patient management and treatment protocols. For functional movement disorders, neuroimaging is instrumental in unraveling the pathophysiology behind such multifaceted diseases, rather than appealing to earlier psychological explanations of conversion disorders, newer work centers on neurobiological models with emotional processing and self-construal. Advanced imaging techniques have uncovered essential information about the brain's functional connectivity and structural integrity, as well as subtle changes that occur with these illnesses. These findings corroborate the notion that functional movement disorders are not merely psychological processes but consist of flawed neural processes. By shedding light on the neurological pathways of such disorders, neuroimaging fosters an improved understanding and encourages the development of targeted treatment protocols, thereby improving patient outcomes and QoL (Edwards et al., 2019). Lastly, biomarkers have become an essential component of the diagnostic process of several neurological disorders, particularly in the assessment of PD. As approached by initiatives like the National Institute of Neurological Disorders and Stroke Parkinson's

Disease Biomarker Program (PDBP), the quest for reliable biomarkers is prompted by an urgent requirement for enhanced diagnostic and predictive measures. Harmonization of biofluid collection methods and clinical evaluations is now at the forefront of enhancing the replicability and validity of biomarkers. While no single marker has yet achieved clinical utility, an integrative approach of using wearable devices and longitudinal observation can potentially uncover the earliest markers of disease onset. Not only do these advances enhance diagnostic sensitivity, but they also enable the stratification of patients for clinical trials, paving the way for new therapeutic interventions (Albin et al., 2017).

12.3.1. Neuroimaging Methods (MRI, CT Scans)

Neuroimaging modalities, such as MRI and CT scans, play a core role within the field of neurology, yielding vital information regarding brain structure and function. MRI employs powerful magnetic fields and radio waves to generate high-quality images of brain tissue, enabling the evaluation of various neurological conditions such as tumors, strokes, and neurodegenerative diseases. CT scans utilize X-rays to create cross-sectional images of the brain and are used for the rapid assessment of acute phenomena like hemorrhage or fracture. Each modality has a specific function: MRI may be the modality of choice because it provides increased soft tissue contrast. At the same time, CT is valued for being quick and easily accessible. This choice of method is essentially a matter of the clinical context, highlighting the need for neurologists to have proficiency in both techniques in order to deliver optimal patient care. A solid foundation in modern neuroimaging techniques, particularly TBI, is essential to enhance diagnostic and prognostic capabilities. Advances in MRI, including structural and functional imaging, have shown immense promise in the detection of biomarkers of TBI outcome. According to recent literature, a combination of volumetric analysis with diffusion tensor imaging makes it possible to assess the integrity and connectivity of the brain comprehensively (Aylward et al., 2012). These multimodal methods allow for subtle alterations in brain networks to be detected, thus guiding patient management and treatment protocols. Neurologists may apply such advancements to advance the comprehension of brain trauma, leading to improved prognostication and rehabilitation efforts based on the complexity of brain recovery.

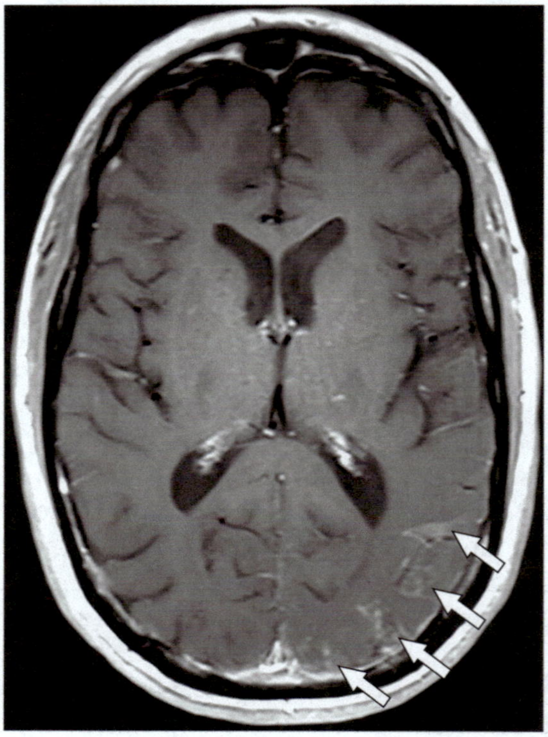

Figure 12.10. Brain MRI obtained at the onset of neurological symptoms. A T1-weighted contrast-enhanced axial image shows leptomeningeal enhancement involving the left occipital and parietal lobes (arrows).

Source: https://www.researchgate.net/publication/326724765/figure/fig1/AS:11431281213960476@1703255986278/Brain-MRI-obtained-at-onset-of-neurological-symptoms-T1-weighted-contrast-enhanced-axial.jpg.

The evolving neuroimaging environment also highlights the importance of education and self-confidence among primary care providers (PCPs) in addressing cognitive disorders. According to one study, PCPs have been observed to show lower confidence levels in interpreting neuroimaging findings compared to neurologists, thereby hindering timely diagnosis and treatment of neurocognitive disorders (NCDs) (Bernstein et al., 2019). Although the majority of PCPs screen cognitively on a routine basis, their hesitation to use imaging results in diagnosis underscores a significant flaw in the continuum of care. By fashioning enhanced training and exposure to diagnostic criteria, neuroimaging can become significantly more potent as a diagnostic resource for NCDs. This interdisciplinary collaboration among PCPs and specialists will eventually yield the highest quality of care for patients, utilizing imaging techniques such as MRI and CT scans to their full potential in neurological practice (Figure 12.10).

12.3.2. Electrophysiological Tests (EEG, EMG)

Electrophysiological tests such as EEG and electromyography (EMG) are in the field of neurology, providing useful data regarding the functioning of the brain and muscles. EEG captures the electrical activity of the brain via electrodes placed on the scalp, allowing clinicians to diagnose conditions such as epilepsy, sleep disorders, and other neurological conditions. This non-invasive method provides real-time information on cortical dynamics. It is therefore extremely useful in evaluating brain reactions to different stimuli, including treatments such as repetitive transcranial magnetic stimulation (rTMS). TEPs-studies have indicated that these signals can follow rTMS-induced effects on cortical excitability, particularly in patient populations such as children with ADHD, and that TEPs can be an effective biomarker to test for therapeutic efficacy as well as safety (Bender et al., 2012). EMG is utilized to quantify the electrical activity of muscles and is crucial to the diagnosis of neuromuscular disorders. By placing electrodes on the skin or by inserting fine needles into muscle tissue, clinicians can examine the electrical signals at muscle contraction and rest. All of this gives critical information regarding the function of the neuromuscular junction, conduction of motor nerves, and the status of muscles, and in the diagnosis of peripheral neuropathy to myopathies. The integration of EEG and EMG information can provide a comprehensive knowledge of the motor pathways and the cortical sources, enhancing the diagnostic role in neurology. EEG and EMG can also be employed synergistically, offering more extensive information on neurological pathology by correlating peripheral motor response to CNS function and hence allowing total patient evaluation.

New work in the field emphasizes the importance of understanding how exogenous rhythmic stimulation, such as rTMS, interacts with endogenous brain rhythms, as evident in EEG studies. New findings suggest that brain oscillations are central to the computations of the brain, with studies showing that sensorimotor cortex activity can be modulated by carefully timed rTMS, particularly at the individual's peak beta frequency. These observations reflect the interaction between the externally applied stimuli and the brain's intrinsic rhythmicity, as the amplitude of EEG responses is heightened when stimulation is delivered at the subject's own frequency (Akam et al., 2016). Such knowledge is critical to optimize therapeutic intervention in neurology because understanding such dynamics may determine the timing and intensity of intervention, like rTMS, and thereby optimize their efficacy in treating many neurological disorders (Figure 12.11).

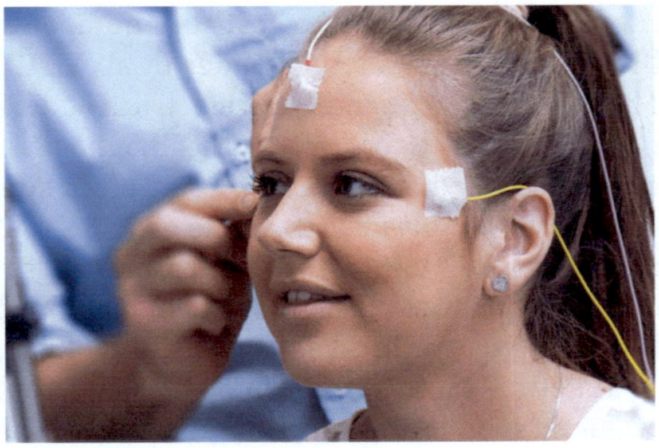

Figure 12.11. Electrophysiology testing.

Source: https://qei.org.au/wp-content/uploads/2019/02/qedic-procedures.png.

12.3.3. Neuropsychological Assessments

Neuropsychological examinations are a critical aspect of neurology that provide valuable information regarding cognitive functions and their relation to the brain's condition. They consist of a set of norm-referenced tests designed to quantify various facets of cognitive functions, including memory, attention, problem-solving, and language. By utilizing both qualitative and quantitative measures, clinicians can better understand how neurological conditions, such as traumatic brain injuries or neurodegenerative diseases, affect an individual's cognitive prowess. Furthermore, these evaluations help distinguish between different types of cognitive impairment, allowing for targeted interventions and tailored treatment plans.

The implicit information gained from neuropsychological testing not only informs diagnosis but also facilitates monitoring the effectiveness of therapeutic methods over time, emphasizing the inherent value of such assessments to neurological practice. The use of neuropsychological testing in clinical practice extends beyond mere diagnosis; it also encompasses evaluating cognitive change over time. Because neurological disorders often take progressive courses, ongoing evaluation can track declining cognition, help recognize changes indicating the need for intervention or a change in treatment plan. Neuropsychological evaluation can also encourage coordination among care providers, patients, and caregivers and enable coordinated management of neurological disorders.

Clinicians can use such an evaluation to provide education on cognitive symptoms and their effects on daily functioning. By creating such awareness, families and even the patients themselves can better deal with the challenges posed by cognitive impairment, securing a better life for those affected. Recent developments in neuroimaging techniques, adding to neuropsychological testing, further complete the picture, incorporating correlations between cognitive performance and the neurological architecture underlying it, while traditional testing relies solely on behavioral responses.

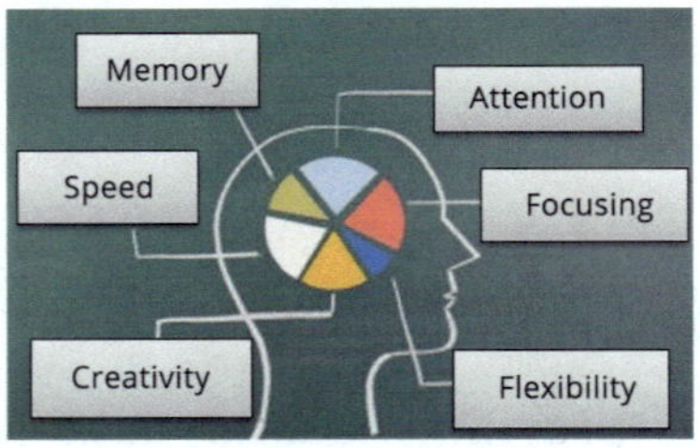

Figure 12.12. Illustration of neuropsychological assessment.

Source: https://www.kemalarikan.com/wp-content/uploads/2018/10/neuropsychological-assessment-i.jpg.

This pairing not only enhances diagnostic accuracy but also informs therapy. For example, awareness of the target brain regions for diseases like Alzheimer's disease can target interventions to preserve or impede the degradation of cognitive abilities. Regarding the future of neurology, integrating neuropsychological testing with technological innovations like neuroimaging is a significant step toward individualizing neurological treatment to specific requirements. This integrative approach not only optimizes treatment outcomes but also fundamentally changes how clinicians view and address cognitive well-being among clients (Powell et al., 2014; Elliott et al., 2018) (Figure 12.12).

Test Your Knowledge

1. What are the main differences between MRI and CT scans in terms of their use, strengths, and limitations in neurological diagnosis?
2. How does an EEG help in diagnosing neurological disorders?
3. In what clinical situations would neuropsychological assessments be particularly valuable, and what cognitive functions do they evaluate?

12.4. Treatment Approaches in Neurology

Learning Outcome

1. Discuss pharmacological treatments in neurology
2. Understand surgical interventions in neurology
3. Describe neurological rehabilitation therapies

The landscape of treatments in neurology has transformed extensively, embracing conventional and revolutionary methods. Neurologists prefer to focus more on a holistic model of pharmacological therapy, physical treatment, and behavioral interventions. This integrative methodology is aimed at tailoring therapies according to patient profiles, considering the exact symptoms and conditions of each. Traditional pharmacologic treatments, traditionally the first line, are directed to specific neurological diseases with drugs that manage symptoms and modify the illness. For instance, antiepileptics play a crucial role in seizure control, and neurotransmitter modulators play critical roles in conditions such as depression or Parkinson's disease. This first view proposes a model supplemented by lifestyle interventions and alternative treatments, thus substantiating the necessity of an integrated approach in treating neurological disorders. In physical therapy and rehabilitation, new methods have come to the forefront. More specifically, dance therapy has emerged as a fascinating alternative treatment modality for patients suffering from diseases such as PD. This form of therapy not only promotes physical movement but also cognitive function and social interaction, in keeping with the holistic dimensions of neurological impairment. In its research, dance therapy has been highly successful in enhancing walking and balance in patients and is a rehabilitative strategy that exceeds conventional paradigms of treatment. With the evaluation of spatial-temporal gait parameters, it can be observed that interventions such as dance therapy can help effect remarkable improvements in cognitive and motor performance among patients with postural instability. These non-pharmacologic interventions are thus a part of long-term neurologic management and offer evidence of the utility in combining creative therapies with conventional interventions (Agnetti et al., 2012). Expanded treatment paradigms also include research on the application of neurostimulation techniques, such as deep brain stimulation (DBS), that offer new avenues for the management of chronic neurological conditions. DBS, a procedure involving the implantation of electrodes in the specific areas of the brain to modulate neuronal activity, is recognized to relieve agonizing manifestations of ailments like essential tremor and treatment-refractory depression. This approach focuses on advances in neurology beyond symptom control, aiming to restore function at the neuro level. The integration of neurotechnological innovations, such as transcranial magnetic stimulation (TMS) and biofeedback, also reflects the call for personalized care pathways. As these technologies develop, they have the potential not only to enhance patient outcomes but also to redefine treatment protocols in neurology, creating a more individualized and streamlined model of care (N/A, 2018).

12.4.1. Pharmacological Treatments

Pharmacological therapies in neurology have been significantly transformed in recent decades due to progress in understanding neurological diseases and their pathophysiologic mechanisms. They comprise a wide range of drugs intended to be symptomatic relief, to modify disease course, and enhance the QoL for patients with diseases such as epilepsy, MS, Parkinson's disease, and Alzheimer's disease. The development of neuropharmacological drugs increasingly relies on new research approaches, as more studies use experimental models to evaluate therapeutic effects and safety. In particular, the zebrafish model organism system has emerged as a valuable asset in drug development and the screening of new therapeutics. It has provided useful insights into neurodegeneration and facilitated the accelerated growth of pharmacological interventions aimed at curing these complex diseases (Nasevicius et al., 2015). Nevertheless, use of pharmacologic treatments in neurology is fraught with challenges, the prime among them being patient selection and personalized treatment. The genetic makeup of the patient, comorbidities, and specific characteristics of the disease must be considered while selecting the best pharmacologic treatment. Further, side effects of the majority of neurological medications have the potential to create significant management problems, which demand vigilant monitoring and adjustment of therapeutic regimens. Clinicians must collaborate in decision-making with patients, ensuring they are aware of the potential benefits and risks of prescribed treatments. This not only improves treatment adherence but also facilitates the patient-centered approach to care, addressing the various ethical issues associated with pharmacological interventions in neurology (Whitaker et al., 2018).

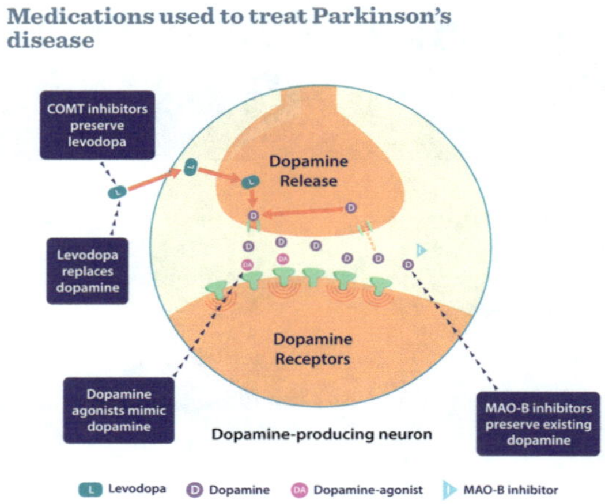

Figure 12.13. Medications used to treat Parkinson's disease.

Source: https://parkinsonsdisease.net/wp-content/uploads/2017/04/Medications-Used-To-Treat-Parkinson%E2%80%99s.jpg.

With the advancing field of neurology, new pharmacological interventions need to be discovered to optimize patient outcomes. Investigations continue to find new targets for therapy and routes of drug delivery with the hope of decreasing side effects and improving efficacy. The integration between pharmacotherapy and other forms of therapy, such as psychotherapy and physical therapy, is increasingly recognized as essential for the integrative treatment of neurological disorders. Notably, the convergence of novel technology techniques, such as nanomedicine and personalized medicine, holds potential for enhancing pharmacological therapy in neurology. Through interdisciplinary collaboration and monitoring innovation progress, the topic can potentially go a long way in enhancing pharmacological treatment to its fullest, ultimately improving the lives of neurologically challenged individuals (Nasevicius et al., 2015) (Figure 12.13).

12.4.2. Surgical Interventions

Neurosurgical procedures encompass a chain of operations used in the treatment of numerous neurological disorders. Neurosurgical procedures can be extremely powerful relative to outcomes among patients, particularly when dealing with cerebral palsy, epilepsy, and brain tumors. For instance, in cerebral palsy therapy, specific surgical techniques can enhance motor function by eliminating spasticity or correcting structural deformities in the brain. According to the literature, the 1994–2008 systematic review highlights the importance of such surgeries to improve the QoL among children with cerebral palsy, pointing out how specific interventions lead to improved functional outcomes (Bowers et al., 2009). Thus, surgical intervention is a component of an interdisciplinary treatment of neurological conditions, usually constituting the last measure if the conservative regimes fail to yield adequate results. The role of surgical therapy also includes not only the relief of symptoms but also that of prevention in the context of various neurological illnesses, particularly in patients with epilepsy. Epilepsy surgery, such as resective surgery, is meant to eliminate the focal site of seizure activity in the brain, aborting or even eliminating seizures. In LMICs, however, the availability and use of such advanced surgical techniques are significantly compromised. A review of functional neurosurgery practices verifies that while epilepsy is much more common in LMIC, actual surgical application is very low due to a myriad of socio-economic barriers as well as the prohibitive cost of availing surgical care (Fezeu et al., 2018). Overcoming these, thus, requires concerted effort and creativity to ensure that surgical practice fits the singular needs and resources available within LMIC settings. Furthermore, advances in surgical technique need to keep pace with advances in technology and method, particularly in the area of functional neurosurgery. Functional neurosurgery attempts to reconstitute lost function using new techniques such as DBS and responsive neurostimulation. The use of advanced imaging modalities has significantly contributed to the precision of such surgery, allowing for more personalized intervention for every patient. Also, with growing health disparities awareness globally, there is increased emphasis on collaboration building between high-income and LMIC. Such collaborations can facilitate the exchange of knowledge and resources, ultimately improving the accessibility of surgical treatment to patients who can afford it. The combined efforts to bridge the gap between clinical need and resource supply for neurosurgical care are critical to addressing the greater burden of neurological diseases worldwide, which calls for a more balanced health setting (Fezeu et al., 2018).

12.4.3. Rehabilitation Therapies

The field of neurological rehabilitation encompasses a variety of therapies oriented to functional restoration and improvement of QoL in patients with neurological disease. Rehabilitation therapies, including physical, occupational, and speech therapy, are combined to address the multifaceted issues of stroke, TBI, and neurodegenerative disease patients recovering from. Notably, the therapies are not just for rehabilitative purposes but also preventive in nature, with the aim of preventing further deterioration of the patient's condition. Emphasizing multidisciplinary care has proven effective in providing interventions tailored to an individual's specific needs, as whole-person care has been shown to optimize overall outcomes. Their integration is essential for rehabilitation that encompasses not only physical disabilities but also cognitive and psychological dimensions, thereby providing comprehensive care for the patient in the neurological context. Amongst all the modalities utilized in neurological rehabilitation, psychological interventions step into the limelight increasingly as integral elements. They were recently found to contribute to pain relief and improve emotional states in patients with neurological illnesses, while also enhancing compliance with physical interventions. Techniques such as Cognitive-Behavioral Therapy, mindfulness, and Acceptance and Commitment Therapy have proven to reverse pain subtypes in diseases such as MS and post-stroke pain according to the Italian Consensus Conference on Pain in Neurorehabilitation classification. Psychological treatments serve as beneficial supplements to conventional rehabilitation by providing improved, comprehensive, patient-centered care. By breaking psychological barriers, these therapies enable a stronger rehabilitation process, allowing patients to become actively involved in their own recovery. Physical rehabilitation therapies play an important role in the rehabilitation of neurological impaired patients as well, particularly in such neurodegenerative disorders as progressive supranuclear palsy (PSP). Increasing evidence supports the potential of gait rehabilitation, balance training, and personalized exercise programs to enhance functional outcomes in patients with such atypical presentations of Parkinsonism. Notwithstanding this, literature demonstrates heterogeneity within reporting and use of these exercise treatments, with calls for increased documentation of intervention protocols. Use of standardized reporting templates, for example, the consensus on exercise reporting template (CERT), would render these studies more replicable and facilitate the enhancement of the knowledge regarding effective exercise interventions. Such care in reporting detail would not only enhance the evidence base for physical interventions but also facilitate practice harmonization across rehabilitation settings and maximize patient care provision for patients with neurological conditions.

Test Your Knowledge

1. What are the common classes of pharmacological agents used to manage neurodegenerative diseases?
2. How do rehabilitation therapies contribute to functional recovery in patients with stroke or traumatic brain injury?

12.5. The Role of Neurology in Mental Health

Learning Outcome

1. Understand the connection between neurology and psychiatry
2. Discuss the neurological basis of mental disorders
3. Focus on the treatment of co-occurring neurological and psychiatric conditions

Neurology is critical for understanding and addressing mental illness because it acts as the bridge between the brain's biological processes and psychological processes. Advances in neuroimaging tools over the last decade have allowed researchers to visualize changes in brain function and anatomy that are responsible for much of mental illness, including depression and anxiety. These instruments show that disorders that are normally explained as being purely psychological can be identified with specific neurological dysfunction. For example, neurotransmitter imbalances—e.g., serotonin and dopamine—invoke neurological involvement in mood disorders. In addition, knowledge of the importance of neuroplasticity provides an understanding of how treatment can bring about structural and functional changes in the brain, ultimately to facilitate recovery as well as overall mental health improvement. The intersection of psychological factors and neurological disorders is most common in diseases like IBS, which presents the case of how mental health can be the cause of physical disease. Psychological interventions, such as CBT, have been effective in managing IBS symptoms through the regulation of the mind-gut relationship. The relationship underscores the need for an interdisciplinary approach that fuses psychological and neurological perspectives in treating the condition. By the confluence of neurological principles and traditional therapeutic methods, clinicians can create treatment plans tailored to an individual that enhance the efficacy of interventions. Not only does this dual approach reduce symptoms, but it also leads to a deeper understanding of underlying mechanisms, ultimately leading to improved patient outcomes. Moreover, the inclusion of neurological information in mental illness treatment favors the integration paradigm that emphasizes harmony among neurologists, psychiatrists, and psychologists. This integration allows for an integral assessment of patients through both medical and psychological evaluation. By understanding the neurological substrate for mental disorders, clinicians can treat more effectively with evidence-based treatment strategies based on individual presentation. Ongoing research into brain function continues to reveal avenues for new therapeutic approaches. As research progresses, the focus on integrating neurological models into mental health will better capture such sensitive interactions, ultimately leading to more effective patient management (Sothu et al., 2025; Verma et al., 2025).

12.5.1. Connection Between Neurology and Psychiatry

The interface between psychiatry and neurology has become more highlighted, particularly with advances in neuroimaging and neurophysiology, which are enhancing the understanding of the etiology of psychiatric disease. Neurology is primarily concerned with diagnosing and treating cerebral diseases such as stroke, epilepsy, and neurodegenerative diseases. In contrast, psychiatry is concerned with psychiatric diseases such as anxiety, schizophrenia, and mood disorders. However, the overlap between these specialties is significant; psychiatric manifestations are most commonly observed in neurological conditions, illustrating the kind of holistic treatment approach that is required. For instance, certain forms of epilepsy, such as temporal lobe epilepsy, have the potential to produce psychiatric disturbance, illustrating that psychological well-being is an impairment of brain function and that there is a need for interdisciplinary treatment in the management of both aspects of a patient's condition (Barker et al., 2007). Further exploration of the interface between psychiatry and neurology is exemplified by conditions such as depression, which often occurs in patients with cognitive compromise or neurodegenerative illness, e.g., dementia. Research has demonstrated that depression symptoms may act as risk factors or prodromes in older persons with mental impairments. This reflects the complex dynamic between psychological and neurological health, necessitating rigorous assessments that consider both emotional and cognitive factors in patient treatment. There are different hypotheses regarding how depression interacts with dementia, according to a systematic review, and these indicate the multiaspectual nature of the interactions (Baeken et al., 2020).

More research in this area needs to be conducted to design effective interventions and improve patient outcomes in both places. Additionally, the evolution of neuroimaging techniques, such as EEG-fMRI, further reveals precise details of how neurological conditions are transmitted and affect psychological states. Such multi-dimensional imaging has identified potential pathways of neural activity, demonstrating how interference in one part of the brain influences others and has implications for both neurological and psychiatric outcomes. With the convergence of neurophysiological data and psychiatric assessment, clinicians are capable of having a complete picture of a patient's condition, facilitating effective and informed treatment. The detection of these connections underscores the importance of interdisciplinarity among psychiatrists and neurologists, ultimately leading to more thorough patient treatment that addresses the full spectrum of brain activity and behavior (Barker et al., 2007) (Figure 12.14).

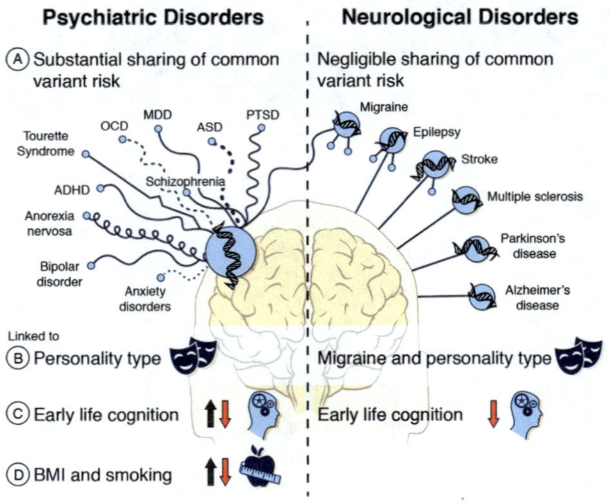

Figure 12.14. Genetic link between psychiatric and neurological disorders.

Source: https://mbi.ufl.edu/files/2018/06/Mathews-figure-for-post-2-600x498.jpg.

12.5.2. Neurological Basis of Mental Disorders

Understanding the neurobiological basis of mental illnesses is imperative to the development of effective treatment strategies and improving the QoL for affected individuals. Recent advances in neuroscience reveal that psychiatric diseases are more likely to be described as resulting from specific neural circuits, imbalances of neurotransmitters, and disruptions in brain structures. For instance, diseases such as depression and anxiety have been associated with dysregulation in serotonin and dopamine systems, hence highlighting the involvement of biochemical processes in modulating emotions. In addition, this neurochemical model accounts for why pharmacologic treatment, e.g., SSRIs or atypical antipsychotics, can constitute an effective therapeutic process for such disorders. Furthermore, the identification of mental illness as a legitimate medical issue can serve to reduce stigma, creating access to an enlightened citizenry that will accept those who are dealing with these conditions (Brodniak et al., 2000).

The correspondence between nervous system activity and mental well-being continues to be explored in the realm of psychomotor theory, which posits that mental states and body motion are inextricably intertwined through a feedback process in the mind-brain-body system. This model demonstrates that symptoms of psychiatry are found concomitantly with disturbances of movement, and neurological disorders are found to provoke symptoms of the psyche, suggesting a reciprocal relationship. Coordination between the mental and motor processes signifies shared neural substrates underlying this relationship, emphasizing how disturbances in one system can deleteriously affect the other. Understanding of this process provides valuable insight into the complexity of the treatment of mental illness because treatment modalities may have to consider the psychological as well as motor component, and promote integrative treatment approaches that honor the wholeness of the psychomotor system (Tan et al., 2007).

Early recognition and treatment of mental illness are also significant in preventing potential long-term consequences. Educational programs designed to de-stigmatize mental illness in various settings, including the workplace, can be instrumental in creating awareness and fostering early recognition. Through the supply of symptom recognition tools and encouragement of access to mental health treatment, it is possible to create a culture that promotes and pursues mental wellness. Including mental health education within organizations not only boosts productivity but also positively influences overall employee morale. All these can ultimately work together to create an environment where mental health is openly addressed and discussed with the same care as physical health, significantly improving the QoL for those afflicted with mental disorders (Brodniak et al., 2000).

12.5.3. Treatment of Co-occurring Neurological and Psychiatric Conditions

Management of co-existing neurological and psychiatric disease is a complex issue that necessitates a whole-person approach. Neurological diseases such as Parkinson's disease often occur in conjunction with psychiatric disease, and consequent compounded symptoms complicate diagnosis and treatment. For instance, Parkinson's patients can experience depression or anxiety, which exacerbate their motor symptomatology as well as their overall QoL. These converging issues call for a collaborative care model blending both psychiatric and neurological insight. The clinicians must adopt an interdisciplinary model in which mental health practitioners and neurologists talk and collaborate effectively to provide holistic patient care. Such integration not only optimizes the efficacy of treatment but can even mitigate the stigma that precedes discussing mental health when dealing with neurological illnesses. Similarly, new treatments are being created as promising interventions for patients with comorbidities. Dance therapy, for example, has been shown to improve cognitive and motor functioning in patients with Parkinson's disease because it encompasses both physical exercise and social interaction, thus addressing the psychological element of treatment (Brodniak et al., 2000). This is an argument for therapies other than the normal application of medications, and aiming towards rehabilitation procedures that cater to both the neurological and psychiatric dimensions. Therapies like dance therapy not only encourage physical well-being but also allow for emotional expression and connection, both of which are crucial in enhancing the overall condition of patients. The blend of physical and mental stimulation inherent in such therapies would provide a more balanced treatment approach, radically improving patients' QoL. In addition, the work environment is an essential setting in which to treat mental illness, particularly in people who have neurological disorders and who face stigma and ignorance in work settings (Brodniak et al., 2000). Investing in mental health educational programs at work can empower employees to get help for early warning signs and build a culture of concern, which reduces the isolation of those struggling with co-occurring disorders. Organizations that make such investments benefit not only their employees but also overall productivity by promoting a healthy work environment. Therefore, initiatives to de-mythologize mental illness problems and expand support networks in the workplace are vital to efficient management and care of individuals with the double load of neurological and psychiatric disorders. This holistic approach is essential in fostering an environment that prizes both body and mind wellness.

Test Your Knowledge

1. How do neurological disorders contribute to the development or exacerbation of psychiatric symptoms?
2. What are some common mental health disorders that have a known neurological basis?
3. What treatment approaches are effective in managing patients with both neurological and psychiatric symptoms?

12.6. Advances in Neurological Research

Learning Outcome

1. Describe the term neurogenetics and its implications
2. Deal with innovations in neurotechnology
3. Focus on future directions in neurological studies

The field of neurological science has undergone significant development, particularly concerning the intricate relationship between sensory impairment and mobility among the elderly. An exemplary research study has highlighted the contribution of visual impairment to physical mobility, showing that older adults with self-reported eye disease exhibit compromised mobility performance and increased fear of falling (FOF) avoidance behavior. The 455 community-residing participants in the study show that higher FOF avoidance is more likely to have greater mobility impairment among participants. Against expectations, the study also shows that visual acuity, as a separate factor, is not significantly associated with mobility outcomes. It suggests an intricate interaction of psychological and physiological factors requiring further research. Clinicians are thus forced to adopt broad-based assessments beyond the usual visual acuity tests, which may enhance the management of the risk of falls among the elderly, as laid out in the study's definitive report (Andrew et al., 2017). In addition, recent research on stroke has found new facts regarding how white and grey matter damage differ with periods of development. Whereas classical research described predominantly grey matter injury, compelling evidence today highlights the supreme role of white matter disease in ischemia. The novel focus of research highlights age-specific vulnerabilities of cellular components like axons and oligodendrocytes during ischemic attacks. For instance, pre-term infants exhibit a characteristic vulnerability to pathologies like periventricular leukomalacia (PVL), whereas older cohorts are faced with special demands posed by altered ischemic responses. Awareness of such developmental variations is crucial for personalizing therapeutic interventions and improving effective stroke treatments to enhance clinical practices specific to each life stage. This evolving perception necessitates rethinking of the unified mechanisms of stroke and encourages emerging streams of research in neurology (Muscat et al., 2013). In addition, the integration of advanced imaging techniques and molecular biology with neurology research has fueled our understanding of several neural disorders. Techniques such as fMRI and diffusion tensor imaging enable unprecedented visualization of brain structure and function, allowing us to identify unique biomarkers associated with neurological diseases. They enable more comprehensive investigations of neurodegenerative diseases such as Alzheimer's and Parkinson's, opening up insights into disease progression and into therapeutic targets. Further, improvements in genetic and epigenetic research are unraveling the complex interactions between genetic predispositions and environmental factors in the development of neurological diseases. As technologies continue to evolve, they will improve diagnostic accuracy, inform treatment models, and ultimately improve patient outcomes in neurology. The proliferation of multidisciplinary approaches is a milestone in neurological studies, with implications for new potential for innovation and better patient care among victims of many neurological diseases.

12.6.1. Neurogenetics and Its Implications

Neurogenetics, the cross-disciplinary field of genetics and neuroscience, has assumed a key role in knowing the genetic basis of neurological disorders. By investigating how some mutations in genes affect the functioning of neurons, researchers are discovering pathways that shed light on schizophrenia, bipolar disorder, and autism. These discoveries have far-reaching implications for the design of targeted therapies as well as the formulation of tailored treatment regimens. For instance, genetic marker identification can be beneficial in predicting susceptibility and disease progression, allowing clinicians to customize treatment according to one's genetic constitution. Understanding the neurobiological substrate of such disorders enhances the potential for discovering novel pharmacological targets and ultimately broadening the reach of traditional neurology to precision medicine. Neurogenetics is also instrumental in untangling the complexities of drug use disorders, particularly alcohol dependence. Research shows that people who are genetically predisposed may have different neurobiological responses to alcohol that influence their susceptibility towards abusive drinking behaviors. With the use of scales such as the Temperament and Character Inventory (TCI), researchers can explore interactions between personality traits, severity of craving, and genes relating to alcohol use disorder (AUD). The findings from these studies indicate the necessity of incorporating genetic evaluations into treatment plans to improve recovery rates. As our understanding grows with advances in the genetic factors involved in addiction, it is becoming clearer that a genetic component must be considered when developing extended treatment strategies for patients who suffer from substance use disorders (Attilia et al., 2014). In addition to psychiatric and substance abuse disorders, neurogenetics is revolutionizing the landscape of genetic illnesses such as DMD. As it informs not only the prognosis but also the suitability of new therapies to correct specific mutations, accurate genetic testing becomes imperative. The recent discovery of molecular therapies designed to replace or restore dystrophin function has revolutionized the treatment of DMD by clinicians. Technologies like multiplex ligation-dependent probe amplification (MLPA) make it possible to identify patients who can benefit from exonic-skipping therapies. New technologies like CRISPR-Cas9 also bring much promise to future interventions. With advances in neurogenetics, it continues to be a core pillar in the quest for personalized medicine, and it brings hope for improved treatment for patients with genetically determined neurological disorders (Bello et al., 2016) (Figure 12.15).

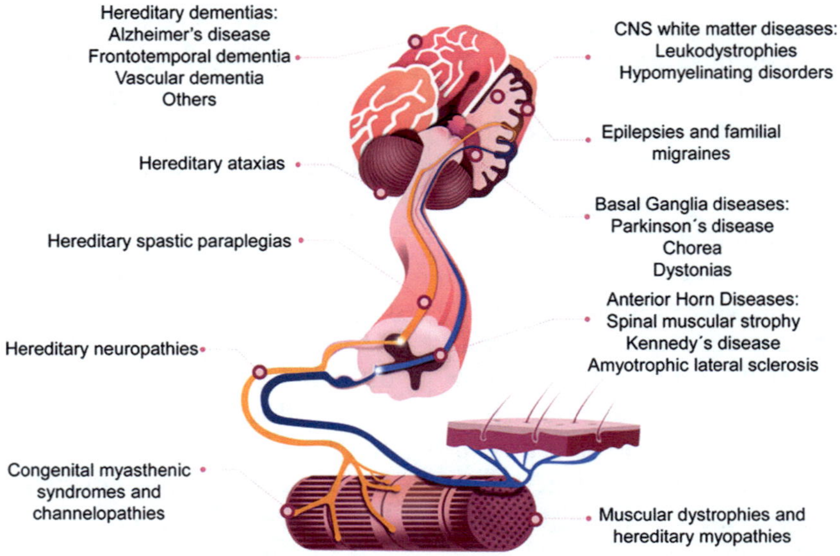

Figure 12.15. Major groups of neurogenetic conditions according to the topographical diagnosis.

Source: https://www.researchgate.net/publication/365244955/figure/fig1/AS:11431281225529555@1708769430416/Major-groups-of-neurogenetic-conditions-according-to-the-topographical-diagnosis.jpg.

12.6.2. Innovations in Neurotechnology

Neurotechnology advancements are a watershed in our understanding and interaction with the human brain. Among the developments is the innovation of brain-computer interfaces (BCIs), a highly significant innovation that provides a one-to-one interface between the brain and devices outside the brain. The application of BCIs is vast, ranging from medical therapy for individuals with motor disabilities to the enhancement of cognitive abilities and healthy humans. Above all, the combination of machine learning algorithms with neural signals not only allows for improved control of prosthetic limbs but also promises the future possibility of converting thoughts into functional commands. While scholars consider the implications of such technologies, it is increasingly clear that the intersection of neurotechnology and ethics requires close examination, particularly regarding privacy and mental autonomy, highlighting a critical need for regulatory standards to control their application responsibly. The ethical objections to neurotechnology advancements are not just about enhancing capabilities; they are also raising fundamental questions about the nature of personal information. At the heart of it is the idea of Conceptualizing Mental Data, which expounds the notion that thoughts are not merely aspects of one's personality but also intimate personal data. The implications of this framework are especially relevant in the context of the General Data Protection Regulation (GDPR), which has the aim of putting robust controls on personal data. With BCIs even having the potential to decode thoughts, the challenge is to separate beneficial uses of neurotechnology from the risk of exploitation. Such a challenge necessitates a careful examination of legal frameworks to protect people's rights, highlighting the need for interdisciplinary collaboration among neuroscientists, ethicists, and policymakers to successfully navigate the new era of neurotechnology (Fonseca et al., 2023). Moreover, as neurotechnology is altering every area of society, from the criminal justice system, the ethical issues intensify. Neurointerventions, particularly in assessing culpability or rehabilitation, introduce additional dimensions involving accountability and autonomy. Data indicate that social attitudes toward these interventions are influenced by both cultural factors and perceptions of justice, foreseeing a broad disparity in acceptance levels. Medicinal clinicians who participate in these procedures are most often faced with ethical dilemmas, walking the thin line between patient dignity and societal safety. While such innovations need to be utilized for rehabilitation and fair sentencing, absolute care must be exercised regarding the effects of reducing an individual's mental autonomy. This underscores the necessity of strong ethical guidelines as neurotechnology becomes more deeply embedded within legal frameworks (Whitaker et al., 2018) (Figure 12.16).

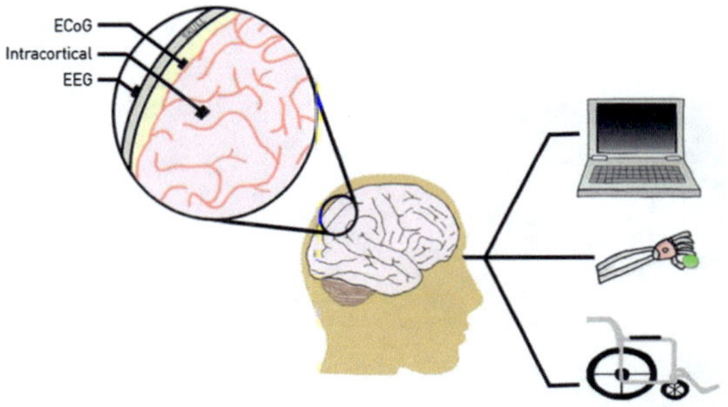

Figure 12.16. Types of brain-computer interfaces and their uses. There are three types of BCIs. They can be non-invasive, such as EEG (measured on the scalp), invasive, such as ECoG (measured on the cortex), and intracortical.

Source: https://www.researchgate.net/profile/Shujhat-Khan/publication/335892770/figure/fig1/AS:804287135375361@1568768404878/Types-of-brain-computer-interfaces-and-their-uses-There-are-3-types-of-BCIs-They-can-be.jpg.

12.6.3. Future Directions in Neurological Studies

With advancing neurology, the future of neurological research is fast shifting towards integrating novel technologies with traditional methodologies. The ongoing overlap of neuroimaging, genetics, and computational analytics is opening avenues for explaining and understanding complicated neurological disorders like never before. For instance, multi-institutional collaborative research efforts such as the Enhancing Neuroimaging Genetics through Meta-Analysis (ENIGMA) Stroke Recovery working group try to explain the interaction of brain structure and function in survivors of strokes. With a pool of data from over 2100 participants in multiple countries, this work is a leap forward in helping to decipher brain-behavior dynamics that underlie recovery processes. By emphasizing scalable data acquisition and multisite harmonization, this research aims to hone our understanding of stroke mechanisms and improve rehabilitation techniques, a testament to big data's potential in transforming neurological research and informing clinical practices (Assogna et al., 2020). With concomitant advances in neuroimaging and the addition of robust clinical trial evidence, neurological research will be affected in the future, particularly in treatment strategies for recurrent neurological events. The findings of trials like RESTART, which demonstrate the potential benefit of antiplatelet therapy in reducing extracerebral hemorrhage risk, highlight the importance of including brain imaging features in clinical decision-making. Specifically, determining how cerebral microbleeds influence brain traits can make therapy more efficient and safer for patients. This area of research also reflects the tremendous promise of personalized medicine in neurology, where treatments are developed to be patient-specific based on brain imaging and patient traits, thus holding promise for much better interventions in the treatment of complex neurological disorders (Abano et al., 2019). Also, the future of neuroscientific research will likely embrace interdisciplinary collaborations involving neuroscience with AI and machine learning. These technologies promise to automate data analysis and even predict patient outcomes through large datasets from varied sources. As computational models get increasingly sophisticated, they could potentially enable researchers to combine enormous amounts of neuroimaging and genetic data better to understand diseases like Alzheimer's and Parkinson's. To do that, however, would require setting ethical standards to enable the use of patient data responsibly, particularly as concerns privacy and informed consent. Thus, the definition of these guidelines will be instrumental in establishing a platform where technological advancement can enhance clinical neurology without compromising ethical standards, thereby increasing the efficacy of future neurological research.

Test Your Knowledge

1. What is neurogenetics, and how has it advanced our understanding of hereditary neurological disorders?
2. Describe some recent innovations in neurotechnology and their applications in diagnosing or treating neurological diseases.
3. What are some key challenges and future directions in neurological research aimed at improving patient outcomes?

SUMMARY

The field of neurology is being regularly updated, with both traditional and non-traditional approaches to patient care. The integration of palliative care principles into neurology, particularly in the treatment of chronic diseases such as Parkinson's disease, is a significant advancement in the care of neurological conditions. From the perspective of palliative care, doctors are not only able to treat the physical symptoms of such diseases but also the psychological and spiritual facets of patients and families. All such a comprehensive approach can do to improve the QoL and therapeutic response for patients suffering from disabling neurologic disorders is highlight an essential shift in perspective beyond curative interventions alone to those with a focus on patient-centered interventions and symptom management, as illustrated in research accounts on palliative care for PD (Bekelman et al., 2017). In addition, neurology is a complex problem, and fixing it will demand interdisciplinary work from healthcare providers. Both methodological and observational studies matter in this case since they aid in determining the needs of individuals with neurological disorders. Utilizing assessment tools developed from those used for other long-term ailments, neurologists will be able to tailor interventions better to overcome the individual barriers posed by diseases like Parkinson's. Notably, as the specialty increasingly learns from experience in managing other health disorders, neurologists are being asked to help facilitate greater collaboration in research. These collaborative efforts can lead to a more robust understanding and better interventions, ultimately benefiting patients with a variety of neurological disorders (Bekelman et al., 2017). Lastly, ongoing progress in neurology underscores the importance of translating clinical practice to increasingly extensive aspects of patient management. As described in other research, the potential benefits of including long-term follow-up care can provide valuable information about treatment efficacy, once more favoring a more advanced treatment approach. Tracking outcomes, such as adopting successful treatments over extended periods, allows healthcare professionals to maximize their interventions and improve patient compliance. By deploying technologies and methods from proximal science, the neurology community is poised to advance its understanding of patient care dynamics, promoting innovations that not only respond to current medical needs but also enhance long-term well-being.

Neurology is a wide category of CNS disorders with considerable QoL implications for patients. Among these conditions, PD stands out in that both motor and non-motor symptoms are involved. Non-motor symptoms like depression, anxiety, and cognitive impairment have come to be increasingly recognized as strong predictors of well-being in PD patients. The non-motor symptoms scale (NMSS) provides a validated instrument to assess the frequency and severity of these symptoms, highlighting the importance of global assessments beyond conventional subjective motor symptoms. By accurately categorizing non-motor symptom burden (NMSB), clinicians can tailor interventions to maximize patient care and direct treatment planning. This supports the idea that effective management of neurological illness requires a more than one-dimensional perspective in understanding patient needs and experiences (Antonini et al., 2013). MS is an excellent case of the complex interplay between neurological disease and QoL. This disabling disease is characterized by fluctuating symptomology, not just disrupting routine, but also causing significant emotional and interpersonal challenges. While individuals adjust to the implications of the disease, psychological intervention plays an important part in facilitating adaptation and managing distress. A trial of CBT versus supportive listening demonstrates the possible value of psychological treatment for the management of early MS. These trials underscore the importance of integrating mental health strategies into the overall domain of neurological care, overcoming psychosocial barriers that affect compliance with treatment and overall life satisfaction. The conclusions derived from this study can help inform best practices and aid in making better therapeutic interventions available to patients confronted with the uncertain prognosis of their illness (Bogosian et al., 2009). Finally, neurology encompasses a variety of conditions that require advanced treatment and care approaches for patients. The acknowledgment of non-motor symptoms in illnesses like Parkinson's, and the psychological aspects of MS, underscores the sheer importance of interfacing care models. Future approaches must not only tackle the biological aspects of the disorders but also integrate emotional and cognitive elements into the treatment model. By prioritizing multidimensional strategies, healthcare experts can help improve patient outcomes and QoL for victims of neurological disease. All this is fundamental to establishing neurology as a medical discipline and making therapeutic interventions as integrated and beneficial as possible.

KEY TERMS FROM THIS CHAPTER

- Alzheimer's disease
- Avoidance behavior
- Brain-computer interfaces
- Cognitive functions
- Cognitive rehabilitation
- Electrophysiological tests
- Exercise interventions
- General Data Protection Regulation (GDPR)
- Health system
- Anatomical investigations
- Brain trauma
- Cognitive disorders
- Cognitive impairment
- Electrophysiological methods
- Ethical dilemmas
- Extensive system
- Guillain-Barré syndrome (GBS)
- Intellectual functions

CRITICAL THINKING QUESTIONS

1. **What is the characteristic clinical feature of Parkinson's disease?**
   a. Spasticity
   b. Resting tremor
   c. Hyperreflexia
   d. Sensory loss
2. **Which diagnostic test is considered the gold standard for confirming multiple sclerosis?**
   a. CT scan
   b. EEG
   c. MRI of the brain and spinal cord
   d. PET scan
3. **Which neurological disorder is characterized by demyelination of the central nervous system?**
   a. Amyotrophic lateral sclerosis (ALS)
   b. Multiple sclerosis (MS)
   c. Myasthenia gravis
   d. Peripheral neuropathy
4. **Which diagnostic technique is most useful in evaluating peripheral nerve function?**
   a. MRI
   b. EEG
   c. Nerve conduction study (NCS)
   d. Lumbar puncture
5. **Which of the following is the most common cause of peripheral neuropathy worldwide?**
   a. Diabetes mellitus
   b. Vitamin B12 deficiency
   c. Guillain-Barré syndrome
   d. Chronic alcoholism

Short Answer Questions

1. What are the hallmark clinical features of Parkinson's disease, and how do they differ from those of Alzheimer's disease?
2. Which neurological disorders commonly present with demyelination, and what are their typical symptoms?
3. What are the primary diagnostic imaging techniques used in neurology, and when is each most appropriate?
4. How does electroencephalography (EEG) contribute to the diagnosis of seizure disorders?
5. What pharmacological treatments are currently used to manage symptoms of multiple sclerosis?
6. When are surgical interventions considered for patients with neurological disorders, and what are some examples?
7. How do rehabilitation therapies support recovery and improve quality of life in stroke patients?

Answers to Critical Thinking Questions

1. (b); 2. (c); 3. (b); 4. (c); 5. (a)

REFERENCES

1. Salman, R. A., Minks, D. P., Mitra, D., Rodrigues, M. A., Bhatnagar, P., Du Plessis, J. C., Joshi, Y., Dennis, M. S., Murray, G. D., Newby, D. E., Sandercock, P. a. G., Sprigg, N., Stephen, J., Sudlow, C. L. M., Werring, D. J., Whiteley, W. N., Wardlaw, J. M., White, P. M., Baigent, C., . . . Thomas, K. (2019). Effects of antiplatelet therapy on stroke risk by brain imaging features of intracerebral haemorrhage and cerebral small vessel diseases: subgroup analyses of the RESTART randomised, open-label trial. *The Lancet Neurology*, *18*(7), 643–652. https://doi.org/10.1016/s1474-4422(19)30184-xAdams, R., Akassoglou, K., Akenami, M. A., Albright, A. V., et al. (2018). A perspective of coagulation dysfunction in multiple sclerosis and in experimental allergic encephalomyelitis. https://core.ac.uk/download/195777098.pdf (accessed on 27th June 2025).
2. Agnetti, V., Aiello, E., De Natale, E., Deriu, F., et al. (2012). Effects of dance therapy on balance, gait and neuro-psychological performances in patients with Parkinson's disease and postural instability. https://core.ac.uk/download/16749566.pdf (accessed on 27th June 2025).
3. Agostini, M., Alfonsi, E., Aloisi, A. M., Alvisi, F., et al. (2016). Psychological treatments and psychotherapies in the neurorehabilitation of pain: Evidences and recommendations from the Italian consensus conference on pain in neurorehabilitation. https://core.ac.uk/download/54538696.pdf (accessed on 27th June 2025).
4. Akam, T., Bauer, M., Blankenship, A., Brittain, J., Brown, P., Cecere, R., et al. (2016). Causal evidence that intrinsic beta frequency is relevant for enhanced signal propagation in the motor system as shown through rhythmic TMS. https://core.ac.uk/download/30710882.pdf (accessed on 27th June 2025).
5. Albin, R., Alcalay, R. N., Babcock, D., Bowman, F., et al. (2017). Parkinson's disease biomarkers: Perspective from the NINDS Parkinson's Disease Biomarkers Program. https://core.ac.uk/download/187423794.pdf (accessed on 27th June 2025).
6. Anderson, T. J., Añor, S., Barcelona, D., Cardinal Herrera University, C. E. U., Ehlers, R., et al. (2015). Development of learning objectives for neurology in a veterinary curriculum: Part II: Postgraduates. https://core.ac.uk/download/36778153.pdf (accessed on 27th June 2025).
7. Andrew, L., Davis, T., & Johnson, C. (2017). The impact of visual impairments on mobility performance in community-dwelling older adults. https://digitalscholarship.unlv.edu/cgi/viewcontent.cgi?article=3923&context=thesesdissertations (accessed on 27th June 2025).
8. Antonini, A., Brooks, D. J., Brown, R. J., Martinez-Martin, P., et al. (2013). A proposal for a comprehensive grading of Parkinson's disease severity combining motor and non-motor assessments: Meeting an unmet need. https://core.ac.uk/download/16220107.pdf (accessed on 27th June 2025).
9. Assogna, F., Baugh, L. A., Bhattacharya, A. K., Bigjahan, R., et al. (2020). The ENIGMA Stroke Recovery Working Group: Big data neuroimaging to study brain–behavior relationships after stroke. https://core.ac.uk/download/322929945.pdf (accessed on 27th June 2025).
10. Attilia, M. L., Battagliese, G., Berman, M. O., Blum, K., et al. (2014). Neurophysiological measures and alcohol use disorder (AUD): Hypothesizing links between clinical severity index and molecular neurobiological patterns. https://core.ac.uk/download/158327904.pdf (accessed on 27th June 2025).

11. Aylward, S. R., Gerig, G., Hovda, D. A., Irimia, A., et al. (2012). Neuroimaging of structural pathology and connectomes in traumatic brain injury: Toward personalized outcome prediction. https://core.ac.uk/download/323078685.pdf (accessed on 27th June 2025).

12. Baeken, C., Engelborghs, S., & Wiels, W. (2020). Depressive symptoms in the elderly: An early symptom of dementia? A systematic review. https://core.ac.uk/download/287939499.pdf (accessed on 27th June 2025).

13. Baker, D., Baneke, P., Brown, D., Browne, P., et al. (2012). Setting a research agenda for progressive multiple sclerosis: The International Collaborative on Progressive MS. https://core.ac.uk/download/30697961.pdf (accessed on 27th June 2025).

14. Barker, G. J., Duncan, J. S., Hamandi, K., Laufs, H., et al. (2007). Combined EEG-fMRI and tractography to visualize propagation of epileptic activity. https://core.ac.uk/download/1688790.pdf (accessed on 27th June 2025).

15. Bateman, K., Chavada, G., Cornblath, D. R., Cornblath, D., et al. (2017). International Guillain-Barré Syndrome Outcome Study (IGOS): Protocol of a prospective observational cohort study on clinical and biological predictors of disease course and outcome in Guillain-Barré syndrome. https://core.ac.uk/download/82893361.pdf (accessed on 27th June 2025).

16. Bekelman, D., Carter, J., Carter, J. H., Fox, S., et al. (2017). Palliative care and Parkinson's disease: Meeting summary and recommendations for clinical research. https://core.ac.uk/download/151161689.pdf (accessed on 27th June 2025).

17. Bello, L., & Pegoraro, E. (2016). Genetic diagnosis as a tool for personalized treatment of Duchenne muscular dystrophy. https://core.ac.uk/download/84921853.pdf (accessed on 27th June 2025).

18. Bender, S., Freitag, C. M., Helfrich, C., Pierau, F., et al. (2012). Monitoring cortical excitability during repetitive transcranial magnetic stimulation in children with ADHD: A single-blind, sham-controlled TMS-EEG study. https://core.ac.uk/download/14527403.pdf (accessed on 27th June 2025).

19. Bernstein, A., Geschwind, M., Higgins, J. J., Kramer, J. H., et al. (2019). Dementia assessment and management in primary care settings: A survey of current provider practices in the United States. https://core.ac.uk/download/323074480.pdf (accessed on 27th June 2025).

20. Bianco, A., Nunes, A., Gaillard, C., Bardi, G., Bates, K., Al-Jamal, K. T., Kostarelos, K., et al. (2013). Functionalized carbon nanotubes in the brain: Cellular internalization and neuroinflammatory responses. https://core.ac.uk/download/29416218.pdf (accessed on 27th June 2025).

21. Bogosian, A., Janssens, A., Stuifbergen, A., Williams, A., Wearden, A. J., Stuifbergen, A. K., Beck, A. T., et al. (2009). Protocol for the saMS trial (supportive adjustment for multiple sclerosis): A randomized controlled trial comparing cognitive behavioral therapy to supportive listening for adjustment to multiple sclerosis. https://core.ac.uk/download/pdf/8648829.pdf (accessed on 27th June 2025).

22. Bowers, R., ISPO (Funder), & Ross, K. (2009). A review of the effectiveness of lower limb orthoses used in cerebral palsy. https://core.ac.uk/download/9024488.pdf (accessed on 27th June 2025).

23. Brand, A., Clare, L., Hindle, J. V., Hoare, Z., et al. (2018). Goal-orientated cognitive rehabilitation for dementias associated with Parkinson's disease—A pilot randomized controlled trial. https://core.ac.uk/download/305121520.pdf (accessed on 27th June 2025).

24. Brodniak, W., Czabala, J. C., Dudek, B., International Labor Office, et al. (2000). *Mental Health in the Workplace: Situation Analyses, Poland.* https://core.ac.uk/download/5129369.pdf (accessed on 27th June 2025).

25. Brust, J., Creeley, C., Feldman, R., Grandjean, P., Herken, H., Panzica, G., Parent, M., et al. (2014). Neurotoxicity. https://core.ac.uk/download/286729125.pdf (accessed on 27th June 2025).

26. Chan, M., Hendry, M., Heng, I., Hu, Z., et al. (2014). MObile technology for improved family planning: Update to randomized controlled trial protocol. https://core.ac.uk/download/pdf/29050330.pdf (accessed on 27th June 2025).

27. Cronin-Golomb, A., Ellis, T. D., Otto, M. W., Reynolds, G. O., et al. (2015). The therapeutic potential of exercise to improve mood, cognition, and sleep in Parkinson's disease. https://open.bu.edu/bitstream/2144/30887/3/nihms735592.pdf (accessed on 27th June 2025).

28. Dalakas, M. (2018). Advances in the diagnosis, immunopathogenesis and therapies of IgM-anti-MAG antibody-mediated neuropathies. https://core.ac.uk/download/155271624.pdf (accessed on 27th June 2025).

29. Dawson, J., Lees, K. R., Quinn, T. J., Walters, M. R., et al. (2008). Variability in modified Rankin scoring across a large cohort of observers. https://core.ac.uk/download/110085.pdf (accessed on 27th June 2025).

30. Edwards, M. J., Roelofs, J. J., & Teodoro, T. (2019). Neuroimaging in functional movement disorders. https://core.ac.uk/download/187718363.pdf (accessed on 27th June 2025).

31. Elliott, E., Langhorne, P., & Quinn, T. J. (2018). Cognitive and mood assessment tools for use in stroke. https://core.ac.uk/download/132212026.pdf (accessed on 27th June 2025).

32. Ethell, I. M., Garcia, M., Koeppen, J., Leish, J., et al. (2016). Astrocytic Ephrin-B1 regulates synapse remodeling following traumatic brain injury. https://core.ac.uk/download/323067166.pdf (accessed on 27th June 2025).

33. Fezeu, F., Henderson, F., Larson, P. S., Melmer, T., et al. (2018). Challenges and solutions for functional neurosurgery in developing countries. https://core.ac.uk/download/323062978.pdf (accessed on 27th June 2025).

34. Fonseca, D. M. de B. (2023). Brain-computer interfaces and the decoding of thoughts as personal data of the mind. https://core.ac.uk/download/614518123.pdf (accessed on 27th June 2025).

35. Gaiseanu, F. (2020). Information based hierarchical brain organization/evolution from the perspective of the informational model of consciousness. https://core.ac.uk/download/322492692.pdf (accessed on 27th June 2025).

36. Giubilei, F. (2016). Beyond cholinesterase inhibition: Anti-inflammatory role and pharmacological profile of current drug therapy for Alzheimer's disease. https://core.ac.uk/download/98347745.pdf (accessed on 27th June 2025).

37. Gomes, M. M., Nard, A. E., & Santos, R. P. (2023). Neurophysiology in between the interests of Dom Pedro II of Brazil, and Charles Brown-Sequard. https://core.ac.uk/download/596312396.pdf (accessed on 27th June 2025).

38. Hoeglinger, G. U., & Stamelou, M. (2013). Atypical parkinsonism: An update. https://core.ac.uk/download/29414452.pdf (accessed on 27th June 2025).

39. Holth, J. K., Holtzman, D. M., Mahan, T. E., Robinson, S., et al. (2017). Altered sleep and EEG power in the P301S Tau transgenic mouse model. https://core.ac.uk/download/83101033.pdf (accessed on 27th June 2025).

40. Kay, K. A. (2015). Relapsing-remitting multiple sclerosis: Advances in disease-modifying therapies. https://open.bu.edu/bitstream/2144/13960/10/Kay_bu_0017N_11509_WEB.pdf (accessed on 27th June 2025).

41. McGinley, J. L., Morris, M. E., Slade, S. C., Underwood, M., et al. (2019). Exercise and progressive supranuclear palsy: The need for explicit exercise reporting. https://core.ac.uk/download/286359414.pdf (accessed on 27th June 2025).

42. Muramoto, O. (2018). Solving the Socratic problem—A contribution from medicine. https://core.ac.uk/download/186330370.pdf (accessed on 27th June 2025).

43. Muscat, R., Valentino, M., & Zammit, C. (2013). The spectrum of ischemia-induced white matter injury varies with age. https://core.ac.uk/download/46602551.pdf (accessed on 27th June 2025).

44. N/A. (2017). *2017 Commencement for Sidney Kimmel Medical College, Jefferson Graduate School of Biomedical Sciences, and Jefferson School of Population Health*. https://core.ac.uk/download/129191763.pdf (accessed on 27th June 2025).

45. N/A. (2018). *Outlook Magazine, Winter 2018*. https://core.ac.uk/download/212868990.pdf (accessed on 27th June 2025).

46. Nasevicius, A., Vaccaro, A., Schaffer, A. E., Rennekamp, A. J., Stewart, A. M., Schmid, B., Russell, C., et al. (2015). New zebrafish models of neurodegeneration. https://core.ac.uk/download/36778410.pdf (accessed on 27th June 2025).

47. Powell, D., & Schlotz, W. (2014). Ambulatory assessment in neuropsychology: Applications in multiple sclerosis research. https://core.ac.uk/download/80685934.pdf (accessed on 27th June 2025).

48. Riese, F., Savaskan, E., Tible, O. P., von Gunten, A., et al. (2017). Best practice in the management of behavioural and psychological symptoms of dementia. https://core.ac.uk/download/90215920.pdf (accessed on 27th June 2025).

49. Sae-Sia, W., Songwathana, P., & Sukraeny, N. (2013). Quality of life (QoL) in patients with traumatic brain injury (TBI): A literature review. https://media.neliti.com/media/publications/154444-EN-quality-of-life-qol-in-patients-with-tra.pdf (accessed on 27th June 2025).

50. Sothu, K., Kori, A., & Patil, S. (2025). Review on diagnosis, treatment and medication for dysmenorrhea for young to old age women. *Journal for Research in Applied Sciences and Biotechnology*. https://www.semanticscholar.org/paper/adcbc429147af4d90257c93de00830b7e85ea5d5 (accessed on 27th June 2025).

51. Tabrizi, S. J., & Wild, E. J. (2007). The differential diagnosis of chorea. https://core.ac.uk/download/1748286.pdf (accessed on 27th June 2025).

52. Tan, U. (2007). The psychomotor theory of human mind. https://core.ac.uk/download/pdf/86857.pdf (accessed on 27th June 2025).

INFECTIOUS DISEASES: TYPES, PATHOPHYSIOLOGY, DIAGNOSIS, AND TREATMENT OPTIONS

13

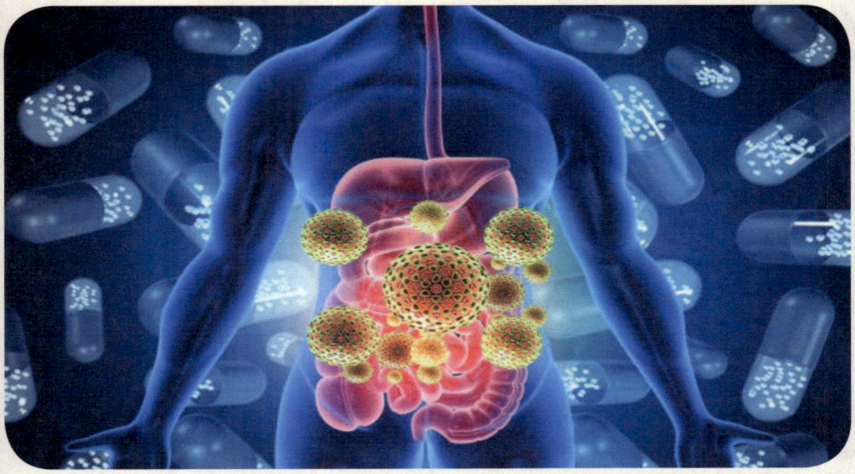

LEARNING OBJECTIVES

After studying this chapter, you will be able to:

1. Explain the types of infectious diseases
2. Discuss the pathophysiology of infectious diseases
3. Understand the diagnosis of infectious diseases
4. Describe treatment options for infectious diseases
5. Focus on prevention and control measures
6. Define the global impact of infectious diseases

Introduction

Understanding infectious diseases is an important aspect of general medicine, involving intricate relationships between pathogens and their human hosts. Infectious diseases are a significant cause of morbidity and mortality globally, demanding a solid grasp of their pathophysiology, epidemiology, and treatment. As clinicians encounter a range of infectious causes—from bacteria and viruses to fungi and parasites—they must acquire diagnostic skills and treatment approaches for individual conditions. This multidisciplinary field not only calls for knowledge of microbiology but also for incorporating infectious disease principles into public health practice. By addressing these diseases using an interdisciplinary approach, practitioners can optimize patient outcomes and reduce the overall disease burden on healthcare systems. An important aspect of infectious disease knowledge is the recognition of the dynamics of transmission. Different routes, including respiratory droplets, direct transmission, and vector-borne transmissions disseminate pathogens. Knowledge of these transmission modes is important in avoiding outbreaks and instituting efficient control measures. For example, a practice study of CP among primary care doctors highlights that many practitioners are unaware of specific syndromes, and this may lead to suboptimal management and more complications in patients with such syndromes (Calhoun et al., 2009). Moreover, the distinction between colonization and infection is essential because it determines appropriate interventions that can prevent unjustified use of antibiotics and combat the increasing threat of AMR. Apart from being aware of the clinical manifestation of infections, another wide-ranging approach is also the utilization of diagnostic tests for excluding or confirming infections. Based on research findings, utilization of urine cultures in hospital settings lacks sufficient backup tests for pyuria, which can lead to misdiagnosis and futile treatment practices (Carson et al., 2017). Hence, it is very much essential to improve the diagnosis accuracy in order to deliver appropriate management to UTI and other infectious disease patients. Improving diagnostic algorithms and staff training among healthcare workers can contribute to the healthcare community's active role in the successful management of infectious diseases. Finally, integrating these elements into medical practice and education can create a stronger, educated healthcare workforce to combat the challenges posed by infectious diseases.

Definition and Scope of Infectious Diseases

Infectious diseases form a broad range of medical conditions caused by pathogenic microbes, including bacteria, viruses, fungi, and parasites. They are characterized by their ability to provoke transmissions, which consequently lead to outbreaks affecting both individuals and the public in significant quantities. Infectious disease definitions constantly evolve with the discovery of new pathogens and increasing medical knowledge. This evolution does not just consist of classical vectors of infection but also the co-evolution between environmental and microbial resistance. The infectious disease ontology (IDO) is a significant resource for classifying and understanding diseases, focusing on their variability and the complexity of treatment and prevention (Bresell et al., 2009). This ontology enhances the understanding of the context for the development of infectious diseases, facilitating more productive interaction and research in the field of general medicine. The scope of infectious diseases is broad, infecting millions of individuals worldwide, predominantly in low- and middle-income nations where there may be scarce healthcare facilities. Infectious diseases are not merely clinical conditions; they are embedded within intricate socio-cultural and economic settings. Recent research emphasizes the need to incorporate social sciences into the study of these diseases, as they tend to identify societal factors driving disease spread and outcomes (Anyamba et al., 2011). Neglected tropical diseases (NTDs), for example, demonstrate the magnitude to which socioeconomic determinants directly influence the prevalence and control of health conditions, validating the need for interdisciplinary research in effectively understanding and combating these infections. As such, the convergence of different scientific disciplines in the development of comprehensive prevention and treatment approaches for infectious diseases is required to address both biomedical and socio-environmental determinants of health. In accordance with the definition and extent of infectious diseases, it is necessary to consider the technological developments driving infectious diseases research. With data sharing and interoperability becoming the priority in biomedical research, inclusion of ontologies is increasingly regarded as an advantage. Formal ontologies allow systematic annotation and structuring of vast quantities of infectious disease data, enabling more effective communication of results and development of interventions (Bresell et al.,

2009). As researchers try to clarify the complex interactions between hosts and pathogens, the need for robust computational systems comes into sharp relief. Ultimately, a technology-focused, transdisciplinary approach is necessary for our extension of knowledge and management of infectious disease, so that action is optimized and transferable across a variety of health environments (Figure 13.1).

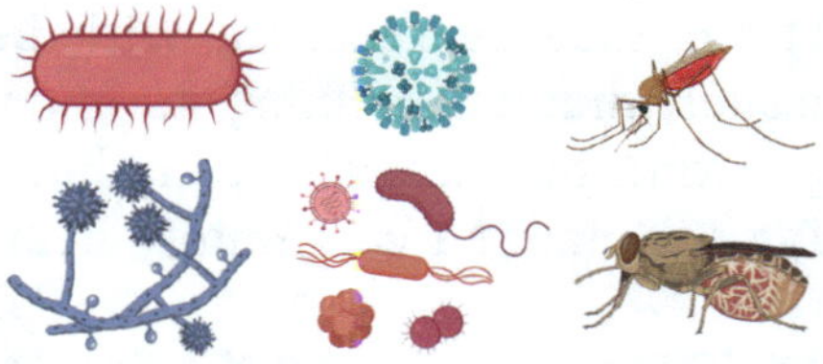

Figure 13.1. Diagram showing infectious diseases.

Source: https://microbenotes.com/wp-content/uploads/2024/04/Infectious-Diseases.jpeg.

Historical Context and Evolution of Infectious Disease Medicine

The past history of infectious disease medicine is one of sophistication in the interaction of scientific discovery and societal response. Since the identification of microorganisms by scientists such as Louis Pasteur and Robert Koch in the 19th century, the medical profession has started to change its concept of the causation of disease. This period marked the transition from miasma theory, where disease was linked to noxious air, to germ theory, enabling the advances in hygiene and the development of vaccines. Once these ideas gained traction, public health measures like quarantine, isolation, and immunization campaigns were developed, marking a groundbreaking change in the way societies dealt with infectious diseases. The social reaction to emergent pathogens, and the social stigma associated with diseases such as TB and cholera, also played an important part in the shaping of public health policy, recognizing the broader cultural atmosphere in which scientific advancement was embraced. The late 20th and early 21st centuries saw a new period characterized by a chain of viral epidemics and antibiotic-resistant illness. The evolving paradigm of infectious diseases was underscored by the emergence of HIV/AIDS, which challenged medical practitioners to their limits and to the forefront of extensive societal implications regarding stigma as well as treatment access. Furthermore, the emergence of drug-resistant microorganisms such as methicillin-resistant Staphylococcus aureus (MRSA) also underscored the limitations of previous medical achievements. As recent research has observed, media reports of MRSA tend to externalize responsibility by assigning blame for infection transmission to unsatisfactory hygiene practices within healthcare settings, rather than appreciating their biological complexity (Joffe et al., 2006). This shift reveals a necessary site of engagement between medical science and lay knowledge, underscoring the necessity of an integrated approach to infectious disease management. Even though the biomedical mode remains the default in infectious disease research, increasing awareness of the need for interdisciplinary models addressing social dynamics of disease spread is being met. Research into NTDs, for instance, points out the deficiencies of an exclusive biomedical orientation, revealing a perpetuating cycle where social science contributions are absent despite the richness of the diseases (Anyamba et al., 2011). While healthcare systems grapple with the multidisciplinary nature of infectious diseases, there is a need to close the gap between social sciences and biological research. Such a convergence not only enhances our understanding of disease mechanisms but also informs effective public health interventions. Developing a unifying methodology that incorporates diverse scientific perspectives will be crucial in addressing both known and newly emerging infectious diseases in an ever-evolving global environment.

Importance of Studying Infectious Diseases in Modern Medicine

Infectious disease knowledge is at the heart of the practice of modern medicine, particularly in light of increasing globalization and the rapid spread of pathogens. The rising incidence of infectious outbreaks solidifies the necessity for doctors to stay abreast of epidemiology, microbiology, and emerging pathogens. With the study of infectious diseases, medical practitioners are better able to diagnose, identify, and treat diseases that might otherwise turn epidemic. In addition, this pool of knowledge is essential in public health programs targeting the containment of infection spread, safeguarding community health, and creating efficient prevention measures. The multidisciplinary nature of infectious disease study guarantees a deep understanding of not just the pathogens themselves but also the socio-economic, cultural, and other factors that influence their spread patterns. An inherent aspect of infectious disease research is its ability to drive the creation of vaccines, which has been central in reducing morbidity and mortality rates in populations. Vaccination programs have long been successful in preventing the spread of some diseases, such as measles and polio, thereby pointing to the necessity of continued research on new and existing vaccines. Moreover, the development of infectious diseases via antibiotic resistance necessitates innovation in treatment and prevention strategies by medical practitioners and researchers. This kind of creative thinking is most frequently a result of public and private sector collaboration, as seen in Public-Private Partnerships for drug development and discovery research to tackle infectious diseases globally (Brown et al., 2009). Such collaborations are essential in advancing the field and keeping solutions as dynamic as ever-evolving challenges. Lastly, the research of infectious diseases is key to addressing the unique health needs of specific groups, like veterans who may be exposed to multi-faceted health risks. The United States Department of Veterans Affairs has developed comprehensive research programs for this population, recognizing the necessity of looking into the interaction of infectious diseases with chronic health issues due to combat experience (N/A, 2014). By expanding the field of infectious disease study to encompass veteran healthcare and social reintegration, medical practitioners can develop specialized interventions that consider the intricacies of this population's health. This highlights the intimate interlinking of infectious disease research with broader health issues, thus underlining its importance not only within the clinical setting but also in enhancing societal and community health.

13.1. Types of Infectious Diseases

Learning Outcome

1. Understand bacterial infections and their characteristics
2. Describe viral infections and their transmission methods
3. Discuss fungal and parasitic infections and their impact on health

Infectious diseases can be classified into various types based on their causative agent, mode of transmission, and nature of infection they produce. Bacterial infections, for instance, are infections produced by pathogenic bacteria such as TB and streptococcal infections. Targeted antibiotic therapy adequately treats these infections. Conversely, viral infections such as influenza and HIV involve more complex mechanisms because the viruses require host cells to replicate. The treatments and prevention processes for various types of pathogens are diverse, which emphasizes the importance of specific diagnostic techniques in hospitals. Moreover, the emergence of antibiotic-resistant bacteria has contributed to the challenge of treating bacterial infections, and hence the significance of continuous surveillance and innovative therapeutic regimens in infectious disease medicine. Fungal and parasitic infections are other groups within the category of infectious diseases. Fungal infections, such as candidiasis and aspergillosis, preferentially affect immunocompromised individuals and require antifungal agents for their treatment. Their prevalence has risen due to factors such as the increased use of immunosuppressive therapy and invasive procedures in medicine. Parasitic diseases like malaria and giardiasis are significant public health problems, especially in the tropics and subtropics. They are most often spread through vectors, with it entailing control barriers distinct from those for viral and bacterial diseases.

The social context in which these diseases are transmitted is most important; as has been described, emergent properties, such as the concept of hope, can influence public health interventions and treatment outcomes (Anderson et al., 2015), again demonstrating the convergence of social determinants and infectious disease epidemiology. Emerging infectious diseases point to the dynamic nature of pathogens and the potential impact on global health. These diseases, often the result of zoonotic transmission or environmental shifts, have become more apparent over recent decades, with examples such as Ebola and Zika viruses. New technology enables the rapid identification and characterization of such emerging pathogens, which can lead to effective public health interventions in a timely fashion. But as the infectious disease landscape evolves, there is an increasingly urgent necessity for robust data management systems. Ontology integration in biomedicine is a revolutionary development that allows for organizing and sharing infectious disease data. IDO offers an organized method for structuring and standardizing data, ultimately improving interoperability and collaboration in infectious disease research and treatment (Bresell et al., 2009). The change reflects the impact of technological innovation on addressing the complexity of modern infectious diseases.

13.1.1. Bacterial Infections and Their Characteristics

Bacterial infections constitute a significant challenge in the practice of general medicine and infectious diseases due to their diversity and pathogenic processes. Gram-positive and Gram-negative bacteria, for instance, differ in their structure and significantly contribute to their virulence and the immune response they elicit in the host. The presence of a dense peptidoglycan layer in Gram-positive bacteria makes them resistant to certain environmental pressures but susceptible to antibiotics like penicillin. Gram-negative bacteria with a sparse peptidoglycan layer and an outer membrane are more resistant to most antibiotic treatments and can secrete endotoxins, making them even harder to treat. An awareness of these fundamental differences is critical in framing appropriate therapeutic interventions and lowering the risk of grave bacterial infection outcomes. The relevance of bacterial infections runs deep, not only in the personal health consequences but also in public health. For instance, specific bacterial pathogens like those responsible for respiratory infections have been linked with elevated morbidity and mortality, particularly in immunocompromised patients. According to a study that examined respiratory disorders among HIV-infected patients, the incidence of respiratory infections remains far greater than that of their uninfected counterparts despite the introduction of highly active antiretroviral therapy (HAART). This is illustrated by data showing an odds ratio of 2.4 for incident respiratory infections in HAART-naive HIV-infected individuals before HAART, which decreases to 1.5 after HAART initiation but remains significantly elevated (Johannessen et al., 2013). Understanding these dynamics is central to effective clinical management and disease prevention initiatives. In addition to the biological cause of bacterial infections, clinician compliance with antimicrobial therapy guidelines is also a controlling factor in the diseases. Research in analyzing drug compliance with prescribing guidelines for common infections indicates that adherence rates vary depending on the specific bacterial infections. For example, compliance rates for lower respiratory tract infections are much higher at 79%, but drop significantly for UTIs only at 40% (Alvarez et al., 2005). The difference may be explained by a number of patient and disease factors, including the rate of co-morbidities, as well as defensive prescribing by the doctors to achieve short-term success with treatment, but not long-term stewardship of antibiotics. Enhanced compliance with evidence-based guidelines is essential to controlling antibiotic resistance and maximizing patient outcomes when faced with bacterial infections (Figure 13.2).

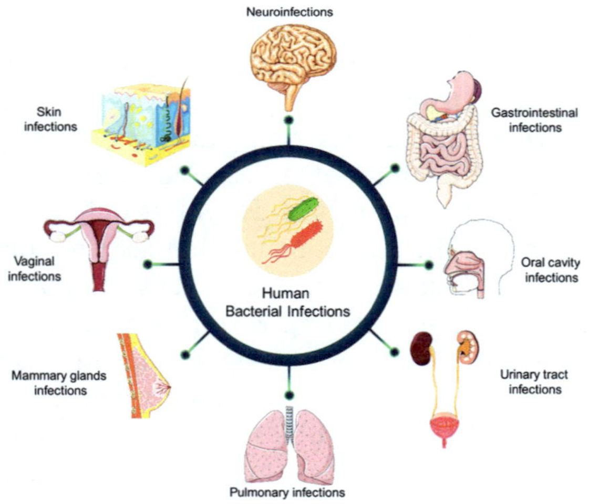

Figure 13.2. The most common human bacterial infections.

Source: https://www.researchgate.net/publication/345239299/figure/fig1/AS:963553309769728@1606740419087/Most-common-human-bacterial-infections.png.

13.1.2. Viral Infections and Their Transmission Methods

Viral infections pose a significant public health threat, with diverse transmission patterns rendering control and prevention difficult. Multiple modes, including direct contact, air, and vector transmission, facilitate the rapid dissemination of viruses among populations. The modes of transmission can vary significantly between viruses, necessitating a public health response. For example, the respiratory viruses like influenza are easily transmitted by aerosols generated by sneezing or coughing and must be handled carefully in crowded settings. However, viruses like HIV rely on direct contact with blood or sexual contact, and this highlights the necessity for targeted education programs among high-risk groups. With the advent of sophisticated diagnostic equipment, such as clinical metagenomic next-generation sequencing (mNGS), understanding the transmission patterns of such viruses becomes increasingly precise, enhancing our scope of disease control (Chiu et al., 2019). Besides this, sexual and blood-borne viral diseases have also garnered considerable attention in maternal health settings. Prenatal testing for sexually transmitted infections (STIs) and blood-borne viruses (BBVs) is critical, given the vertical transmission risk of infective agents from mother to child. The Department of Health (DOH) in Western Australia has highlighted the importance of comprehensive STI testing, such as chlamydia, during antenatal care. Although early audits showed that the majority of pregnant women were being tested for severe STIs like HIV and syphilis, the rates of chlamydia testing were alarmingly low (Combs et al., 2008). These findings reinforce the need for closer adherence to updated recommendations on testing, potentially lessening the risks of viral infections among maternal and perinatal health. The contagious dynamic of viral infection transmission underscores the need for continuous education and intervention strategies. Public health campaigns not only educate clinicians but also engage high-risk groups in understanding modes of viral transmission specific to their risk category. The integration of new technology like mNGS into routine clinical practice can enhance the detection and characterization of viral pathogens, ultimately leading to the formulation of preventive and therapeutic strategies.

Moreover, plugging gaps identified in practice, such as chlamydia antenatal screening, are also needed to enhance health outcomes in vulnerable groups. Overall, an integrated scientific approach, balanced by effective public health interaction, can lead to dramatic reductions in the transmission and impact of viral infections in various populations (Figure 13.3).

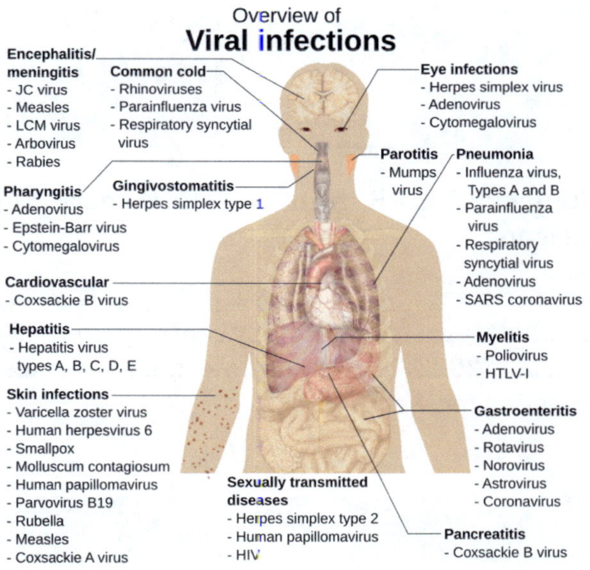

Figure 13.3. A simplistic overview of the main viral infections and the most notable species involved.

Source: https://upload.wikimedia.org/wikipedia/commons/thumb/c/c2/Viral_infections_and_involved_species.svg/800px-Viral_infections_and_involved_species.svg.png.

13.1.3. Fungal and Parasitic Infections and Their Impact on Health

The significance of parasitic and fungal infections on public health cannot be overstated, as they significantly contribute to the global disease burden. Fungal infections, particularly more prevalent in immunocompromised individuals, have severe health consequences and tend to require prolonged treatment. These infections not only cause morbidity but also mortality, particularly in individuals with weakened immune systems due to HIV/AIDS, cancer therapy, or other diseases. However, parasitic infections by helminths, for example, have infected over a billion individuals worldwide and resulted in enormous performance losses in livestock as can be witnessed in agricultural settings. The link between health and agricultural productivity emphasizes the social aspect of infections, including broader economic and social systems in the cycle of disease-poverty (Andam et al., 2025). In addition, dynamic interactions among parasitic and fungal infections and host immunity explain the complexity of health impacts associated with these pathogens (Figure 13.4).

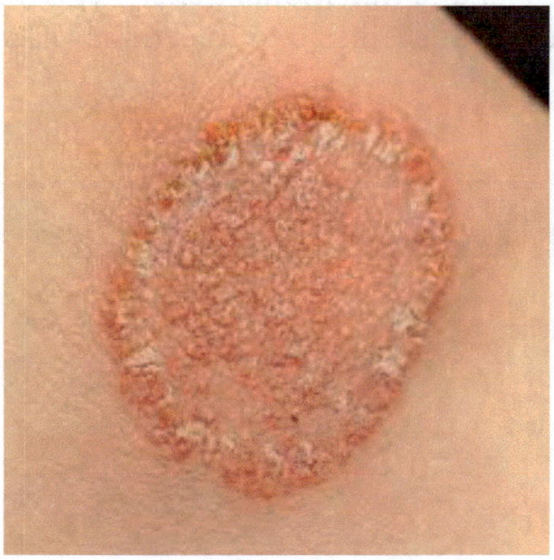

Figure 13.4. Fungal infection (tinea/ringworm).

Source: https://rasaderm.com/wp-content/uploads/2025/04/FUNGAL-.jpeg.

It has been shown through studies that chronic exposure to parasites can downregulate and evade host immunity, making individuals vulnerable to co-infection with other diseases, such as fungi. Aging may also create immune changes that increase this vulnerability, as older people are capable of having defective adaptive immunity. Evidence currently available indicates that adaptive immunity, which is critical in combating infections, is significantly compromised in aging and accounts for greater parasite burdens in elderly persons who might also be under a secondary fungal infection burden (Babayan et al., 2018). This condition poses a multilayered challenge to health systems because it requires targeted intervention to contain both infections and optimize outcomes among the vulnerable population. Further, the socio-economic effect of parasitic and fungal infections extends to influence farming activities, both directly and indirectly impacting health. In the region where farming is a significant source of income, health challenges emanating from infections lead to work absenteeism, diverting family resources towards caregiving, and eroding long-term agricultural productivity. For instance, unsanitary food harvesting and storage practices not only increase the likelihood of mycotoxin formation but also lead to nutritional deficiencies, making individuals susceptible to infections (Andam et al., 2025). The cycle highlights the imperative need for intersectoral agricultural and health policies that target these intersections of health to develop resilience in rural families. Treatment of fungal and parasitic diseases in general medicine requires considering these diseases in the context of broader health, economic stability, and agricultural production, thereby emphasizing the need for general healthcare policy (Figure 13.5).

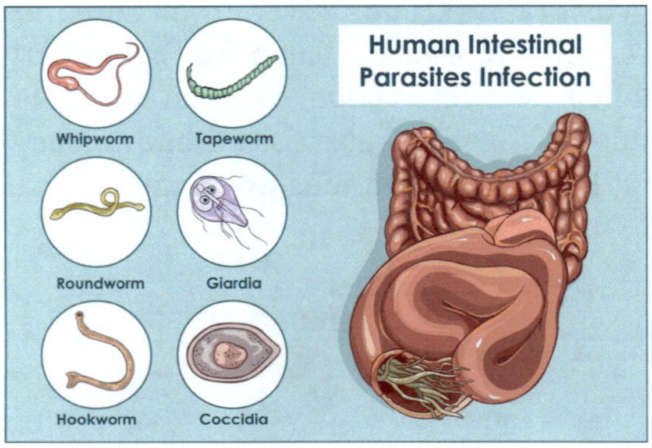

Figure 13.5. Human intestinal parasites infection.

Source: https://www.manhattangastroenterology.com/wp-content/uploads/2022/05/Human-Intestinal-Parasites-Infection.jpg.webp.

Test Your Knowledge

1. What are the key characteristics that distinguish bacterial infections from viral infections in terms of structure, symptoms, and treatment?
2. How are viral infections typically transmitted, and what factors influence their spread within populations?
3. What are some common bacterial infections, and how are they diagnosed and treated?

13.2. Pathophysiology of Infectious Diseases

Learning Outcome

1. Understand mechanisms of infection and host response
2. Explain the factors influencing disease severity and progression
3. Define the role of the immune system in combating infections

Pathophysiology of infectious diseases represents an interactive, dynamic process of host-pathogen interactions that affects disease course and outcome as well as clinical presentations. The pathogens initially infect the host's tissues using a variety of mechanisms to evade the immune system while they gain infection. Bacterial pathogens, for example, may employ biofilm formation or virulence factor release to facilitate their survival in harsh environments. These interactions may lead to varied clinical presentations, ranging from focal infections to inflammatory responses in the body, such as in sepsis. Pathophysiology also entails the host's innate and adaptive immune response, which are evoked in an attempt to clear the pathogens causing infections. More understanding of these interactions is needed in order to effectively develop , practical diagnostic and therapeutic methods, as well as public health interventions, in order to contain the spread of infectious diseases. In bacterial infections, the role of environmental determinants cannot be underestimated either. Sanitation, water quality, and population density are determinants that have a significant impact on the prevalence of infectious diseases. For instance, diarrheal disease research highlights the central role played by home sanitation and access to clean water as determinants of critical significance to health outcomes. Interestingly, young populations in developing countries are disproportionately affected by such diseases due to poor infrastructure and educational facilities. The addition of literature relating to such contextual determinants allows us to more clearly outline infectious disease pathophysiology and overall determinants of health and enable specific interventions that address the unique concerns of specific groups, as in the evidence that suggests the relevance of school hygiene in India (Dutta et al., 2012). Further, recent research on chronic infection illustrates how varying levels of medical doctor awareness of disease classification and therapy lead to suboptimal patient outcomes. For instance, in chronic prostatitis/chronic pelvic pain syndrome (CP/CPPS), primary care physicians demonstrated in most cases a lack of know-how regarding proper treatment protocols, even though the condition is prevalent.

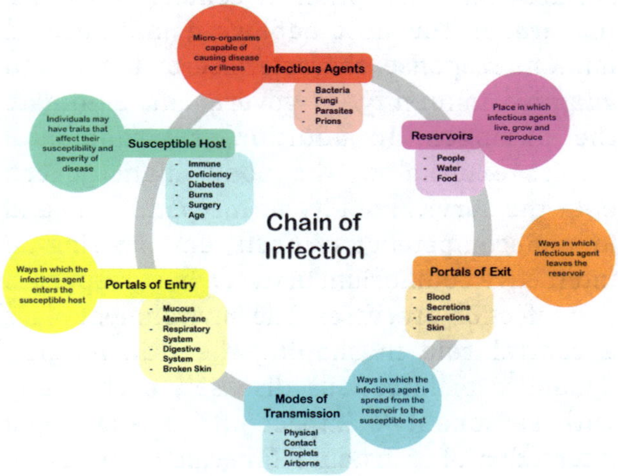

Figure 13.6. Chain of infection.

Source: https://psu.pb.unizin.org/app/uploads/sites/100/2019/04/Chain_of_Infection.png.

This isolation highlights the importance of continuous education in medical practice to equip clinicians with the capacity to handle prevalent infectious diseases convincingly. Such programs of education are vital based on the fact that management typically entails EBP, to which local standards need to be confirmed. Hence, bridging the distance between infectious disease expertise and clinical practice becomes vital in maximizing patient outcomes and care, thus the overall public health response to these chronic issues (Calhoun et al., 2009) (Figure 13.6).

13.2.1. Mechanisms of Infection and Host Response

The mechanisms by which pathogens and the associated host reactions initiate infection are complex and multifaceted, an evolutionary co-adaptation of infectious agents and their hosts. Pathogens use a variety of strategies to enter host tissue, evade the immune response, and proliferate. For instance, many bacteria have virulence factors, such as adhesins and toxins, which assist in attachment to epithelial surfaces and disruption of cellular functions. In parallel, the host deploys a multifaceted immune response, characterized by innate and adaptive immunity, to govern and eliminate the pathogen. In addition, environmental factors external to the body might govern both the survival ability of the pathogens and immunocompetence of hosts, emphasizing an interactive equilibrium between host responses and infection processes. The environment plays a central role in shaping the transmission dynamics of infectious diseases, particularly with seasonality's impact on host-pathogen interactions. For instance, for schistosomiasis in humans, environmental factors such as hydrology and temperature directly impact schistosome life cycles. Mathematical models that explore these interactions have begun incorporating time-varying environmental factors and have demonstrated how these factors shape disease outbreaks and transmission capacity. These models suggest that more understanding of ecological determinants can inform control strategies for vector-borne disease. These findings underscore the importance of integrating ecological perspectives into public health planning and the need for adaptive management in infectious disease epidemics across various settings (Remais et al., 2010). In addition, biological rhythms have started to appear as an essential aspect of host-parasite relationships. Experiments have demonstrated that the immune response exhibits temporal patterns due to circadian and other biological rhythms, which reflect changes in pathogen activity. The host response rhythm may generate divergent effects on infection dynamics, suggesting that the timing of infections and treatments may be the determining factor in their efficacy. As both host and pathogen learn to accommodate such rhythms, they engage in an ongoing arms race of evolutionary tactics, inclining towards survival and transmission (Helm et al., 2015). Understanding the role of biological rhythms in infectious disease dynamics offers new avenues for therapeutic interventions and prevention strategies, and it deepens our knowledge of host-pathogen interactions within the broader public health paradigm.

13.2.2. Factors Influencing Disease Severity and Progression

It is significant in the context of infectious diseases to understand complex factors influencing disease severity and pathogenesis. Multifactorial thinking is relevant in terms of biological, environmental, and psychosocial determinants. First among these is the biological basis of genetics and sexual dimorphism, in which sex and gender are central to moderating immune response and health outcome. The inclusion of gender medicine in clinical practice underscores the imperative for tailored healthcare in which treatment protocols take into consideration sex-differentiated reactions to infection. These practices enhance the specificity of clinical interventions, enabling practitioners to tailor approaches based on distinct biologic and psychosocial profiles and thus aim at alleviating susceptibility and optimizing therapeutic effects (Bellini et al., 2019). Furthermore, psychosocial determinants play a crucial role in the modulation of disease progression, influencing immune function as well as overall health. There is growing evidence that adverse psychosocial stressors impair immune function, which could exacerbate infectious diseases like TB. It has been observed that stress dampens vaccine effectiveness and infection susceptibility. Conversely, supportive and stable social psychosocial environments can boost immune function and support recovery processes. The findings identify the need to add psychosocial assessments to routine clinical examinations to provide more inclusive management of infectious diseases, potentially enhancing clinical outcomes (Boccia et al., 2019). Last but not least, environmental factors cannot be overlooked in disease severity and development assessment. Socioeconomic status, access to healthcare, and place are all key to an understanding of differential outcomes of disease.

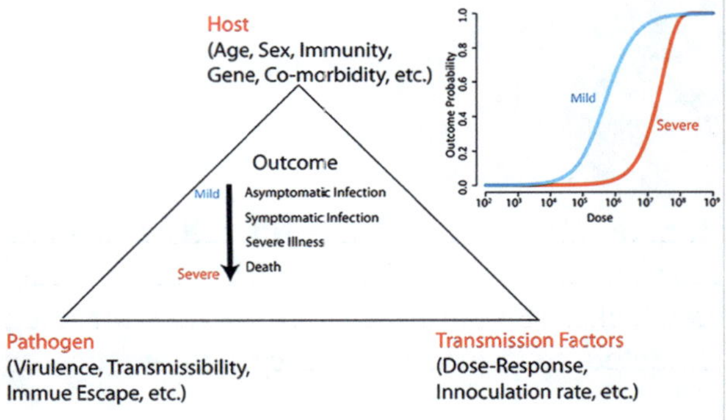

Figure 13.7. A model of interacting host, pathogen, and transmission factors affecting the outcome of exposure to an infectious pathogen.

Source: https://www.frontiersin.org/files/Articles/1391719/fpubh-12-1391719-HTML/image_m/fpubh-12-1391719-g001.jpg.

Individuals living in resource-poor settings experience a greater burden of infectious diseases due to restricted access to medical care, sanitation, and education. In addition, environmental risk exposures—such as pollution or crowding—can add to the susceptibility for infection. Public health activities aimed at lessening disease severity are vital in resolving these social determinants. By employing an integrative approach of targeting biological, psychosocial, and environmental determinants, healthcare professionals can develop multifaceted intervention strategies to combat infectious diseases and improve population health outcomes (Figure 13.7).

13.2.3. Role of the Immune System in Combating Infections

The immune system plays a central role in combating infection through a multi-faceted response that includes innate and adaptive factors. The innate immune response is the body's front line of defense and includes physical barriers such as skin and mucous membranes, and cellular responses that respond against pathogen invasion. When infection occurs, innate immune cells like macrophages and neutrophils are quickly mobilized to recognize and kill invading microorganisms by phagocytosis and the release of antimicrobial molecules. A quick response is necessary to contain and regulate infections until the adaptive immune system can effectively mount a more precise reaction tailored to the respective pathogen involved. The adaptive immune response is a critical factor in eliciting a specific response to individual pathogens, based on lymphocyte activation and proliferation, particularly by T and B cells. In response to antigen exposure, T cells become differentiated into subsets that help to regulate the immune response and directly kill infected cells. At the same time, B cells create antibodies that attach to pathogens, tagging them for elimination and interfering with their capacity to infect host cells. This advanced interrelation between cells enables the immune system to create immunological memory, leading to a more immediate and potent response when encountering the same pathogen in the future. This ability to adapt not only aids in the eradication of infections but also illustrates the relevance of vaccination in strengthening this defense mechanism. However, the effectiveness of the immune response can be compromised by various factors, including antibiotic resistance in organisms such as MRSA. As the immune response fails to combat infection, drug-resistant forms of the organism complicate treatment processes, leading to increased morbidity and mortality. MRSA has also altered perceptions regarding the organism by the general populace, with the organism characterized as a 'superbug', eroding trust in modern medicine. With the decline in the rate of new antibiotic discovery, predominantly due to financial and regulatory limits, healthcare systems must rethink their infection management strategy, emphasizing the critical role of effective immune defense, as well as prudent use of antibiotics, to combat the twin threats of infectious disease and AMR (Joffe et al., 2006; Coukell et al., 2016) (Figure 13.8).

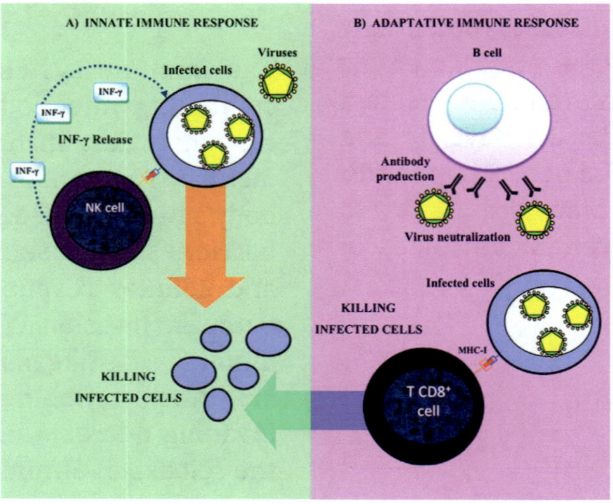

Figure 13.8. Immune response against viruses. (A) Innate immune response: NK cells recognize cells infected by viruses in an antigen-independent manner, exert cytotoxic activities, and rapidly produce large amounts of IFN-γ to eliminate infected cells. (B) Antibody production directed against viral antigens. T CD8^{+} cells eliminate virus-infected cells and secrete cytokines such as TNF-α and IFN-γ.

Source: https://www.researchgate.net/publication/321958898/figure/fig3/AS:573902322454532@1513840384850/mmune-response-against-viruses-A-Innate-immune-response-NK-cells-recognize-cells.png.

Test Your Knowledge

1. What are the key steps in the pathogenesis of an infectious disease from pathogen entry to symptom development?
2. How does the innate immune system respond to an initial infection, and what role does it play in controlling pathogen spread?
3. How do pathogens evade the host immune system to establish chronic or recurrent infections?

13.3. Diagnosis of Infectious Diseases

Learning Outcome

1. Discuss clinical evaluation and patient history
2. Understand laboratory tests and imaging techniques
3. Focus on challenges in diagnosing infectious diseases

Effective diagnosis of infectious diseases is crucial to ensure appropriate management and treatment are offered. The diagnostic process begins with a comprehensive clinical examination where the physician takes the patient's history and presentation. This is a highly critical step because it guides other diagnostic investigations, which may include laboratory studies such as blood culture, polymerase chain reaction (PCR), and imaging. For example, bacterial pneumonia, while commonly diagnosed in dogs, presents differently in cats and must therefore be approached uniquely when considering symptoms and underlying conditions. Such vigilance is crucial in arriving at the proper diagnosis and follow-up treatment protocols that consider potential complications and prevention, thereby improving patient outcome and management strategy in the long run (Dear et al., 2020). Diagnostics have radically improved our ability to identify infectious agents due to advances in technology. Most impressive among these are molecular techniques such as PCR and NGS, which have revolutionized the speed and accuracy of pathogen identification. They allow detection of difficult-to-culture pathogens and thereby facilitate the timely administration of effective therapy. Diagnosis and treatment of TB are excellent examples of the importance of such advances. Following a 1993 WHO declaration of a global TB emergency, affordable interventions like directly observed treatment short course (DOTS) have improved identification and treatment, lowering mortality rates significantly. Yet the emergence of MDR and extensively drug-resistant (XDR) strains makes the situation more complex, with the necessity for more effective diagnostic support systems (Abubakar et al., 2012). The global challenge posed by diagnosing infectious diseases emphasizes the importance of robust country-wide health infrastructure and active surveillance. In low-resource environments, suboptimal laboratory capability undermines the detection of MDR and XDR TB, being the most significant barrier to proper case management and control. Enhanced investment by national health programs is critical to improve diagnostic capability for the timely detection and treatment of drug-resistant cases. Additionally, addressing operational issues, such as routine surveillance and drug susceptibility testing, is essential in order to prevent the growing threat of drug-resistant infections. As international health programs continue to evolve, prioritizing better diagnostics will be pivotal in advancing improved health outcomes and reducing the infectious disease burden worldwide and planning for a better response to future epidemics (Abubakar et al., 2012).

13.3.1. Clinical Evaluation and Patient History

Clinical evaluation of patients suffering from infectious diseases begins with a proper patient history, and this is essential for correct diagnosis and treatment. Clinicians must first know the patient's demographics, their past illnesses, and even the nature and duration of symptoms. Detailed questionnaires can also identify significant factors such as recent travel history, exposure to infectious pathogens in the past, or prior vaccination. A well-structured patient history recognizes all probable risk factors specific to infectious diseases, allowing for early intervention. Social determinants of health also enhance the assessment process, informing clinicians of the socioeconomic setting impacting a patient's overall health as well as pathogen exposure. Following the initial patient history, clinicians must conduct a complete physical examination to assess manifestations of infectious diseases. The assessment typically involves evaluating principal indicators like vital signs, skin lesions, and pulmonary findings to create a clinical picture that guides further diagnostic testing. Be sure to note evidence of systemic infection, such as fever, lethargy, or lymphadenopathy, which suggests the presence of a causative infectious pathogen. Besides, correlating clinical data with the history can reveal specific trends in certain infections, such as pneumonia, where there should be ample history of the patient's respiratory status and past infections.

The completeness of examination and history taking helps the physicians avoid missing crucial details that are crucial for proper diagnosis and management. Also, the intersection of patient history and clinical evaluations typically sheds light on areas of remediation in medical training and treatment effectiveness. For instance, in the context of infectious diseases, this intersection will subject fellows-in-training to gaps in knowledge for managing complex cases. As underscored in futuristic models to close the remediation gaps in fellowship programs, these talks highlight the importance of including continuous feedback loops to enhance clinical competence in diagnosing and treating infectious diseases (Escota et al., 2020). Closing the gaps in knowledge not only enhances the individual practitioner's ability but ultimately improves patient care quality by making treatment decisions based on thorough workups and patient histories. In addition, information regarding specific management for individual infections, such as canine bacterial pneumonia, also validates the need for a detailed examination of every patient (Dear et al., 2020) (Figure 13.9).

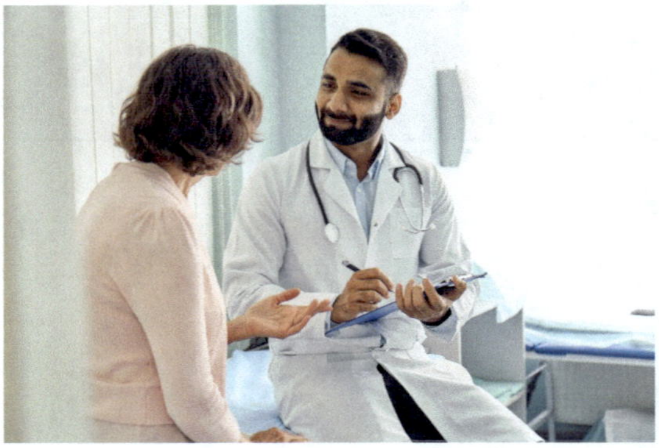

Figure 13.9. Doctor taking the patient's history for the diagnosis of infectious diseases.

Source: https://www.news-medical.net/images/Article_Images/ImageForArticle_23874_16963341179465915.jpg.

13.3.2. Laboratory Tests and Imaging Techniques

In general medicine, laboratory tests and imaging techniques are the core of diagnosis and treatment of infectious diseases. Proper detection of pathogens is necessary since it dictates treatment modalities and prevents infection transmission. Laboratory tests, including serological tests and cultures, enable clinicians to detect specific antibodies or microbial agents in patient samples. These techniques are complemented by molecular techniques, such as PCR, which offer rapid and sensitive detection of infectious pathogens. Emerging developments in diagnostic technology provide improved accuracy and speed, revolutionizing the potential for diagnosing diseases such as bacterial and viral infections. As a result, clinicians can initiate specific therapies sooner, eventually improving patient care. Imaging procedures, nonetheless, are precious complements to the laboratory examinations in the diagnosis of infectious diseases. Radiologic imaging, such as X-rays, ultrasound, and CT scans, can determine the scope and nature of infectious processes in the body. Such modalities are useful when laboratory examinations may be unhelpful or if a secondary complication is suspected. Advanced imaging can detect abscess formation, pneumonia, or osteomyelitis and indicate whether clinical decision-making should be interrupted with additional invasive procedures or surgery. By integrating imaging modalities with laboratory information, the diagnostic yield is enhanced, and a complete assessment of the patient's condition is facilitated. The focus on this multidisciplinary approach highlights the importance of utilizing an array of tools in infectious disease management. As infectious diseases evolve, so does the methodology of diagnosis. Present efforts have centered on the necessity to initiate collaboration between laboratory and clinical practitioners toward the development of standardized protocols and definitions for the diagnosis of invasive fungal diseases (IFDs).

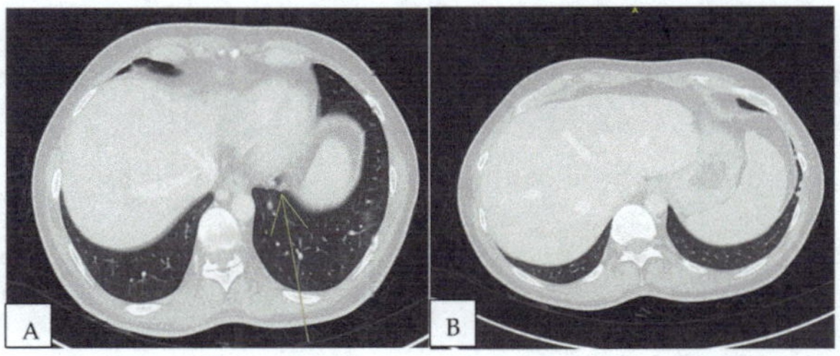

Figure 13.10. Total-body CT scan revealed non-specific pulmonary consolidations. Other diseases could explain these observations, such as sarcoidosis, neoplasm, or other infectious diseases (TB, NTM, herpesviruses, cryptococcosis). (A) Nodule in the retrocardiac area (yellow arrow); (B) two nodules in the subpleural area.

Source: https://www.researchgate.net/publication/391114293/figure/fig1/AS:11431281469841924@1748404484540/Total-body-CT-scan-revealed-non-specific-pulmonary-consolidations-Other-diseases-could.tif.

As noted in research efforts led by specialist working groups, updated definitions of proven, probable, and possible IFD should now include populations not traditionally considered. The contract highlights the need to ensure strict laboratory diagnosis in patient populations with heterogeneity, particularly due to new diagnostic tools and criteria that are established (Akan et al., 2019). Developing laboratory procedures and imaging technologies to identify infectious diseases can further contribute to improving public health programs by enabling timely interventions across various patient populations (N/A, 2004). Higher levels of diagnostic capacity provide the opportunity for improved surveillance, epidemiology, and ultimately, more effective control measures against infectious diseases (Figure 13.10).

13.3.3. Challenges in Diagnosing Infectious Diseases

Infectious disease diagnosis faces challenges due to the complexity of human biology, the diversity of pathogens, and limitations in available diagnostic facilities. As the infections can have syndromes overlapping one another, discrimination between numerous diseases can require advanced clinical acumen and laboratory investigations. The traditional methods, like culture and serology, are too time-consuming and do not provide timely results, particularly in outbreaks or where instant decision-making is necessary. In addition, the emergence of multi-drug-resistant pathogens, such as multi-drug-resistant tuberculosis (MDR-TB) in India, further adds complexity to the diagnostic situation. The life cycles of the pathogens demand an equally dynamic public health system that can respond rapidly to changing epidemiological patterns and diagnostic needs, calling for speedy development and adaptability to improve control activities and ultimately patient outcomes (Engel et al., 2025). The integration of advanced technologies into diagnostic practice is necessary but difficult. Clinical mNGS, for instance, is an advanced technology that can revolutionize infectious disease diagnosis; its ability to sequence microbial and host-derived genetic material makes it possible to perform thorough pathogen detection without culture. Nonetheless, the application of mNGS in medical environments is still hindered by issues such as high technological expenses, infrastructural capital outlays, and the need for specialized training of medical staff. Furthermore, these technologies must also contend with regulatory environments and yield clinically meaningful interpretations that can positively affect patient outcomes. The potential of mNGS to address issues like AMR and enhance diagnostic accuracy highlights its potential, along with the broad range of challenges that need clarification for successful integration into standard practice (Chiu et al., 2019). Secondly, socio-cultural background significantly contributes to determining diagnostic practices, which leads to additional challenges in managing infectious diseases. Health beliefs and practices are very heterogeneous between populations, and both affect the likelihood of presenting for care as well as symptom interpretation. Cultural stigmas related to illnesses in most of the world are enough to dissuade individuals from obtaining early diagnoses, further hindering the public health response. Structural impediments like the availability of health infrastructure, trained personnel, and access to healthcare often render manifest the problems with diagnostics. For health systems to operate effectively in the prevention of infectious diseases, there is a need for a deep understanding of such socio-cultural forces, as well as the integration of new technological inventions. This multi-pronged approach not only enhances diagnostic accuracy but also guarantees greater acceptance and utilization of health services among different segments (Chiu et al., 2019; Engel et al., 2025).

Test Your Knowledge

1. Why is a thorough patient history and clinical evaluation essential in the initial diagnosis of infectious diseases?
2. What are the most commonly used laboratory tests for identifying infectious agents, and how do they differ in application?
3. What challenges do clinicians face when diagnosing infections with nonspecific symptoms or overlapping clinical presentations?

13.4. Treatment Options for Infectious Diseases

Learning Outcome

1. Understand antibiotics and antiviral medications
2. Explain the role of supportive care and symptomatic treatment
3. Focus on emerging therapies and resistance issues

The treatment context of infectious disease has radically transformed in the last decades, with the demand for more effective approaches to combat these conditions, which are widespread as a threat to health. In the case of HIV, the choice of treatment can have profound implications for maternal and child health. Option B$^+$ has emerged as a game-changing strategy that favors long-term antiretroviral therapy (ART) among HIV-infected pregnant women. This strategy effectively reduces the risk of mother-to-child transmission (MTCT) both during pregnancy and breastfeeding. Evidence from Ghana indicates that although Option B$^+$ costs more, its long-term benefit in reducing infections and improving quality-adjusted life years in both mothers and children renders it a cost-saving intervention that warrants widespread use in settings with limited resources (Agyarko-Poku et al., 2015). Other than HIV, the management of AMR is becoming increasingly urgent with the declining efficacy of traditional antibiotics. The treatment of AMR requires an interdisciplinary strategy incorporating judicious antibiotic use, rigorous surveillance interventions, and robust infection prevention and control (IPC). There is evidence that understanding the effect of current policies to combat AMR remains dynamic, and there is a high priority for a consolidated body of evidence. For instance, human and veterinary health policy initiatives for promoting responsible use must be tailored to the unique challenges of each region. This makes sense in light of the requirement for rigorous cost-effectiveness and generalizability analyses of projected interventions in all income groups and sectors, particularly in LMICs (Aarestrup et al., 2015). Furthermore, an interdisciplinary approach termed One Health is being adopted in infectious disease control with growing frequency. It recognizes the interconnectedness of human, animal, and environmental health, enabling more effective coordinated efforts towards controlling emergent illnesses. Through coordination between these disciplines, stakeholders can create responsive policies that address not only the immediate issues brought about by infectious agents but also consider the complexity of health systems. This approach is particularly effective in combating zoonotic diseases, those that pose serious global health risks. The One Health application is an investment by all sectors and acknowledges the individual health realities of a country. Ultimately, the integration of these methods into one is a proactive move towards an integrated and efficient system for the treatment of infectious diseases within the framework of overall general medicine.

13.4.1. Antibiotics and Antiviral Medications

Antibiotic and antiviral drug use is a matter of great concern in infectious disease control because the two types of drugs work through distinct modes to destroy pathogens. Antibiotics are generally administered to kill or inhibit bacterial growth, and antiviral drugs are aimed at preventing viral replication within host cells. The emergence of antibiotic resistance, due to misuse and overuse, complicates the treatment of bacterial infections and poses a significant public health problem. Recent studies, for example, the one assessing the impact of quick multiplex respiratory panels, show that innovative diagnostic solutions are anticipated to reduce unnecessary antibiotic prescriptions, thus decreasing the likelihood of resistance (Bang et al., 2019). Additionally, the application of antivirals has gained important attention in the realm of new viral threats, and increased awareness about their use and effectiveness in clinical settings is necessary. Apart from their therapeutic uses, , as well as both antibiotics and antiviral medications, have been incorporated into broader health security measures. World governments are now realizing the importance of such drugs in their preparation for future bioterrorism and pandemics (Elbe et al., 2014). This kind of pharmaceuticalization of security reflects a shift in the understanding of health in international politics, interweaving security and public health initiatives with national security imperatives. The stockpiling of antiviral medications, such as Tamiflu for pandemic flu, illustrates the extent to which these medications are considered essential for the safeguarding of populations from the threat of infection. Thus, the union of medicine and security warrants sincere attention to the complexities of drug creation, delivery, and the ethical considerations in the stockpiling of such precious resources. While the boundary between antibiotics and antivirals is certain, their function is often dependent on evolving research and practice. The landscape of treating infectious diseases is changing rapidly, as new therapies and combination regimens keep emerging. Antimicrobial stewardship programs are present in various health centers to maximize the appropriate use of antibiotics, thereby keeping them effective and reducing harm as a result of resistance. At the same time, antiviral drug research is broadening, with emphasis on pan-spectrum drugs having the potential to offer effective therapy in a variety of viral infections. This two-way emphasis on maintaining the effectiveness of antibiotics and advancing antiviral research highlights the significance of innovative approaches to treating infectious diseases. By promoting proper use and continuous development of both antibiotic and antiviral medications, the medical field will be better placed to combat the issue of contagious diseases confronting a more interconnected world (Figure 13.11).

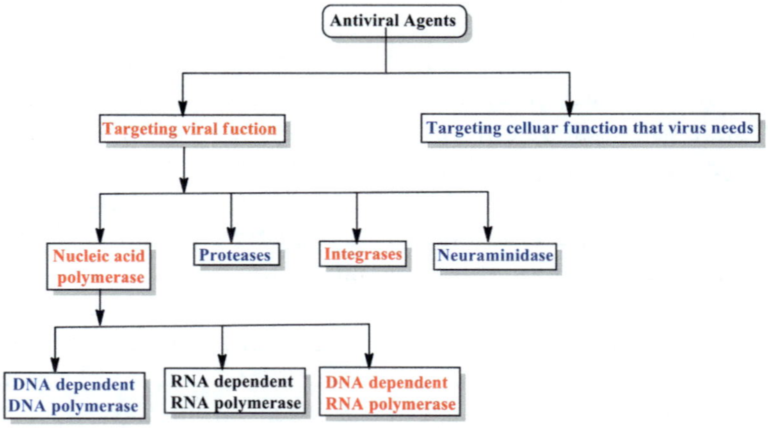

Figure 13.11. Common inhibitory action of antiviral drugs.

Source: https://www.intechopen.com/chapters/80145.

13.4.2. Supportive Care and Symptomatic Treatment

Supportive care plays a crucial role in the management of infectious diseases, primarily since it is composed of an extensive range of interventions aimed at alleviating symptoms and improving the patient's QoL. Supportive care can include fluid resuscitation, control of pain, and nutritional support, all ideally tailored to the patient's requirements. Supportive management for viral infections or pneumonia may be necessary when curative treatment is limited or ineffective. It is particularly so among vulnerable populations, such as those undergoing stem cell transplantation, where infections like histoplasmosis remain a confounding factor despite antifungal prophylaxis. It is not possible to overstate the necessity for prompt identification of these infections and supportive management, as evidenced by cases where timely treatment led to spectacular improvement in clinical symptoms once adequate pharmacotherapy, e.g., itraconazole for pulmonary histoplasmosis (Agrawal et al., 2020), was initiated. Symptomatic treatment is also a component of infectious disease treatment, focusing on relieving specific symptoms without regard for eradicating the causative pathogen. This approach is most critical where full recovery can be postponed, or where the cause presents a limited target for treatment. Effective symptomatic management may involve the use of analgesics, antiemetics, or symptom-specific therapies, which significantly enhance patient comfort and concordance. Ebola virus disease is one of such clinical illnesses that presents a range of incapacitating symptoms, including GI distress and severe weakness, which makes it challenging to manage the patient in resource-poor settings. Collection and analysis of clinic information from epidemics are vital to streamlining symptomatic treatment protocols and case management on a large scale. Organizations that care for such patients need to optimize practice on a regular basis to maximize outcomes for future epidemics (Grolla et al., 2012). The synergy between supportive care and symptomatic treatment lends itself to improved management of infectious disease. This multi-dimensional consideration allows the medical caregivers to cope with the complex needs of the patients, particularly in severe infections. Such infections as Ebola carry high mortality risk and varied clinical presentations that will easily overwhelm the healthcare system. Incorporating supportive treatments as part of a comprehensive treatment plan, therefore, increases the chances of patient survival and QoL.,. Further, disease-specific best practices and recommendations should continue to develop from ongoing research and clinical data, ensuring that supportive care and symptomatic management remain abreast of new infectious threats. Overall, the incorporation of these methods is reflective of the growing seen patient-centered approach for all medicine, in particular within infectious disease contexts.

13.4.3. Emerging Therapies and Resistance Issues

With the evolving nature of infectious diseases, developing therapies for emerging resistant strains has been the main priority. The biggest challenge is that currently available antibiotics are no longer potent against resistant pathogens that evolved due to excessive drug exposure and inadequate drug application. This is not only specific to medicine but also a challenge in agricultural applications. For instance, organic stock farming seeks to reduce the use of pharmaceutical drugs but also faces its own set of challenges related to emerging animal welfare and disease resistance issues. This agricultural practice not only impacts the well-being of the animals but also has the potential to compromise food safety and public health by establishing infectious loops between livestock and humans alike, generating further concerns about the effectiveness of existing therapeutic interventions (Eijck et al., 2006). It is necessary to investigate alternative therapies that complement conventional approaches or offer novel options to effectively address resistance problems. New technologies in therapeutic modalities, such as phage therapy and monoclonal antibodies, show promise to break through bacterial resistance patterns.

Additionally, the use of prebiotics and probiotics within therapies also shows promise in enhancing the ruggedness of the microbiome and thereby reducing the risk of infection and resultant antibiotic treatment. However, the vast majority of these new therapies are hampered by limited strong evidence of their efficacy and feasibility. These gaps must be addressed through continued clinical trials so that interventions are not only practical but safe and implementable within the health system (Eijck et al., 2006). Resistance issues are compounded by socio-economic determinants that create conditions for the dissemination of NTDs. The intersection of poverty, urbanization, and environmental change is largely contributing to the recurrence and persistence of these diseases, bringing them to the center of public health. In many cases, government and healthcare infrastructure is not equipped with the resources necessary to respond appropriately, fueling a cycle of contagion that is unchallenged. Strengthening community consciousness and building capacity among vulnerable groups is the solution to enabling health and averting NTD risk. By alerting people to the complex socio-economic and environmental connection, health promotion messages can be better structured to facilitate successful disease control programs and contribute to improved overall health status among communities.

Test Your Knowledge

1. What factors determine the selection of an appropriate antibiotic or antiviral medication for treating a specific infectious disease?
2. How does antibiotic resistance develop, and what practices contribute to its rise in both community and healthcare settings?
3. In which clinical situations is supportive care the primary treatment approach for infectious diseases, and what does it typically include?

13.5. Prevention and Control Measures

Learning Outcome

1. Describe vaccination strategies and public health initiatives
2. Focus on infection control practices in healthcare settings
3. Explain the role of education and awareness in the prevention of infectious diseases

Effective prevention and control measures are most critical in managing infectious diseases, particularly in endemic and emerging pathogen settings. Vaccination is one of the primary strategies used globally to contain contagious diseases by nearly eradicating the prevalence of infectious diseases due to the formation of herd immunity. Not only does vaccination confer protection to individuals, but it also stops disease transmission at the population level. Public health programs should provide equal access to vaccination since unequal vaccination coverage can cause epidemics and further complicate control measures. In addition, ongoing education about the efficacy of the vaccine and the value of immunization is fundamentally important in countering myths that tend to undermine public compliance. The increased use of immunization programs has been found to effectively control diseases, aligning with global health targets to control or eliminate infections like polio and measles, ultimately saving lives and reducing healthcare costs. Beyond vaccination, proper surveillance systems also play a fundamental role in preventing and controlling infectious diseases. Effective surveillance enables the timely detection of outbreaks and disease trends, allowing for prompt action to prevent the spread of diseases. Adding technology and analysis to surveillance systems maximizes their effectiveness, enabling public health professionals to identify patterns and risk factors for disease transmission. Moreover, global collaboration in surveillance exercises is required, especially where resources are scarce, to derive an overall scenario of global disease dynamics. This collaboration is seen in initiatives like the Global Health Security Agenda, whose aim is to increase preparedness against emerging infectious disease threats. Lack of adequate surveillance causes the disease to spread before intervention measures can be put in place, resulting in increased morbidity and mortality, especially among vulnerable populations (Abubakar et al., 2012). Infectious disease complexities are resolved by adopting a more holistic approach that includes quality health infrastructure and community interventions. Control actions must include not only clinical intervention but also health education, sanitation, and the availability of clean water, as these factors significantly influence the dynamics of disease spread. Community participation is crucial; specifically tailored education programs for specific groups can prepare individuals to take preventive action in maintaining their own health and others' health. Properly trained healthcare personnel must also be equipped to identify infectious disease signs and offer public education on prevention, thereby strengthening the health environment. The implementation of the International Health Regulations lays specific emphasis on coordinated global interventions towards infectious disease, emphasizing the importance of preparedness for public health emergencies triggered by environmental and climatic variations (Ivanova et al., 2017). In this context, establishing a coordinated global health system becomes imperative to continue long-term prevention and control strategies.

13.5.1. Vaccination Strategies and Public Health Initiatives

The implementation of vaccination programs is an integral part of public health initiatives to control infectious diseases. Effective vaccinations are designed to induce herd immunity in populations and significantly reduce the incidence of vaccine-preventable conditions. These approaches should be well-planned and implemented in various settings, from urban healthcare facilities to rural communities where accessibility can be limited. The combined effort of governments, health professionals, and community organizations is essential in enhancing vaccination coverage. For example, particular programs among high-risk groups such as health workers and elderly persons with comorbidities should be accorded the highest priority to effectively curb the spread of diseases. In this way, populations are protected from being infected with diseases, thereby minimizing the total healthcare burden and making the community more resistant to infectious diseases. To even better optimize vaccination strategies, there must be periodic review and refinement of public health policy. These mechanisms allow an understanding of geographic differences in disease incidence and rates of immunization. By critically analyzing vaccine programs, one finds a starkly high degree of geographical variation; regions with strong health infrastructures are more likely to have higher vaccination rates compared to regions with weak systems. The Italian experience is a mirror to this trend, with regional prevention plans (RPPs) capturing varying strategies but highlighting the necessity of greater dissemination of best practices among the regions. That addresses the need not only to implement these plans but to make them robust enough to evolve according to local needs and situations. Increased communication between health authorities and the public has the potential to make public health programs more effective by encouraging higher vaccination rates among different population subgroups (de Belvis et al., 2015).

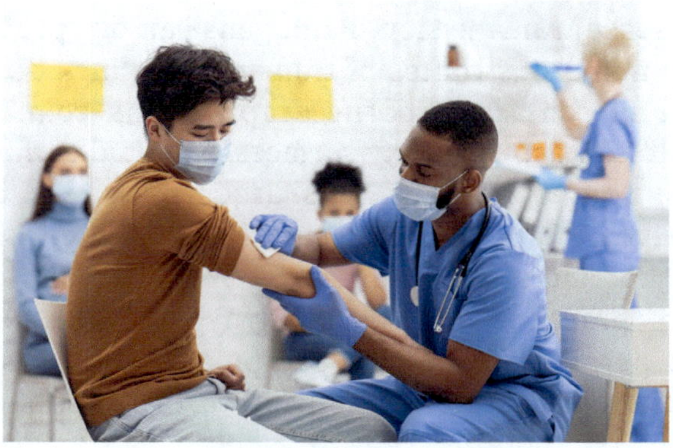

Figure 13.12. Young man getting vaccination in hospital.

Source: https://newsinhealth.nih.gov/sites/newsinhealth/files/2021/August/aug-2021-capsule1-young-man-getting-vaccination-hospital-cropped.jpg.

Multi-sectoral alliances also emerge as a critical factor in the achievement of vaccination strategies and public health programs. New partnerships among health ministries, schools, and non-governmental organizations can lead to more cohesive healthcare campaigns. Community involvement at the local level will reduce misinformation and vaccine hesitancy that often undermines immunization drives. For instance, zoonoses such as rabies have been found to have educational potential on animal-to-human disease transmission that can result in positive impacts within communities. Localized awareness and training place a strong emphasis on building public response to health threats (Bourhy et al., 2012). By integrating these mutualistic models within public health systems, the process of vaccination can become increasingly effective, thereby promoting the greater goal of reducing the infectious disease burden on the globe (Figure 13.12).

13.5.2. Infection Control Practices in Healthcare Settings

Good infection control practices are necessary in the healthcare setting to limit infectious disease transmission. Pathogens can be spread by numerous routes of transmission, including direct contact, airborne droplets, and coming into contact with dirty surfaces. As noted earlier, a stronger framework is urgently needed to drive IPC policy, particularly when fighting AMR (Aarestrup et al., 2015). What is required are practices such as hand hygiene, the use of personal protective equipment (PPE), and adherence to sterilization protocols. It should be strictly enforced to reduce healthcare-associated infections. Having a culture of abiding by these practices is a prerequisite to ensuring a safe environment for healthcare workers and patients alike. Continuous training and education of healthcare professionals are key to closing knowledge and practice gaps, thereby enhancing overall safety in health facilities. Infection control requires surveillance, which tracks infection rates and pathogen strains systematically. With the aid of data analysis, healthcare institutions can identify trends, evaluate the effectiveness of current IPC interventions, and respond proactively to potential risks. Involving surveillance data in decision-making may enhance the efficacy of interventions that are tailored to a particular environment, treating the individual issues existing across diverse healthcare environments (Aarestrup et al., 2015). For example, antibiotic stewardship programs can be built on surveillance outcomes to mitigate the colossal rise in antimicrobial-resistant infections. Furthermore, fostering collaboration among multidisciplinary teams will lead to more comprehensive infection control strategies, ensuring that policies are adhered to at all levels of care. Successful surveillance hinges on its ability to inform EBP and support resource management. Acceptance of the multifaceted problems of infection control in healthcare settings emphasizes the importance of interdisciplinary care. One Health is particularly relevant, as it emphasizes the interconnectedness of human health, animal health, and the environment. The collective perspective ensures that infection prevention policies across sectors are coordinated and integrated, addressing the complexities of AMR. There is a need for coordination, especially in low-income settings where the infectious disease burden is high and health resources are limited. Strategies need to encompass not only clinical practice but also community outreach to enhance awareness of infection prevention practices. When healthcare systems put such comprehensive measures into place, they are in a position to improve resilience to infections while ultimately saving lives and promoting public health (Figure 13.13).

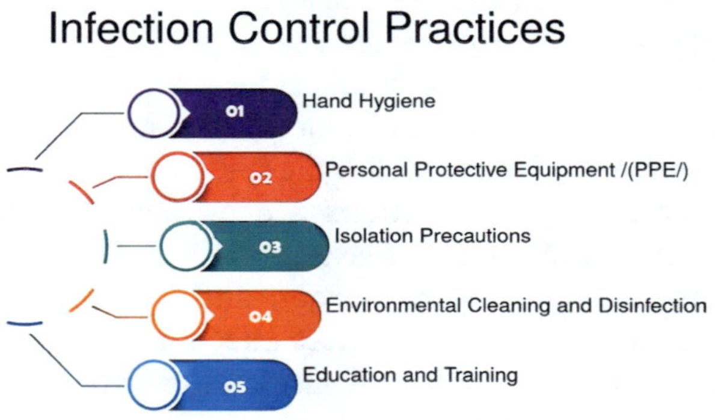

Figure 13.13. Infection control practices.

Source: https://fastercapital.co/i/Caregiver-safety-protocols-Essential-Safety-Measures-for-Caregivers--A-Comprehensive-Guide--Infection-Control-Practices.webp.

13.5.3. Role of Education and Awareness in Prevention

Awareness and education are essential elements of infectious disease prevention, as they empower individuals and communities with the necessary information to effectively be cognizant of and combat such diseases. Effective education programs can raise people's level of awareness regarding the modes of transmission, symptoms, and preventive measures for various infectious diseases. For instance, the principles of One Health promote inter-sectoral coordination among sectors like human health, animal health, and environmental health to conceptualize a holistic approach to disease management. This enhances support for communication between specialists of different fields—such as medicine and veterinary science—so that they can communicate and trust each other, thereby constituting a robust defense mechanism against zoonotic diseases that strike both humans and animals (Buttigieg et al., 2015). Further, targeted educational programs can have a tangible effect on public sentiment regarding vaccination and preventive health practices. As seen in a study at Shaikh Zayed Medical College, awareness among medical students regarding the swine flu virus showed that most of them knew its causative agent and mode of spread. But an evident lack of knowledge on vaccination indicates an urgent need for education (Bakhtawar et al., 2020). As future health practitioners, such students require not only facts but also the ability to encourage preventive measures in their respective communities. Such training can inspire public health movements that reduce the incidence of infectious diseases and promote overall health among communities. In addition to formal education structures, public health campaigns become crucial elements in encouraging awareness and preventive measures among populations. Effective messaging attuned to the cultural climate of the community can increase receptivity and stimulate risk-reducing practices. Education campaigns on hand hygiene, food safety, and the benefits of vaccination can, for example, enhance health literacy and individual agency. Together with access to healthcare resources, these campaigns can allow individuals to take proactive steps towards managing their own health, thus reducing the infectious disease burden. As human populations face the threats of emerging and re-emerging diseases, the push for prevention through education and awareness remains the pillar of effective public health strategy.

Test Your Knowledge

1. How do vaccination strategies contribute to the prevention of infectious diseases at both individual and population levels?
2. How do herd immunity and vaccine coverage rates influence the success of public health vaccination programs?

13.6. Global Impact of Infectious Diseases

Learning Outcome

1. Understand epidemiology and statistics of infectious diseases worldwide
2. Discuss the socioeconomic effects of infectious disease outbreaks
3. Focus on global health organizations and their role in combating infections

The global infectious disease burden is a pressing matter that cuts across geopolitical divides and can have implications on public health, economic stability, and social structures worldwide. Contagious diseases such as malaria, HIV/AIDS, and TB have inflicted enormous burdens throughout history, predominantly on middle- and low-income countries. As of 2023, the WHO estimates that infectious diseases account for a significant percentage of mortality in regions where healthcare services are often inadequate to respond effectively. New emerging contagious diseases, driven by climate change and globalization, have a greater potential to disrupt societies and economies. Our interconnected world makes a local outbreak an immediate global issue, thus underlining the imperative of robust global collaboration and efficient public health measures to address these issues in time. In addition, the shift in the global health policy emphasis mirrors the advancing epidemiological transition, where NCDs are now a significant public health problem across much of the world. But infectious diseases remain a fundamental threat, particularly to those groups that are most at risk. The growing burden of NCDs, responsible for 35 million annual deaths, disproportionately weighs on LMICs and thus highlights the need for urgent and focused interventions. Such trends in epidemiology pose unique governance challenges, necessitating ongoing coordination between agencies to develop effective strategies. Comprehensive global health policies, like the development of strict food labeling laws and advertisement control, have been proposed to cover these twin epidemics. The problems, however, are related to complexity and multifactorial determinants that require innovative governance interventions, engaging the private sector and civil society in preventive health measures, as outlined by Gostin et al. (2013). Finally, professional and academic training in infectious diseases should be directed towards addressing existing challenges of contagious and NCDs. The Infectious Diseases Society of America recognized that effective educational models are required to enhance the strength of prospective clinicians in this field—reminders at the 2018. The National Fellowship Program Directors Meeting placed focus on remediation measures if fellows experience difficulties during their training. Particular areas of focus included the addition of feedback mechanisms, performance management, and career development, ultimately aiming to develop a more resilient workforce. By implementing competency-based approaches in education and training, program directors can effectively prepare healthcare professionals to address the diverse health needs posed by infectious diseases, as elaborated by Escota et al. (2020). Highlighting the need for ongoing learning and adjustment, this framework emphasizes the vital function of education in addressing international health issues and enhancing health outcomes overall.

13.6.1. Epidemiology and Statistics of Infectious Diseases Worldwide

Epidemiologic and statistical research on infectious diseases is a core component of general medicine that provides useful information regarding the distribution and determinants of disease. Understanding the incidence and prevalence of infectious diseases worldwide allows public health professionals and researchers to mobilize resources and implement interventions properly focused. Furthermore, epidemiologic information allows for the detection of risk groups and informs preventive strategies targeted to contexts. Analysis of these numbers can reveal trends that account for the socio-economic and environmental determinants governing the transmission of infections by geographical location. Graphing such trends consolidates global health policy and encourages the formulation of interventions aimed at reducing morbidity and mortality rates of infectious diseases, ultimately promoting public health priorities worldwide. Network theory has become increasingly prominent in the field of epidemiology, offering novel insights into the patterns of transmission of infectious diseases within populations. By studying the links between individuals and groups within a network, researchers can better understand the dynamics of transmission of various pathogens. This technique provides a method for identifying the most important nodes or individuals whose behavior may significantly affect disease spread, making it an extremely useful tool in public health planning. The coupling of statistical modeling and network analysis enhances the accuracy of modeling the spread of contagious diseases and forecasting future trends. Recent studies demonstrate that by including network characteristics in epidemiological models, we can achieve more insight into contagion patterns. Thus, epidemiology's contact with network theory is a step towards sophisticated analysis in the understanding and control of infectious diseases (Danon et al., 2010). Globally, data related to infectious diseases are not only a tool for assessment but also serve as an impetus for international cooperation to face health crises. Such organizations as the WHO make use of detailed epidemiological data in order to monitor outbreaks and coordinate responses across international borders. By constructing databases that summarize conclusions from numerous studies, such organizations facilitate cooperative efforts to generate vaccination programs and treatment guidelines suited to different epidemiological settings. Furthermore, the use of advanced statistical methods facilitates the analysis of surveillance data, identifying high-risk areas and guiding public health interventions. Understanding the interdependence of countries in controlling infectious diseases requires recognizing how shared data and resources are critical to establishing future outbreak resilience. Hence, ongoing emphasis on good epidemiological practice is still required to construct enhanced global health security and effectively respond to infectious disease threats (London School of Hygiene and Tropical Medicine, 2013) (Figure 13.14).

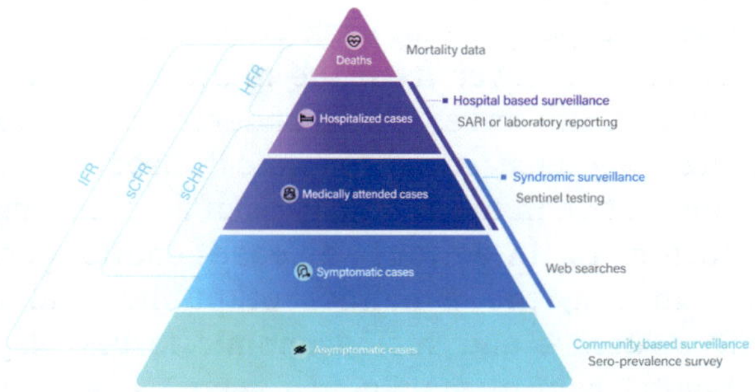

Figure 13.14. The burden pyramid of infectious disease and epidemiological severity parameters. The clinical spectrum of communicable diseases and the possible surveillance system at each level.

Abbreviations: SARI: Severe acute respiratory infection; IFR: infection fatality rate; sCFR: symptomatic case fatality rate; sCHR: symptomatic hospitalization rate; and HFR: hospitalization fatality rate.

Source: https://www.researchgate.net/publication/365399605/figure/fig1/AS:11431281212132946@1702545997591/The-burden-pyramid-of-infectious-disease-and-epidemiological-severity-parameters-The.tif.

13.6.2. Socioeconomic Effects of Infectious Disease Outbreaks

Socioeconomic effects of infectious disease outbreaks extend far beyond acute health emergencies, profoundly affecting economic stability, social structure, and healthcare institutions. Emerging infectious diseases have the potential to cause significant disruptions to labor markets because individuals become ill or are quarantined. For instance, during epidemic breaks, production drops significantly due to employee absenteeism, leading to delays in production and decreased economic output. Further, economic burdens become unbearable as healthcare costs skyrocket, leaving people and families to contend with the expense of treatment and prolonged care. This financial burden can further aggravate disparities, particularly in developing countries where resources are limited, as people may lack adequate support systems to recover from the multiple impacts of such health crises. Thus, understanding and addressing such socioeconomic consequences is imperative in the formulation of an enduring solution to infectious disease challenges. In addition, the dynamics of public health infrastructure and socioeconomic forces play a pivotal role in managing infectious disease pandemics. Countries with robust healthcare systems are likely to perform better when they can act effectively, thereby limiting the spread and impacts of diseases. Conversely, nations such as India with a disconnected public health system face increased challenges in avoiding infections like multidrug-resistant tuberculosis (MDR-TB) (Gamon et al., 2013). This effect is not merely on the health side but also has an economic impact, as poor nations can be affected multiple times due to their inability to implement on-time interventions. Strengthening health systems, enhancing accessibility, and improving health literacy have the potential to facilitate effective control of infectious diseases, thereby ensuring economic stability and social cohesion in times of outbreaks. The current interconnectedness of the world created by modern transport fosters the fast spread of infectious diseases, highlighting the need for coordinated international response mechanisms. Models examining the global pandemics' international dynamics emphasize the vital role air transport must play in transmitting diseases (Barrat et al., 2007). Examining mobility patterns and potential measures of containment, it is apparent that outbreaks can lead to widespread socioeconomic disturbance across national borders. The implications are particularly pertinent for less developed nations with limited healthcare resources, which cannot manage increased healthcare burdens and prevent economic meltdown. Implementing cooperative measures, such as travel restrictions and balancing the distribution of therapeutic resources, is vital to lessening the socioeconomic impact of outbreaks. A holistic strategy that balances health and economic equilibrium is critical in mitigating the challenges presented by infectious diseases with an increasingly interconnected global community.

13.6.3. Global Health Organizations and Their Role in Combating Infections

The role of global health institutions in fighting infections has never been more critical as AMR increasingly threatens public health. Organizations such as the WHO and the Global Fund have plans in place that not only cover short-term infection prevention but also prioritize long-term measures. These groups help develop new diagnostics, vaccines, and treatments tailored to individual needs, highlighting the imperative of flexibility in responding to infectious diseases. Forging ahead is the threat of AMR fueled by the abuse of antibiotics in human and veterinary medicine, which results in resistance that transcends boundaries. The demand for international cooperation and good governance is actualized by mutual structures to resist pressure, emphasizing that losses in one country can lead to disasters elsewhere worldwide. The comprehensive approach ensures that efforts to improve healthcare infrastructures are not only prioritized but also appropriately funded and executed. The agreement with the intricacy of international health corruption is a vital element that ensures efficiency in health organizations combating infections. Corruption is a principal barrier, diverting funds intended for the development of health and dissolving trust in healthcare systems. The economic impact of corruption in global health has been tremendous, with estimated losses reaching billions of dollars. Global health institutions are therefore increasingly fixated on anti-corruption policies as part of their agenda against infection. Through the involvement of a multidisciplinary team of specialists, such organizations develop effective responses to the specific challenges represented by corruption-related problems in health, thus protecting investments in disease control and prevention. Embedding anti-corruption into health approaches not only strengthens the support for public health programs but also enriches the governance machinery necessary to achieve sustainable health gains against infectious diseases. Besides, the contribution of innovation toward the development of new treatments for infectious diseases cannot be overestimated. Global health organizations are key to mobilizing investment in R&D needed to address the shortages in current treatment regimes. With the advent of AMR and multidrug resistance, the need for innovative solutions to meet the challenge of evolving pathogens is more urgent than ever. Effective responses require international cooperation between public and private sectors in a concerted effort to stimulate R&D and access new technologies. This requires concerted efforts to enhance surveillance systems, spread educational materials, and facilitate robust regulatory systems that guarantee judicious use of antibiotics. By such collective efforts, global health agencies not only combat the impact of infections but also develop enhanced immunity against future infections, paving the way for healthier populations worldwide (Clare et al., 2016; Bhagwandin et al., 2017).

Test Your Knowledge

1. How does epidemiological data help in understanding the global burden and distribution of infectious diseases?
2. What are some of the major infectious diseases that continue to have significant global impact, and in which regions are they most prevalent?

SUMMARY

In assembling the central questions of the chapter General Medicine for Infectious Diseases, it is evident that a composite model is critical to the success and avoidance of infectious diseases. Growing complexity from sources such as AMR and varying healthcare access necessitates a robust, interdisciplinary system. A priority for improved vaccination protocols and research in diagnostic methods can have a significant impact on the trajectory of disease control. Secondly, recognizing the intersections of socioeconomic determinants and health disparities is vital in policy formulation aimed at enhancing preventive care and treatment accessibility. The continuous mutation of pathogens, especially MDR pathogens, underscores the need for targeted research and intervention strategies to mitigate public health threats, drawing on lessons learned from previous outbreaks and available epidemiological data. Furthermore, with the changing global infectious disease landscape, the role of educative efforts continues to be paramount in equipping health workers as well as communities at large. Awareness of the implications of other treatments, such as phytotherapy in organic agriculture, provides important information about knowledge gaps that must be filled through research (Eijck et al., 2003). This translates to a broader need for integrating approaches that focus not only on conventional medicine but also on complementary methods. Capacity development through sustainable agriculture and livestock production practices can, in turn, indirectly affect human health by preventing the transmission of zoonotic diseases. Therefore, establishing intersectoral research platforms that bridge the divide between veterinary and human medicine has the potential to be gigantic in preventing infectious disease outbreaks at the source. Overall, the intricate interplay between contagious disease and the health systems that deal with it demands concerted efforts from everyone. As the success of WHOs activities has shown, especially against TB, functional systems like DOTS can be highly effective even though problems still persist with MDR disease (Abubakar et al., 2012). This underlines the necessity for proper integration of surveillance and response to looming health crises. Additionally, ongoing research and policy reform aimed at improving health coverage among vulnerable populations need to be given greater importance. Our future knowledge of infectious diseases will not be based solely on clinical interventions but will depend on the interplay between public health programs, community engagement, and cross-border collaboration if we hope to effectively counteract the impacts of infectious diseases in an increasingly integrated world.

In the field of general medicine, particularly regarding infectious diseases, there is a need to identify the intricate determinants through which water, sanitation, and hygiene (WASH) influence health outcomes. Preventing diarrhea, improving maternal and newborn well-being, and enhancing learning achievement through better school attendance are significant focal areas. These topics encompass the main areas of concern where infectious diseases are interlinked, highlighting the utmost significance of WASH interventions. Recent partnerships with UNICEF have helped identify important outcomes associated with various life stages, which are heavily influenced by proper sanitation and access to clean water. Improving WASH systems not only addresses the present health needs but also supports long-term development goals for improving QoL among vulnerable populations, thus making it a strategic focus of the fight against infectious diseases in general medicine (Mills et al., 2016). In addition, the enormous sociocultural implications of the risks around infectious diseases should be taken into consideration. For instance, when researching Chittagong live bird trading network, it is possible to observe that measures of biosecurity are founded on past events rather than future anticipation of outbreaks. This kind of temporal risk management influences responses of individuals and communities to threats such as avian influenza. The notion of the Black Swan theory is most relevant in this context; unexpected situations are often followed by logical explanations that discount the importance of successful preventive actions. Such a mindset may hinder progress in biosecurity investment and readiness, demanding more forceful intervention in addressing future infectious disease threats (Appadurai et al., 2018). Finally, the normalization of disease risk in standard practices is an obstacle to public health efforts. Individuals indulging in riskier behaviors might not perceive a need for rigorous biosecurity efforts because they have experienced no outbreaks in the past, thus providing them with a false sense of security. Normalization can lead to complacency and, ultimately, erode the efforts of controlling infectious diseases. Education and outreach within a community are essential to reframe risk perceptions and remind people of the benefits of prevention. By understanding and reacting to the social, cultural, and behavioral dimensions of infectious disease, general medicine is able to develop more practical interventions that not only respond to current threats, but also prepare populations for unforeseen challenges in the future.

KEY TERMS FROM THIS CHAPTER

- Adaptive immunity
- Antimicrobial molecules
- Bacterial infections
- Biomedical research
- Blood-borne viruses (BBVs)
- Chronic prostatitis
- Community health
- Diagnostic algorithms
- Drug susceptibility testing
- Environmental health
- Formal ontologies
- Fungal infections
- GI distress
- Health consequences
- Healthcare system
- Immunosuppressive therapy
- Infected cells
- Infectious disease ontology (IDO)

CRITICAL THINKING QUESTIONS

1. Which of the following is a viral infection?

a. Tuberculosis
b. Malaria
c. Influenza
d. Ringworm

2. Which immune cells are primarily involved in the early innate response to bacterial infections?

a. B cells
b. T-helper cells
c. Eosinophils
d. Neutrophils

3. What class of drugs is primarily used to treat bacterial infections?

a. Antivirals
b. Antifungals
c. Antibiotics
d. Anthelmintics

4. Which of the following is a gram-positive coccus?

a. Neisseria gonorrhoeae
b. Streptococcus pneumoniae
c. Salmonella typhi
d. Vibrio cholerae

5. Antiretroviral therapy is used in the treatment of:

a. Hepatitis A
b. Tuberculosis
c. Influenza
d. HIV/AIDS

Short Answer Questions

1. What are the key differences between bacterial, viral, fungal, and parasitic infections in terms of structure, transmission, and treatment?
2. Give examples of diseases caused by each major type of infectious agent and describe their typical clinical presentations.
3. How do pathogens invade the human body and trigger an immune response?
4. What are the primary diagnostic tools used to identify infectious diseases, and how do they vary depending on the type of pathogen?
5. Why is taking a thorough patient history important in diagnosing infectious diseases, especially in regions with endemic conditions?
6. How are antibiotics, antivirals, antifungals, and antiparasitic drugs selected based on the specific infectious agent?
7. What are the major challenges in treating infectious diseases, including drug resistance and limited access to care in some regions?

Answers to Critical Thinking Questions

1. (c); 2. (d); 3. (c); 4. (b); 5. (d)

REFERENCES

1. Dar, O. A., Hasan, R., Schlundt, J., Harbarth, S., Caleo, G., Dar, F. K., Littmann, J., Rweyemamu, M., Buckley, E. J., Shahid, M., Kock, R., Li, H. L., Giha, H., Khan, M., So, A. D., Bindayna, K. M., Kessel, A., Pedersen, H. B., Permanand, G., . . . Heymann, D. L. (2015). Exploring the evidence base for national and regional policy interventions to combat resistance. *The Lancet, 387*(10015), 285–295. https://doi.org/10.1016/s0140-6736(15)00520-6Abubakar, I., Atun, R., Chakaya, J., Cox, H., et al. (2012). Drug-resistant tuberculosis—Current dilemmas, unanswered questions, challenges and priority needs. https://core.ac.uk/download/9839026.pdf (accessed on 27th June 2025).
2. Agrawal, V., Brinda, B. J., & Farag, S. S. (2020). *Histoplasma capsulatum* infection in an allogeneic hematopoietic stem cell transplant patient receiving voriconazole prophylaxis. https://core.ac.uk/download/299809034.pdf (accessed on 27th June 2025).
3. Agyarko-Poku, T., Long, E. F., Paintsil, E., VanDeusen, S., et al. (2015). Cost effectiveness of option B plus for prevention of mother-to-child transmission of HIV in resource-limited countries: Evidence from Kumasi, Ghana. https://core.ac.uk/download/323078115.pdf (accessed on 27th June 2025).
4. Akan, H., Alexander, B. D., Andes, D., Azoulay, E., et al. (2019). Revision and update of the consensus definitions of invasive fungal disease from the European Organization for Research and Treatment of Cancer and the Mycoses Study Group Education and Research Consortium. https://core.ac.uk/download/287649722.pdf (accessed on 27th June 2025).
5. Alvarez, A., McCaig, D. J., Bearden, D. T., Ibrahim, E. H., Brown, E. M., European Antimicrobial Resistance Surveillance System, Haaijer-Ruskamp, F. M., et al. (2005). Limited effect of patient and disease characteristics on compliance with hospital antimicrobial guidelines. https://core.ac.uk/download/pdf/12919553.pdf (accessed on 27th June 2025).
6. Andam, K. S., Asenso-Okyere, K., Chiang, C., Thangata, P., et al. (2025). Interactions between health and farm-labor productivity. https://core.ac.uk/download/pdf/6237651.pdf (accessed on 27th June 2025).
7. Anderson, R. M., Aunger, R., Banaji, M., Barnett, T., Denton, D., et al. (2015). Some considerations concerning the challenge of incorporating social variables into epidemiological models of infectious disease transmission. https://core.ac.uk/download/36778292.pdf (accessed on 27th June 2025).
8. Anyamba, A., Bauer, A., Chang, A., Dodoo, A., Escalante, A., Flahault, A., Nederhof, A. J., et al. (2011). Social sciences research in neglected tropical diseases 2: A bibliographic analysis. https://core.ac.uk/download/337135.pdf (accessed on 27th June 2025).
9. Appadurai, A., Bouma, A., Lakoff, A., Martinot, A., Kleinman, A. M., Kousky, C., Lowe, C., et al. (2018). Competing biosecurity and risk rationalities in the Chittagong poultry commodity chain, Bangladesh. https://core.ac.uk/download/161515025.pdf (accessed on 27th June 2025).
10. Babayan, S. A., Duprez, J. S., Selman, C., Sinclair, J., et al. (2018). Chronic helminth infection burden differentially affects hematopoietic cell development while ageing selectively impairs adaptive responses to infection. https://core.ac.uk/download/151395611.pdf (accessed on 27th June 2025).

11. Bakhtawar, M., Haq, M. U., Iftikhar, S., Rizwan, A., et al. (2020). Awareness of swine flu among the medical students of Shaikh Zayed Medical College Rahim Yar Khan. https://media.neliti.com/media/publications/302010-awareness-of-swine-flu-among-the-medical-8b23412a.pdf (accessed on 27th June 2025).
12. Bang, H., Hon, S., May, L., Mooso, B., et al. (2019). Rapid multiplex testing for upper respiratory pathogens in the emergency department: A randomized controlled trial. https://core.ac.uk/download/323070651.pdf (accessed on 27th June 2025).
13. Barrat, A., Valleron, A. J., Vespignani, A., Galvani, A. P., Barthelemy, M., & Colizza, V. (2007). Modeling the worldwide spread of pandemic influenza: Baseline case and containment interventions. https://core.ac.uk/download/pdf/7527473.pdf (accessed on 27th June 2025).
14. Bellini, T., Bonaccorsi, G., Bramanti, B., Carè, A., et al. (2019). "Bridging the gap": Everything that could have been avoided if we had applied gender medicine, pharmacogenetics and personalized medicine in the gender-omics and sex-omics era. https://core.ac.uk/download/286075866.pdf (accessed on 27th June 2025).
15. Bhagwandin, N., Jenner, A., & Kowalski, S. P. (2017). Antimicrobial resistance (AMR) and multidrug resistance (MDR): Overview of current approaches, consortia and intellectual property issues. https://core.ac.uk/download/215505935.pdf (accessed on 27th June 2025).
16. Boccia, D., Dowd, J. B., Fletcher, H., Hayward, A. C., et al. (2019). A systematic review of the impact of psychosocial factors on immunity: Implications for enhancing BCG response against tuberculosis. https://core.ac.uk/download/286270876.pdf (accessed on 27th June 2025).
17. Bourhy, H., Gaidet, N., & Molia, S. (2012). Mission to Indonesia to participate to the 1st Indonesia-France Seminar in Medicine & Public Health and investigate potential collaborations on animal health: 2nd–9th of November 2012. http://agritrop.cirad.fr/567354/1/document_567354.pdf (accessed on 27th June 2025).
18. Bresell, A., Djebbari, A., Doms, A., Ruttenberg, A., Valouev, A., Yu, A. C., Grinde, B., et al. (2009). Infectious disease ontology. https://core.ac.uk/download/131212652.pdf (accessed on 27th June 2025).
19. Brown, C. J., & Frame, P. (2009). Communities of practice in the public-private-partnership sector for neglected diseases drug development: The importance of mindset mapping. https://core.ac.uk/download/1639972.pdf (accessed on 27th June 2025).
20. Buttigieg, M. (2015). A review of the One Health concept: Increasing awareness and collaboration between the Maltese medical and veterinary professionals. https://core.ac.uk/download/46603760.pdf (accessed on 27th June 2025).
21. Calhoun, E. A., Clemens, J. Q., Kusek, J. W., Litwin, M. S., et al. (2009). Primary care physician practices in the diagnosis, treatment and management of men with chronic prostatitis/chronic pelvic pain syndrome. https://core.ac.uk/download/323079649.pdf (accessed on 27th June 2025).
22. Carson, A. L., Jackups, R., McMullen, K. M., Munigala, S., et al. (2017). Inpatient urine cultures are frequently performed without urinalysis or microscopy: Findings from a large academic medical center. https://core.ac.uk/download/83100994.pdf (accessed on 27th June 2025).
23. Chiu, C. Y., & Miller, S. A. (2019). Clinical metagenomics. https://core.ac.uk/download/323062552.pdf (accessed on 27th June 2025).

24. Clare, J., Lewis, M., Mackey, T. K., et al. (2016). The disease of corruption: Views on how to fight corruption to advance 21st century global health goals. https://open.bu.edu/bitstream/2144/31130/1/mackey_disease.pdf (accessed on 27th June 2025).

25. Combs, B. G., Giele, C. M., Kwan, K. S. H., Mak, D. B., et al. (2008). Audit of antenatal testing of sexually transmissible infections and blood borne viruses at Western Australian hospitals. https://core.ac.uk/download/61303469.pdf (accessed on 27th June 2025).

26. Coukell, A., Shore, C., Jungman, E., Talkington, K., Kothari, P., & Urahn, S. K. (2016). A scientific roadmap for antibiotic discovery: A sustained and robust pipeline of new antibacterial drugs and therapies is critical to preserve public health. https://core.ac.uk/download/75785719.pdf (accessed on 27th June 2025).

27. Danon, L., Ford, A. P., House, T. A., Jewell, C. P., et al. (2010). Networks and the epidemiology of infectious disease. https://core.ac.uk/download/1381886.pdf (accessed on 27th June 2025).

28. Danso-Appiah, A., Utarini, A., Crampin, A. C., Pond, B., Paul, B. D., Babu, B. V., Braga, C., et al. (2009). Social research on neglected diseases of poverty: Continuing and emerging themes. https://core.ac.uk/download/338058.pdf (accessed on 27th June 2025).

29. de Belvis, A. G., De Vito, C., Federici, A., La Torre, G., et al. (2015). Policy and planning of prevention in Italy: Results from an appraisal of prevention plans developed by regions for the period 2010–2012. https://core.ac.uk/download/54520402.pdf (accessed on 27th June 2025).

30. Dear, J. D. (2020). Bacterial pneumonia in dogs and cats: An update. https://core.ac.uk/download/286361309.pdf (accessed on 27th June 2025).

31. Dutta, A., Meijers, H., Ramani, S. V., & Frühauf, T. (2012). Determinants of the prevalence of diarrhoea in adolescents attending school: A case study of an Indian village school. https://core.ac.uk/download/75783133.pdf (accessed on 27th June 2025).

32. Eijck, I., & Kijlstra, A. (2006). Animal health in organic livestock systems: A review. https://core.ac.uk/download/10924572.pdf (accessed on 27th June 2025).

33. Eijck, I., Groot, M., Kasteel, D., Kijlstra, A., et al. (2003). Analysis of black holes in our knowledge concerning animal health in the organic food production chain. https://core.ac.uk/download/10919416.pdf (accessed on 27th June 2025).

34. Elbe, S. (2014). The pharmaceuticalisation of security: Molecular biomedicine, antiviral stockpiles, and global health security. https://core.ac.uk/download/30610244.pdf (accessed on 27th June 2025).

35. Engel, N. (2025). Flexibility and innovation in response to emerging infectious diseases: Reactions to multi-drug-resistant tuberculosis in India. https://core.ac.uk/download/pdf/6941410.pdf (accessed on 27th June 2025).

36. Escota, G., & Melia, M. T. (2020). The struggling infectious diseases fellow: Remediation challenges and opportunities. https://core.ac.uk/download/322802240.pdf (accessed on 27th June 2025).

37. Esteves Mills, J., & Cumming, O. (2016). The impact of water, sanitation, and hygiene on key health and social outcomes: Review of evidence. https://core.ac.uk/download/75761114.pdf (accessed on 27th June 2025).

38. Gamon, M. (2013). Multidrug-resistant tuberculosis in India: Solving a problem by reconstructing the public health infrastructure. https://core.ac.uk/download/67755957.pdf (accessed on 27th June 2025).

39. Gostin, L. O., & Thomas, B. P. (2013). Tackling the global NCD crisis: Innovations in law and governance. https://core.ac.uk/download/70375002.pdf (accessed on 27th June 2025).

40. Grolla, A., MacNeil, A., Tuffs, A., Georges, A. J., Casillas, A. M., Jeffs, B., Le Guenno, B., et al. (2012). Clinical manifestations and case management of Ebola hemorrhagic fever caused by a newly identified virus strain, Bundibugyo, Uganda, 2007–2008. https://core.ac.uk/download/pdf/10674394.pdf (accessed on 27th June 2025).

41. Helm, B., & Martinez-Bakker, M. (2015). The influence of biological rhythms on host–parasite interactions. https://core.ac.uk/download/42361213.pdf (accessed on 27th June 2025).

42. Ivanova, E., Kircheva, A., Kolarova, M., Konstantinov, I., et al. (2017). Sea epidemiology in teaching maritime medicine–Prevention of infectious diseases, being subject to international health regulation and controlled by WHO. https://core.ac.uk/download/389005121.pdf (accessed on 27th June 2025).

43. Joffe, H., & Washer, P. (2006). The hospital 'superbug': Social representations of MRSA. https://core.ac.uk/download/1670700.pdf (accessed on 27th June 2025).

44. Johannessen, A., Lindberg, A., Chaturvedi, A. K., Morris, A., Phillips, A. N., Balbi, B., Celli, B. R., et al. (2013). The impact of HAART on the respiratory complications of HIV infection: Longitudinal trends in the MACS and WIHS cohorts. https://core.ac.uk/download/12214715.pdf (accessed on 27th June 2025).

45. Lillestolen, D. (2018). Infections not fought: Antibiotic resistance in underserved communities. https://core.ac.uk/download/158970352.pdf (accessed on 27th June 2025).

46. London School of Hygiene & Tropical Medicine. (2013). *Annual Report 2013*. https://core.ac.uk/download/19452766.pdf (accessed on 27th June 2025).

47. N/A. (2004). *Campus & Alumni News*. https://open.bu.edu/bitstream/2144/22309/1/BostonUniversityMedicine2004v13n1_web.pdf (accessed on 27th June 2025).

48. N/A. (2014). *Research Advances: January 2014*. https://core.ac.uk/download/75777581.pdf (accessed on 27th June 2025).

49. Remais, J. (2010). Modelling environmentally-mediated infectious diseases of humans: Transmission dynamics of schistosomiasis in China. https://core.ac.uk/download/323082019.pdf (accessed on 27th June 2025).

INDEX

C

D

E

F

G

H

I

J

K

L

M

N

O

P

Q

R

S